The Nervous System and Behavior

MICHAEL D. MANN, Ph.D.
ASSOCIATE PROFESSOR
DEPARTMENT OF PHYSIOLOGY AND BIOPHYSICS
UNIVERSITY OF NEBRASKA MEDICAL CENTER
OMAHA, NEBRASKA

The Nervous System and Behavior

M. D. Mann

1981

HARPER & ROW, PUBLISHERS
PHILADELPHIA
Cambridge
New York
Hagerstown
San Francisco
London
Mexico City
São Paulo
Sydney
1817

The authors and publisher have exerted every effort to ensure that drug selection and dosage set forth in this text are in accord with current recommendations and practice at the time of publication. However, in view of ongoing research, changes in government regulations, and the constant flow of information relating to drug therapy and drug reactions, the reader is urged to check the package insert for each drug for any change in indications and dosage and for added warnings and precautions. This is particularly important when the recommended agent is a new and/or infrequently employed drug.

10 9 8 7 6 5 4 3 2 1

Printed in the United States of America. For information address Medical Department, Harper & Row Publishers, Inc., East Washington Square, Philadelphia, Pennsylvania 19105

Library of Congress Cataloging in Publication Data

Mann, Michael D

The nervous system and behavior.

Bibliography:

Includes index.

1. Neurophysiology. I. Title. [DNLM: 1. Nervous system—Physiology. 2. Behavior. WL 102 M282n]

QP361.M36 152 81-258

ISBN 0-06-141576-6 AACR1

To Sally, with love, thanks and joy

Contents

Preface

This treatment of neurophysiology was developed, in part, from lectures given to the medical students at the University of Nebraska College of Medicine. An attempt has been made to integrate clinical material throughout the presentation mainly as examples to illustrate the principles of normal operation of the nervous system. It was never the intention of the author to make this a textbook of clinical neurology, a compendium of diseases of the nervous system, or a "how-to" book for the neurological exam. The pattern recognition aspect of neurology, the recognition of frequently encountered syndromes, is best learned in the clinic or at the bedside and it is best taught by the clinician. It was the author's intention to present the normally functioning nervous system to the student to give him a "feeling" for how the nervous system works and what it can and cannot do and to equip him with basic concepts to be used in dealing with newly recognized disease processes involving the nervous system.

This book is unique amongst basic textbooks of neurophysiology in the incorporation of new and, to some extent, controversial concepts of the nervous system based upon recent data. The classic viewpoint (what most textbooks present) is presented, but in many cases the discussions are elaborated in order to give the student a better idea of how the system works. Not every controversy involves new ideas; many currently "new ideas" were actually espoused by the great physiologists, like Sir Claude Bernard (1813–1878), Henry Head (1861–1940), and John Hughlings Jackson (1835–1911). The author's view is that it serves medicine no benefit to repeat (and perpetuate) concepts that most of recent experience with the nervous system repudiates. Rather, the benefit for medicine is derived from making it possible for the medical student to be amongst the leaders in the changing clinical world. A knowledge of basic concepts and a "feel" for the nervous system are necessary in promoting innovation in patient care. Because a good deal of the scientific controversy in modern neurophysiology is included in this treatment, it may also serve as an introductory textbook for graduate students provided that it is supplemented by readings in the literature. References are supplied to get the curious student started in further study.

It is assumed that the reader of this book has an understanding of basic physics or, at least, basic electricity. The electrophysiology of nerve and muscle cells is presented in enough detail that even a student with a weak background should be able to master this material if he applies himself. It is also assumed that the student has studied neuroanatomy. The anatomy of various systems and structures is reviewed briefly, but not in sufficient detail to achieve a full understanding. There are a number of good textbooks of neuroanatomy available to the student. A good treatment for the medical student can be found in Barr ML: The Human Nervous System, An Anatomic Viewpoint, 3rd ed. Hagerstown, MD, Harper and Row, 1980. The student who wants more detailed treatment or a bit more of the "flavor" of neuroanatomic research can consult Brodal A: Neurological Anatomy In Relation to Clinical Medicine, 3rd ed. New York, Oxford Univ. Press, 1981.

The organization of the book is a bit different from that of most neurophysiology textbooks. The text begins with an overview of the nervous system and its roles in an organism and a preview of the topics in the remainder of the book. Instead of launching then immediately into a discussion of the properties of excitable membranes, the text discusses human behavior as the entity neurophysiology attempts to explain. Chapter 2 is a presentation of psychophysics and movement. The properties of excitable membranes are discussed in Chapter 3. Included are discussions of the structure and properties of excitable membranes, the origins and characteristics of the membrane potential and the action potential, and nerve conduction. Chapter 4 is a general discussion of receptor mechanisms and information coding that is elaborated for each specific sensory system in Chapters 5 to 11.

Chapters 12 to 14 present discussions of the properties of peripheral nerves, the mechanisms of synaptic transmission, and the mechanisms of muscle contraction, partly for their own intrinsic interest and partly as building blocks for the discussions of reflex activity in the nervous system (Chapter 15) and of the initiation and control of movement (Chapter 16). Chapter 17 presents a discussion of both spinal and supraspinal control mechanisms in the autonomic nervous system.

Chapters 18 and 19 present introductions to two topics seldom seen in introductory textbooks of neurophysiology for medical students. These topics are neurotrophic functions and growth and repair in the nervous system. The former topic is one that is of current interest, representing information derived almost entirely from research done in the last 15 to 20 years. The topics of growth and repair are fundamental to medical practice, and it surprises the author that they are so seldom discussed in medical texts.

The origin of cerebral cortical evoked potentials and the electroencephalogram, their properties, and their usefulness to experimental physiology and clinical practice are discussed in Chapter 20. The role of the cerebral cortex in relationship to subcortical structures in learning, emotion, consciousness, and personality and the divergence of function of the two hemispheres are the subject of Chapter 21. The final chapter ties the textbook together, harkening back to the overview, and presenting reasons for a more optimistic view of the possibilities of successfully treating neurologic problems. It is emphasized that the clinician's view of how the nervous system works determines what he will do for the patient.

One major goal of any introductory course is to familiarize the student with the vocabulary of the field. The author has presented the extended glossary at the end of the text for quick reference to that vocabulary. Most of the terms appear in boldface when they are first introduced in the text. In most cases, a student who can define and properly use every term in this glossary will have mastered the subject matter of this book.

Neurophysiology is a developing field and is currently undergoing a metamorphosis. In the history of the field, the period from 1920 to 1975 can be characterized as one of intense interest in electrophysiology, but the recent history is dominated by neurochemical approaches. One reason for this shift is the inability of electrophysiology to provide all of the answers to questions about the nervous system. It is doubtful that neurochemistry, by itself, can provide them either. What is certain is that there are more questions unanswered than answered! The student may be struck by the frequency of occurrence of phrases like "we do not know" in this text. He must understand that the nervous system is extremely complex. There are those who doubt that the human brain can ever understand itself. Although the author does not share this opinion, he must often say "we do not know what the answer is"!

MDM
Omaha, Nebraska, 1980

Acknowledgments

The author wishes to acknowledge the assistance of the medical students at the University of Nebraska Medical Center in the development of clear exposition of many of the ideas in the text. It was answering their questions that indicated areas where the text was unclear. The author also wishes to thank the following people for their valuable comments on parts of the manuscript: R Beuerman, FJ Clark, G Doetsch, V Dionne, KA Follett, KW Horch, JA McMillan, GH Pollack, AL Towe, CF Tyner, and J Wagoner. Special thanks are due to Arnold Towe under whose tutelage many of the ideas were developed. The assistance of D Martin and KA Follett in preparing some of the illustrations is also acknowledged. The author also wishes to acknowledge the special assistance of his wife, Sally, in reading, editing, typing, and encouraging the development of the manuscript.

The Nervous System and Behavior

1

Neurophysiology: An Overview

Neurophysiology is a study of **neurons, nerves,** and **nervous systems,** what they do, and how they do it. A neuron is a cell that is specialized in two of the fundamental properties of living matter, namely **excitability** and **conductivity.** Excitability is the ability to respond to changes in the environment; conductivity is the ability to convey an impulse or action potential from one part of the cell to another. In most neurons the portion of the cell that carries action potentials away from the cell body is called the **axon** or **nerve fiber.** Some axons are short, a few micrometers in length; some axons are long, in man up to 6 feet in length. A nerve is a bundle of these axons originating in various cells. Finally, a nervous system is the aggregate of all nerve cells within a single organism. It happened that, in the course of evolution, all but the simplest animals have resorted to the use of a nervous system of some sort to organize and carry out their behaviors. So it is that the study of the nervous system, in other words **neurophysiology,** is fundamental to the study of behavior.

In the discussion of any phenomenon as complex as the nervous system, it is nearly impossible to present every topic in appropriate sequence without mentioning some ideas, events, or structures out of order. A brief overview of the topics to be discussed may help the reader maintain a sense of order even when topics are mentioned before they are discussed in detail. The nervous system is composed of billions of individual nerve cells, each having its own membrane that separates electrical charges; in biologic tissues those charges are in the form of ions. The result is that each cell has a resting membrane voltage, or potential, that acts as a source of potential energy for the workings of the cell. Membrane voltages of nerve cells can change with time, and these changes can be communicated as signals to other nerve cells or to effector organs such as glands and muscles. In fact, this is one of the major activities of the nervous system.

If the distances for communication are short, the local changes in voltage can be communicated directly; however, because the nerve membrane is a poor conductor of electricity, the local voltage signals would not span distances greater than a millimeter or two. Thus, a special communication device, the action potential, is used to communicate over great distances, in large animals over many meters. The action potential is well suited to this purpose because of its short duration (0.5 msec or so) and rapid conduction (at 1–120 m/sec) without decrement. The short duration of the action potential allows it to recur at high frequencies, up to 500/sec.

Cells communicate with each other by way of special junctions, called synapses. Synapses are of two types: chemical and electrical. At chemical synapses, the voltage signal in one cell triggers the release of a chemical transmitter substance onto another cell. This transmitter substance can either increase the activity of the receiving cell, that is, increase the likelihood that it will discharge action potentials, or it can decrease the activity of the receiving cell, that is, decrease the likelihood that it will discharge action potentials. We refer to the former effect as excitation, to the latter effect as inhibition. Electrical synapses do not use transmitter substances but communicate changes in membrane voltage directly, and they usually only involve excitation. In mammals, chemical synapses seem to form the majority of synaptic junctions.

The receiving cell is usually influenced synaptically not by one other cell but by many. It integrates the excitatory and inhibitory influences from a number of other cells and, based on this integration, generates its own signals that, in turn, influence other cells. Understanding this integrative property of nerve cells is extremely important in understanding how the nervous system behaves normally and how it malfunctions. Some cells require a lot of synaptic influences to generate an output; others do not. Most nerve cells require a lot of synaptic input to generate an output; muscle cells do not. A single action potential arriving at the synaptic junction of a nerve on a muscle, the neuromuscular junction, always causes the muscle to generate a single action potential of its own and to contract.

Some nervous structures, the receptors, are specialized to receive signals from the external environment or from the internal environment, that is, signals about the condition of the body itself. Receptors use the potential energy of their membrane voltages to respond to these environmental signals and to generate coded signals of their own that tell the rest of the nervous system what has been sensed in the environment. The signals are normally trains of action potentials that vary in pattern or frequency depending upon the qualities of the environmental signals. These action potential signals are sent over axons into the central nervous system (CNS). Sometimes part of the code of the signal is determined by which particular axon or which particular pathway in the central nervous system it traverses. Signals in particular pathways are often associated with particular sensory events. Much of the study of neurophysiology is a consideration of how sensory systems code sensory information.

Movements are generated within the central nervous system, both as direct, automatic responses to sensory signals (the reflexes) and as responses to the environment, more independent of particular sensory signals. The spinal cord plays a big role in both kinds of movements, both because it supplies the only effective connection between the nervous system and skeletal muscles and because it contains the neural machinery that generates most of the reflex activity and other more complicated activity, such as walking. However, the spinal cord does not normally work independently of the rest of the nervous system. Important deficits in movement and behavior occur with disruption of activity at a great many places in the nervous system. These deficits can range anywhere from small changes in fine tuning of movements, which occur following damage to the pyramidal tract, to lack of coordination and synergy of muscle contraction, which occur with lesions of the cerebellum, to complete absence of any normal activity, which occurs with small vascular lesions of the brain stem.

The "higher functions"—learning, emotion, speaking, thinking—presumably are produced using the same cellular processes that are involved in simple reflex behavior but involving these processes in many different structures.

In dealing with the nervous system, it is natural to ask why animals, including man, have resorted to the use of nerves instead of some other mechanism for directing their activities. It is not difficult to conjure up a variety of alternate schemes, some of which are, in fact, found in nature, but it soon becomes clear that for large organisms, the only practical way, other than a nervous system, to stimulate a distant part of the body is through the use of chemical substances, called hormones, that are carried in the blood.

Let us briefly compare both nervous and hormonal systems with respect to some of the essential features of the nervous system. A primary function of both the nervous system and the hormonal system is to communicate information from one part of the body to another. Nerve cells are capable of carrying a signal from the toe of a 6-foot man to his cerebral cortex in about 25 msec, that is, in about 25/1000 of a second. If a hormone were secreted into the blood at the toes, it would not be able to reach the cerebral cortex in less than 17 seconds. *Speed* is at a premium in the behavior of most animals, and clearly the speed advantage lies with the nervous system. Can you imagine what would happen to a cat whose righting reflex was mediated by hormones? A hormone secreted by the vestibular apparatus, which senses orientation, would reach the muscles of the neck, where righting begins, in let's say about 2 seconds. In earth's gravity, an object falls 64 feet in 2 seconds. This means that a cat would not be able to right itself if dropped from less than 64 feet above the ground. Clearly, the performance of normal cats exceeds this level. Of course, where speed is not essential, such as in the regulation of growth, the hormonal system works perfectly well and, indeed, is used for that purpose. The same functions served by hormonal systems in a slow organism, or one that does not need rapid responses, may be served by a neural system in an organism that does need to respond rapidly. For example, the sensitivity of the eye is variable in most organisms in such a way that, in bright light, it is less sensitive and, in dim light, it is more sensitive. In relatively slow-moving crustacea that do not respond rapidly to changes in light intensity, this sensitivity is under hormonal control, whereas in man and relatively fast-moving insects that do need to respond rapidly to changes in light intensity, the same mechanism is controlled by the nervous system. Another major function of the nervous system is to *coordinate* precisely the contraction of the various muscles in the body. The hormonal systems also play a role in coordination, but only for activities that do not require close timing or abrupt onset and offset. The nervous system uses action potentials to send signals. Because these action potentials last only a fraction of a second and travel at high speeds, movements can be started and stopped in a fraction of a second. In contrast, hormones have half-lives of seconds or minutes and travel about a thousand times more slowly, because they must be conveyed to the tissues through the vascular system, and, therefore, cannot start actions quickly or end them quickly. On the other hand, where speed of response is not essential, hormones can adequately coordinate activity in many tissues in different places, as they do, for example, in the case of the events surrounding ovulation. Where prolonged activity is required, hormones again have the advantage. They can act for a long time, because hormones have long half-lives compared to those of action potentials. To do the same job, prolonged nervous activity would be required, which means continuous generation of action potentials at perhaps higher metabolic costs.

Another difference between nervous control and hormonal control lies in the number of target organs activated at one time. If a given behavior requires the action of several organs to provide a generalized response, a hormonal system may be well suited, but if only one or a few organs are required to respond in a specific manner, then nervous control is better suited. Were it necessary to regulate every movement of a normal human by hormonal control, a hormone combination would be required for every movement and receptor sites would be required for several hormones on the same organ. Otherwise, an organ would not know what kind of response to give: small or large, fast or slow. Clearly, the number of hormones would be immense and the system impractical. On the other hand, if it were necessary to regulate growth with the nervous system, it would require a neural connection to each cell of the body, also an impractical condition. The nervous system does participate in some generalized responses as we shall see when we consider the autonomic nervous system later, but, in general, the nervous system provides highly specific control of only one or a few organs.

Another essential function of the nervous system is to collect and **integrate** sensory information, that is, to combine, analyze, and process information about the environment both inside and outside the body in order to execute an appropriate response. Because the common denominator of activity in all sensory systems is changes in electrical potential, it is no problem to add them together. It is easy to sum electrical potentials. If integration were to be accomplished by a chemical system, the matter would be much more complicated. One would, for example, want to distinguish visual events from auditory events, so each sense must use a separate hormone. Then there is the problem of how to add them together, something like adding apples and oranges; molecules would have to combine chemically, and then different cells would be required to respond to all possible ways of combining the hormones. This kind of chemical integration does occur in hormonal systems, for example, in the control of fat cell activity; however, the number of hormones involved and the total repertoire of responses of the organ are limited compared to the number of different ways a neuron can respond and the total behavior of an organism. On the level of the whole organism, the thorny problem for chemical integration is how to handle something like mathematical computations. It is no doubt obvious by now that nervous control of behavior does provide certain advantages over all the alternatives. These are (1) increased speed of performance, (2) increased precision of performance related not only to speed and control of onset and offset, but also to the way neurons are connected to the organs, and (3) economy of chemistry with no need to synthesize large numbers of hormones. Nervous control of behavior is least efficient in the initiation and organization of generalized or prolonged responses.

Up to this point, we have dealt with the nervous system and neurons as if their only function were to produce action potentials. Most textbooks, in fact most neurophysiologists, deal with the nervous system as if this were true. There is now a lot of evidence of other functions. For example, removing the innervation of a striated muscle results ultimately in wasting or atrophy of the muscle. This implies that the contact of the nerve is required for the muscle to maintain its integrity. Furthermore, the nerve determines, at least to some extent, the contractile properties of the muscle. The characteristic rate of contraction of a muscle can be altered in a systematic way by denervating it and reinnervating it with the nerve from a different muscle. It also appears that it is the neuron that induces the formation of myelin around the axon by the Schwann cells. In addition, the axons probably supply nutrients or some other factors vital to the maintenance of myelin.

Another function of neurons is secretion. Most neurons communicate with each other by way of chemical transmitter substances. These substances are synthesized in the cell body of the neuron, probably stored in the Golgi apparatus, and then transported down the axon. There are two rates of transport in this orthograde direction: One is rapid of the order of 410 mm/day (this is among the fastest rates of intracellular transport for all cells in the body), and the other is relatively slow, of the order of 1 to 12 mm/day. In the terminal portion of the axon, the transmitter substance is stored for later release by action potentials onto nearby neurons, whose activity it influences in characteristic ways. In addition, it is now known that axons transport substances in the retrograde direction, that is, from the terminals back to the soma, at a rate of 40 to 100 mm/day. The terminal portions of the axon pick up substances from their environment; proteins are taken up by nerve terminals and transported back to the soma where they may be used as they are in making other compounds, broken down and used in further synthesis, or eliminated as waste products.

There is also the possibility that neurons may play a role in disease control processes. For example, sectioning the trigeminal nerve or a part of it for the treatment of chronic pain or for any other reason is often followed by an outbreak of herpes zoster virus infection in the area of the face served by that nerve. Some investigators believe that the virus may be controlled by uptake into the neurons and that when the neurons are damaged they release their captive viruses into their terminals in the skin. This notion receives some support from the recurrence of cold sores (herpes viral infections) at the same site or at nearby sites over a period of many years. There, of course, may be other explanations, but the possibility exists that the nerves play some role in disease control.

How important these nonspike activities of the neurons are to the functioning of the nervous system is not known. It is possible that they are a major route for interneuronal communication. It is also possible that they are only manifestations of basic cellular metabolic processes. The near future may hold the answer.

How did the nervous system of the human come about? The nervous system is subject to evolutionary pressures in the same way as any other part of an organism. Its structure may be altered or added to in order to allow the species to survive in a changed or new environment that requires a new life style. Thus, we might expect to be able to trace the evolution of nervous systems in fossil records. This has proved difficult to do because nervous tissue is soft, and it is not preserved the way bones are. However, we do have some idea of the development of nervous systems. The first organisms were probably single cells like the ameba. Because single-celled animals have all of the characteristics of living matter, they must have conductivity and excitability. In this way, these first single-celled organisms were the first nervous systems, doing many of the things that more complex systems do. As animals became more complex, it became more efficient to differentiate cells into functional types. Different tissues appeared and, with them, nerve cells. At first, nerve cells may have been poorly organized, perhaps in loose bundles with no obvious order; later they associated more closely in organized groups called ganglia. Still later the ganglia became interconnected and coalesced to form what we know as the spinal cord and brain stem. In the course of phylogeny, some new groups of cells or nuclei were added; later, in different animals, these nuclei increased in size and complexity, whereas others decreased or stayed the same. The cerebral cortex made its first appearance in evolution among the reptiles and then gradually changed in size and complexity to reach its current configuration in the human brain.

The phylogenetic development of the nervous system may be characterized by analogy to the wooden blocks you played with as a child. At first, there were just a few blocks strewn on the floor, but you quickly put them in order to form a framework, then you reached into the box and picked out a few more blocks, and added them to your construction as they were needed. The basic foundation remained, you just added more blocks on top. In the same way, the framework of the spinal cord evolved with its basic neural connections that provide the **reflexes.** As environments changed, for example from wet to dry as previously aquatic species emerged onto the land, pressures were applied to the species, forcing them to change their behavior or die out. In many successful species, this meant modification of the basic framework in the spinal cord and brain stem, and in some cases, the addition of new structures. Each new structure was capable of modifying the activity of the basic framework. Even in the human brain, so-called higher centers, such as the cerebral cortex, work by modifying the activity of lower centers, but these higher centers are not capable of controlling behavior by themselves. It is this modification of the basic reflex activity and not direct control of muscle contraction that leads to the fluid, continuous activity characteristic of the higher mammals, including man.

To summarize, the functions of the nervous system are as follows:

Communication
Sensation
Integration
Coordination
Movement or secretion
Behavior

In our study of the nervous system, we consider these functions more or less in this order. By the term communication, we mean simply getting information from one place in the body to another, usually by transmission of nerve impulses. To understand this process, we must know how impulses are generated and propagated, that is, how nerves carry signals and transmit information to other nerve cells, muscles, and glands. The study of sensation involves consideration of what features in our environment can be sensed, of the different organs used to sense, of the process of transduction, that is, converting energy (be it mechanical, thermal, or light) into a form that can be used by the nervous system, namely, the action potential, and of how these processes finally lead to a sensation. This last topic includes some consideration of how the activity of the nervous system relates to what we sense. Integration is the combination and comparison of information from various sensory organs and from memory to be used in making decisions about behavior. Movement and secretion are, of course, the end products of all the machinations of the nervous system, and when numerous movements or secretions are assembled together into complex patterns that are modifiable by experience over time, the result is termed behavior. It is the understanding of behavior that is the final goal of neurophysiology and, as such, it is the topic about which the least can be said, in the inclusive sense. We discuss stereotyped behaviors like the scratch-reflex of the dog or a sneeze in man, and a few, more complex behaviors such as sleeping, speaking, and learning, but what we can say about them is extremely superficial compared to the complexity of behaviors that exist. We are not even close to understanding the learning process, nor the coordination that allows a swift to fly at 140 miles per hour through a slit in a wall only slightly larger than its body. Neither can we say very much about the mechanisms of personality or of consciousness. Though our understanding of these phenomena is in its infancy, new "facts" are being turned up all the time; and existing knowledge is, at the same time, perplexing and fascinating.

2

Human Behavior

Before one can even begin an attempt to account for behavior in terms of activities of the nervous system, one must have some idea of what behavior is. The early psychologists began by studying the mind or mental processes, but, in an attempt to put psychology on a more solid scientific footing, abandoned the study of the mind and concentrated on the study of behavior. In fact, most modern psychologists probably define psychology as the study of behavior. They define behavior as the "*observable* responses of an organism" (Kendler, 1963). In most modern psychology textbooks, the topic of mind is not even mentioned because the mind is not observable. A quick scan of the table of contents shows the following topics: sensation, perception, learning, motivation, talking, frustration, conflict, personality, social behavior, emotion, and abnormal behavior. It is surprising that movement is seldom discussed as a behavior *per se*.

Looking back over the list of topics in the preceding paragraph, it is striking how few of these behaviors are actually observable. Sensation and perception are not observable by anyone else except the person experiencing them. Learning, motivation, conflict, frustration, and emotion are also not observable; we merely infer their existence from the behavior of the person *after* they occur. A person says he has seen something. That is the behavior we observe; the talking of the person, not his sensation or perception. An animal's behavior changes in a training situation, and we infer that it has learned. What we observe are the consequences of learning and motivation. Is it less reasonable to infer the other workings of the mind: thinking, calculating, and reasoning? We should not be surprised that a great deal of progress has not been made in understanding these phenomena; it is always more difficult to deal on a scientific basis with inferences or constructs than with directly observable events like movement. A thorough discussion of behavior would require several volumes, but a discussion of sensation and movement is presented as groundwork for later discussions of their neurophysiology.

PSYCHOPHYSICS

The study of sensation probably began with the first man or perhaps even before him, but the scientific consideration of sensation began in the 1800s, when physicists and mathematicians began to wonder if a sensation could be treated like any other "physical" phenomenon. That is, they wondered, "Could sensation be quantified?" This early interest in sensation was the first step in the formation of neurophysiologic understanding of sensation. The science of **psychophysics** was developed to determine just what can be sensed. Elaborate methods have been developed to measure sensation, but a detailed description of these methods is beyond the scope of this presentation. We will confine our discussion to what these methods tell us about sensation.

We all are aware of various aspects of our world through our senses. These senses are mediated by structures, called **receptors,** that are specialized to be particularly sensitive to some form of energy, either light, mechanical, thermal, or chemical energy. Eyes are receptors sensitive to light energy. Ears are receptors for mechanical energy in the form of sound vibrations and so on. Stimuli are simply presentations of energy to sensory receptors. One important aspect of a stimulus is its strength or intensity. Not every intensity of a particular form of energy can be sensed by a human. The minimum strength required to cause a sensation is called the **threshold:** Below this threshold level there is no sensation.

The term "threshold" may cause some confusion because of its multiple usages in the field of neurophysiology. We use the term threshold in the sense just defined. To refer to the minimum *change* in stimulus strength required to elicit a different sensation, we employ the term "difference threshold" or its psychologic equivalent "difference limen." One should not confuse these concepts with the level of depolarization from the resting membrane potential at which the action potential is initiated. We refer to this as the **critical firing level.**

In Table 2-1 are listed some threshold values for various sensory modalities. The table will give you an idea of the exquisite sensitivity of our sensory receptors and the units used to specify thresholds. (The units of measure will be further dealt with when we consider each sense separately.) Take vision for example. The absolute threshold for many visual receptors (*i.e.,* the minimum energy required to excite a visual receptor) is one photon, a single particle of light. (You may recall, light has properties of both waves and particles. Here it is useful to think of light as particles.) Now look at audition. The threshold for vibration of the eardrum, that is, the minimum distance the eardrum must move for a sound to be heard, has been estimated at 10^{-8} cm or about half the diameter of the hydrogen ion. Auditory systems are extremely sensitive to pressure vibrations in the air. Engineers would give their right arms to be able to design instruments as sensitive as these that have developed in nature.

The thresholds are listed in the table as if they were constants, but in fact they are only representative values. The actual threshold values depend upon three factors: (1) the method used to measure them, (2) the individual being tested, and (3) the environment in which the thresholds are measured. Some people are more sensitive than others to certain stimuli. Sensitivity often varies with age, and in women sensitivity can vary with time during the menstrual cycle. Distracting a subject's attention elevates the threshold measured on any person by any method.

Although thresholds for sensation are useful in determining the minimum energy a person can respond to, they tell us little about the range of stimulus strengths we can sense. For example, what happens to our perception when the strength of a stimulus is increased by some amount? You might say, "That's simple, the magnitude of the sensation evoked increases," and in general, that is true if the increase in stimulus strength is great enough. But, if we expect to gain an understanding of the underlying physical mechanisms, more precise information is needed. There are a number of ways that sensation can be related to stimulus strength. For instance, there could be a linear relationship between the amount of stimulus energy (S) and the sensation or, in psychologic terms, the response (R), such that equal increments in stimulus strength yield equal increments in the magnitude of

TABLE 2-1. THRESHOLDS FOR SOME STIMULI IN VARIOUS MODALITIES

MODALITY	THRESHOLD
Vision	Intensity: (absolute) 1 photon Wavelength: 400 nanometers Acuity: 0.5 seconds of visual angle against a background of brightness of clear daylight sky
Audition	Movement of eardrum: 10^{-8} cm
Olfaction	Ethyl ether: 5.83 mg/liter of air Artificial musk: 0.00004 mg/liter of air
Taste	Sucrose (sweet): 0.02 molar NaCl (salt): 0.035 molar Quinine sulfate (bitter): 0.0000004 molar
Somesthesia	Pressure: Back of hand, 12 grams/mm^2 Pain: Back of hand, 100 grams/mm^2

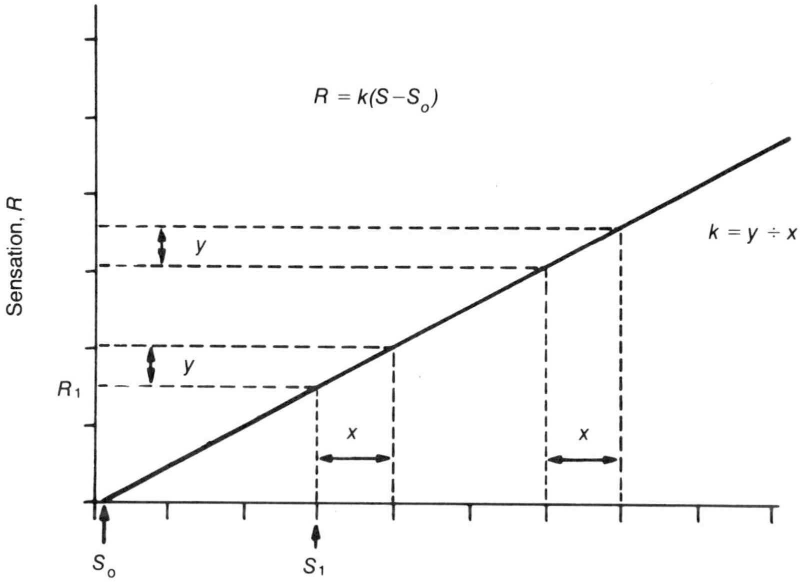

FIG. 2-1. A plot of a linear relationship between stimulus strength (S) and response magnitude (R) as expressed by the equation $R = k\ (S - S_0)$ where S_0 is the threshold stimulus strength. In a linear relationship, equal changes in stimulus strength (x) yield equal changes in response magnitude (y) no matter what the values of strength and magnitude.

the sensation. The graph of Figure 2-1 shows a linear relationship of the form $R = k\ (S - S_0)$. R is the magnitude of the sensation plotted on the y axis or ordinate. S is the stimulus strength plotted on the x axis or abscissa. The term k is a constant, and it is the slope of the straight line. Its value can be computed by dividing the value y by the value x in the illustration. It should be noted that the line intercepts the abscissa at the value S_0. Because the abscissa corresponds to $R = 0$, that means that when $S = S_0$ there is no sensation, that is, $R = 0$. There is a range of stimulus values, $S < S_0$, that is not sensed. Therefore, S_0 is the threshold value of the stimulus and is here treated as if it were a constant. Actually, the threshold is not a constant, as we have said. We therefore arbitrarily set the threshold at that value of stimulus strength that gives a sensation in 50% of its presentations. The magnitude of the sensation, R, evoked by any stimulus, S, that is above threshold, can be determined by reading up from the stimulus value on the abscissa to the corresponding point on the plot, then across to the ordinate. Notice that equal increments in stimulus strength, "x," produce equal increments in sensation, "y," no matter what the absolute values of S and R might be. This is the principal feature of a linear relationship. Changes in stimulus strength are accurately signaled over the whole range of strengths. The main disadvantage of a linear relationship is that only a relatively small range of strengths can be accommodated because of limitations on the maximum and minimum rates at which neurons can discharge. As we shall see, in many senses the advantage of linearity, namely, discriminability, has been sacrificed in order to sense a greater range of strengths.

Let us examine other possible relationships and see how one goes about testing whether a relationship between a stimulus and the resulting sensation is linear or nonlinear. Let us compare the heaviness of two weights as our sample problem. One way to do the experiment is to put a weight into each of a subject's hands and ask whether one weight is heavier. Suppose we begin with two 100-gram weights. If the subject is normal, he will say that the weights are equally heavy. Now, add small amounts of weight to one hand until the subject can first discriminate that one weight is heavier than the other. We find that we need to add 2 grams. When the subject can first detect a difference, we call the difference between the two weights the just-noticeable-difference, or *JND*. We cannot measure sensation directly because it is covert and we cannot lay a ruler to it. We therefore must express equal increments in sensation in terms of the changes in stimulus energy that produce them. The *JND* is thus a standard unit of measure of sensation and represents, in actuality, the amount by which stimulus strength must be changed to produce a different sensation, an example of a **difference threshold.**

With a 100-gram weight, the *JND* was 2 grams. Expressed as a fraction, the ratio of the *JND* to the standard weight, *S*, is 2 divided by 100, or $JND/S = .02$. Now we repeat the experiment, starting with 150-gram weights in each hand. We find that the subject cannot detect a difference until 3 grams have been added. Now the *JND* is 3 grams instead of 2 as before. However, the ratio of the *JND* to the standard weight, that is, JND/S, is still .02 (3/150). No matter what standard is chosen, within limits, we find that the ratio $JND/S = .02$. This means that the amount of weight that must be added for the subject to detect a difference is a *constant proportion* of the standard weight—not a constant increment as the linear relationship would require. The ratio of *JND* to the standard is called the **Weber fraction.** It turns out that for most sensations, the Weber fraction is a constant over a moderate range of intensities. However, at the upper and lower extremes of stimulus strength, the Weber fraction is no longer constant. Although this is of theoretical importance, it need not concern us at this point.

Using the observations that for many of our senses there is a threshold stimulus strength below which we sense nothing and that the ratio of the *JND* to the standard, *S*, is a constant, we can develop the law that relates sensation to stimulus strength (Table 2-2). For example, let us assume a threshold value of 2 and a Weber fraction (that is, the *JND* to *S* ratio) of 0.2. Because the Weber fraction is constant, we will use it as our basic measure. The table lists *JND* steps and the corresponding stimulus strengths for our example. The stimulus strength for each succeeding *JND*, the values for which are shown in the second column, was computed by multiplying the previous *S* value by the Weber fraction, 0.2, and adding it to the previous *S* value. Thus, from a standard value of 2 (the threshold), the stimulus must be increased by 0.4 units to 2.4 for a change in sensation to be perceived. With a standard of 2.4, the stimulus must be increased by 0.48 units to 2.88, and so on. When plotted, the values of *JND* versus stimulus strength yield the curve shown in Figure 2-2. If the *logarithms* of the stimulus values are compared as shown in the third column of the table, the differences between successive log values are the same, namely, 0.0792. If we plot the *JND* versus log *S* instead of the *S* value itself, we get a straight line of slope *k*. Figure 2-3 shows that this is true. The data from Figure 2-2 are replotted with the magnitude of the sensation again plotted on the ordinate. This time, however, we have plotted the logarithm of the stimulus values on the abscissa. A major feature of the logarithmic relationship is that each log unit represents an equal *percentage* (constant proportion) change in the value of *S*. Notice that equal changes in sen-

TABLE 2-2. DEVELOPMENT OF THE LOGARITHMIC RELATION FROM THE WEBER FRACTION*

JND STEPS	STIMULUS VALUES	LOG STIMULUS	INCREMENT OF LOG
0	2	0.3010	
1	2.4	0.3802	0.0792
2	2.88	0.4594	0.0792
3	3.456	0.5386	0.0792
4	4.147	0.6178	0.0792
5	4.9764	0.6969	0.0792

* $JND = kS$, $k = 0.2$, $S_0 = 2$.

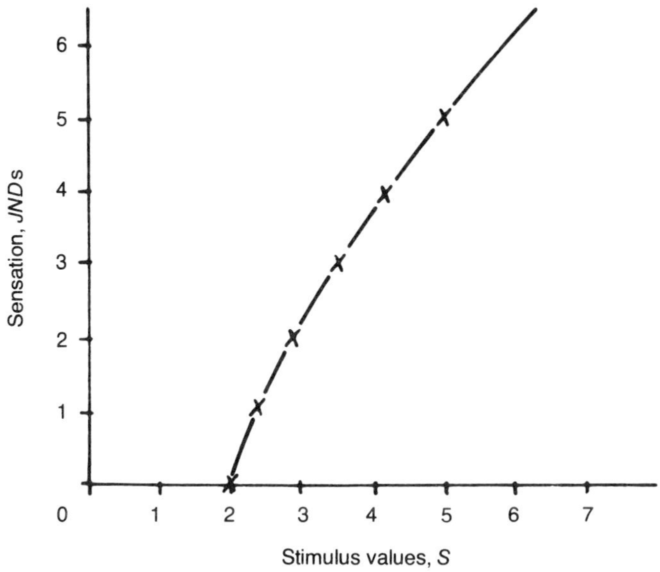

FIG. 2-2. The logarithmic relationship between stimulus strength and response magnitude. The sensation values are plotted against stimulus values in Table 2-2.

FIG. 2-3. Logarithmic relation. Data presented in Table 2-2 are replotted, this time plotting the log stimulus values instead of the values themselves, yielding a linear relationship whose equation is $R = k \log (S/S_0)$. The thing to notice here is that equal percentage changes in stimulus strength result in equal changes in response no matter what the values of strength and magnitude.

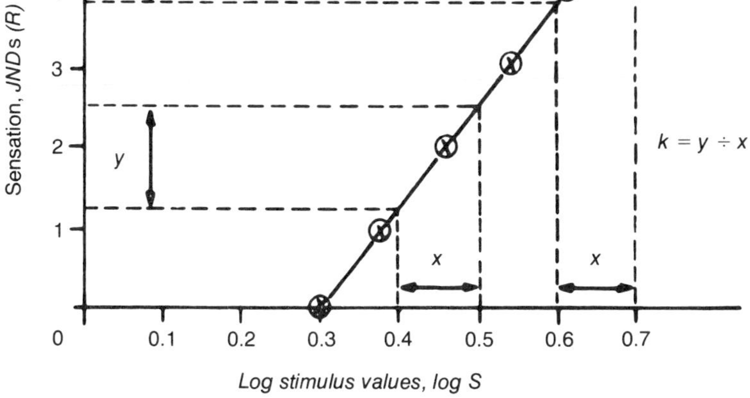

sation, "y," are produced by equal percentage changes in strength, "x."

A general relationship between stimulus strength and response magnitude for most senses then is the log function, $R = k \log (S/S_0)$, where R is the magnitude of the response, S is the stimulus strength, k is a constant for the particular sense, and S_0 is the threshold stimulus strength again treated as if it were a constant. You can prove to yourself that S_o is indeed the threshold. Rearrange the basic equation to the form $R = k \log S - k \log S_o$. If S_o is the threshold, then when $S = S_o$, R should equal zero. The magnitude of the sensation is a linear function of the log of the stimulus strength. This log relationship is usually referred to as the **Weber–Fechner function** or simply the **Fechner function.**

As mentioned earlier, the logarithmic relationship holds fairly well for midrange values of stimulus strength, but breaks down near threshold and maximal values. Because of this failure, the relationship between sensation and stimulus strength is often better fitted by a power function. With a power function law, sensation is related to stimulus strength raised to some power. Mathematically, a power function is represented by the equation $R = (S - S_o)^k$. In Figure 2-4A are plotted three power functions with different powers or exponents. They are k is equal to 1, k less than 1, and k greater than 1. In the case of $k = 1$, the power function is a straight line, the lines are curved upward for powers greater than 1, and downward for powers less than 1. It should be pointed out that all three curves pass through the origin; thus, the threshold, S_o, is set at zero. However, this is usually not the case; S_o usually has some nonzero value! The power function $R = (S - S_o)^k$ can be rearranged to the form, $\log R = k \log (S - S_o)$. This is the equation for a straight line. Therefore, if the values of sensation and stimulus intensity are plotted on log–log coordinates, a straight line results. The slope of this line is the exponent k. The power function relationship says that equal percentage changes in stimulus strength give equal percentage changes in the magnitude of the sensation.

But what is the biologic significance of these complicated relationships between sensation and stimulus? Why have organisms evolved in this way? We will demonstrate the biologic significance of logarithmic and power relationships by using an example. The average human can detect vibration of the palm of the hand over a range of frequencies from 2 to 400 cycles per second (or Hertz, Hz). A typical response curve is shown in Figure 2-5. In this graph, the amplitude of the vibration at threshold, expressed in micrometers, is plotted on the ordinate, and the frequency of the sine wave vibration stimulus, on the abscissa. The lowest threshold occurs at about 200 Hz, but the range of frequencies detected lies between 2 Hz and 400 Hz. With a standard frequency of 200 Hz, the measured *JND* for frequency of vibration is about one-tenth of the period or 0.5 msec (0.1×5 msec). This means that the period of the sine wave must be changed by 0.5 msec in order for the change in frequency to be detected. The 0.5-msec change in period corresponds to a 20-Hz change in terms of frequency. A frequency of 220 Hz is distinguishable from 200 Hz, but any frequency in between 220 and 200 Hz is not distinguishable from 200 Hz. A 2-Hz stimulus has

FIG. 2-4. Examples of power functions of the form $R = (S - S_o)^k$ for values of the constant k less than, equal to, or greater than 1. In **A,** stimulus values are plotted directly against response values, whereas in **B,** both stimulus and response values are plotted as logarithms.

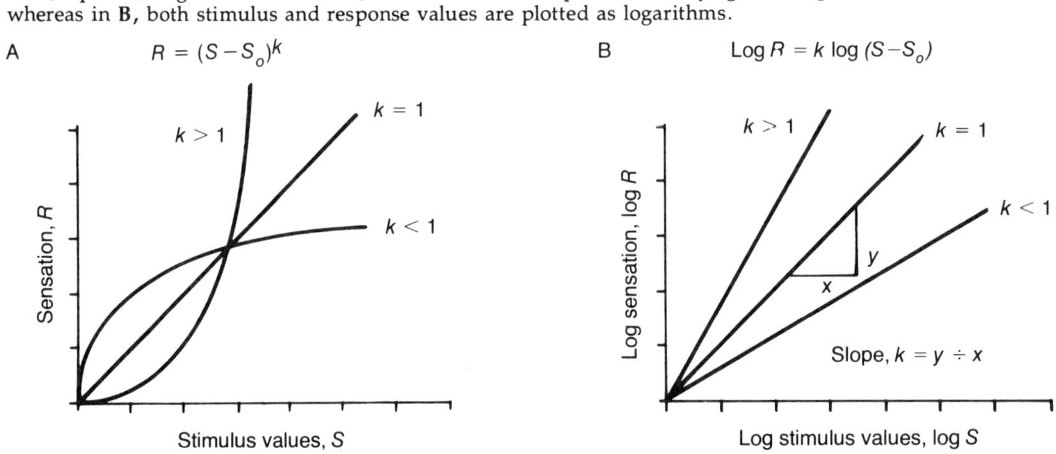

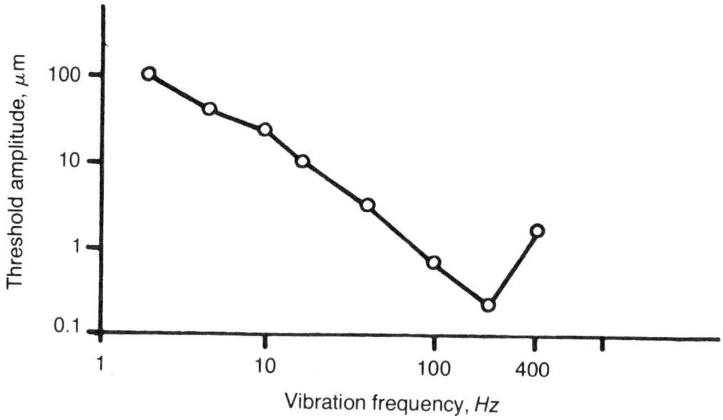

FIG. 2-5. The threshold displacement for vibration of the palm of the hand is plotted against the frequency of the vibration. (Mountcastle VB, LaMotte RH, Carli G: J Neurophysiol 35:122–136, 1972)

a period of 500 msec, whereas the period of a 400-Hz stimulus is 2.5 msec. These periods differ by 497.5 msec, which is divisible into 995, 0.5-msec intervals.

If the sensation of vibration frequency were a linear function of period length over the whole range of frequencies, a subject could distinguish 995 different frequencies. We have seen that the nervous system deals in action potentials, tiny voltage changes that last about 0.5 to 1 msec. If nerves from the skin were to signal a 2-Hz vibration by discharging 1 impulse/second, then the signal for 400 Hz would have to be nearly 1000 impulses/second. If each impulse lasts 1 msec, it is impossible for a neuron to squeeze more than 1000 impulses into a second. In actual fact, most neurons cannot discharge more than 400 to 500 impulses/second. This would create a problem for coding for the nervous system. However, the sensation of vibration frequency is not related directly to the stimulus period, but rather to a percentage of the period by the Weber fraction, $JND/S = 0.1$. Therefore, the number of frequencies that can actually be distinguished over the range from 2 to 400 Hz is only about 59, but the range of frequencies is greater than could be had by a linear relationship. A neuron discharging 1 impulse/second for a 2-Hz stimulus would only need to discharge 50 impulses/second to signal a 400-Hz vibration. This is an easy task for most neurons.

Thus, what the logarithmic or power relationship does is to expand the range of stimulus values that the person can sense, but the cost is a loss in ability to discriminate. This is made clear by examining the summary of the previous example in Table 2-3. If we limit the range of stimulus values by allowing only the values that can be signaled by a neuron (assuming an upper limit of 500/sec for axonal discharge rate), then the range of values a subject could sense if there were a linear function would be 2 to 4 Hz. (Remember that the *JND* is expressed in periods, not frequencies! 500 msec − 500 intervals (0.5 msec) = 250 msec or 4 Hz) The range for the logarithmic function would be

TABLE 2-3. COMPARISON OF THE PROPERTIES OF LINEAR AND LOGARITHMIC RELATIONS

PROPERTY	LINEAR $R = k\ (S - S_o)$	LOGARITHMIC $R = k \log (S/S_o)$
Range of stimulus values encodeable (500/sec)	2–4 Hz	2–1.5 × 10^{23} Hz
Number of discriminable frequencies in the range 2–400 Hz	995	59

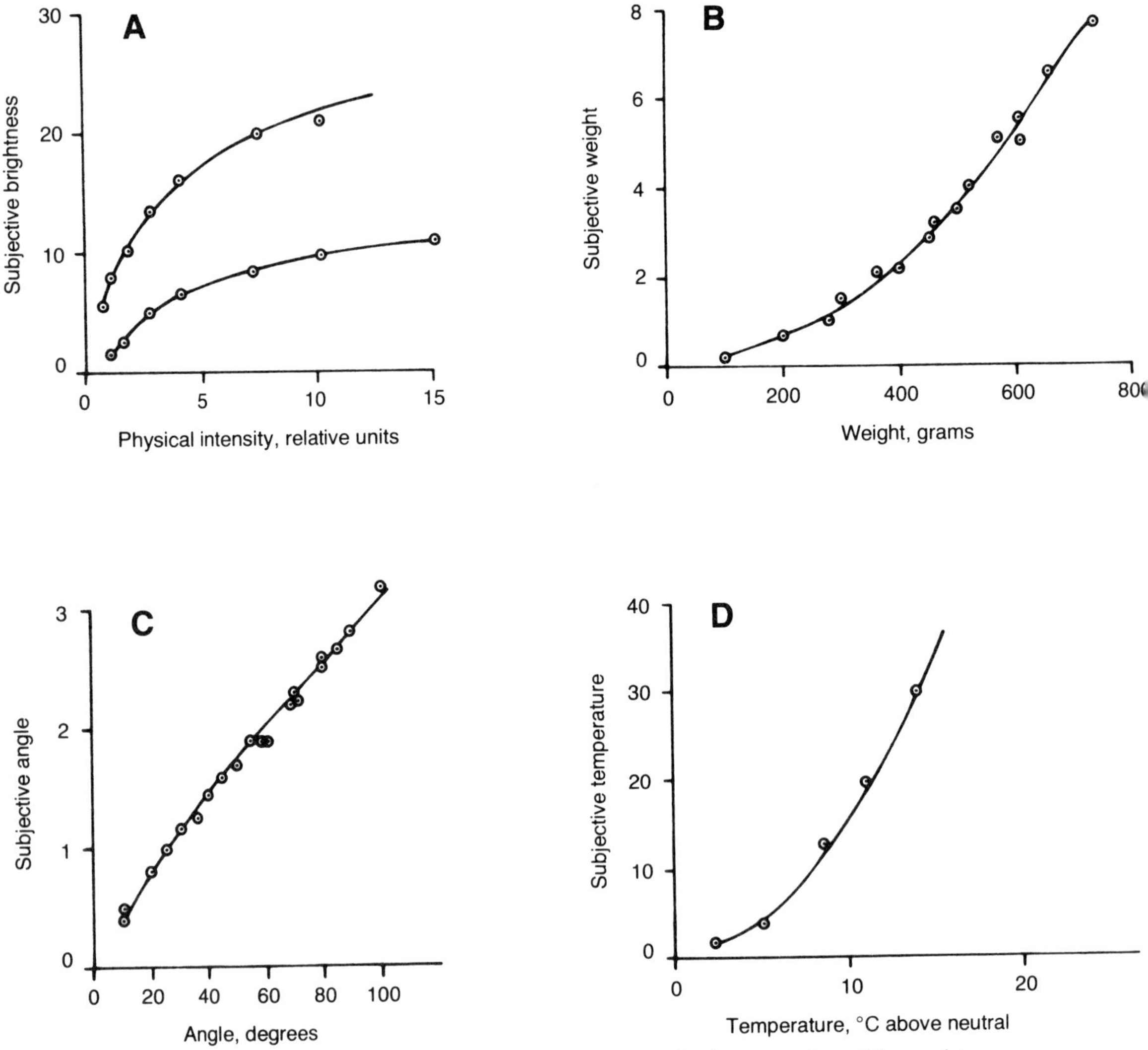

FIG. 2-6. Relationship between stimulus and response magnitudes for four sensations. Linear plots of stimulus magnitude (abscissa) against perceived magnitude (ordinate). **A.** Subjective brightness of lights of 672 nm (red) wavelength and 554 nm (green) wavelength at different strengths. **B.** Perceived magnitude of a lifted weight. **C.** Perceived angle between two surfaces felt with the hands. (Ekman G: Some aspects of psychophysical research. In Rosenblith WA [ed]: Sensory Communication. Cambridge MA, MIT Press, 1961) **D.** Geometric mean for 12 observers of perceived warmth of a stimulus applied to the inside of the forearm plotted against temperature in degrees centigrade above the threshold (Stevens SS: The psychophysics of sensory function. In Rosenblith WA [ed]: Sensory Communication. Cambridge MA, MIT Press, 1961)

2 to 1.5×10^{23} Hz. At the same time, the number of discriminable frequencies in the range of human perception would be 995 in the linear case and only 59 in the logarithmic case. On the average, the stimulus frequency must be changed by a greater amount to be judged as different in the case of a logarithmic relationship than would be the case if there were a linear relationship between sensation and stimulus strength. This is less true at lower frequencies than at higher ones. Of course, this analysis applies only to cases in which the exponent of the power function is less than one. When the exponent is greater than one, sensitivity is greater than for a linear relationship, but the range of stimulus values sensed is even smaller.

So far, we have dealt mainly with abstractions, but now we can examine some con-

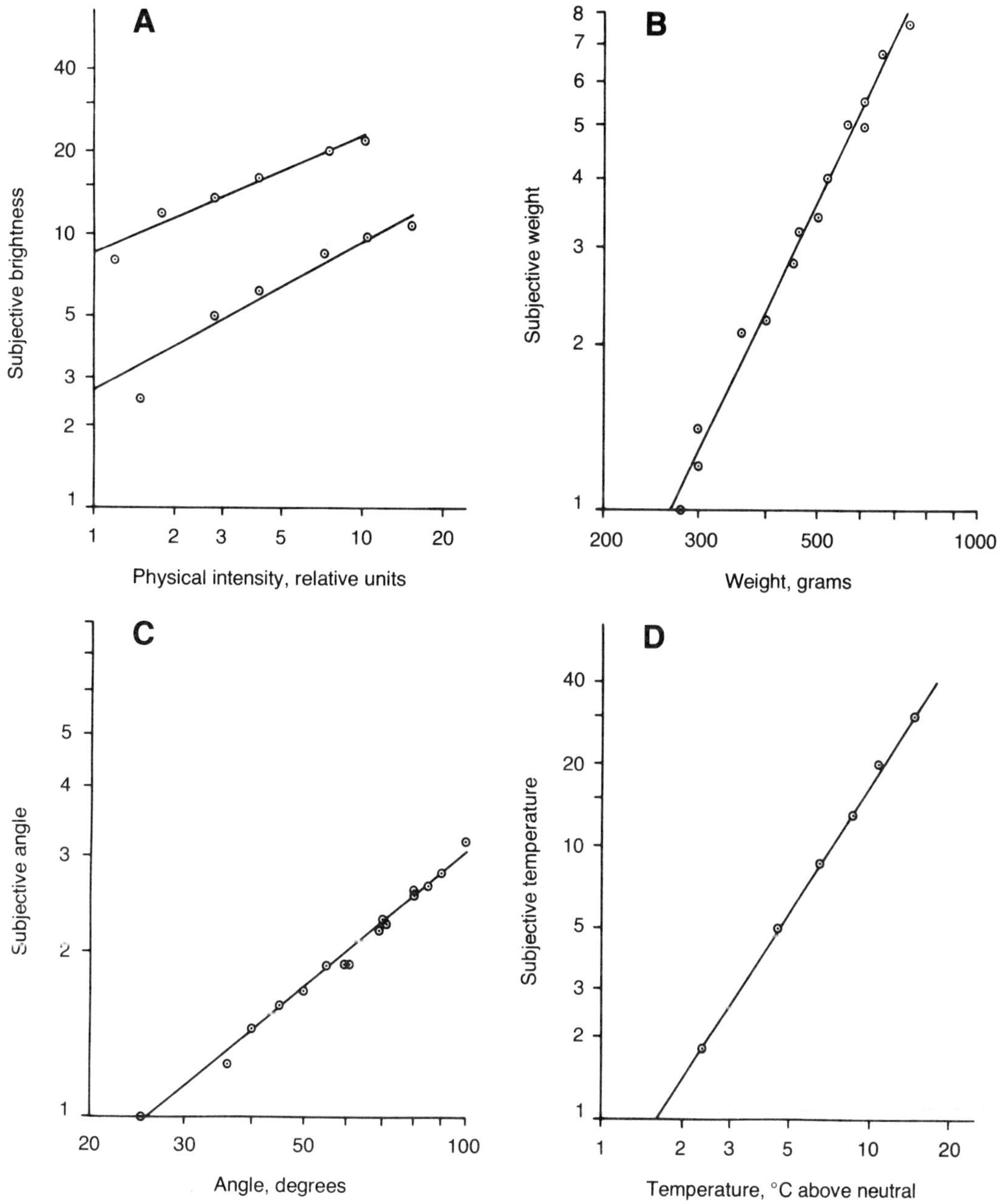

FIG. 2-7. Relationship between stimulus and response magnitudes for four sensations. Log plots of stimulus magnitude (abscissa) against log perceived magnitude (ordinate). Same conventions and sources as Figure 2-6.

crete examples of sensory thresholds. Linear plots of stimulus–response relationships for various sensations are shown in Figure 2-6. Upward concaved plots are shown for the perceived weight of a lifted object (Fig. 2-6B) and sensations of warmth (Fig. 2-6D). Downward concaved relations are shown for subjective brightness of lights of 554 nm (green, upper curve in A) and 672 nm (red, lower curve) and perceived angle between two surfaces felt with the hands (Fig. 2-6C). Figure 2-7 shows log–log plots for the same data as in Figure 2-6. Notice that the curves that are concaved upward result in lines with slopes greater than one (B,D), whereas those that are concaved downward result in

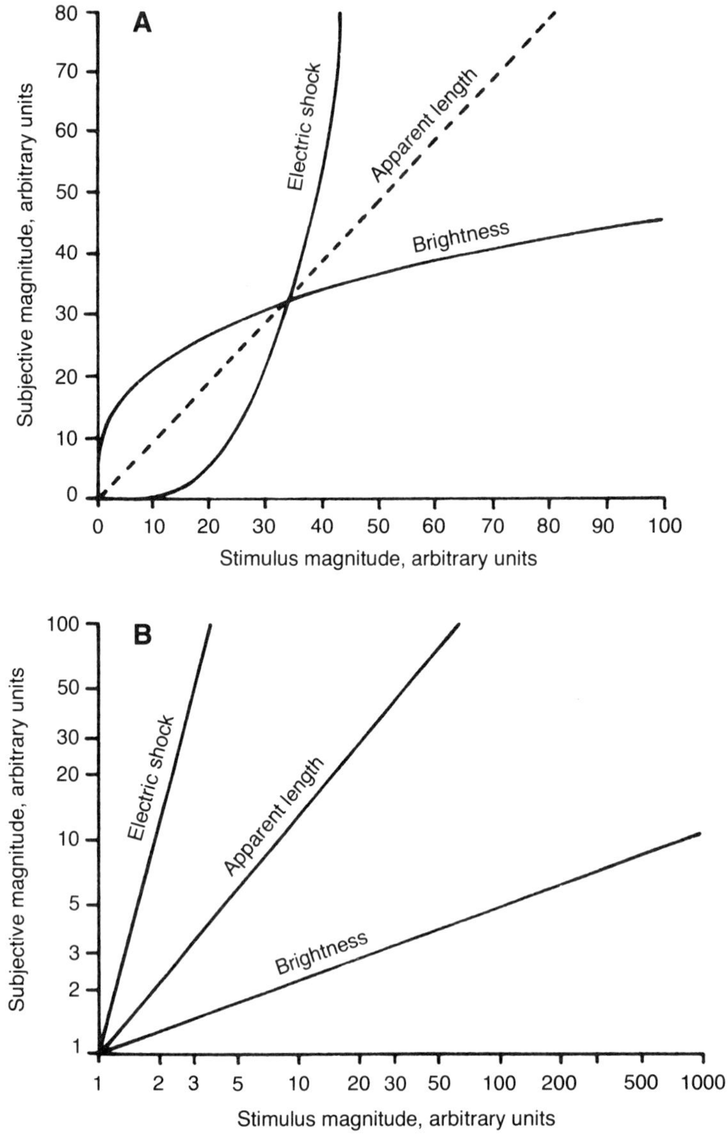

FIG. 2-8. Relationship between stimulus and response magnitude for electric shock, visually estimated length, and brightness. **A.** Linear plot of stimulus strength (abscissa) versus response magnitude (ordinate). **B.** Log–log replot of data in **A.** (Stevens SS: The psychophysics of sensory function. In Rosenblith WA [ed]: Sensory Communication. Cambridge MA, MIT Press, 1961)

lines with slopes less than one (A,C). The exponents of the power functions fitted to these data are 0.363 (red) and 0.356 (green) for brightness curves, 1.6 for perceived weight, 0.28 for perceived angle, and 1.6 for warmth.

Other examples of stimulus–response relationships are shown in Figure 2-8. In A are shown on the same linear axes, relationships between subjective magnitudes and stimulus magnitudes for sensitivity to electrical shock, visually estimated length, and brightness. These are concave upward (electric shock), concave downward (brightness), and nearly linear (apparent length). The resulting exponents of the descriptive power functions are 3.5 for shock, 0.33 for brightness, and 1.4 for length. These are the slopes of the lines in Figure 2-8B that are log–log replots of the data in A.

Exponent values for power functions for various sensory experiences, varying over a fairly wide range, are summarized in Table 2-4. The lowest value in the table is 0.28, the highest, 3.5. Most values are near 1.0, that is, nearly, but not quite linear. Different exponent values are sometimes obtained for the same variables, the exact value depending upon how the experiment is conducted and, therefore, the exact sensitivity measured. For example, when the magnitudes of sensations evoked by electrical shocks are measured using 60-Hz alternating current, the relationship is a simple power function with an exponent of 3.5, as shown in Figure 2-8. On the other hand, when single electrical pulses are used instead of alternating current, the relationship is a double power function, one extending from 0 to 2 mA with exponent 1.8 and one extending from 2 to 50 mA with exponent 0.9. Probably, two different sensations are being measured in these two studies. We will see, when we consider the sensory modalities, how some of these psychophysical functions may be related to processes in the central nervous system.

Let us summarize our discussion of psychophysics. Psychophysics is the science of measuring sensations and their thresholds. Thresholds vary depending upon the method of measurement and the individual. The magnitude of sensation increases as the stimulus energy is increased. The just-noticeable-difference is the amount of increase in stimulus strength needed in order for a person to perceive that a change has occurred. For most sensations, the *JND* is a constant fraction of the standard of comparison over a moderate range of stimu-

TABLE 2-4. REPRESENTATIVE EXPONENTS OF POWER FUNCTION RELATING PSYCHOLOGIC MAGNITUDE TO STIMULUS MAGNITUDE*

SENSATION	EXPONENT	STIMULUS CONDITIONS
Loudness	0.6	Binaural
Loudness	0.54	Monaural
Brightness	0.33	5° target—dark-adapted eye
Brightness	0.5	Point source—dark-adapted eye
Saturation	1.2	Reflectance of gray paper
Smell	0.55	Coffee odor
Smell	0.6	Heptane, citric acid
Taste	0.8	Saccharin
Taste	1.3	Sucrose
Taste	1.3	Salt
Temperature	1.0	Cold—on arm
Temperature	1.6	Warmth—on arm
Vibration	0.95	60 Hz—on finger
Vibration	0.6	250 Hz—on finger
Duration	1.1	White-noise stimulus
Repetition rate	1.0	Light, sound, touch, shocks
Angle†	0.28	Felt angles
Length	1.4	Visual estimation of line length
Finger span	1.3	Thickness of wood blocks
Pressure	1.1	Static force on skin of palm
Weight†	1.6	Lifted weights
Heaviness	1.45	Lifted weights
Force of handgrip	1.7	Precision hand dynamometer
Autophonic level	1.1	Sound pressure of vocalization
Pain‡	0.9	Electrical shocks to tooth pulp
Electrical shock	3.5	60 Hz, through fingers
Electrical shocks§	1.8, 0.9	Single pulses

* All values from Stevens SS: The psychophysics of sensory function. In Rosenblith WA [ed]: Sensory Communication. Cambridge, MA, MIT Press, 1961

† Ekman G: Some aspects of psychophysical research. In Rosenblith WA [ed]: Sensory Communication. Cambridge, MA, MIT Press, 1961

‡ Schwartz P: J Exp Psychol 45:288–293, 1953

§ Rosner PS, Giff WR: Contrib Sensory Physiol 2:169–221, 1968

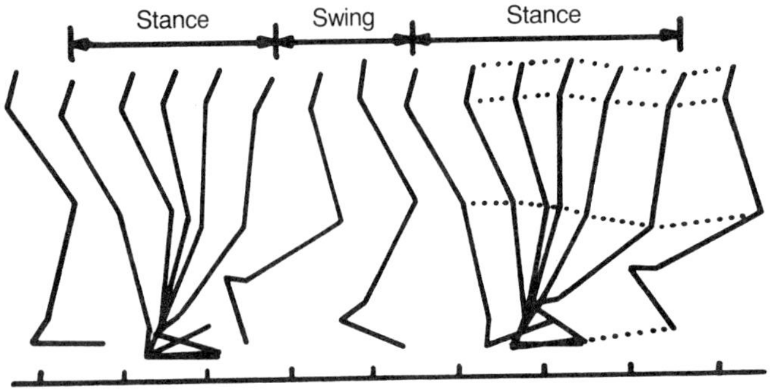

FIG. 2-9. Stick figures representing lower limb of a normal man walking on level ground at a rate of 90 steps/min. Approximate boundary positions for stance and swing phases are indicated. (Brunnstrom S: Clinical Kinesiology, 3rd ed. Philadelphia, FA Davis, 1972)

lus values. Finally, the relationship between the magnitude of a sensation and the stimulus strength most often is a power function. This allows a greater range of stimulus strengths to be sensed, but decreases the discriminability of two different stimulus strengths at low powers and a greater discriminability with a smaller range at high powers.

MOVEMENT

The range of movements that a human can produce is really extraordinary. He can move both rapidly and with great endurance, attaining speeds of 10 m/sec over a distance of 100 m. Among animals this is not a speed record by any measure; there are animals both faster and slower. The swift is capable of speeds of 62 m/sec through the air and the cheetah of 29 m/sec over land. Yet, although a man cannot outrun an antelope or kangaroo in a short distance (antelopes and kangaroos are capable of speeds of 18 m/sec for short distances), Australian aborigines are able to run them down over long distances. Modern man is capable of running nonstop more than 180 miles at an average speed of 2.7 m/sec (6 miles per hour). In water, a human can achieve a speed of 2 m/sec for short distances (100 meters). He can jump into the air more than 2 meters and leap at the end of a run nearly 9 meters; he can throw a hammer more than 75 meters (250 feet) and lift over his head more than 236 kg (521 pounds).

Obviously, these movements were achieved by athletes or highly practiced individuals and, therefore, they are not representative of the abilities of the average human. Figure 2-9 shows a movement of the average human, walking at the rate of 90 steps/min. The figure shows two complete stepping cycles for walking by a normal man. Stepping is divisible into two phases: a stance phase and a swing phase, both of which are indicated in the figure. The stance phase begins when the foot hits the ground (footfall) and ends when it is removed again, whereas the swing phase begins when the foot leaves the ground and ends when it makes contact again. Propulsion in the forward direction is achieved near the beginning of the stance phase when the joints of the limb are extending. The force they exert upon the substrate is not applied exactly vertically but obliquely, the horizontal component producing forward movement.

Figure 2-10 shows the rotation of the hip, knee, and ankle joints during the first cycle of stepping after a subject is given a "go" signal. Shortly after the signal, the toe leaves the ground and the ankle, hip, and knee joints are all flexing, as the leg is lifted. Before the end of the swing phase, the ankle and the knee begin to extend in preparation for contact of the limb with the ground, whereas the hip joint remains flexed until well into the stance phase, when it begins to extend as the leg moves backward with respect to the body. Just after the beginning of the stance phase, the ankle begins to flex as the leg begins its backward movement

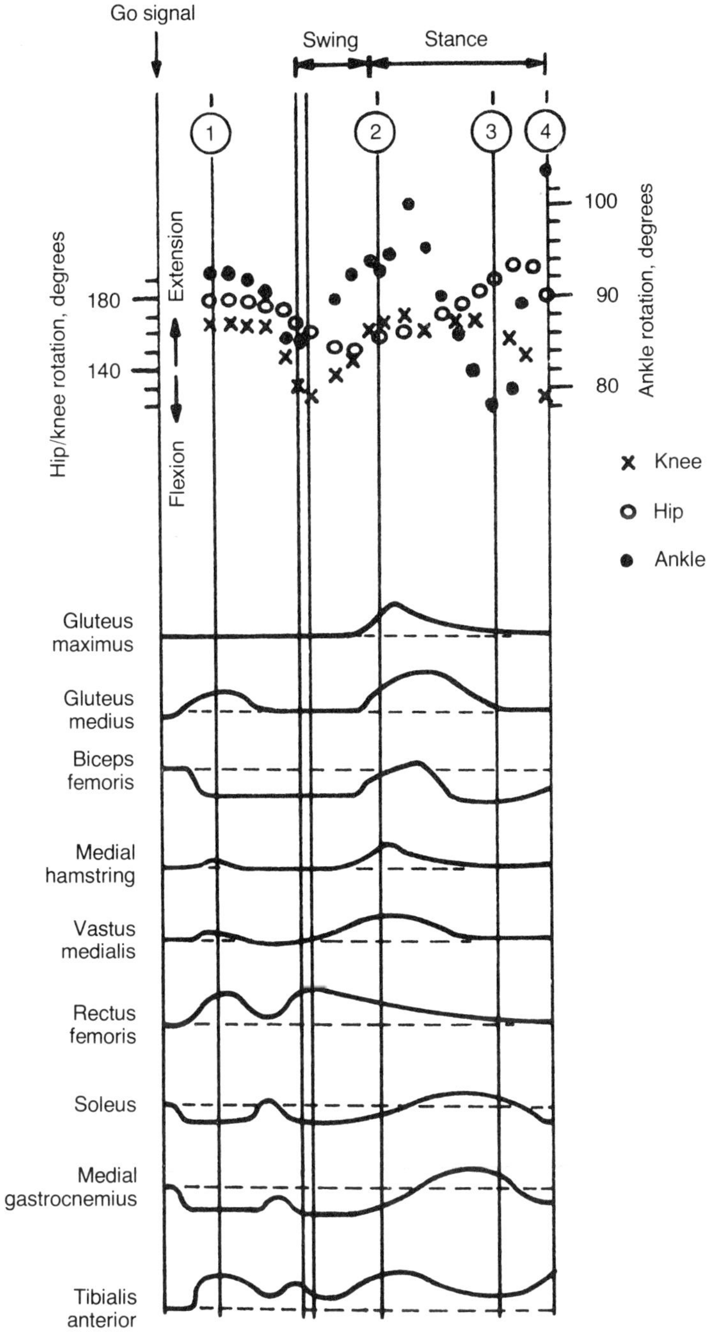

FIG. 2-10. Rotation of joints and muscle contraction during the stepping cycle in man. **Upper:** Angular motion of the ankle, knee, and hip joints during the step cycle. All movements are calibrated from a standard anatomic position: hip and knee at 180° and ankle at 90°. The subject began stepping at the "go" signal. Swing and stance phases are marked; circled numerals indicate: **1.** beginning of ankle rotation, **2.** foot flat on ground, **3.** heel off, and **4.** toe off. **Lower:** Envelope of the EMG activity of various muscles of the limb during the stepping cycle. **Dashed lines** indicate baseline EMG activity. (Herman R, Cook T, Cozzens B et al: Control of postural reactions in man. In Stein RB, Pearson KG, Smith RS, et al [eds]: Control of Posture and Locomotion. Advances in Behavioral Biology, Vol. 7. New York, Plenum Press, 1973)

and finally it extends again, lifting the heel away from the ground. The knee does not begin to flex again until the heel is removed from the ground, at which time the ankle and hip begin to extend. The three joints do not move in phase; the ankle leads the knee that leads the hip. The pattern of movement in Figure 2-10 occurs in all normal people.

The durations of the swing and stance phase vary with the speed of stepping, but the duration of the stance phase is always longer than that of the swing phase. As the stepping speed increases, the duration of the stance phase decreases, but the duration of the swing phase stays about the same, on the order of 0.5 sec, still remaining shorter than the stance phase. The two limbs move such that the toe of one limb leaves the ground, beginning its swing phase, when the center of mass of the body is nearly directly over the other foot, at the foot flat position in Figure 2-10. The hip and shoulder on the same side of the body move out of phase, such that when the hip is extending, the shoulder is flexing. The contralateral shoulder moves in phase with the hip.

The swing phase begins with increased activity in the gluteus medius, rectus femoris, and tibialis anterior muscles and decreased activity in the biceps femoris, soleus, and medial gastrocnemius muscles, as shown at the bottom of Figure 2-10. In the trace beside the name of each muscle, an upward deflection indicates an increase in the activity of the muscle and a downward deflection indicates a decrease. The decrease in activity of the soleus and medial gastrocnemius occurs suddenly 130 to 210 msec after the go signal and leads the increased activity in the antagonistic muscles (muscles with opposite action at the same joint) by 20 to 60 msec. Just before the beginning of the stance phase, all of the muscles whose activity is shown in the figure begin to increase their activity, that is, all but the rectus femoris that is decreasing its activity. Most muscles have more than one period of activity or inactivity during a single stepping cycle. In fact, an increase or decrease in the activity of the gastrocnemius and soleus and the reciprocal decrease or increase in the activity of their antagonist, the tibialis anterior, occurs four times during the time from quiet stance to toe off. The reciprocal relationship between activities in antagonistic muscles is necessary to allow the joint to rotate. We will see later that much is known about the neurophysiology of the stepping cycle, but much still remains to be learned about how the stepping cycle is initiated and how it is modulated to compensate for differences in terrain or for the presence of obstacles. We are also beginning to get a picture of what goes on in the nervous system during simple movements of the arms (see Chap. 16), but of more complicated movements, such as playing the piano, we know little.

Psychologists treat movements as if they were all responses to stimuli and therefore individual, isolatable units. This results from the stimulus-response paradigms of the behaviorist's theoretical framework and appears to be related to the insistence that behavior be observable. However, not all behavior is observable; animals and people do things that are unseen and can only be inferred from their later behavior. The author is reminded of a story told to him by Dr. Arnold Towe of the University of Washington. During a visit to the San Diego Zoo, Dr. Towe was watching the orangutan, who was lounging with his feet up and his head resting in his hands, much like an executive behind a desk. The orangutan was gazing about him but appeared to be paying no particular attention to another man standing nearby, smoking a cigar. The orangutan got up and began walking slowly around the cage in a spiral path that eventually brought him near the man with the cigar. When he was near enough, the orangutan's hand shot out and he grabbed the cigar before the man could react. The orangutan then resumed his "executive" posture, this time smoking the cigar as he had observed the man doing. Clearly, the orangutan had been paying careful attention to what was happening around him, but this attention was not observable and therefore, for the psychologist, could serve as neither stimulus nor response.

This example also serves to illustrate that behavior is not a series of disjointed stimuli and responses to them. Rather, it is a continuous flow system in which stimuli are constantly present and changing and behavior is continuous and continuously modifiable by both changing stimuli and previous behavior. This conceptual framework has made little impact on the thinking of physiologists, perhaps because we do not have an adequate way of dealing with flow systems in our thought processes.

OTHER BEHAVIORS

A simple catalog of human behaviors would fill several volumes, but even simple ones like perception and movement are not easily explained, as we shall see. More complex behaviors pose another type of problem for both the psychologist and the physiologist—that is, the problem of definition. What do we mean by emotion, motivation, personality, or frustration? What is thinking? Do animals do it? If so, how can we tell when they are doing it? Until we can get adequate answers to these questions, it is doubtful that any real progress can be made toward understanding these behaviors. Still, some progress has been made, as we shall see in Chapter 21.

SUGGESTED READING

Herman R, Cook T, Cozzens B, Freedman W: Control of postural reactions in man. In Stein RB, Pearson KG, Smith RS, Redford JB [eds]: Control of Posture and Locomotion. Advances in Behavioral Biology, Vol. 7. New York, Plenum Press, 1973

Herman R, Wirta R, Bampton S, Finley FR: Human solutions for locomotion. I. Single limb analysis. In Herman RM, Grillner S, Stein PSG, Stuart DG [eds]: Neural Control of Locomotion. Advances in Behavioral Biology, Vol. 18. New York, Plenum Press, 1976

Kendler HH: Basic Psychology. New York, Appleton-Century-Crofts, 1963

Stevens SS: Psychophysics, New York, John Wiley, 1975

3

Properties of Excitable Membranes: The Membrane Potential and the Spike

In attempting to account for behavior in relationship to the nervous system we should first turn our attention to what a single neuron does. Then, having the properties of single neurons in mind, we can proceed to put neurons together, studying their properties in networks.

MEMBRANE STRUCTURE

Neurons, like most living cells, have the full complement of intracellular organelles—nucleus, endoplasmic reticulum, Golgi apparatus—but it is the membrane of neurons that has received the most attention in scientific investigations. Other parts of nerve cells are beginning to occupy more prominent positions in ideas about nerve function (*e.g.*, see Chap. 18 on trophic functions), yet the rapid events typical of nerve cells are membrane events.

Like all cells, neurons are bounded by a membrane, the plasma membrane or plasmalemma. It is in many ways like the membranes of all animal cells, being composed of lipids (40%) and proteins (60%). The lipids of membranes are usually amphipathic, that is, their molecules have both polar and nonpolar regions. The polar regions are hydrophilic, meaning that in water the lipids orient themselves on the surface so that the polar ends are in water and the nonpolar ends project into the air as shown in Figure 3-1. Because the cell membrane separates two aqueous fluids, the extracellular fluid and the intracellular fluid or cytoplasm, the lipids of the membrane align themselves in two parallel rows, with polar ends toward the aqueous fluids and nonpolar ends facing each other, as shown in Figure 3-2. This arrangement, called a lipid bilayer or bimolecular leaflet, forms the skeleton of the membrane and is approximately 5 to 10 nm (1 nm = 10^{-9} meters) thick. Electron-microscopic views of membranes showed them to be uniformly trilaminar in appearance with two dark stripes separated by a lighter region. This appearance led to a model of the membrane, the so-called unit membrane, that was composed of the lipid bilayer covered completely on both inner and outer surfaces with protein molecules. More recent evidence suggests that globular proteins are actually intercalated into the bilayer with perhaps up to 80% of the surface being bare of proteins.

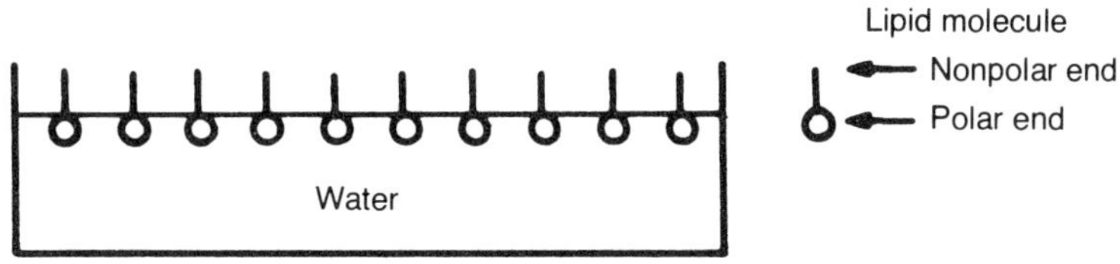

FIG. 3-1. Orientation of lipid molecules in an aqueous medium. When placed in water, lipid molecules line up on the surface with the polar ends in the water and the nonpolar ends out of the water.

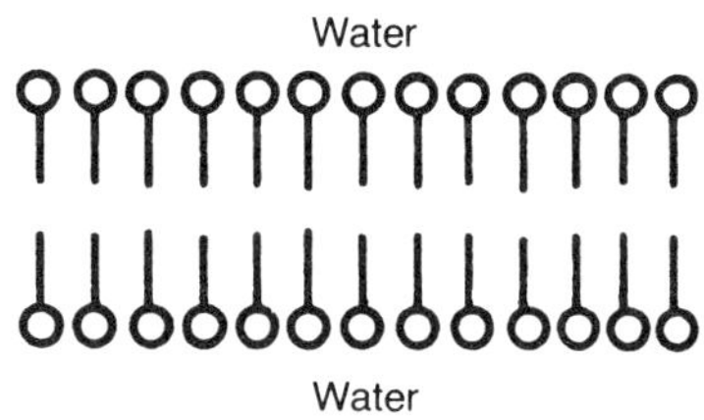

FIG. 3-2. Lipid bilayer between two aqueous phases. Lipids placed in a solution containing two phases (like intra- and extracellular fluids) form a bilayer with polar ends away from each other and nearer the aqueous phases and nonpolar ends toward each other and away from the aqueous phases.

FIG. 3-3. Fluid mosaic model of membrane. Lipid bilayer forms a fluid sea in which protein molecules float either on the surface, as extrinsic or structural proteins, or within the fluid, as intrinsic proteins. Channels are thought to be aggregates of intrinsic proteins, in contact with both intra- and extracellular fluids, surrounding a water-filled pore through which ions pass. Voltage-gated channels open when the transmembrane potential changes and chemically gated channels open when they are contacted by a transmitter molecule, indicated here as acetylcholine. (de Robertis E: Science 171:963–971, 1971)

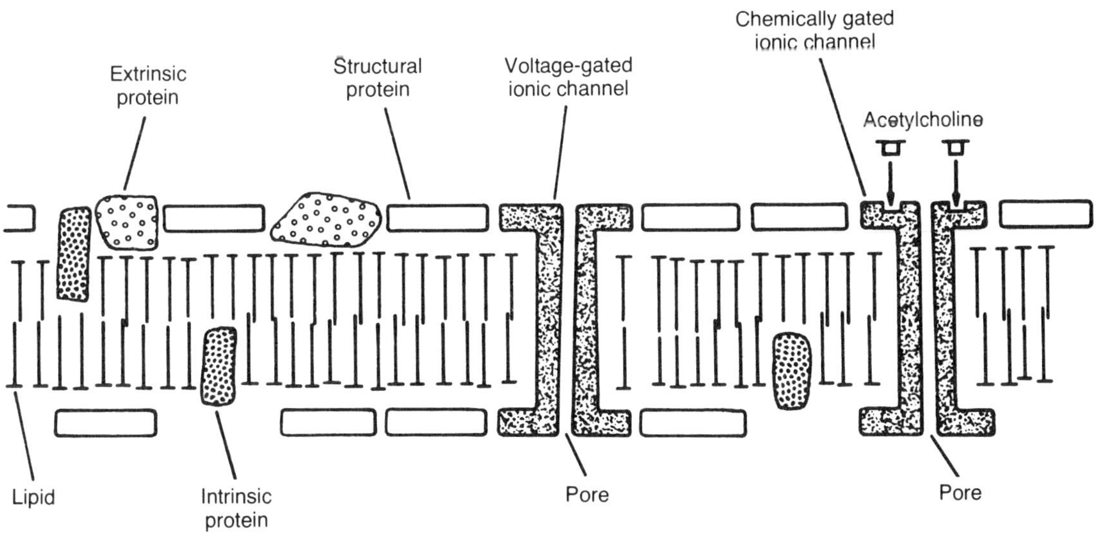

More hydrophilic proteins are only weakly associated with the lipids, and they remain near the surface of the membrane. These are often called peripheral proteins. Proteins that are more hydrophobic may extend across much of the bilayer; these are the intrinsic proteins. When the proteins have hydrophilic ends and large hydrophobic regions, they may extend completely through the lipid bilayer and jut out into the adjacent fluids (Fig. 3-3).

The lipid bilayer is considered to be a fluid in or on which the proteins float. Many of the proteins appear to have relatively free movement; others appear to be firmly attached to a substructure and therefore do not move. Certainly, the polarization of neurons, with axons and dendrites having distinct, relatively fixed functions and properties, suggests that some of the proteins must be fixed. On the other hand, the apparent migration of acetylcholine receptors (binding sites for the transmitter substance) away from a previous end-plate region (point of synaptic contact with motoneurons) in denervated muscle and their reaggregation upon reinnervation suggests that the mobility of proteins within the membrane may be limited by forces external to the cell.

What distinguishes one membrane from another is the nature of the proteins in the membrane. In nerve, there appear to be five functional types of membrane proteins. These are structural elements, enzymes, **receptors, channels** or **pores,** and **pumps.** The structural proteins may be involved in holding cells together at junctions, stabilizing other proteins within the membrane, or maintaining some aspects of subcellular structure. Enzyme proteins facilitate chemical reactions, and presumably those located in or on the membrane are involved in chemical reactions involved in membrane function. The membrane of the cell must be able to recognize particular molecules (*e.g.*, transmitter substances) and bind selectively with those molecules. Receptor proteins provide binding sites of high affinity and selectivity. Charged molecules do not pass readily through lipid media; thus, the membrane must contain specific channels through which ions can move to enter or leave the cell. These channels are provided by certain protein molecules. As we shall see shortly, the concentrations of different ions are not the same inside and outside the cell and yet the membrane is leaky to these ions. To maintain these differing ion concentrations that are fundamental to neuron function, pumps expend energy to expel certain ions from the cell and bring other ions into the cell. The pump proteins are intimately involved in this process. It is not necessary that a given protein molecule serve only one of the functions above. In fact, at the neuromuscular junction, the same protein is thought to act as a receptor for acetylcholine and a channel protein for both Na^+ and K^+ ions. Channels and pumps are discussed in more detail later.

MEMBRANE PERMEABILITY

The nerve membrane is permeable to a large number of compounds and ions. In general, lipid-soluble substances move through the membrane more rapidly than lipid-insoluble substances, and smaller molecules move through more rapidly than larger ones. Medium and large molecules move through the membrane only if they are lipid-soluble, but small molecules move through whether they are lipid-soluble or not. The existence of pores or channels through the membrane was postulated to explain how lipid-insoluble substances could diffuse through a lipid membrane in which they cannot dissolve. No one has yet seen a pore under the microscope but it seems likely that the pores are tortuous pathways through protein molecules or between them. It appears that there is a spectrum of pore diameters and permeabilities, some admitting most ions smaller than a certain maximum size and others selectively permitting only particular ions to pass through. Divalent ions usually pass through less readily than monovalent ions. For monovalent ions, the permeability of the membrane is $Cs^+ > Rb^+ > K^+ > Na^+ > Li^+$ and $I^- > Br^- > Cl^- > F^-$. These sequences are not determined strictly by molecular weight or diameter; Na^+ ions are 30% smaller in diameter than K^+, yet the membrane is 20 to 30 times more permeable to K^+.

This surprising result is explained in part by the tendency of ions to be hydrated. There is an attractive force between the positive charge of the ion and the negative end of the water dipole, so that water molecules accumulate around the ion, forming a shell. The radius of the hydration shell for sodium is larger than that for potassium; it has an effectively larger diameter. As we shall see, the two ions share some channels and also have separate channels in the membrane, and the ease with which they pass through the membrane is a function of

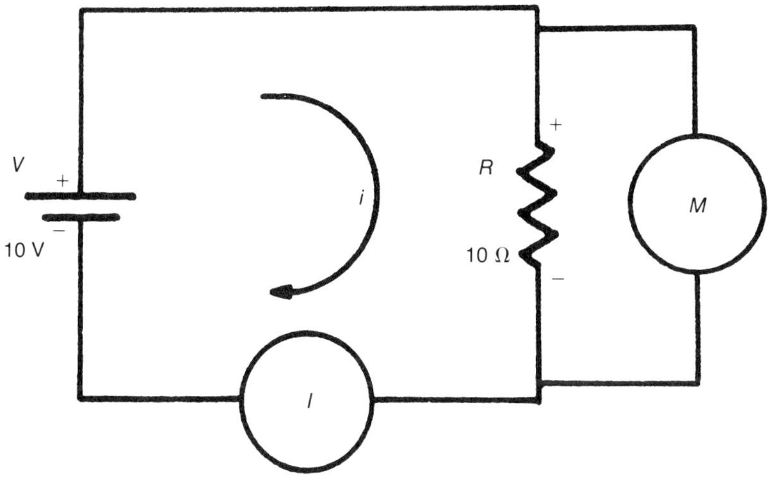

FIG. 3-4. A simple resistance circuit. A battery, V, is used to apply a voltage of 10 V across a resistance, R, of 10 Ω. The voltage and current in the circuit are measured using a voltmeter, M, in parallel with R and an ammeter, I, in series with R. In this case, the voltmeter reads 10 V, with polarity as indicated by +,− signs, and the ammeter reads 1 A.

interactions with parts of the channel structure and the positions of water molecules within the channel.

ELECTRICAL PROPERTIES OF MEMBRANES

The nerve cell membrane behaves like an electrical circuit containing resistance and capacitance. To understand its behavior it is important to review the behavior of electrical circuits. First, let us recall a few definitions. A voltage or potential difference is a separation of unlike charges in space; the greater the amount of charge separated, the larger the voltage, V, and the greater the tendency for the charges to flow toward each other. Voltage is always measured at one point with respect to another point. The unit of voltage is a volt, V. A flow of electrical charges is a current, i, measured in coulombs/sec or amperes, A. Resistance is a measure of the difficulty with which current flows in a circuit; the greater the difficulty, the greater the resistance, R. The unit of resistance is the ohm, Ω. The reciprocal of the resistance is called the conductance, g, a measure of the ease with which a current flows in a circuit. The unit of conductance is the mho.

Current, voltage, and resistance are related to each other by Ohm's law: $i = V/R$. This relationship for simple resistive circuits says that for a given resistance, the current increases linearly with the voltage or the current driven by a particular voltage depends upon the resistance. Of course, Ohm's law can be rewritten $i = gV$, where $g = 1/R$. We will have occasion to use this form later.

Consider the simple circuit in Figure 3-4. The circuit contains a voltage source, V, indicated by the battery and a resistance, R. Kirchhoff's law states that current flows only in complete or closed circuits. The circuit shown is complete. Because we have a potential difference and a resistance, we know there will be current in the circuit that can be measured by an ammeter, I. That current can be calculated from Ohm's law as follows:

$$V = 10 \text{ V}$$
$$R = 10\ \Omega$$
$$i = V/R = 1 \text{ A}$$

The current flowing through the resistor produces a voltage drop (a difference in electrical potential) across the resistor that can be measured by the meter, M, a voltmeter. We can assume that the meters are perfect (real meters seldom are), that is, no current flows through them and they do not influence the operation of the circuit; thus, the entire voltage, V, is imposed across R. The measured voltage drop across R will be

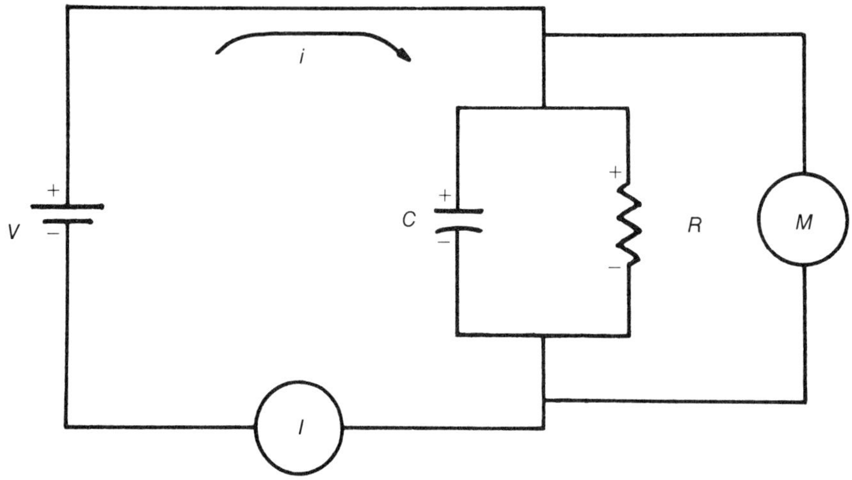

FIG. 3-5. A simple resistance–capacitance circuit. The same circuit as in Figure 3-4, but with a capacitor, C, placed in parallel with the resistance, R. The voltages across the resistance and the capacitance are the same as the battery voltage, V, and the same as read by the voltmeter, M. The polarity of the voltages is as indicated by +,− signs.

10 V with the polarity of the voltage as shown. The wires of the circuit have a very low resistance, so there will be essentially no voltage drop due to the wires (from Ohm's law again, $V = iR$; if $R = 0$, then $V = 0$) and the potential will be the same at the upper ends of the resistor and the battery. The same argument applies to the lower ends.

The direction of current flow in the external circuit, that part of the circuit outside the battery, is taken, by convention, to be the direction a positive particle would move. Actually, current in this type of circuit is carried by electrons, but the direction of current flow is opposite to their movement, that is, from + to −. Notice that, in order to complete the circuit, current flows from − to + within the battery (the internal circuit). We will see that most charge carriers for membrane events are positively charged ions, or cations; currents, by convention, will flow the way they move.

A capacitor is a device that is capable of separating and storing charge. Usually a capacitor is made of two parallel conducting plates separated by a nonconductor or dielectric material. The capacitance of a capacitor is symbolized by C and related to voltage by $C = Q/V$, where Q is the charge. The unit of capacitance is the farad. The larger the capacitance, the larger is the amount of charge that must be added to the plates to bring the voltage between them to a given value. Looked at in another way, the larger the capacitance, the larger will be the amount of charge stored on the plates for a given voltage between them. We speak of increasing the charge stored on a capacitor as "charging the capacitor" and decreasing the charge stored as "discharging the capacitor."

Introduction of a capacitor, as in Figure 3-5, changes the behavior of the circuit. No electrons actually flow between the plates of a capacitor because of the dielectric material between them, but when the battery is connected in the circuit, positive charges build up on the upper plate and are drawn off of the lower plate, producing a voltage between the plates. The charge flowing onto or off of a plate is a current, the capacitor current, i_c. This current is related to capacitance and voltage by the equation $i_c = C\, dV/dt$, where dV/dt is the rate of change of voltage between the plates. Before the battery is hooked up, the voltage is zero and unchanging; therefore, $dV/dt = 0$ and $i_c = 0$. When the battery is hooked up, the plates start to charge and continue until the voltage between the plates equals V. At this time, dV/dt again becomes zero and $i_c = 0$. Thus, current only flows "through" the capacitor when the voltage is changing.

If there were no resistance in the circuit of Figure 3-5, the battery could be disconnected, and the voltage between the plates of the capacitor would remain at V (at least

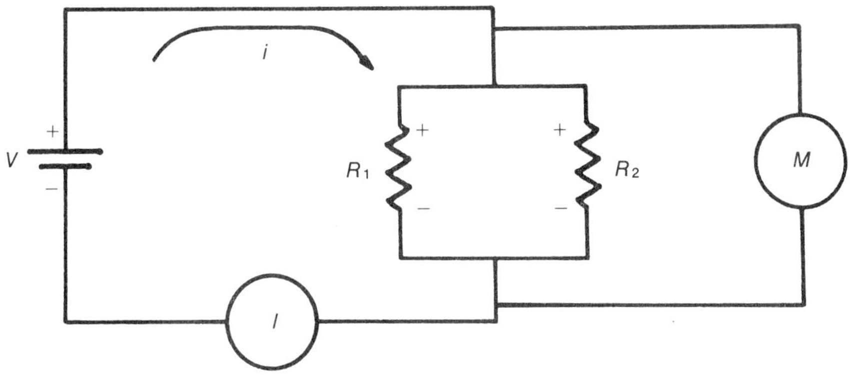

FIG. 3-6. A simple parallel resistance circuit. The two resistances, R_1 and R_2, are in parallel, that is, they share the same input and combine their outputs. The voltmeter, *M*, still reads the value of the battery, *V*.

FIG. 3-7. Effects of varying resistance on circuit voltage. **A.** A battery and a resistor are shown in each of two parallel circuits. With the configuration shown, the voltmeter, *M*, will read 85 V, point **b** positive with respect to point **d. B.** The same circuit as in **A**, but with the resistors interchanged, leads to a voltmeter reading of 35 V, point **b** negative with respect to point **d.** The polarity and voltage have been changed by simply changing the resistances.

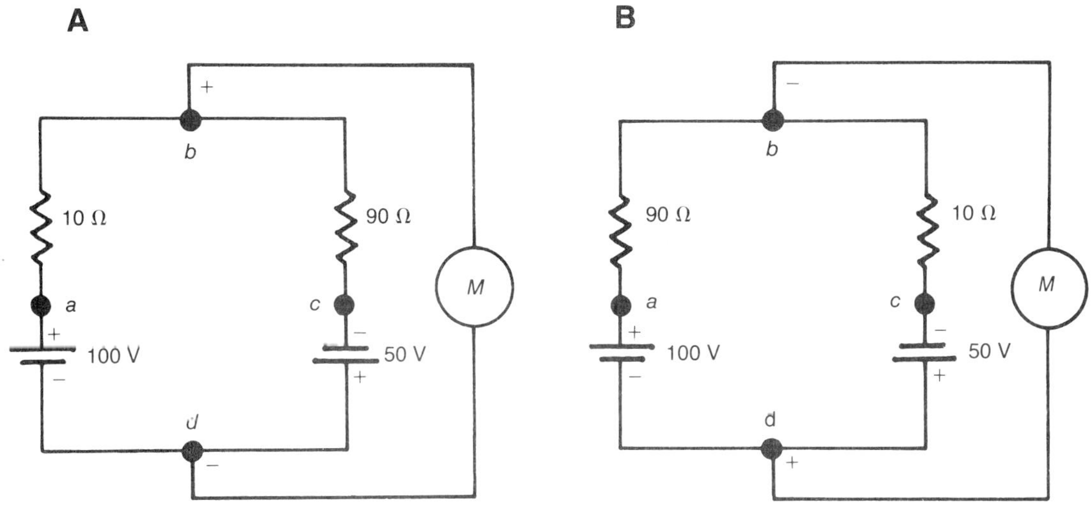

for a perfect capacitor). The resistor provides a current pathway through which the capacitor can discharge. The larger *R* is, the less current will flow per unit of time and the less rapidly the capacitor voltage will fall. In fact, the time for discharge varies directly with both *R* and *C*. The time required for the voltage to attain $(1 - 1/e)\ \Delta V$ or about $\frac{2}{3}\ \Delta V$ (ΔV is the total voltage change) is called the **time constant,** τ, and is given by the equation $\tau = R \times C$. If *R* is expressed in ohms and *C* in farads, then τ will be expressed in seconds. In circuits, such as that in Figure 3-5, without rectification, the charging and discharging time constants are equal. (Here, rectification is used in the engineer's sense of a lower resistance to current flow in one direction than the other through a circuit element.) As we shall see, the membrane has rectifying properties that make them unequal.

In electrical circuits, resistances in series simply add. Thus, *R* in Figure 3-4 can be replaced by two resistors of value *R*/2 in series without changing the properties of the circuit. However, parallel resistances are another matter. Consider the parallel resistive circuit in Figure 3-6. The potential difference across both R_1 and R_2 will be the same, namely V. Thus, the current through R_1 will be $i_{R_1} = V/R_1$ and that through R_2 will be $i_{R_2} = V/R_2$. The total current will be as follows:

$$i = \frac{V}{R_{\text{total}}} = i_{R_1} + i_{R_2} = \frac{V}{R_1} + \frac{V}{R_2}.$$

Dividing by V gives

$$\frac{1}{R_{\text{total}}} = \frac{1}{R_1} + \frac{1}{R_2}$$

Thus, in a parallel resistive circuit, resistances add reciprocally. Capacitors in parallel each store charge; therefore, more charges are stored for the same voltage. In parallel, $C_{\text{total}} = C_1 + C_2$. When capacitors are in series, each sees a voltage that is smaller and thus stores fewer charges. In series,

$$\frac{1}{C_{\text{total}}} = \frac{1}{C_1} + \frac{1}{C_2}$$

Two additional circuits are worth considering before beginning our discussion of membrane events. These are shown in Figure 3-7. The batteries in Figure 3-7A are both driving current in the same direction, thus the voltage between points a and c will simply be the sum of the two battery voltages, 150 V, with point a being positive with respect to point c. The total resistance of the circuit (the resistors are in series) is 100 Ω. Therefore, the current in the circuit is 150 V/100 Ω or 1.5 A. When 1.5 A flows through 10 Ω, a potential drop of 1.5 A × 10 Ω or 15 V is produced, point a being positive with respect to point b. The potential difference between points b and d, the value shown on the meter, will be 100 V − 15 V or 85 V, with point b being positive with respect to point d. Calculation of the voltage using the 90-Ω resistor portion of the circuit must yield the same value and can be done as an exercise.

Figure 3-7B is the same as 3-7A except that the values of the resistors are interchanged. The current in the circuit is still 1.5 A and the potential drop across 10 Ω is still 15 V, but this time the meter will read 50 V − 15 V or 35 V, with point b being negative with respect to point d. Again, by symmetry, the calculation for the 90-Ω resistor will give the same value. Note that the potential difference between points b and d is changed in magnitude and polarity simply by changing the resistance (or conductance), without altering the battery voltages. This observation will become important later when we consider the origin of the action potential.

Electrically, the nerve axon behaves like a very poor conductor of electricity. The axoplasm, the cytoplasm in the axon, has a very high resistance. For the squid axon, the longitudinal resistivity is about 30 to 60 Ω cm. This is extremely high compared with a copper wire of the same diameter, which has a resistivity of only 1.8×10^{-6} Ω cm. The main reasons for this difference in resistance are that the density of charge carriers is smaller (ions in cytoplasm are less dense than electrons in copper wire) and their mobility is less (ions in solution move much less readily than electrons in copper wire). The voltage drop (loss) along 1 cm of cytoplasm is about 10^7 times greater than that occurring along 1 cm of wire.

The membrane of a neuron behaves like a resistor, that is, when current is passed through the membrane, a voltage drop occurs that is predictable from Ohm's law. Values of membrane resistance are usually expressed as area specific resistance in Ω cm^2. (Membrane resistance decreases with increases in membrane area; therefore it is measured in ohms × cm^2, whereas membrane capacitance increases with increases in area and is expressed as μF per cm^2.) Motoneurons of the lobster have a membrane resistance of 2300 Ω cm^2.

The neural membrane also behaves like a capacitor, that is, it is capable of separating and storing charge. The capacitance of most neural membranes is of the order of 1 μF/cm^2, meaning that the membrane can separate and store a charge of 1×10^{-6} coulomb/volt of potential across the membrane per cm^2. Thus, the membrane can separate charges due to 10^{-12} mole of univalent ions/volt (Faraday's constant: 96,516 coulombs/mole of univalent ions). We will see shortly that the membrane does in fact separate considerable charge.

The effects of membrane resistance and capacitance are shown in Figure 3-8. The drawing shows the setup of the experiments. A pair of micropipette electrodes are inserted through the membrane of the axon. The pipettes are made of 1 to 2-mm glass capillary tubing drawn out into a fine tip (less than 1 μm in diameter) and filled with

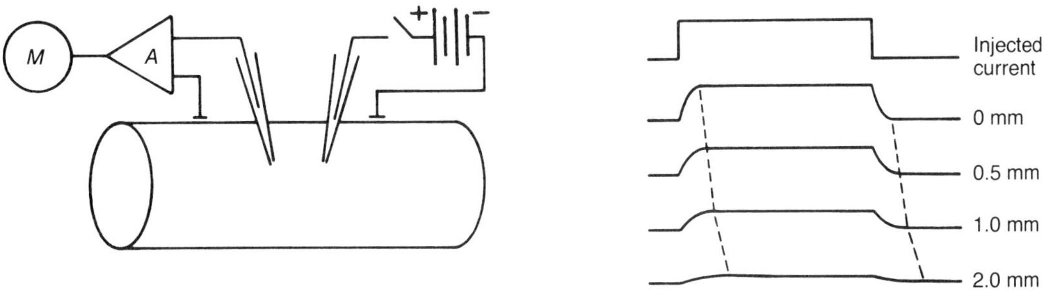

FIG. 3-8. Effects of membrane resistance and capacitance on membrane voltage. Recording setup shows two micropipette electrodes penetrating an axon membrane, one used for stimulation **(right)** and the other for recording **(left)**. The transmembrane potential is recorded between the micropipette inside the axon and another electrode outside the axon, using amplifier A and an oscilloscope, M. The stimulating current flows from the second micropipette, out through the membrane, and back, through another external electrode, to the battery. The distance between the micropipette electrodes can be varied. On the right are the monitor of the injected current in the upper trace and the transmembrane voltage in successively lower traces when the electrodes are 0, 0.5, 1.0 and 2.0 mm apart. The gain of the amplifier is the same in all voltage traces.

FIG. 3-9. Resistance–capacitance model of the membrane. The outside of the membrane is at the **top**, the inside at the **bottom** of the figure. A single short segment of membrane is shown at the left and two consecutive segments at the right. Membrane resistance is indicated by R_m, membrane capacitance by C_m, and the longitudinal resistance of the intracellular fluid by R_i.

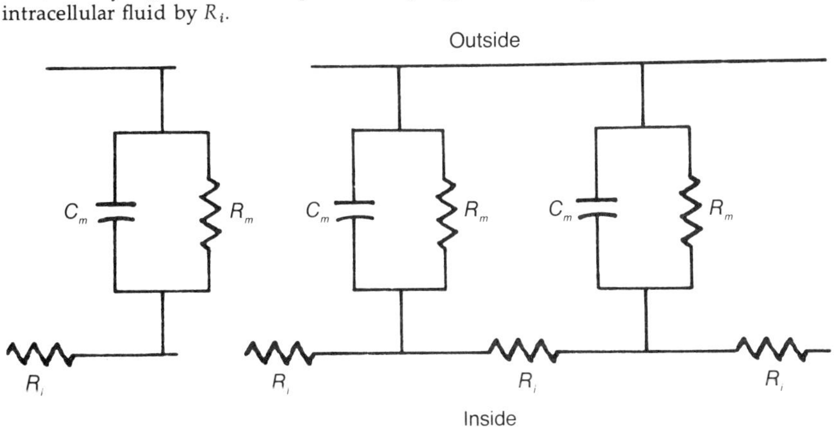

a conducting solution such as KCl. A fine wire is inserted into each of the pipettes, and one is connected to a stimulator that produces a square current pulse while the other is connected to the input of an amplifier. The other amplifier input contacts the extracellular fluid and thus the transmembrane voltage is amplified and can be displayed on an oscilloscope. When a square current pulse, such as that shown in the upper trace, is passed through the membrane, the recording system sees a voltage such as that shown in the second trace. The recorded voltage rises more slowly than the current to a maximum and then, after the current is turned off, the voltage falls slowly back to its initial value. The greater the distance between the stimulating and recording electrodes, the more slowly the voltage will rise and the smaller will be the maximum value (lower traces in Fig. 3-8). This experiment illustrates why the time constant of the membrane should be measured at the site of current injection; values at other sites will be inaccurate because of the influences of membrane length. Values for τ for neurons range from 0.5 to 5.0 msec.

It is useful in attempting to understand the properties of the nerve membrane to construct a circuit model as done in Figure 3-9. We know that the membrane has both resistance and capacitance and that the intracellular and extracellular fluids both have a resistance. We can symbolize these as R_m, C_m, R_i, and R_o, respectively. The longitudinal resistance, whether inside the axon or out, is inversely related to the area of the pathway over which current can flow. Although the intracellular area is small and bounded by the axis cylinder, the interstitial medium is large. The extracellular resistance is therefore much smaller than the intracellular resistance and it can be neglected. The figure shows the membrane resistance, R_m, in parallel with the membrane capacitance. This arrangement is shown repeated in each adjacent patch of membrane. These patches are linked by the intracellular fluid resistance and the extracellular fluid resistance, the latter treated here as zero. The changes in the membrane voltage are the result of current flow through the membrane only, but to reach each patch of membrane the current must flow through the intracellular fluid resistance. The intracellular resistances are in series so the farther a given patch is from the source of the current the larger will be the effective intracellular resistance and the greater the attenuation of the voltage ($V = iR$).

The distance along the membrane at which the imposed voltage, V, has been attenuated to $1/e \times V$ is called the **space constant,** λ. Because $e = 2.72$ or about 3, λ is the distance along the membrane at which V has fallen to about ⅓ of its initial value. The space constant is related to axon resistances as $\lambda = \sqrt{R_m/(R_o + R_i)}$, where R_m is the transmembrane resistance, and R_o and R_i are external and internal longitudinal resistances, respectively. For most neurons, λ is about 2 mm. Thus, if information to be transmitted is expressed as a membrane voltage and this voltage is conducted passively or electrotonically along the neuron, distances over 5 mm would be well outside the conduction ability of the membrane; 5 mm away from its source, the voltage would be essentially zero.

The membrane capacitances shown in Figure 3-9 are in parallel so the farther away from the current source the greater is the capacitance. The greater the capacitance and resistance of a circuit, the greater is the time constant and the more slowly voltage changes occur. It is not surprising, in view of these drastic attenuations and distortions over short distances, that neural transmission occurs by a specialized process, the self-regenerative action potential.

MEMBRANE IONIC ENVIRONMENT

The nerve membrane is capable of storing, transmitting, and releasing electrical energy and yet it contains no metallic conductors. Neither are such metallic conductors found in the intra- or extracellular fluids. It is, therefore, unlikely that membrane currents represent flows of free electrons, but it is to the electrolytes, the ions, that we must look for carriers of membrane currents.

The intracellular fluid consists of an aqueous solution containing relatively large amounts of potassium, but small amounts of chloride, sodium, calcium, and magnesium. In addition, it contains some organic anions (negatively charged molecules) to which the membrane is impermeable, that is, they cannot leave the cell. Table 3-1 shows both intracellular and extracellular concentrations of ions for the giant axon of the squid mantle (a cylinder of membrane about 0.5 mm in diameter), frog muscle fibers, and motoneurons in the cat spinal cord. Relative to intracellular fluid, extracellular fluid is rich in sodium, chloride, calcium, and magnesium, but poor in potassium.

DIFFUSION

The behavior of ions in solution is such that these differences in concentration across the membrane could not long be maintained unless the membrane formed an effective barrier between the two aqueous phases or some energy-requiring process existed to maintain them. Let us examine the behavior of ions in solution in some detail. If we place some salt, NaCl, into one of two compartments separated by a removable partition, as shown in Figure 3-10A, and add equal volumes of water to both compartments, we can determine how solutes move in solutions. Within a few minutes after removal of the partition, the solutions in both compartments will contain salt and the solutions will have the same concentrations. The salt must have moved throughout the compartments; this movement is called **diffusion.**

TABLE 3-1. IONIC ENVIRONMENTS OF THE MEMBRANE

PREPARATION	ION	CONCENTRATION (mM) INTRA-CELLULAR	EXTRA-CELLULAR	RATIO EXTRA-CELLULAR/ INTRA-CELLULAR	ϵ(mV)
Squid axon*	K^+	400	20	0.05	−75.5
($V_r = -70$ mV)	Na^+	50	440	8.80	+54.8
	Cl^-	40	560	14.00	−66.5
	Ca^{2+}	0.4	10		
	Mg^{2+}	10	54		
	Organic anions	~110			
Frog muscle†	K^+	140	2.5	0.02	−98.5
($-100 < V_r < -70$ mV)	Na^+	10	117.5	11.75	+62.1
	Cl^-	2.5	120	48.00	−97.5
	Ca^{2+}	4.9	2.1		
	Mg^{2+}	14.0	1.2		
	HCO_3^-	12.4	26.6		
	Organic anions	~74	~13		
Cat motoneuron‡	K^+	150	5.5	0.04	−81.1
($-80 < V_r < -60$ mV)	Na^+	15	150	10.00	+58.0
	Cl^-	9	125	13.89	−66.3

* Kuffler SW, Nichols JG: From Neuron to Brain. Sunderland, MA: Sinauer Assoc., 1976
† Conway EJ: Physiol Rev 37:84–132, 1957
‡ Coombs JS, Curtis DR, Eccles JC: J Physiol (Lond) 130:326–373, 1955

FIG. 3-10. Diffusion and diffusion potentials. **A.** A container, with a removable partition, contains water. Ordinary table salt, NaCl, is added to side 1 and then the partition is removed. After a time, NaCl is found in equal concentrations on both sides. **B.** A container, divided by a membrane permeable to sodium but not chloride, is filled with water. NaCl is added to side 1. Na^+ diffuses to side 2, but chloride cannot. **C.** An excess of positive charge, carried by Na^+, builds up on side 2, leaving an excess of negative charge, carried by Cl^-, on side 1, that is, a voltage builds up between the two sides.

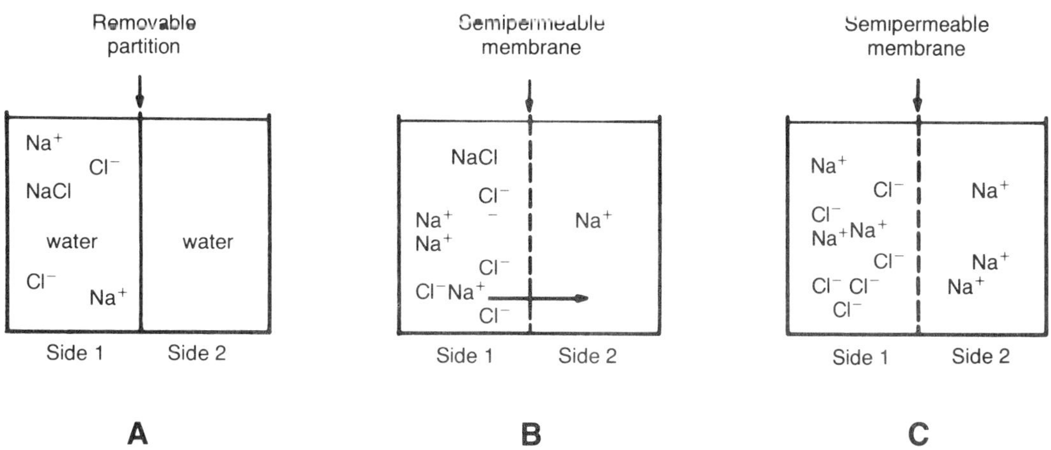

Molecules in solution at temperatures above absolute zero are in random motion. The direction of motion of any one molecule can be changed by collision with another molecule or the side of the vessel, but once in motion the molecule will travel in a straight line until a collision occurs. The higher the temperature, the greater is the velocity of movement; the higher the concentration of the solution, the greater is the likelihood of a collision. Some collisions will result in molecules moving toward the interface between the two compartments and crossing it. The probability that a given molecule will cross the interface is therefore proportional to both temperature and the concentration of the solution. Thus, the **flux** from one compartment to the other, J, is given by:

$$J = kC \tag{1}$$

where k is a constant for a given temperature and C is the concentration in the compartment *from* which the flux is occurring.

In Figure 3-10A, the side where the salt was put is numbered 1; the other side is numbered 2. Therefore, the flux from side 1 to side 2, J_{12} is

$$J_{12} = kC_1 \tag{2}$$

where C_1 is the initial concentration of salt on side 1. As soon as some molecules have crossed the interface, the concentration on side 2 begins to increase, and there is an increasing likelihood of a molecule recrossing the interface back to side 1. This probability is related to temperature and concentration—this time, to the concentration on side 2, C_2. Thus, the back flux, J_{21}, is given by

$$J_{21} = kC_2 \tag{3}$$

The net movement or net flux, J_N, between the two compartments at any time is simply the difference between the two one-way fluxes, J_{12} and J_{21},

$$J_N = J_{12} - J_{21} = kC_1 - kC_2 = k(C_1 - C_2) \tag{4}$$

Diffusion is simply a net flux. The net flux is positive when $C_1 > C_2$, so the diffusion is from a region of higher concentration to a region of lower concentration, down the concentration gradient. The net flux is proportional to $C_1 - C_2$ or proportional to the concentration difference between the two compartments.

Equilibrium is defined as the condition of no net flux, $J_N = 0$. When $J_N = 0$, $J_{21} = J_{12}$. Expressed in words, the equation means simply that the two one-way fluxes are equal at equilibrium, but neither flux need be zero. Even at equilibrium molecules can move from one compartment to the other, but equal numbers must move in both directions. Only the *net* flux need be zero. Equation 4 can be solved for $J_N = 0$ as follows:

$$0 = J_N = kC_1 - kC_2, \text{ or } kC_1 = kC_2, \text{ or } C_1 = C_2 \tag{5}$$

Thus, equilibrium occurs when the concentrations in the two compartments are equal. Until equilibrium is reached, there will be a net flux from side 1 to side 2 proportional to the concentration difference.

If we introduce a membrane, permeable to NaCl, between the compartments and repeat the experiment, the result will be the same. The net flux will be proportional to the difference in concentration between the two compartments with the constant of proportionality equal to the permeability coefficient, p, of the membrane for NaCl or $J_N = p(C_1 - C_2)$.

EQUILIBRIUM POTENTIALS

Thus far, we have not considered the effect of ionic charge on movement of the ions in solution. In Figure 3-10B, the compartments of the vessel are again separated by a membrane, but this time let us suppose that the membrane is permeable only to sodium. If we now add salt to one compartment as before, there will be a diffusion of sodium ions (recall that NaCl ionizes almost completely in water) from side 1 to side 2 (as before) because of the concentration gradient. Chloride would move with sodium to preserve electrical neutrality, but it cannot penetrate this membrane. As sodium crosses the membrane, an excess of positive charge (sodium is a positively charged ion or cation) builds up on side 2, leaving an excess of negative charge on side 1 due to unpaired chloride ions. This separation of charge is by definition a voltage. We speak of this voltage as being an electrical gradient. The excess of positive charge acts as a repellent to further movement of sodium across the membrane (like charges repel) or, alternatively, the excess negative charge on side 1 attracts sodium ions back across the membrane (unlike charges attract). The greater the accumulation of sodium ions and excess positive charge on side 2, the greater will be the repulsive force against further diffusion. This is the principle of operation of a concentration cell; voltage is generated by differences in concentration across a semipermeable membrane.

At some point, the concentration force promoting diffusion of sodium ions will be exactly balanced by the electrical force preventing diffusion and a condition of equilibrium will result, in which $J_N = 0$. This is called **electrochemical equilibrium.** The value of the membrane potential at electrochemical equilibrium for a particular ion is called the **equilibrium potential** for that ion and is abbreviated ϵ. A subscript is added to show the ion at equilibrium, in the case of sodium, ϵ_{Na^+}.

The situation in our vessel at electrochemical equilibrium is shown in Figure 3-11. The chemical (concentration) gradient for sodium is oriented from side 1 to side 2; the electrical gradient is oriented from side 2 to side 1. At equilibrium, the chemical force, tending to move ions to side 2, and the electrical force, tending to move ions to side 1, are equal in magnitude but opposite in direction. One way of looking at the magnitudes of these forces is in terms of the amount of work required to prevent movement of ions. The total work, W_t, is the sum of the chemical work, W_c, and the electrical work, W_e, or

$$W_t = W_c + W_e$$

At equilibrium, $W_t = 0$ because there is no net movement. Thus,

$$W_c = -W_e. \qquad (6)$$

From thermodynamics,

$$W_c - RT \ln \frac{[Na^+]_1}{[Na^+]_2},$$

where R is the gas constant; T, the absolute temperature; $[Na^+]_1$ is the sodium concentration on side 1; and $[Na^+]_2$ is the sodium concentration on side 2. This is the work required to maintain the concentration gradient. At chemical equilibrium $[Na^+]_1 = [Na^+]_2$ and $W_c = 0$; no work need be done to maintain equal concentrations.

The work necessary to move ions against the electrical gradient is

$$W_e = ZF\epsilon,$$

where Z is the valence of the ion, F is Faraday's constant, and ϵ is the potential difference between the two compartments. Substitution for W_e and W_c in equation 6 yields

$$W_c = -W_e = -RT \ln \frac{[Na^+]_1}{[Na^+]_2} = ZF\epsilon \ .$$

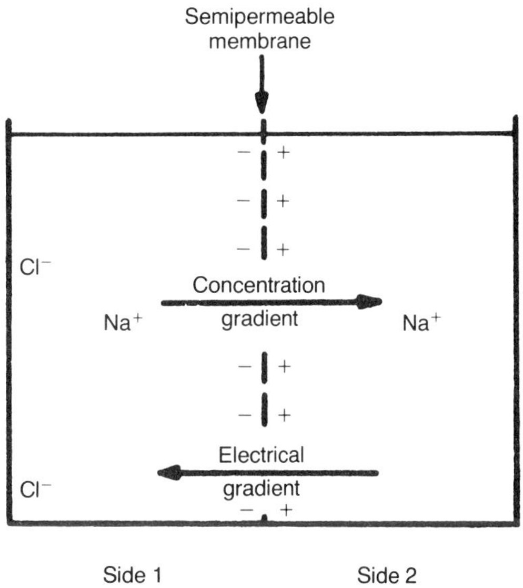

FIG. 3-11. The equilibrium condition of the experiment in Figure 3-10*B* and *C*. Electrochemical equilibrium develops in which the Na^+ concentration gradient, indicated by the **upper arrow,** is just balanced by the electrical gradient, indicated by the **lower arrow.** At this point, there is no net flux of Na^+ to either side.

Rearranging terms:

$$\epsilon = \frac{-RT}{ZF} \ln \frac{[Na^+]_1}{[Na^+]_2}.$$

This equation is known as the **Nernst equation.** Substitution of values for the gas constant, Faraday's constant, and physiologic temperature allows the Nernst equation to be simplified, using logarithms to base 10, to the form:

$$\epsilon_{Na^+} = -\frac{58}{Z} \log_{10} \frac{[Na^+]_1}{[Na^+]_2}.$$

The Nernst equation not only specifies the transmembrane voltage necessary to maintain a given concentration difference, it also specifies the voltage that will result from maintenance of a given concentration difference, that is, it specifies the voltage that will result from a concentration cell. In its most general form, the Nernst equation is written:

$$\epsilon_X = \frac{-58}{Z} \log \frac{[X]_1}{[X]_2}, \qquad (7)$$

where X is any ion.

THE MEMBRANE POTENTIAL

Looking back at Table 3-1, we can see that essentially all ions experience a concentration gradient across the cell membrane. This is true for the squid axon, the frog muscle, and the cat motoneuron. Thus, in all cells sodium, chloride, calcium, and magnesium ions experience a chemical driving force toward the inside of the cell, that is, if the concentrations were the only factors involved in determining ion distributions, all of these ions would diffuse into the cell. The only diffusible ion that experiences a reverse gradient, from inside to outside of the cell, is K^+.

These concentration gradients should form concentration cells, and one would expect to find a potential difference (or voltage) between the inside and outside of a living cell. But, what should be the value and polarity of the potential? These can be calculated from Ohm's law and the Nernst equation. Any current flowing across the membrane will result in a voltage drop, predictable from Ohm's law:

$$i = gV$$

That current will have to be carried by ions because the membrane contains no metallic conductors, so the total current will be equal to the sum of the currents carried by each ion:

$$i = i_{K^+} + i_{Na^+} + i_{Cl^-} + i_{HCO_3^-} + i_{Mg^{2+}} + i_{Ca^{2+}} \cdots$$

The current carried by any ion is determined by its driving force and the conductance of the membrane to it. The driving force is determined by the deviation of the membrane voltage from the equilibrium potential for the ion. Thus:

$$i_{K^+} = g_{K^+}(V_m - \epsilon_{K^+})$$
$$i_{Na^+} = g_{Na^+}(V_m - \epsilon_{Na^+})$$
$$i_{Cl^-} = g_{Cl^-}(V_m - \epsilon_{Cl^-})$$

and so on, where V_m is the **membrane potential.** Ohm's law can now be rewritten in the form:

$$i = g_{K^+}(V_m - \epsilon_{K^+}) + g_{Na^+}(V_m - \epsilon_{Na^+}) + g_{Cl^-}(V_m - \epsilon_{Cl^-}) + \cdots \quad (8)$$

Because of their very low concentrations, Ca^{2+} and Mg^{2+} ions contribute only slightly to the membrane potential, though they play a significant role in the functioning of both nerve and muscle, as we shall see. We shall ignore these ions for the present. We want to determine the value of V_m in equation 8 above. To do this, we have to know the values of the equilibrium potentials for the various ions. Let us choose the squid giant axon for our example and calculate the equilibrium potentials from values in Table 3-1. It is customary in neurophysiology to express membrane potentials as **potential inside the cell with respect to outside.** Therefore, the Nernst equation takes the form:

$$\epsilon_X = -\frac{58}{Z}\log_{10}\frac{[X]_{inside}}{[X]_{outside}} \quad (9)$$

Substituting values for K^+, we get:

$$\epsilon_{K^+} = -\frac{58}{+1}\log_{10}\frac{400}{20} = -58\log_{10} 20 = -75.5 \text{ mV}$$

Thus, K^+ will be in electrochemical equilibrium at a 20/1 concentration ratio (inside/outside) when the inside is 75.5 mV negative with respect to the outside. At any potential less negative than this value, K^+ will leave the cell; at any potential more negative than this value, K^+ will enter the cell. We can calculate the equilibrium potentials for both Na^+ and Cl^- in a similar way:

$$\epsilon_{Na^+} = -\frac{58}{+1}\log_{10}\frac{50}{440} = +58\log_{10}\frac{440}{50} = +58\log_{10} 8.80 = +54.8 \text{ mV}$$

$$\epsilon_{Cl^-} = -\frac{58}{-1}\log_{10}\frac{40}{560} = -58\log_{10}\frac{560}{40} = -58\log_{10} 14 = -66.5 \text{ mV.}$$

In cell membranes, the conductance to chloride ions is high. Nerve membrane conductance to chloride is slightly lower than for potassium, but muscle membrane has a higher conductance to chloride than to potassium. Because of the high conductance, chloride is able to redistribute itself across the membrane by simple diffusion in response to changes in the membrane voltage. Thus, the chloride ion will always be at equilibrium in the vicinity of the resting membrane potential. The contribution of chloride to the membrane potential can be ignored because of its tendency to redistribute itself. Potassium cannot redistribute itself because high intracellular concentrations are needed to balance the charge of the large anions that cannot leave the cell (see Table 3-1). Electrical neutrality of the intracellular fluid is maintained by high intracellular K^+ levels. The low sodium conductance of the resting membrane prevents sodium ions from redistributing.

That leaves us with only K^+ and Na^+ to contribute to the membrane potential. At rest, the membrane is at equilibrium, that is, there is no net transmembrane current flow, so $i = 0$, therefore

$$0 = i = g_{K^+}(V_r - \epsilon_{K^+}) + g_{Na^+}(V_r - \epsilon_{Na^+})$$

or

$$g_{K^+}(V_r - \epsilon_{K^+}) = -\,g_{Na^+}(V_r - \epsilon_{Na^+}),$$

where V_r is the value of V_m at equilibrium and is called the **resting membrane potential.** Rearranging terms,

$$\frac{g_{K^+}}{g_{Na^+}} = -\frac{V_r - \epsilon_{Na^+}}{V_r - \epsilon_{K^+}} \qquad (10)$$

The nerve membrane is permeable to both Na^+ and K^+, but the permeability to K^+ is much higher. The ratio of the conductance of the membrane to K^+ to the conductance to Na^+ varies from 10 to 30 in different cells. If the ratio is taken to be 20, then

$$\frac{20}{1} = -\frac{V_r - \epsilon_{Na^+}}{V_r - \epsilon_{K^+}}.$$

Solving for V_r, we see that

$$V_r = \frac{20}{21}\epsilon_{K^+} + {}^{1}/_{21}\,\epsilon_{Na^+}.$$

Substituting values for ϵ_{K^+} and ϵ_{Na^+} from Table 3-1, we see that $V_r = -69.3$ mV. That is, we expect the membrane potential to be 69.3 mV negative inside with respect to outside. Taking the two extremes of the ratio, namely $^{30}/_{1}$ and $^{10}/_{1}$, yields predicted membrane potentials of -71.3 mV and -63.6 mV. The greater the ratio, that is, the (relatively) more impermeable the membrane is to Na^+, the closer V_r will be to ϵ_{K^+}. Thus, the membrane potential is due mainly to the concentration difference for potassium and is close to ϵ_{K^+}. The greater the relative permeability to Na^+, the farther V_r will deviate from ϵ_{K^+} or the closer it will deviate toward ϵ_{Na^+}.

The accuracy of this theoretical prediction of V_r can be examined by actually measuring the resting membrane potential. This is done using a micropipette electrode as shown in Figure 3-8. When the electrode is in the extracellular fluid, zero potential difference will be recorded because both the microelectrode and the indifferent electrode are in the same fluid and therefore at the same potential. This is shown in the first part (A) of the record of Figure 3-12. In this figure, known as a driving force diagram, positive membrane voltages are plotted above zero, negative voltages below. The positions of ϵ_{Na^+} at $+54.8$ mV and ϵ_{K^+} at -75.5 mV are shown. As the micropipette penetrates the membrane, the potential it records goes negative by 70 mV (section B of the record). If the membrane seals around the electrode, the recorded voltage will stay at -70 mV, the value of V_r, the resting membrane potential. When the micropipette is withdrawn from the cell, the voltage returns to zero (section C of the record). At times, the membrane is badly damaged by the electrode and a membrane voltage less negative than the actual V_r will be recorded, presumably because the concentration gradients are destroyed. Enough cells have been examined to indicate that

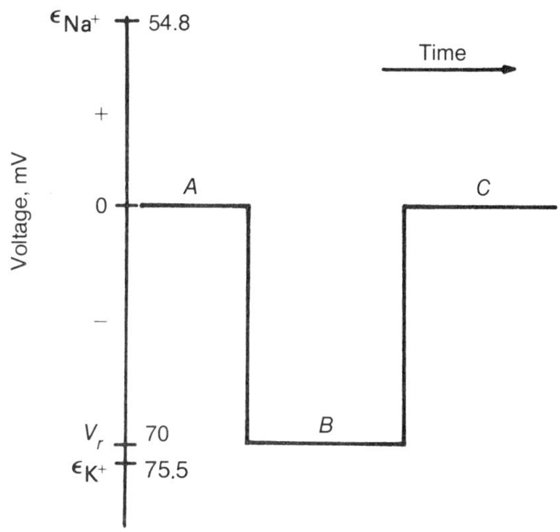

FIG. 3-12. The membrane potential. A graph of the voltage recorded between a movable micropipette electrode and a fixed electrode in the extracellular fluid (ordinate) against time (abscissa). At the origin, both the pipette and the fixed electrode are in the extracellular fluid and the voltage between them is zero **(A).** When the micropipette penetrates the membrane, the voltage changes to -70 mV, inside with respect to outside **(B).** When the electrode is backed out of the cell, the potential returns to zero **(C).** The positions of ϵ_{Na^+} and ϵ_{K^+} are indicated on the ordinate.

the membrane potential of the squid axon is about -70 mV in sea water at normal temperatures. Thus, the preceding theoretical analysis is reasonably accurate. Any inaccuracies that exist may be the result of inaccuracies in the measurement of ion concentrations or they may be due to small contributions from Ca^{2+} or Mg^{2+} to the membrane potentials. A more accurate prediction is obtained when these ions are also included in the analysis. Their contribution, as noted previously, is small.

Not all cells, not even all neurons, have the same resting membrane potential. In all cells, however, the value of the resting membrane potential depends upon ϵ_{K^+} and g_{K^+}/g_{Na^+}. The values of ϵ_{K^+} for the three types of cells in Table 3-1 vary from -75 to -99 mV, and these values are reflected in their membrane potentials. Frog muscle cells have resting potentials of -70 to -100 mV, whereas cat motoneurons vary from -60 to -80 mV. Neurons in the cerebral cortex typically have resting membrane potentials around -50 mV, presumably reflecting either lower values of ϵ_{K^+} or g_{K^+}/g_{Na^+} or both.

If this analysis of the origin of the resting membrane potential is accurate, then the membrane potential should be highly sensitive to changes in the concentration gradient for K^+. That this is the case is shown in Figure 3-13 for frog muscle fibers. As the external concentration of K^+ is raised from 12 mM (moving to the right on the abscissa), the membrane potential falls (moving upward on the ordinate) as predicted from the Nernst equation (the solid line). At lower $[K^+]_o$ values, the role of Na^+ becomes greater because of the greater driving force (greater deviation of ϵ_{Na^+} from V_r), and the points deviate from the Nernst relation. Increasing the internal K^+ concentration has similar consequences for the membrane potential. Similar alterations in external sodium ion concentration produce little change in V_r because of low sodium conductance.

The existence of Na^+ and K^+ concentration gradients suggests an **electrical equivalent circuit.** The concentration gradients can be viewed as concentration cells or batteries whose voltages are the equilibrium potentials for the ions at these concentrations. We may, therefore, modify the circuit of Figure 3-9 to include the membrane potential. Figure 3-14 includes the Na^+ and K^+ batteries and separate resistances or conductances for the two ions. The Na^+ battery is shown oriented with the negative pole toward the outside and the K^+ battery, with the negative pole toward the inside. These are the orientations of the Na^+ and K^+ equilibrium potentials. We can see how this circuit accounts for the membrane potential by examining the limiting conditions. Suppose R_{Na^+} were infinitely large. All of the voltage across the membrane would then come from the potassium battery, ϵ_{K^+}. If R_{Na^+} were zero, then the contribution to the membrane potential from ϵ_{K^+} would be negligible compared to that from ϵ_{Na^+}. Similarly, if R_{K^+} were infinite, ϵ_{Na^+} would determine the membrane potential. However, neither resistance is infinite or zero; rather the sodium resistance is 20 to 30 times larger than the potassium resistance (remember $g_{Na^+} = 1/R_{Na^+}$), so that the membrane potential is dominated by ϵ_{K^+}, but not equal to ϵ_{K^+}.

THE SODIUM–POTASSIUM PUMP

Few of the ions around the membrane are at electrochemical equilibrium when the membrane is at rest, that is, when $V_m = V_r$. V_r is far from ϵ_{Na^+} and it is not equal to ϵ_{K^+}. Only Cl^- is in equilibrium at V_r. There is a weak tendency for K^+ to move out of the cell and a strong tendency for Na^+ to enter the cell. A rapid equilibration of ionic concentrations is prevented by the low resting sodium conductance of the membrane, but the resting g_{Na^+} is not zero and, therefore, in the absence of any other mechanism, the membrane potential should slowly decline toward zero. As sodium moves into the cell down its concentration gradient, it provides positive charge to balance the internal anions and thus allows K^+ to diffuse out of the cell. As K^+ leaves, its concentration gradient falls and ϵ_{K^+} and V_r become less negative.

There exists, within the membrane, a mechanism for expelling Na^+ and taking up K^+ against their concentration gradients. This mechanism is called the **sodium–potassium pump** or, simply, the **sodium pump.** Obviously, if the ions have a natural tendency to move in one direction, causing them to move in the opposite direction requires the expenditure of energy. The tendency of ions to move down their concentration gradients constitutes a potential

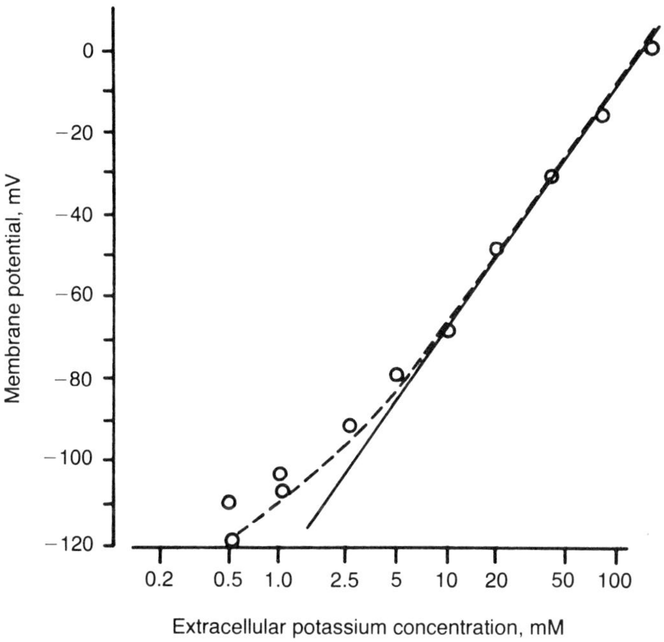

FIG. 3-13. A plot of the measured membrane potential (ordinate) for frog muscle fibers against the extracellular concentration of potassium (abscissa, log scale). Note that the membrane potential becomes more positive as the extracellular K^+ increases (the K^+ gradient falls). The solid line is a plot of the Nernst equation for potassium,

$$V_m = -58 \log \frac{140}{[K^+]_o}$$

which the data points follow down to a concentration of 5 mM. Normal extracellular potassium is about 20 mM. The dashed line is the relationship predicted for a small contribution of sodium ions to the membrane potential at very low extracellular potassium concentrations,

$$V_m = -58 \log \frac{140}{[K^+]_o + 0.1\,[Na^+]_o}$$

(Hodgkin AL, Horowicz P: J Physiol (Lond) 145:405–432, 1959)

FIG. 3-14. An electrical circuit model of the resting membrane. Outside of the membrane is at the **top**, inside at the **bottom**. Shown are the membrane capacitance, C_m; sodium and potassium resistances, R_{Na^+} and R_{K^+}; internal longitudinal resistance of the intracellular fluid, R_i; and the sodium and potassium batteries, ϵ_{Na^+} and ϵ_{K^+}.

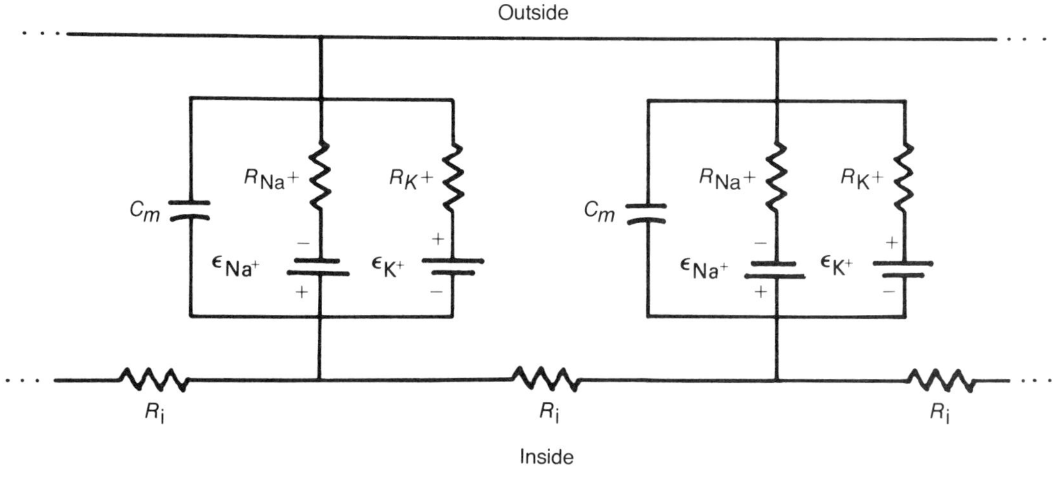

energy (as opposed to kinetic energy) that can be counteracted only by expending at least an equal amount of energy. That this process of pumping ions is, indeed, an active process is indicated by its sensitivity to changes in temperature, that is, cells accumulate more sodium and lose more potassium at low temperature, and by the blockade of the pumping and decline of the membrane potential over a prolonged period when metabolic activity, involving splitting the high-energy phosphate bonds of adenosine triphosphate (ATP), is blocked by the inhibitor ouabain or by cyanide. The extrusion of 3 sodium ions requires the hydrolyzation of 1 molecule of ATP.

The rate of extrusion of Na^+ by the sodium pump is proportional to the internal sodium concentration. For example, at an internal concentration of Na^+ of 50 mM, the Na^+ efflux is about 30 picomoles (pmol)/cm^2/sec in the squid axon, but the rate rises to about 150 pmol/cm^2/sec at an internal concentration of 230 mM. The relationship between pumping rate and the internal Na^+ concentration appears to be linear for some cells (*e.g.*, squid axon) but not for others (*e.g.*, frog muscle).

In most cells, the pumping of sodium ions is linked to the pumping of potassium. In fact, extrusion of sodium can be reduced by as much as 70% in the absence of potassium in the extracellular fluid. A pump that exchanges one Na^+ for one K^+ will not produce a net charge transfer, and therefore there will be no change in membrane potential as a result of pump activity. This is called a **nonelectrogenic pump.** However, if the amount of Na^+ transported exceeds the amount of K^+ transported, a potential will develop as a result of the net transfer of charge. This is called an **electrogenic pump.** An electrogenic pump can add to potentials set up by diffusing ions and cause the ions to redistribute themselves in order to restore equilibrium. The activity of electrogenic pumps can therefore affect ion distributions and membrane potentials either through action on concentration gradients or by altering the membrane potential. In any event, at equilibrium the net fluxes due to pump activity or to any other forces, must still be zero. Active fluxes (pump-related) must exactly balance passive fluxes (diffusional).

The sodium pump of erythrocytes has a Na^+/K^+ transport ratio that is nearly one, that is, it is essentially nonelectrogenic. In the squid axon, the ratio can be as high as 3 or as low as 1, depending upon whether the intracellular Na^+ concentration is high or low. Thus, the transport ratio need not be fixed, but can vary, providing a mechanism for a relatively constant K^+ transport rate and a variable sodium transport rate.

There is some evidence that suggests that the transport system may involve Na^+–K^+-activated ATPases (enzymes that hydrolyze ATP) within the membrane. These have a greater affinity for Na^+ and a lesser affinity for K^+ at the inner surface of the membrane and a lesser affinity for Na^+ and greater affinity for K^+ at the outer surface. They hydrolyze ATP at a rate dependent upon the Na^+ and K^+ concentrations. The actual physical mechanism by which the ions are moved is unknown, but the suggestion has been made that the ATPase is an intrinsic protein that perhaps rotates after picking up intracellular Na^+ and extracellular K^+. In this new orientation or conformation, the affinity for the transported substance is reduced and Na^+ is released outside and K^+ inside the cell. Finally, the protein rotates back to its original orientation and affinity, and the process repeats.

It has been estimated that each sodium pump can transport up to 200 Na^+ and 130 K^+ per sec, the actual rate being determined by ion concentrations. Other estimates suggest that, on the average, sodium pumps have a density of 100 to 200 per mm^2 of membrane, but, in some parts of the cell, they can be up to 10 times more dense. Thus, a typical neuron might have a million pumps with a maximum capacity of 200 million Na^+ ions/sec.

The importance of the resting membrane potential is seldom stated explicitly, but its importance cannot be over-emphasized. All living cells, not just nerves and muscles, have a resting membrane potential. It is a ubiquitous property of living matter. The work of nerve and muscle cells depends upon the membrane potential. It acts as an energy store, a source of potential energy from which these cells draw to initiate their characteristic activities, the nerve and muscle action potentials and muscle contraction. The secretion of chemical substances by nerve terminals and glands also depends upon the existence of the membrane poten-

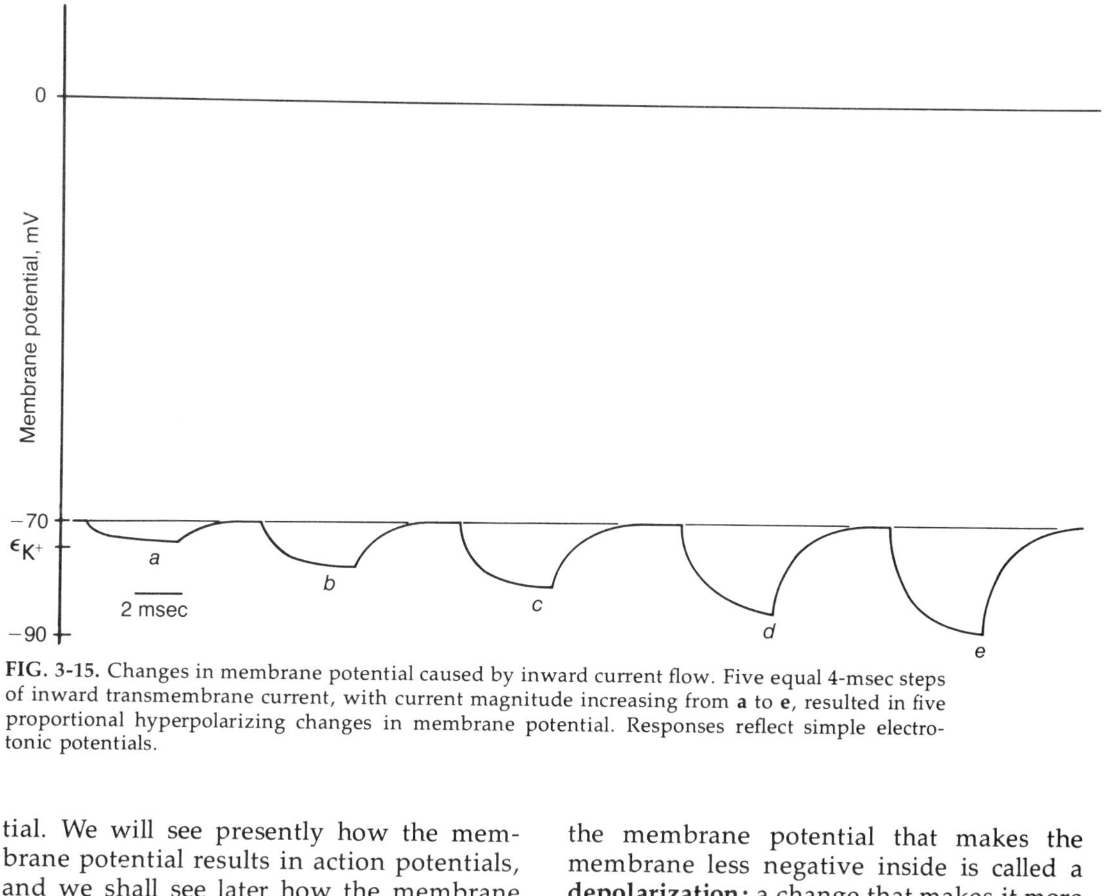

FIG. 3-15. Changes in membrane potential caused by inward current flow. Five equal 4-msec steps of inward transmembrane current, with current magnitude increasing from **a** to **e**, resulted in five proportional hyperpolarizing changes in membrane potential. Responses reflect simple electrotonic potentials.

tial. We will see presently how the membrane potential results in action potentials, and we shall see later how the membrane potential is involved in contraction.

THE ACTION POTENTIAL

In the experiment shown in Figure 3-8, only small amounts of current were passed through the membrane, and these caused only small changes in membrane potential. If greater currents are used some new phenomena show up in the recordings. When current is passed through the membrane from outside to inside (micropipette is cathode), the voltages shown in Figure 3-15 can be recorded from the immediately adjacent membrane. The membrane responds as a simple passive resistance–capacitance circuit. The membrane potential changes more slowly than the applied current as the membrane capacitor charges and discharges. Even with the greatest currents, the membrane still behaves as a simple passive circuit. We speak of the resting membrane as being **polarized** (negative inside with respect to outside). A change in the membrane potential that makes the membrane less negative inside is called a **depolarization;** a change that makes it more negative than V_r is called a **hyperpolarization.** Inward currents, therefore, hyperpolarize the resting membrane.

When current is passed in the other direction across the membrane, from inside to outside, the membrane at first behaves as a simple resistance–capacitance circuit, approximately symmetric with its behavior for inward current. Responses in Figure 3-16 were obtained for the same strength outward currents as were used for the correspondingly lettered responses to inward currents in Figure 3-15. In Figure 3-16, responses in a and b are symmetric with responses in a and b in Figure 3-15. However, c in Figure 3-16 is not symmetric to its counterpart. The response begins like its counterpart, but the response is larger in amplitude and longer in duration. Response d is even more variant; the shape is no longer that of a capacitor being charged. An active process has been initiated by the change in membrane potential that occurred in c and d; it was not initiated by the smaller changes in membrane potential in a and b.

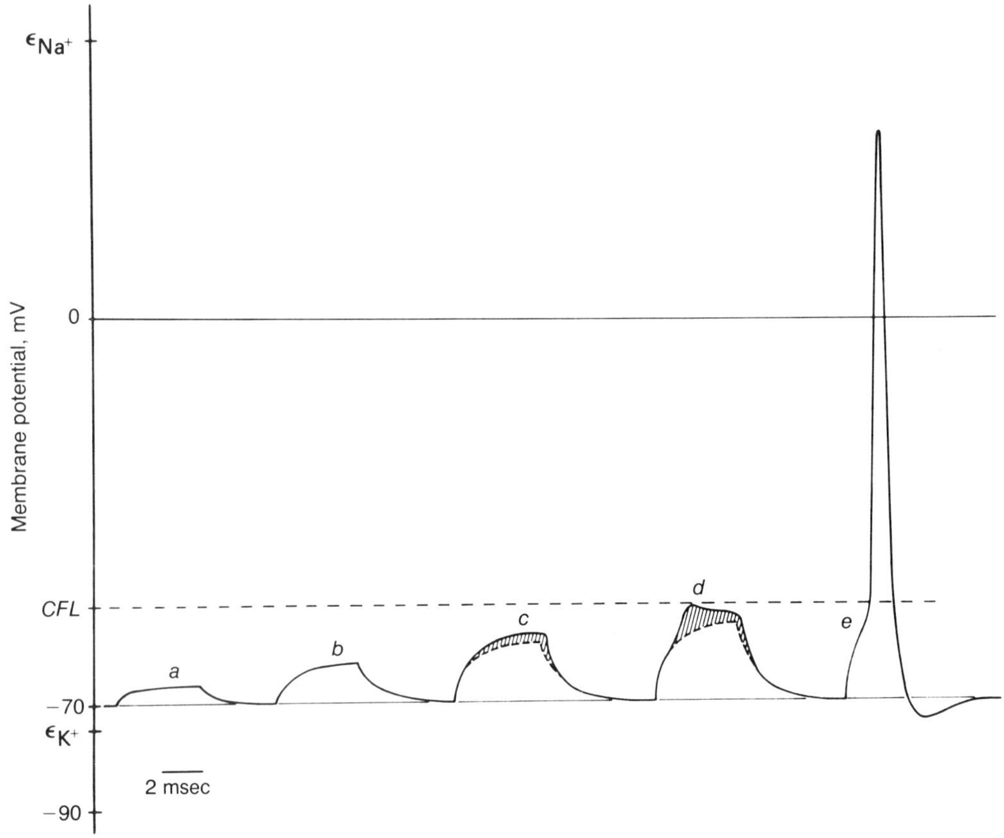

FIG. 3-16. Changes in membrane potential due to outward current flow. Five equal 4-msec steps of outward transmembrane current, with current magnitude increasing from **a** to **e** (and the same magnitudes as for similarly lettered traces in Fig. 3-15), resulted in depolarizing electrotonic potentials in **a** and **b**, electrotonic potentials leading to local active responses (hatched regions) in **c** and **d**, and an electrotonic potential leading to a spike in **e**. **CFL** = critical firing level

When a still stronger current is passed outward through the membrane, the membrane potential begins to change passively (response e in Fig. 3-16); then the active process begins; and finally the membrane polarization continues to diminish rapidly toward zero (the membrane is depolarized) and beyond, becoming positive inside with respect to outside. The membrane polarity actually becomes reversed. After the peak of positivity is reached, the membrane rapidly returns to its original polarity and potential and may proceed to a potential more negative than V_r. Finally, the membrane returns to V_r, the whole event lasting 2 to 3 msec. Actually, the event, from its start at V_r to peak positivity and back to V_r (omitting the period when V_m is more negative than V_r), requires only 0.5 to 1.0 msec, depending upon the neuron. This event is called the **action potential** or simply the **spike.**

Figure 3-17 shows the action potential on an expanded time scale. The various parts of the spike are labeled. The rapid positive change in membrane potential is called the **upstroke,** the **rising phase,** or the **depolarization phase.** The positive portion of the spike is the **overshoot,** and the return to the resting potential is called the **falling phase** or the **repolarization phase.** At the end of the falling phase, the repolarization (reestablishment of the resting polarity) slows down and may pass the resting potential to a value more negative than V_r, that is, the membrane may become hyperpolarized. This is the **hyperpolarizing after-potential** or **after-hyperpolarization.** In some cells, there may also be another phase of depolarization following this, the **depolarizing after-potential** or **after-depolarization.** This phase is usually small, a few mV, and frequently absent.

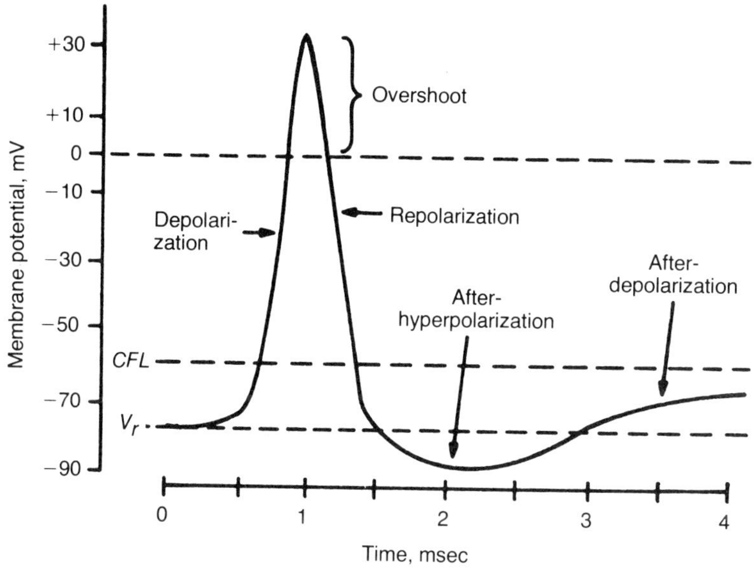

FIG. 3-17. Phases of the action potential. The time course of the spike is shown with depolarization and repolarization phases, overshoot, and hyperpolarizing and depolarizing after-potentials labeled. Also indicated are levels of the resting membrane potential, V_r, and the critical firing level, CFL. Transmembrane voltage is indicated on the ordinate; time is indicated on the abscissa.

The action potential is initiated when the membrane is depolarized *beyond* a certain value. This value varies from cell to cell; it is of the order of 10 to 15 mV, but constant for a given cell and termed the **critical firing level** (CFL). If the membrane is depolarized just to but not beyond the critical firing level, it may either discharge a spike or it may simply return to V_r. The critical firing level is a highly unstable condition. Actually, a minimum rate of change in membrane potential is required to initiate the spike. If the membrane potential is changed very slowly, the critical firing level can be passed without an action potential being initiated. In Figure 3-18, the responses of an axon to stimuli with five different rates of rise are shown. As the rate is increased, the apparent critical firing level becomes more positive, going from 21 mV of depolarization from V_r in a to 28 mV in d. In e, no spike is initiated at all, despite the fact that the membrane is depolarized by more than 30 mV. Actually, during any maintained depolarization that does not cause a spike to occur, the critical firing level becomes more positive. This phenomenon is called **accommodation.** When the depolarization is terminated, the critical firing level returns to its original value. If, however, the minimum rate of change of membrane potential is exceeded, the spike will be initiated as the membrane potential becomes more positive than the critical firing level. Most neural events are rapid, and it is doubtful that the firing level is frequently crossed in natural functioning of the healthy neuron without a spike occurring. There are certain pathologic conditions where this occurs, for example, in certain kinds of epileptic seizures in which there are extremely large changes in membrane potentials at synaptic junctions.

Once the action potential is initiated, it goes to completion. The maximum value of the positive overshoot is a constant (usually about 30 mV) for a given neuron when the spike is initiated starting with the membrane at or near V_r. The amplitude of the spike does not depend upon the size of the stimulus; larger stimuli do not give rise to larger spikes. Longer duration stimuli do not prolong spikes. Therefore, the spike is referred to as an **all-or-none** (often written **all-or-nothing**) event. The fixed size results from the fact that the stimulus triggers events that lead to the spike, but once they are triggered their time course is independent of the stimulus. The consequences of slowly rising stimuli producing accommo-

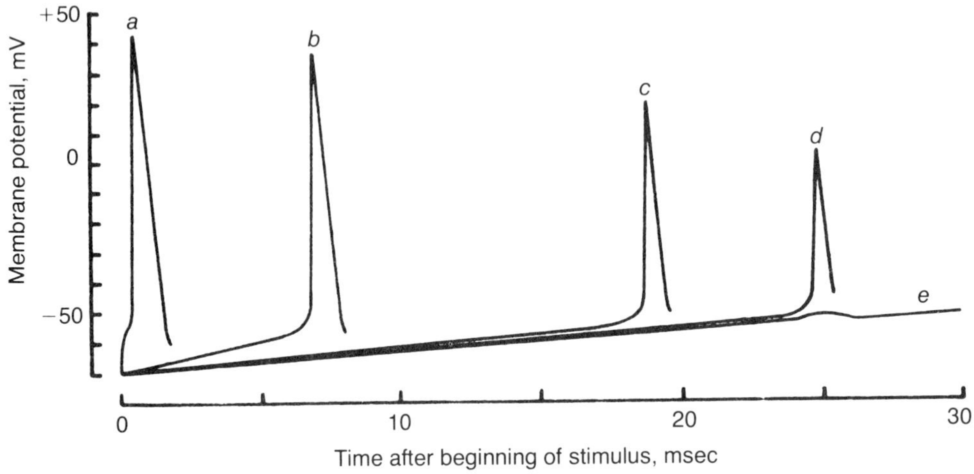

FIG. 3-18. Accommodation of the nerve membrane. Five superimposed traces show the membrane response to linearly varying electrical stimuli with rates of rise decreasing from **a** to **e**. Note that the critical firing level changes from a 21-mV depolarization in **a** to a 28-mV depolarization in **d** and no spike occurs in **e**. Note also that the amplitude of the spike falls with decreasing rise rate. (Frankenhaeuser B, Vallbo AB: Acta Physiol Scand 63:1–20, 1965)

FIG. 3-19. Circuit diagram for the voltage clamp. Transmembrane potential is measured between an intracellular micropipette electrode and an electrode in the extracellular fluid by amplifier 1 and compared with the clamp voltage by amplifier 2. A current, *i*, is generated to bring the membrane potential to the clamp voltage and the current is measured by the ammeter, *I*.

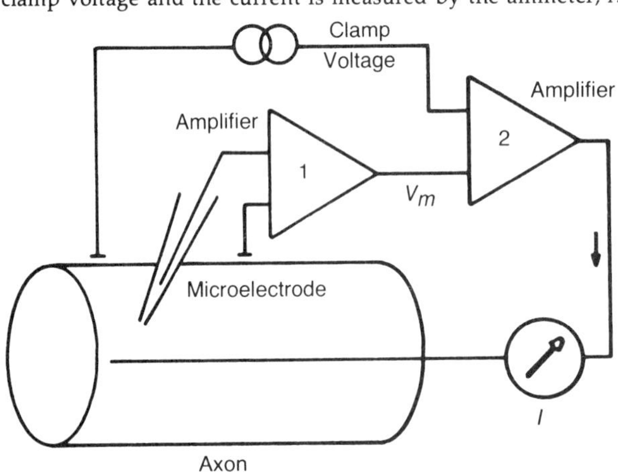

dation (Fig. 3-18) are an apparent contradiction to this all-or-none property; but, as pointed out previously most naturally occurring changes in membrane potential occur rapidly, at rates higher than 4 mV/msec, at which the spike amplitude is reduced by less than 2%.

THE VOLTAGE CLAMP

What are the events that lead to the action potential? Obviously, the change in membrane potential of the spike results from a membrane current, and that current must result from an increase in membrane conductance. If membrane conductance were unchanged, there would be no disturbance of the resting membrane equilibrium. Membrane currents can be measured directly using a device called the **voltage clamp.** The circuit of the voltage clamp is shown in Figure 3-19. The membrane potential of the squid axon or another cell is measured with a micropipette as in previous figures, using amplifier 1. The output of this amplifier is compared, by a second amplifier, with a command signal specified by the experimenter. The command signal indicates the voltage at which the membrane is to be "clamped," the clamp voltage. If the membrane potential is not the same as the command signal, a current is generated by the second amplifier that is appropriate in magnitude and direction to bring the membrane potential to the clamp voltage. If, in the neuron, a current is generated that would result in a change in membrane potential, that change is sensed and countered *as it occurs* by the voltage clamp. In this way, the membrane potential is maintained at the clamp voltage. The current that is generated by the second amplifier, the clamp current, is measured by the ammeter, I. This current is equal in magnitude but opposite in direction to any membrane current.

If the voltage clamp is applied to the squid axon and the membrane voltage clamped at −10 mV (55-mV depolarization), a current flow results, as shown in Figure 3-20B. The effect of the clamp on membrane potential is shown in Figure 3-20A. The membrane simply changes instantaneously from −65 mV (V_r, in this case) to −10 mV, and stays there. This depolarization is more than enough to start the spike mechanism, but, of course, the membrane potential cannot change. At the time when the rapid membrane depolarization of the spike would have occurred, there is a brief outward current (upward deflection in current traces is an outward current), followed immediately by an inward current that reaches a peak at about 0.6 msec and declines to zero by 1.5 msec. This inward current is followed by a prolonged outward current that lasts as long as the membrane is clamped. The brief outward current at the beginning of the record represents the discharging of the membrane capacitance. This current is short because the change in membrane potential, as it moves from V_r to the clamp voltage, is so rapid. Recall that $i_c = C\, dV/dt$ and $dV/dt = 0$ except at the time the clamp is initiated.

It is possible to determine which ions are carrying the currents in a number of ways. First, suppose that the concentration of Na^+ in the extracellular fluid is reduced and the removed Na^+ is replaced by choline, such that $\epsilon_{Na^+} = -10$ mV. Then, when the membrane potential is clamped at −10 mV, $V_m = \epsilon_{Na^+}$ and

$$i_{Na^+} = g_{Na^+}(V_m - \epsilon_{Na^+}) = 0.$$

Therefore, there will be no current due to sodium ions. The resultant voltage-clamp current is shown in Figure 3-20D as a smoothly rising outward current. The inward current is eliminated completely, suggesting that it was carried by sodium ions. Another way to show this is to vary the clamp voltage in an axon with normal ion concentrations. The result of doing this is shown in Figure 3-21. When the membrane is clamped at +26 mV, the inward current is reduced but present, and the outward current is larger than that at a clamp voltage of −10 mV. At a clamp voltage of +39 mV, the inward current is still smaller and the outward current still larger, whereas, at +52 mV (approximately ϵ_{Na^+}), the inward current is eliminated completely. This is what would be expected if the inward current is carried by Na^+ because at +52 mV, $V_m = \epsilon_{Na^+}$ and thus $i_{Na^+} = 0$. When the membrane potential is clamped at +65 or +70 mV, an outward current appears where the inward current used to be, again as expected.

In the driving force diagram of Figure 3-22, V_r, ϵ_{Na^+}, and ϵ_{K^+} are indicated along with the clamp voltages −10, +26, and +65 mV. Recall that the driving force on an ion is $V_m - \epsilon_{ion}$. Therefore, at a clamp voltage of −10 mV (V_m), the driving force on Na^+ is equal to the length of the line in the driving force diagram from ϵ_{Na^+} to the −10 mV clamp voltage. Likewise, the driving force on K^+ is the length of the line from ϵ_{K^+} to the −10 mV clamp voltage. In both cases, the direction of the arrowhead indicates the direction of the driving force, inward for Na^+, outward for K^+. If the sodium conductance increases, there will be an inward i_{Na^+}; if g_{K^+} increases, there will be an outward i_{K^+}.

The magnitudes and directions of the driving forces for both Na^+ and K^+ are similarly indicated by the lengths and directions of the lines to the +26- and +65-mV clamp voltages. Notice that the driving force for K^+ is greater as the clamp voltage becomes more positive and it is always directed outward. We should, therefore, expect the magnitude of the outward current, if it is carried by potassium ions, to become larger as the membrane potential is clamped at

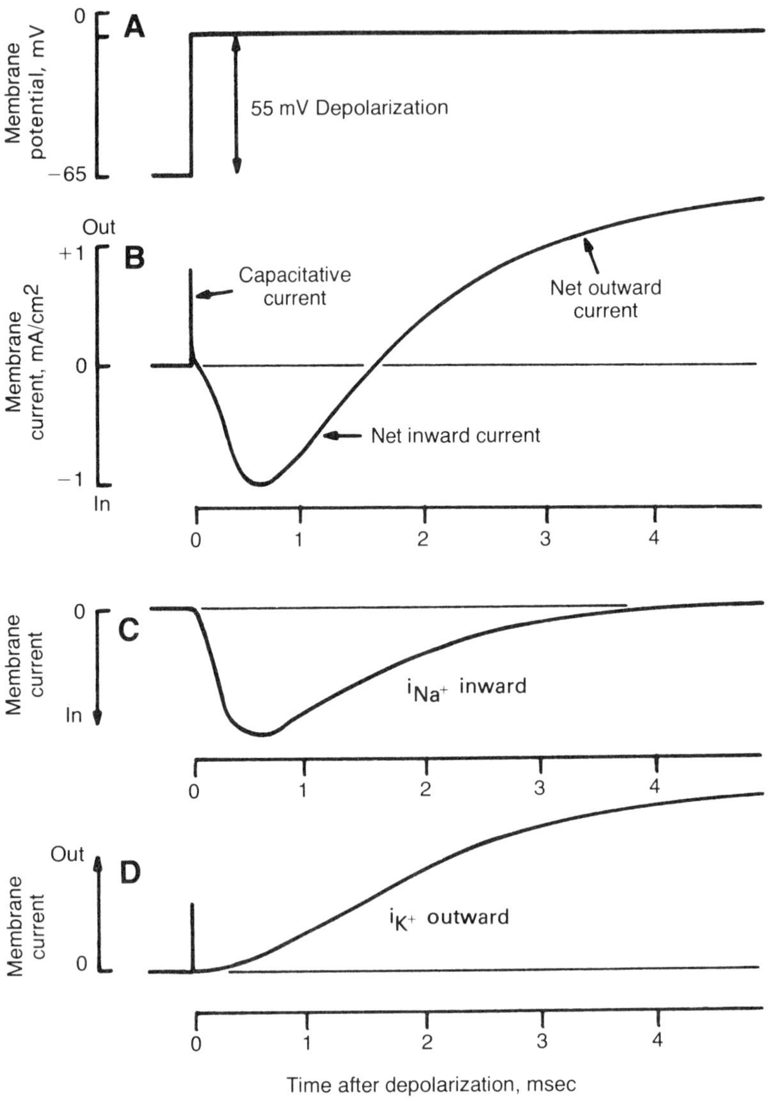

FIG. 3-20. Transmembrane currents during a spike. **A.** The transmembrane potential showing rapid clamp at −10 mV from a resting potential of −65 mV, a 55-mV depolarization. **B.** Total membrane current consists of a brief capacitative current, lasting only a few microseconds, a slower net inward current (downward deflection of the trace is inward current by convention) lasting about 1.5 msec, and a prolonged outward current. Total ionic current can be divided into two components: a transient inward current caused by sodium entry **(C)** and a prolonged outward current caused by potassium efflux **(D)**. (Hodgkin AL, Huxley AF: J Physiol (Lond) 116:449–472, 1952)

more and more positive values. This is seen clearly in Figure 3-21.

The driving force for Na^+ decreases as the clamp voltage approaches ϵ_{Na^+}. When the clamp voltage is more positive than ϵ_{Na^+}, the driving force reverses direction from toward the inside to toward the outside of the membrane. At even more positive values of the clamp voltage, the driving force will increase in magnitude, but its direction will still be outward. At clamp voltages less positive than ϵ_{Na^+}, i_{Na^+} will be an inward current; at values more positive, it will be an outward current, again as seen in Figure 3-21.

We can show that the outward current in

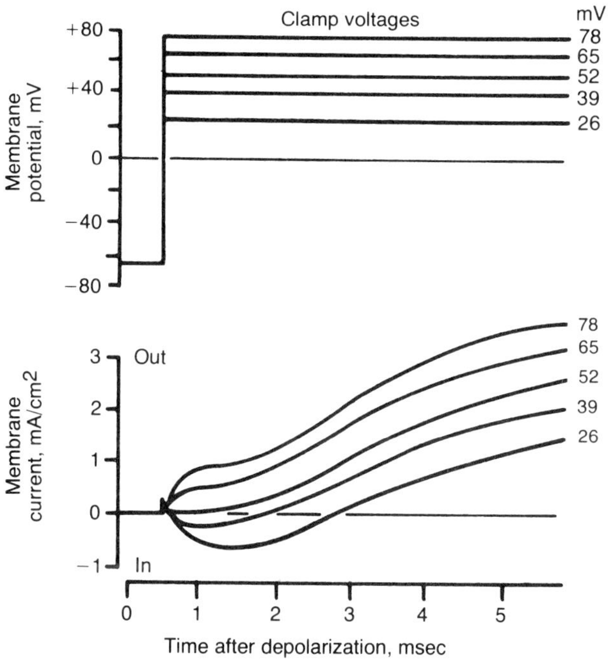

FIG. 3-21. Effect of membrane potential on membrane current. Upper traces show five different clamp voltages, +26 mV to +78 mV, applied to the squid axon. Lower traces show total net current flows for each clamp voltage. As the clamp voltage becomes more positive, the net outward current becomes larger and larger, whereas the net inward current becomes smaller, is zero at 52 mV, and then becomes net outward. (Hodgkin AL, Huxley AF, Katz B: J Physiol (Lond) 116:424–448, 1952)

FIG. 3-22. Driving force diagram. With the membrane voltage clamped at −10 mV, the driving force on K^+ is proportional to the length of the arrow from ϵ_{K^+} to the clamp −10 line at the left of the figure. The driving force on sodium is proportional to the length of the arrow from ϵ_{Na^+} to the clamp −10 line. Directions of the forces are given by the direction of the arrows, upward being outwardly directed, downward, inwardly directed. The center pair of arrows show driving forces on K^+ and Na^+ at a clamp voltage of +26 mV, whereas the right pair shows them for a clamp voltage of +65 mV. Note that all K^+ driving forces are outward; sodium driving forces are inward for −10 and +26 mV, and outward for +65 mV.

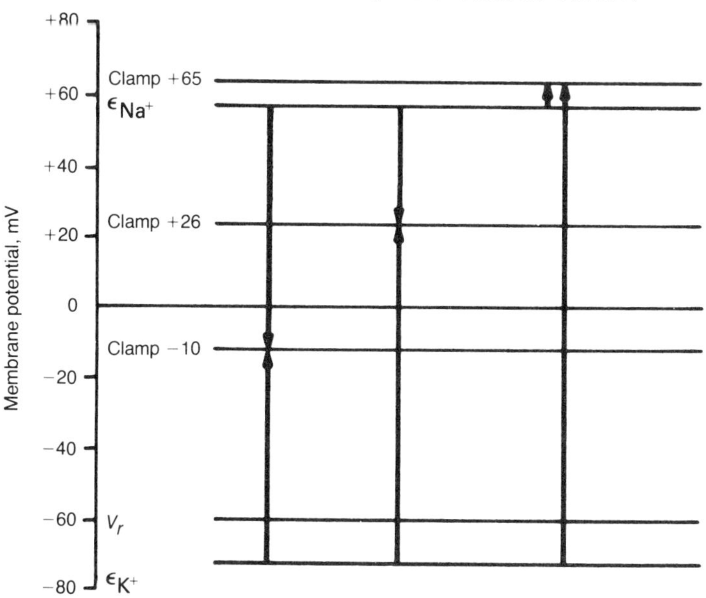

Figure 3-20 is a potassium current in a similar way. If the extracellular K^+ concentration is increased such that ϵ_{K^+} is equal to the clamp voltage, there is no outward current, only inward current (shown in Fig. 3-20C), the sodium current. The sodium current can also be calculated by subtracting the potassium current in Figure 3-20D from the total current in Figure 3-20B. To make this calculation, it is necessary to assume that there is no interaction between Na^+ and K^+ or their conductances. This is probably a good assumption, because, as we shall see, the conductances for the two ions change at different times relative to the action potential, and the outward and inward currents can be blocked independently. Tetrodotoxin (TTX), a toxic substance that occurs naturally in the puffer fish,* blocks the inward sodium current and, with it, the action potential, without changing the outward potassium current. The lethality of TTX is due to its ability to block the action potential. By comparison, tetraethylammonium (TEA) ions block the outward K^+ current without influencing the sodium current.

Having measured both the current flow and the change in membrane potential during the spike, we can compute the changes in membrane conductance from Ohm's law, $g_{Na^+} = i_{Na^+}/(V_m - \epsilon_{Na^+})$. In Figure 3-23, the changes in both sodium and potassium conductances (B) during the spike are shown in relation to the time course of the spike (A). The sodium conductance increases rapidly at the beginning of the upstroke, reaches a peak at the peak of the overshoot of the spike, and then rapidly declines. The potassium conductance increases more slowly, reaches a peak during the falling phase of the spike, and gradually declines back to its initial value.

ACTIVATION AND INACTIVATION

What causes the increase in g_{Na^+} during the action potential? The answer is, the initial depolarization! How? Recall that some of the membrane proteins act as channels or pores through which lipid-insoluble substances can pass. Actually, three types of channels are recognized. Some channels, for example, some K^+ channels, are open all the time and allow ions to pass through the membrane down their electrochemical gradients. Many K^+ channels are open in the resting membrane, but few Na^+ channels are. Other channels are gated, some electrically and some chemically. **Chemically gated channels** are opened by substances called transmitter substances, and they occur in specialized regions of cells where contacts are made with other cells (*i.e.*, at synapses). We will have more to say about them later.

The **voltage-gated channels** are opened when the membrane is depolarized. Because the cell membrane is so thin, the resting potential sets up an electric field across the membrane that has a strength of about 100 kV/cm of membrane thickness! The Na^+ channel, and perhaps similarly the K^+ channel, is probably a cluster of protein molecules embedded in the membrane lipid. The diameter of the channel is estimated at about 8 nm. The charged groups of the proteins within the channel give it a large electric dipole moment and the dipoles tend to align themselves with the huge electric field in such a way as to close the channel. Field strength is altered by depolarization, according to a popular hypothesis, causing the dipoles to reorient and open the channel. At any rate, the channel is opened by depolarization, allowing Na^+ to enter the cell. Sodium entry holds the channel open longer and causes more channels to open, allowing more sodium to enter and more channels to open and so forth. Opening of the channel is called **activation.** Channels appear to open in an all-or-none fashion, each increasing conductance by about 8×10^{-12} mho.

Once the channels are opened, something causes them to close again. This is called **inactivation.** The channels do not, however, go back to their original closed state. The inactivated channel cannot be reopened for a period of time, the time it takes to return to the resting closed condition, and Na^+ conductance during inactivation is even lower than in the resting membrane. The membrane potential has to remain at a value more negative than the critical firing level for a millisecond or so before the chan-

* According to fanciers of puffer fish, the fish are best when eating them makes the lips tingle. The sensation must be similar to that that occurs when novocaine begins to wear off following a trip to the dentist.

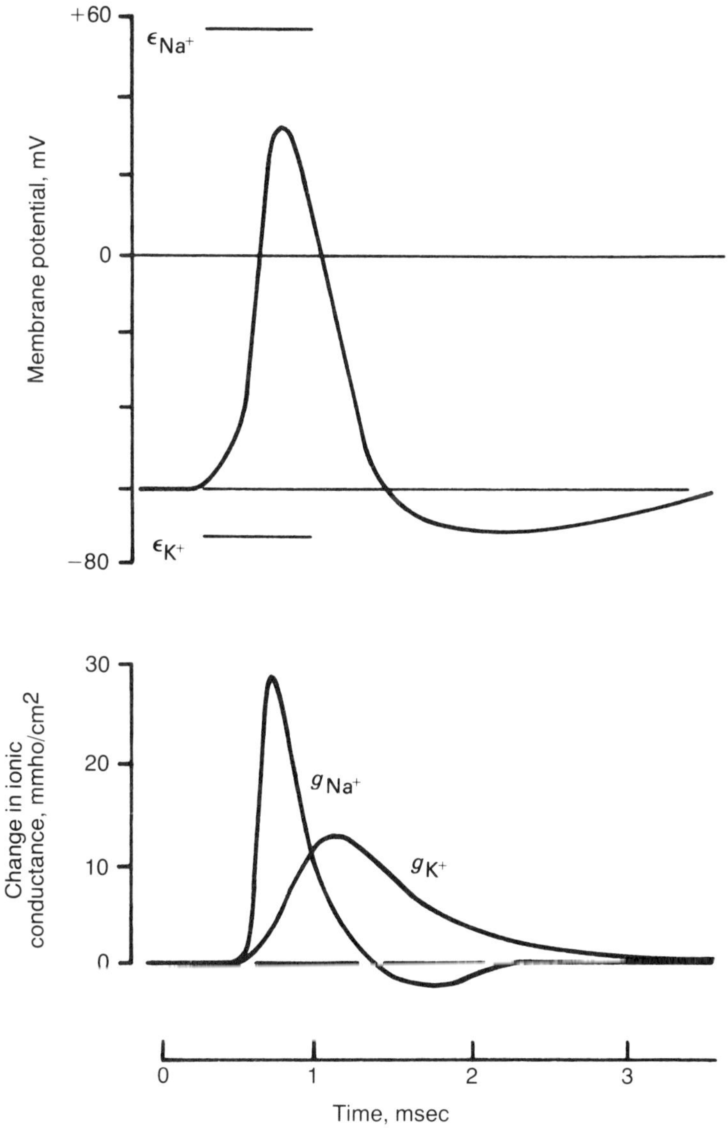

FIG. 3-23. Changes in sodium and potassium conductances during the spike in the squid axon. Upper trace shows the time course of the spike. Lower traces show the earlier rapid increase in g_{Na^+} from near 0 to 30 mmho/cm^2 and the slower return to near zero and the delayed, slower increase in g_{K^+} to more than 10 mmho/cm^2, followed by a slower return to resting levels. (Aidley DJ: The Physiology of Excitable Cells. Cambridge, Cambridge Univ Press, 1971)

nel can be opened again. This accounts for the phenomenon of accommodation: As the membrane is depolarized by a small amount, less than the critical firing level, some Na^+ channels open and then are inactivated, but not enough are opened to generate a spike. More and more channels are opened as long as the depolarization is maintained, but the rate of opening is still too low to lead to a spike. Once a channel is inactivated, it remains inactivated until the membrane repolarizes. If the rate of depolarization is slow enough, many of the Na^+ channels can be inactivated without causing a spike and the critical firing level will be pushed in the positive direction. When most of the channels have been inactivated, no spike can be initiated no matter

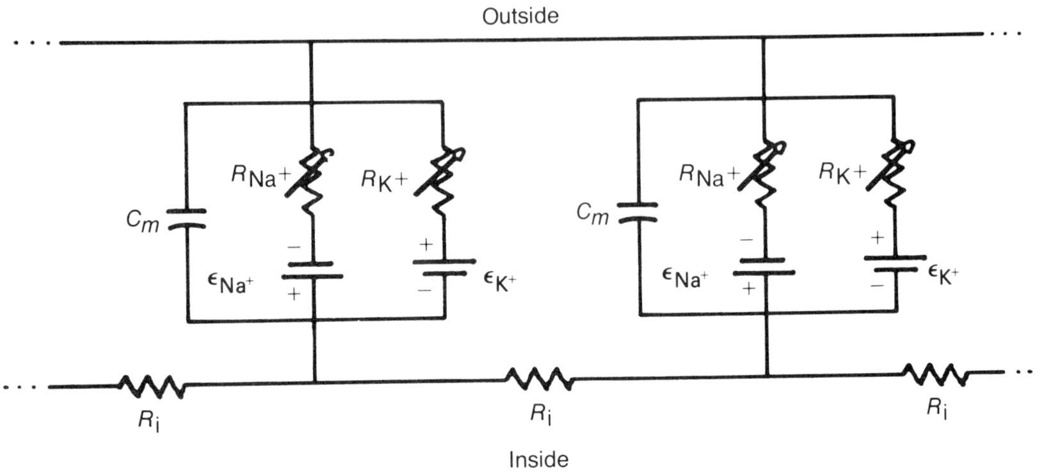

FIG. 3-24. Membrane equivalent circuit. The circuit of Figure 3-14 redrawn to show that conductances (resistances) for sodium and potassium are not fixed, but variable.

how positive the membrane potential becomes.

THE IONIC MECHANISM OF THE ACTION POTENTIAL

How then can we account for the action potential? First, we must update Figure 3-14 to include the variability of the Na^+ and K^+ resistances or conductances. In Figure 3-24, the fixed resistors are replaced with variable resistors, as indicated by the arrows through the resistor symbols. With this change, we can understand the mechanism of generation of the action potential. Initially, before the stimulus is applied to the neuron, g_{K^+} is small, but g_{Na^+} is much smaller, so V_r is near ϵ_{K^+}. The stimulus or, as we shall see, an approaching action potential provides an outward current that passively discharges the membrane capacitance, causing a depolarization of the membrane. When the membrane has been depolarized by a specific amount (a few millivolts), the sodium conductance begins to rise as voltage-gated channels open, allowing some sodium ions to enter the cell down their electrochemical gradient, an inward current. The transfer of positive charge to the inside of the cell results in further depolarization, further increase in conductance as more voltage-gated channels open, and further entry of Na^+ ions.

This cycle of depolarization and increased conductance is sometimes called the **Hodgkin cycle,** and it is schematized in Figure 3-25. The result of this regenerative cycle is that the sodium battery is relatively much more important than the potassium battery in determining the membrane potential, V_m. Perhaps recalling the discussion of the circuits in Figure 3-7 will help to understand how the membrane potential can change so drastically with only a change in membrane conductance (g_{Na^+}). As the sodium battery makes itself felt, the membrane potential moves rapidly toward ϵ_{Na^+}. If nothing changed at this point, g_{Na^+} remained high and g_{K^+} remained low, the membrane would seek a new resting potential predictable from equation 10 and near ϵ_{Na^+}. But now, the inactivation begins; Na^+ channels close and g_{Na^+} drops. At the same time, the depolarization of the membrane has increased g_{K^+} by opening voltage-gated K^+ channels. Figure 3-25 shows this process. Notice that this process is not a regenerative one—increased depolarization leads to increased g_{K^+}, but increased g_{K^+} leads to repolarization, not depolarization. Any change in conductance with a change in voltage is a **rectification.*** The change in g_{K^+} is often called **delayed rectification** because it occurs at a later time than the change in g_{Na^+}. As g_{Na^+} decreases and g_{K^+} increases, the potassium battery again becomes relatively more important in deter-

* This use of the term rectification by biophysicists is quite different from that of electrical engineers, meaning lower resistance to current flow in one direction than the other through a circuit element. Do not confuse these usages.

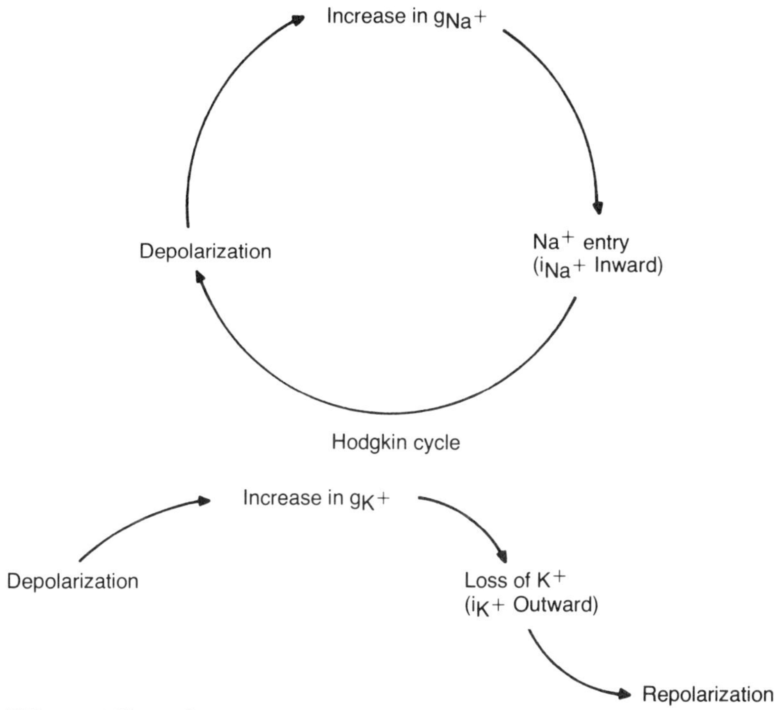

FIG. 3-25. Effects of increasing membrane conductance on the membrane potential. Depolarization leads to increased g_{Na^+}, which leads to sodium entry, which reinforces depolarization in the Hodgkin cycle **(above)**, whereas depolarization leads to increased g_{K^+}, which leads to K^+ efflux, which leads to repolarization **(below)**.

mining the membrane potential and so the potential falls back toward ϵ_{K^+}. This repolarization further reduces g_{Na^+} and the potential change accelerates. The potassium conductance does not inactivate as the sodium conductance does; it simply decreases with repolarization. This ensures that the repolarization occurs completely. Actually, the membrane would repolarize if the sodium conductance inactivated and potassium conductance remained at resting levels, but the repolarization would take longer. The potassium conductance also begins to decrease as the membrane repolarizes, but g_{K^+}/g_{Na^+} is greater than in resting membrane, so the membrane potential passes the resting level and moves even nearer to ϵ_{K^+}. Finally, as g_{K^+} falls back to resting levels, the membrane potential moves back toward V_r as determined by equation 10.

SODIUM DEFICIENCY

We saw previously that the resting membrane potential depends upon the concentration gradient for potassium. If the extracellular Na^+ concentration is slowly lowered, the resting potential hardly changes; usually it becomes less than 10 mV more negative. However, as the extracellular Na^+ is reduced, the peak of the positive overshoot becomes less positive, that is, the amplitude of the action potential decreases, and the spike rises more slowly. When the extracellular Na^+ concentration is lowered below 20 mM, the neuron becomes totally inexcitable and no spikes can be initiated. This results from a reduction in the Na^+ concentration gradient and, therefore, in the sodium current. We have already seen that the sodium current is an integral part of the mechanism of the spike.

MOVEMENTS OF IONS DURING THE SPIKE

If there is a significant ionic current during the spike, ion concentrations both inside and outside the neuron should change. Actually, the ionic shifts through the membrane during the spike are small in relation to the intracellular and extracellular ion concentrations. Measurements of ion movements show that there is a net influx of about 3.7×10^{-12} moles of Na^+ ions/cm^2 of membrane and an equal K^+ efflux during the spike. In large axons, this is about 1/1,000,000 of the resting concentrations. Even in small neurons, the actual ion movement is only 1/1000 of the resting concentration. There is, therefore, only a small change in ion concentration as a result of ion movement during the spike.

The sodium ions that flow in are expelled by the sodium pump, which works not only to maintain resting ion concentrations, but also to restore these concentrations when they are disturbed. Actually, the sodium pump is not important for the individual spike because thousands of spikes can still be initiated in an axon in which the sodium pump has been poisoned with ouabain, cyanide, or dinitrophenol.

PROPAGATION OF THE ACTION POTENTIAL

Obviously, neurons must be able to generate action potentials by themselves, that is, without an experimenter passing current through the membrane. We will see later how sensory stimuli and synaptic transmission from other cells can lead to action potentials; it suffices for now to say that both types of stimuli eventually result in generation of a current outward through the membrane and a depolarization as described above. However, the outward current that results in a spike can also be generated by a spike occurring in an adjacent region of membrane.

Because of Kirchhoff's law (current flows only in complete circuits), the current that flows into the cell during the upstroke of the action potential must flow along the inside of the cell and out through adjacent membrane as shown in Figure 3-26. This outward current discharges the capacitance of the adjacent membrane, leading to a depolarization, an increase in g_{Na^+}, and an action potential. Once the inward ionic current of the spike is started, an outward current will be generated through the next segment of membrane. This process will be repeated in each adjacent segment of membrane throughout the length of the membrane, that is, the action potential will be propagated essentially without decrement along the membrane. The spike itself is an active process, due to the sodium battery, but propagation results from electrotonic (decremental) conduction (a passive process) into nearby membrane segments where a new spike is initiated. If the action potential is initiated in the middle of a length of axon membrane, it will propagate in both directions away from the site of initiation.

One result of propagation is that the action potential pattern as seen plotted in time in Figures 3-17 and 3-23 can just as well be plotted in length along the membrane as shown in Figure 3-26. The spike, shown in the upper panel, A, has been stopped instantaneously in space as it was travelling from right to left. In Figure 3-26B are shown the total membrane current, i_m, the capacitative current, i_c, and the ionic portion of the current, i_i. Obviously, $i_m = i_c + i_i$. The total membrane current is indicated schematically through a section of membrane in C, where arrowheads indicate the direction of current flow, and the closeness of the lines indicates the approximate current density. In D, the equivalent circuit is shown with directions and approximate magnitudes of the membrane, capacitative, and ionic currents indicated by arrows. The changes in conductances are indicated by changes in the lengths of the Na^+ and K^+ resistance symbols. Greater conductance is indicated by a shorter resistance symbol.

Reading from left to right, successive segments of membrane are going through successive phases of the action potential at a given instant in time. Thus, at the time the spike was "frozen" in this position, it had not yet begun at site 1, but outward current (being driven by the inward current at site 3 and nearby) has begun to discharge the membrane capacitance. At site 2, the membrane is depolarized enough to increase g_{Na^+} and, therefore, i_{Na^+}. Between sites 1 and 2 the membrane current is mainly capacitative and outwardly directed, but between sites 2 and 3 the ionic current becomes larger as the Na^+ channels open (Fig. 3-26B). The increased Na^+ conductance is indicated by the shorter resistance symbol at site 2 than at site 1, and at site 3 than at site 2 in D. The sodium conductance has reached its maximum at site 3 and the potassium conductance has increased

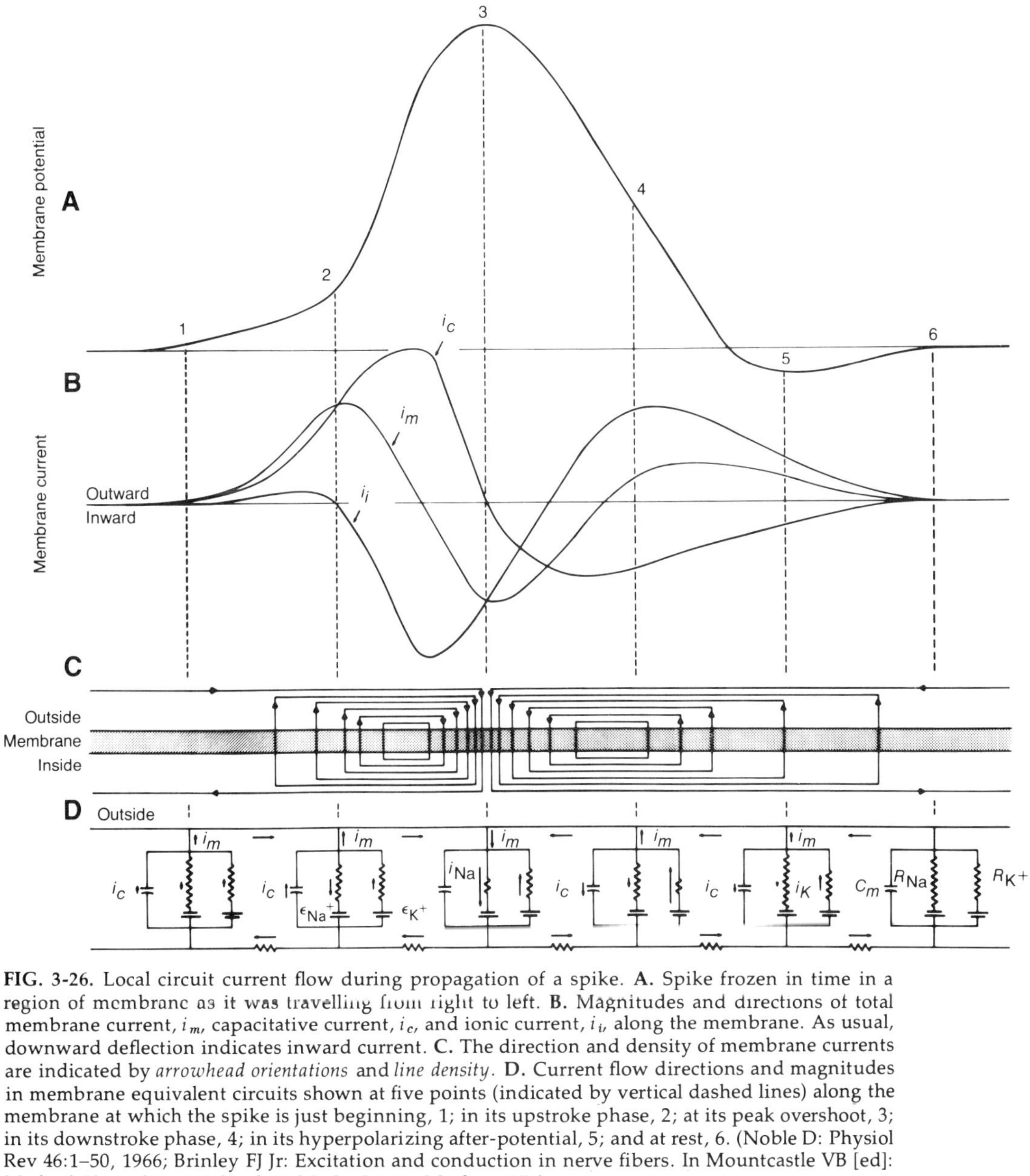

FIG. 3-26. Local circuit current flow during propagation of a spike. **A.** Spike frozen in time in a region of membrane as it was travelling from right to left. **B.** Magnitudes and directions of total membrane current, i_m, capacitative current, i_c, and ionic current, i_i, along the membrane. As usual, downward deflection indicates inward current. **C.** The direction and density of membrane currents are indicated by *arrowhead orientations* and *line density*. **D.** Current flow directions and magnitudes in membrane equivalent circuits shown at five points (indicated by vertical dashed lines) along the membrane at which the spike is just beginning, 1; in its upstroke phase, 2; at its peak overshoot, 3; in its downstroke phase, 4; in its hyperpolarizing after-potential, 5; and at rest, 6. (Noble D: Physiol Rev 46:1–50, 1966; Brinley FJ Jr: Excitation and conduction in nerve fibers. In Mountcastle VB [ed]: Medical Physiology, 13th ed, Vol I, St. Louis, Mosby, 1974)

somewhat (as indicated by the shorter K^+ resistance symbol in D) at the peak overshoot of the spike. The capacitative current is zero at site 3 because $dV/dt = 0$ and thus, $i_m = i_i$.

Sodium inactivation is well underway, but potassium conductance is still high during the repolarization phase at site 4. Total membrane current is small and outwardly directed. Sodium inactivation is complete (as indicated by the long Na^+ resistance symbol in D), but potassium conductance is still higher than normal causing the membrane potential to approach ϵ_{K^+} and generating the hyperpolarizing after-potential at site 5. Both sodium and potassium conductances are normal and the membrane is back at the resting potential at

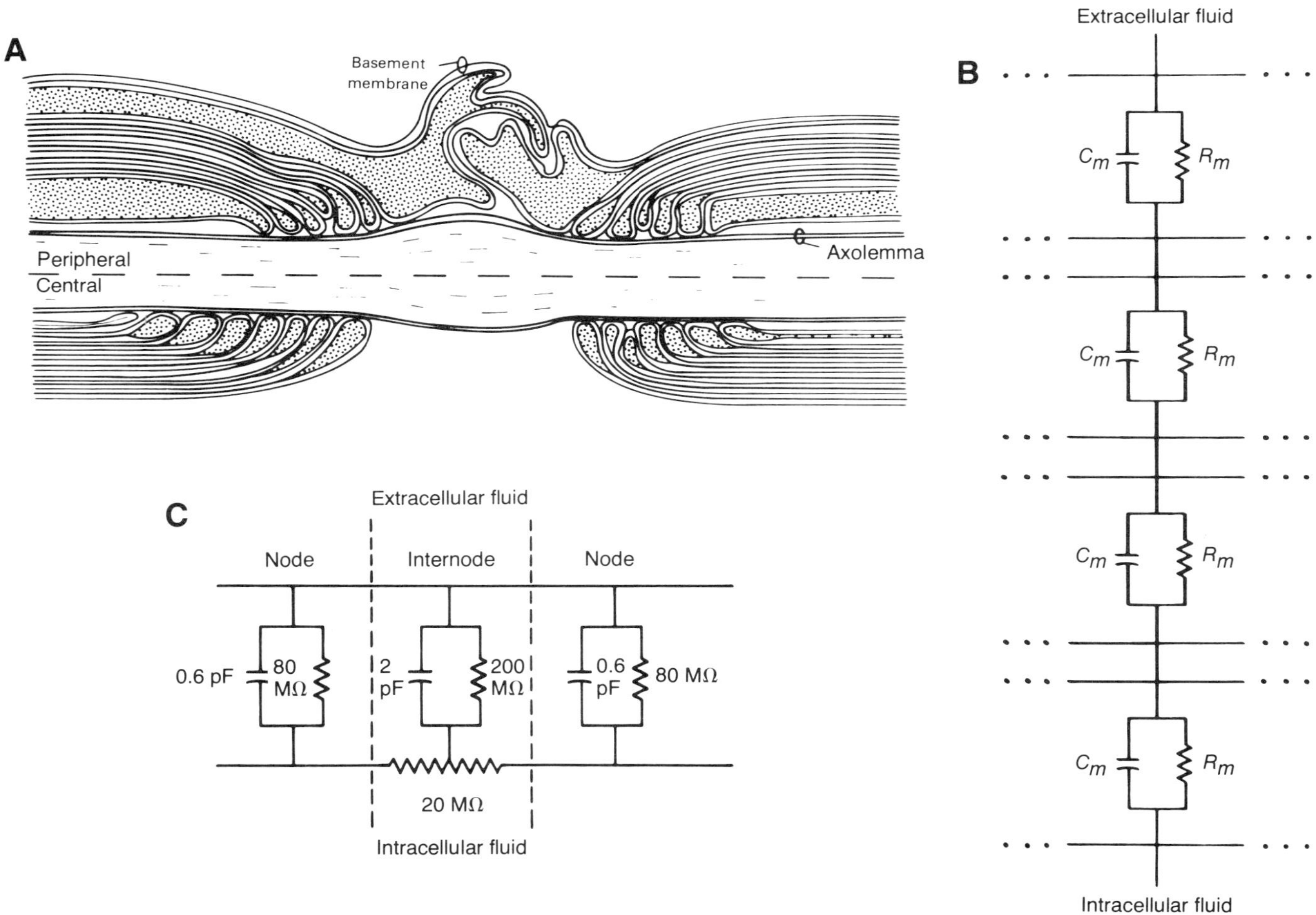

FIG. 3-27. Saltatory conduction in myelinated axons. **A.** Longitudinal section through a small myelinated axon in the peripheral nervous system (*above dashed line*) and in the central nervous system (*below dashed line*). Note difference in structure of nodal region. (Landon DN, Hall S: The myelinated nerve fibre. In Landon DN [ed]: The Peripheral Nerve. London, Chapman and Hall, 1976) **B.** Equivalent circuit for a region of internode, showing how membrane resistances, R_m, and capacitances, C_m, are arranged in series, making resistance very high, capacitance low in the internode. **C.** Equivalent circuit for two nodes and intervening internode with values of membrane resistance, membrane capacitance, and internal longitudinal resistance inserted. (Aidley DJ: The Physiology of Excitable Cells. Cambridge, Cambridge Univ Press, 1971)

site 6. Thus, the sequence of events occurring along the length of the membrane at an instant in time during conduction is exactly the same as that occurring in time at a fixed point on the membrane.

The velocity of the propagation of the spike increases with the magnitude of i_{Na^+} or with the amount of the Na^+ influx. The more current there is available to depolarize adjacent, unexcited membrane after local capacitance is discharged, the faster the adjacent membrane will depolarize to critical firing level and the faster it will generate current to depolarize unexcited membrane next to it, and so on. In order to depolarize adjacent regions of membrane, the inward i_{Na^+} must traverse a volume of intracellular fluid. The resistance of that fluid is a factor in determining how much current actually reaches the adjacent membrane. The resistance to passage of current along the inside of the fiber decreases with the square of the inside fiber diameter; a larger area contains a larger number of potential current pathways. Thus, larger axons will have lower values of R_i and therefore have faster conduction velocities than smaller axons.

It is in propagation, nearly without decrement, that the reason for the existence of the action potential lies. The subthreshold events, that is, the events that occur in response to stimuli that do not bring the membrane to the critical firing level, are not propagated along the axon, but conduct decrementally. Events like those in Figure 3-15 and Figure 3-16a d will produce no effect on the membrane of the cell at a distance of more than a millimeter. The action potential will be of the same magnitude at the site of initiation and at the end of the cell, a meter or even several meters away. When it is necessary to communicate information (neural information) over distances greater than a few hundred micrometers, only the action potential will suffice.

SALTATORY CONDUCTION

The ionic current that flows inward through the membrane results from an active process, the change in sodium conductance. On the other hand, the longitudinal current flow inside and outside the axon is passive, following the rules of electrotonic conduction. If the electrotonic potentials rise faster, that is, if the time constant of the membrane, τ, is decreased, and if they decline less with distance, that is, if the space constant, λ, is increased, the conduction velocity must increase because more current will flow through more distant segments of membrane. The membrane time constant will decrease if the membrane capacitance is reduced, and the space constant will increase if the membrane resistance is increased.

During evolution, animals first exploited increasing axon diameter as a means of increasing conduction velocity, but there is a limit to how large neurons can be; the problem is simply one of bulk. Few giant axons could be accommodated by the squid's body, unless it were greatly enlarged. Fortunately for the squid, it does not need many. The problem becomes even more severe when the nervous system contains more than 10^9 rapidly conducting neurons, as does the human nervous system. Another solution, which uses the principles of electrotonic conduction, requires the cooperation between neurons and glia, the Schwann cells. During development, the Schwann cells wrap themselves around the axons, producing a fatty sheath, composed of layers of membrane and called myelin. Axons with a myelin sheath are said to be **myelinated axons;** axons without a myelin sheath are called **unmyelinated axons.** Each Schwann cell covers (totally surrounds) an area of membrane about 1 mm in length, with a space between adjacent Schwann cells, called the node of Ranvier or simply the node. The region of myelin coverage between two nodes is the internode. Figure 3-27A shows a node (with two adjacent segments of internode) in the peripheral nervous system (above) and the central nervous system (below). The central node is apparently more open to extracellular fluid, but the peripheral node is also bathed in extracellular fluid.

The tightly wrapped layers of membrane prevent contact of extracellular fluid with the axon membrane in the internode, but such contact is provided at the nodes. Overlapping Schwann cell membranes act as series resistances and capacitances as shown in Figure 3-27B. Because resistances in series are simply additive, the total resistance at the internode will be much higher than in unmyelinated membrane or at the node. Because series capacitances add as reciprocals, the total transverse capacitance at the internode will be much lower than at the node. Measurements in the frog axon show that the resistance of the node is only 20 Ω cm², whereas that at the internode is 160,000 Ω cm². Conversely, the capacitance of the node is 3 μF/cm², whereas the internode has a capacitance of .0025 μF/cm². For a 12-μm axon, the node has an area of 20 μm²; the internode has an area of 88 × 10³ μm². Using these areas, the capacitance of a node and internode can be calculated (Fig. 3-27C). The calculated capacitance of the node is 0.6 pF, that of the internode 2 pF (recall that the area of the internode is much larger). At the same time, the measured transverse membrane resistance at the node is 80 MΩ, that of the internode is 200 MΩ, and the internal longitudinal resistance, R_i, is only 20 MΩ.

Because the internode's membrane resistance is so high, most of the longitudinal current generated by a spike occurring at a node will pass along the intracellular fluid rather than outward through the myelin. Although there will still be some loss of electrotonic potential along the internode, the high resistance and low capacitance ensure that the loss will be less than in the same length of unmyelinated axon. The result is that most of the current will flow out through the next node and the current density there will be high, sufficiently high to discharge the membrane capacitance rapidly to the critical firing level, initiating a spike. No action potential can occur in the internode, so the spike jumps from node to node to node. The conduction in myelinated axons is called **saltatory** (from the Latin, to jump). The current density at the node is about 20 mA/cm² (current density in unmyelinated squid axon is seldom greater than 1 mA/cm² under the same conditions), and this is five to seven times greater than that required to bring the membrane to critical firing level. This safety factor ensures that conduction from node to node will occur. In fact, saltatory conduction probably occurs between every other node because there is sufficient current to bring even the second node away from a spike to the critical firing level.

Conduction in myelinated axons is much faster than in unmyelinated axons because the spike, at one point on the membrane, initiates another spike at a point further down the axon (1 or 2 nodes away) by virtue of the longer space constant. The largest unmyelinated fibers in mammals are 2 μm in diameter and conduct at 2 m/sec; the largest myelinated fibers are 22 μm in diameter and conduct at 120 m/sec. Longitudinal, intracellular resistance decreases as the square of internal diameter in myelinated as in unmyelinated axons, so conduction velocity in larger myelinated axons will be higher than in smaller ones. In peripheral nerves, a rough rule of thumb is that conduction velocity of myelinated axons in meters per second is six times the axon diameter in micrometers. This estimate does not work well for axons in the central nervous system.

REFRACTORY PERIODS

Note in Figure 3-26C that current flows outward through the membrane both in front of and behind the advancing action potential. What prevents the action potential from turning around and propagating in the reverse direction? The answer lies in the refractory period. After the peak overshoot of the spike, the Na^+ conductance begins to be inactivated and, by the time the membrane repolarizes to the resting potential, sodium conductance is almost entirely inactivated. The membrane must remain near the resting potential for some time (a millisecond or so) before the sodium channels return to their closed state, ready for activation again. During this time, the sodium conductance cannot be changed substantially by depolarization. Thus, a new spike cannot be initiated no matter how large the depolarization. This phase of inexcitability, called the **absolute refractory period,** is shown in Figure 3-28. It has about the same duration as the spike itself in many cells.

The channels do not all convert to the closed, activatable state at the same time. Therefore, as time passes after the repolarization, more and more channels will be available until all are available. The excitability increases, or, in other words, the threshold falls as a function of time after the spike. The fall in the threshold is shown in Figure 3-28B. Even though a spike can be initiated within 2 or 3 msec after another

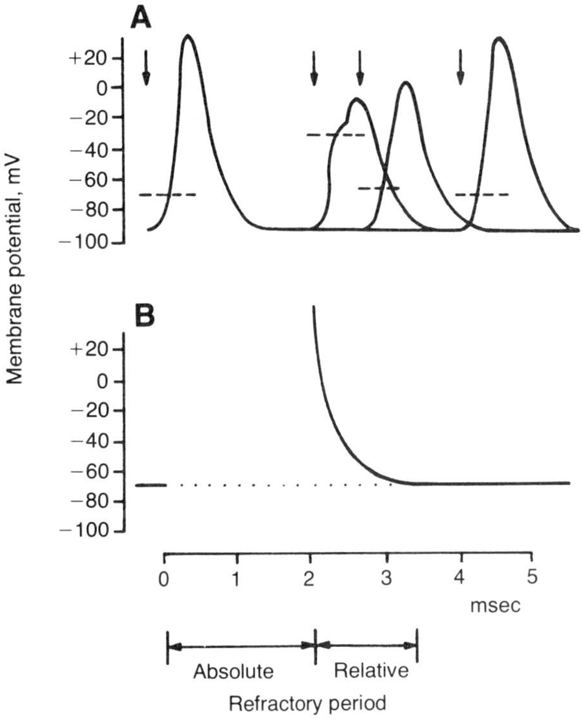

FIG. 3-28. Time course of refractoriness following a spike. **A.** Spikes elicited by pairs of stimuli at different time intervals. The first stimulus of each pair was applied at the leftmost downward arrow. Because pairs are far apart in time, the response to this stimulus always has the same configuration. The second stimulus of the first pair occurred 2 msec after the first stimulus **(second arrow)**, of the second pair occurred about 2.8 msec after the first **(third arrow)**, and of the third pair occurred about 4 msec after the first **(fourth arrow)**. Spikes initiated during the refractory period are stunted and prolonged. **Dashed line** on rising phase of each spike indicates approximate critical firing level. **B.** Time course of change in critical firing level through the refractory periods. Approximate durations of absolute and relative refractory periods are indicated at the bottom of the figure (Dudel J: In Schmidt RF [ed]: Fundamentals of Neurophysiology, 2nd ed. New York, Springer-Verlag, 1978)

spike has occurred, it is only a partial spike because not all Na^+ channels are available to the spike-generating mechanism. This period of reduced excitability is the **relative refractory period.**

The refractory periods, absolute and relative, have two important consequences. First, the refractory period is long enough that the electrotonic and ionic voltages behind the spike have declined to below the critical firing level before the refractory period is over. Thus, the spike cannot turn around and go the other way. Likewise, because two action potentials cannot occupy the same region of membrane at the same time, two action potentials approaching each other along an axon will cancel each other out; neither action potential will pass the point of their meeting. This is called **occlusion.**

Another consequence of the refractory periods is that there is a maximum rate of discharge for the neuron. This rate is limited by the absolute refractory period for strong stimulation and by the relative refractory period for weak stimulation. A neuron that fires a 0.5-msec duration spike with a 1.0-msec refractory period cannot, under any circumstance, fire at a frequency greater than 1000/sec. If the spike and the refractory period are longer the maximum frequency decreases.

INFLUENCES OF OTHER IONS

Ions other than Na^+ and K^+ do not seem to play a major role in generation of the action potential, at least in axons. That is not to say that they cannot affect the action potential, however. Calcium has a complex effect on the action potential threshold. When the extracellular concentration of calcium is lowered, the axon becomes more sensitive to excitation, lowering the threshold for intracellular stimulation and causing the cells to discharge spikes spontaneously. The influence of calcium seems to be to stabilize the membrane. At very low concentrations of Ca^{2+}, less than 1×10^{-5}M, the axon becomes inexcitable by any stimulus intensity, although excitability can be restored by increasing extracellular Ca^{2+} again.

Above-normal extracellular calcium concentrations depress neuron firing at many places in the central nervous system, yet they do not change either resting membrane potentials or membrane resistance. Synaptic potentials, the potentials that occur as a part of transmission between cells, are not influenced by increasing extracellular Ca^{2+}. Magnesium ions have an influence on axon excitability similar to that of calcium, but, as we shall see, the effect of magnesium on synaptic transmission is opposite to that of calcium.

Neurons and muscles in mammals use sodium and potassium conductance changes to generate action potentials, but these are not the only ions that can serve this function. In fact, in crustacean muscles and in the dendrites and, in some cases, somata of neurons in the cerebral cortex, of Purkinje cells of the cerebellar cortex, of neurons in the inferior olivary nucleus, and perhaps of spinal motoneurons in mammals, Ca^{2+} ions take the place of Na^+ in carrying inward current. Calcium conductance is activated by depolarization, but the kinetics of activation are slower than those for sodium; thus the calcium spike develops more slowly and it lasts longer. Like the sodium conductance, the calcium conductance inactivates with time, and potassium conductance increases, repolarizing the membrane. The calcium spike is not blocked by tetrodotoxin as is the sodium spike. Likewise, procaine, which blocks sodium spikes, is without effect on calcium spikes. Tetraethylammonium ions prolong and increase the amplitude of the calcium spike as they do for the sodium spike. The calcium spike is blocked (by competitive inhibition) by other divalent ions, Mn^{2+}, Co^{2+}, Ni^{2+}, but the sodium spike is not. This implies that, although Ca^{2+} can pass through Na^+ channels, it has its own channels in membranes sustaining calcium spikes.

It has been noted that sodium spikes are found where conduction of the action potential is important. Surely, the conduction velocity of the calcium spike would be quite slow; a definite speed advantage would lie with the sodium spike. On the other hand, in primitive, slowly moving animals, there was no particular premium on speed of conduction; calcium spikes probably sufficed. Calcium spikes are found when electrical excitation couples to an effector process, for example, contraction or secretion. The utility of calcium spikes in the dendrites of neurons in the central nervous system is not known. It has been suggested that these calcium spikes are a holdover from more primitive times; yet there is no compelling evidence for this conjecture at present.

INHOMOGENEITY OF THE NERVE MEMBRANE

The existence of sodium spikes in the axon and calcium spikes in the dendrites of some cells in the central nervous system suggests that the membrane of a neuron is not the same all over, from dendrites, to soma, to axon, to axon terminals. Older concepts of the neuron treated the **dendrite** as the receptive part of the cell, receiving either sensory stimuli from the environment or inputs from other cells. The **soma** was an integrative part of the cell, summing inputs from a variety of sources and generating an output based on the sum. Axons were simply conducting cables following the output of the soma but not altering it in any way, whereas the terminals transmitted the action potentials to other neurons or effectors by releasing small amounts of a transmitter substance. More recent concepts of neurons do not delegate such exclusive functions to parts of neurons, but allow broader overlap in function. Still, the differences in the properties of parts of a nerve cell membrane suggest that the membrane is inhomogeneous.

We have seen that the axon membrane contains an abundance of voltage-gated sodium and potassium channels, giving it

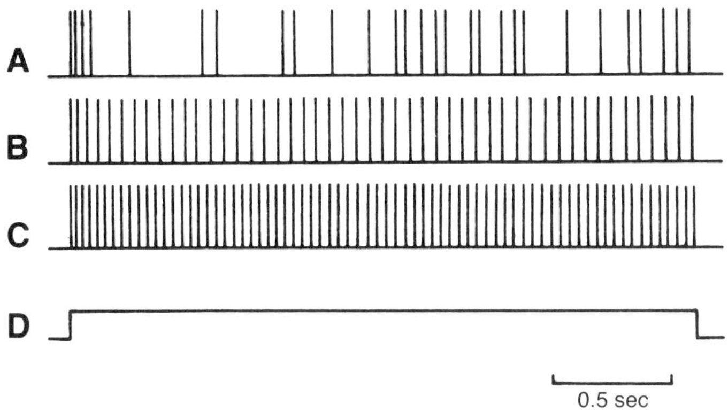

FIG. 3-29. Accommodation in the soma. **A–C.** Intracellularly recorded responses of a motoneuron to prolonged depolarizing current at increasing strength. **A:** 7×10^{-9}A, **B:** 7.7×10^{-9}A, **C:** 10×10^{-9}A. **D.** Monitor of current flow; upward deflection is on. (Granit R, Kernell D, Shortess GK: J Physiol (Lond) 168:911–931, 1963)

the ability to generate action potentials. The density of such channels in axons has been estimated at 1000 per μm^2. Membranes that do not contain voltage-gated channels do not generate spikes. The soma and dendrites of some neurons have few, if any, voltage-gated channels, although neurons that support dendritic and somatic sodium or calcium spikes may have many. The receptor sites on membranes, sites sensitive to sensory stimuli and transmitter substances, do not generate spikes, but they do generate nonpropagated, graded potentials that lead to spikes. As we shall see, the generation of spikes in such membranes would disrupt their ability to encode the qualities of the stimulus.

The dendrites and soma have many chemically gated channels, especially at the sites of contact with other cells at synapses. Some estimates indicate that the number of such channels at synapses is limited only by their maximum packing density. Chemically gated channels are of several types that can be classified either in terms of the chemical transmitter substance that opens them or in terms of their selectivity for certain ions. Some chemically gated channels are opened by acetylcholine, others by norepinephrine and others by other substances. (For a further discussion of the topic of transmitter substances, see Chapter 13.) Channels are seldom absolutely selective. Thus, the acetylcholine-gated channels at the neuromuscular junction, the synapse between the motoneuron and the muscle, allow both sodium and potassium ions, in fact, nearly all ions to pass through. This nonselective change in membrane permeability leads to a depolarization of the muscle membrane (the end-plate potential), a spike, and muscle contraction. At other synapses, the channels open to create a more selective change in membrane conductance for potassium and chloride. Axons themselves contain no chemically gated channels, though the terminals of the axons may contain them at sites of special synaptic contacts, the axo-axonic synapses.

Not only is the density of different kinds of ionic channels different in various parts of the nerve membrane, but the behavior of the same kind of channel is different in different parts of the membrane. If a pair of micropipette electrodes is used to penetrate the cell body of a neuron as in Figure 3-8 and a constant current is passed outward through the membrane, a train of action potentials will be initiated, lasting as long as the current is maintained. Figure 3-29 shows this for three different magnitudes of current through the soma of a motoneuron. In D is shown the monitor of the current that turns on abruptly as the trace deflects upward and off abruptly as the trace deflects downward. At a current magnitude of 7×10^{-9} A, the spike train is a bit irregular, but continues for the duration of the current flow (A). At higher currents (B and C), the trains are regular, and the frequency of discharge (spikes/sec) within the trains is proportional to the current magnitude. This

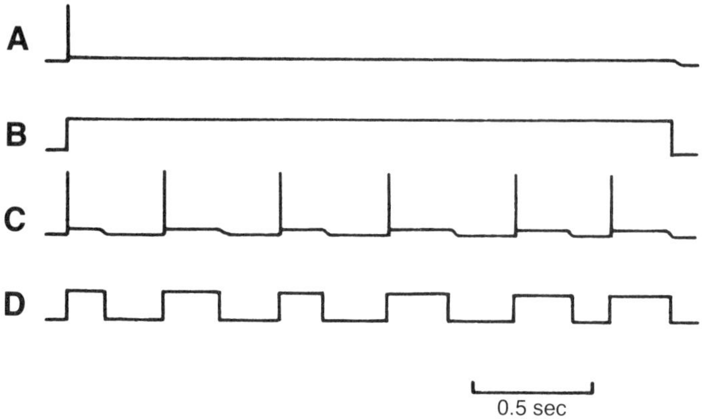

FIG. 3-30. Accommodation in the axon. **A.** Response of an axon to prolonged depolarizing current as shown in **B. C.** Response of the same axon to repeated short pulses of depolarizing current shown in **D.**

kind of behavior is representative of most somata of mammalian neurons, though it is debated whether it is a property of the soma itself or the initial segment of the axon (the transition from soma to axon). For this discussion, we will treat the initial segment as part of the soma.

If the same experiment were done in an axon, each current step would result in a single action potential as the membrane potential crossed the critical firing level. Trains of spikes are never generated in axons unless the currents are excessively (perhaps pathologically) high. This rapid fall in the firing frequency of the axon in spite of the constant stimulus is called **adaptation** and, in the case of the axon, probably results from an extreme accommodation of the membrane. Adaptation also occurs in sensory receptors (as we shall see in Chap. 4) where it may have causes other than accommodation. The adaptation of the axon membrane is illustrated in Figure 3-30. A step of current is indicated in B and the axon's response to that current step is shown in A. Within reasonable limits, larger currents will give only a similar single-spike discharge, although the spike will occur slightly sooner after the start of the largest currents. However, if the current is turned on and off several times within the same time period, as indicated by the repeated upward and downward deflections of the current monitor in D, the axon discharges a spike each time the current comes back on (C), as long as there is sufficient time after the previous spike for the refractory periods to have ended. This kind of behavior is typical of axons in mammalian nervous systems (but not invertebrate systems).

How the sodium channels differ in these two types of membranes is not known, but there is a clear difference in accommodation. Actually, there is no reason for the axon to behave like the soma in response to prolonged outward currents, because axons probably never experience such currents. The axon is basically a follower; it follows what the soma (or initial segment) does. Its spikes are caused by the soma spikes by propagation as described earlier. The soma spikes generate fast current transients that recur with each spike and recurrently initiate axon spikes as in Figure 3-30C. Axons, therefore, always generate trains of spikes identical in their timing (the spikes occur at the same times relative to each other) to those that occur in the soma. The soma, on the other hand, is the pacemaking or spike-generating region of the neuron, responsible for coding information it receives from other neurons (a property the soma shares with sensory receptors, as we shall see in the next chapter). It experiences prolonged current flows (synaptic currents) and must respond to changes in current flow with changes in frequency of discharge. The soma's behavior, like that of the axon, is appropriate to its role in neural function.

The existence of different kinds of ionic channels in different densities in different regions of the neuron's membrane reemphasizes that the fluidity of the lipid membrane is not unlimited. If it were so, then the dendrites would often have properties of axons, the somata often properties of dendrites, and so forth. In cases where an element external to the cell is involved, as at synapses, these elements may influence the aggregation of certain channels near them. Not every case involves an external element; in these other cases, some internal factor must aggregate appropriate channels.

SUGGESTED READING

Cooke I, Lipkin M [eds]: Cellular Neurophysiology. A Source Book. New York, Holt, Rinehart, and Winston, 1972

Eccles JC: The Physiology of Nerve Cells. Baltimore, Johns Hopkins Press, 1968

Hagiwara S: Ca spike. Advan Biophys 4:71–102, 1973

Hodgkin AL: The Conduction of the Nervous Impulse. Springfield IL, Charles C Thomas, 1964

Junge D: Nerve and Muscle Excitation. Sunderland MA, Sinauer, 1976

Katz B: Nerve, Muscle, and Synapse. New York, McGraw-Hill, 1966

Llinás R, Hess R: Tetrodotoxin-resistant dendritic spikes in avian Purkinje cells. Proc Nat Acad Sci 73:2520–2523, 1976

Stevens CF: The Neuron. Sci Am 241:55–65, 1979

Waxman SG: Integrative properties and design principles of axons. Int Rev Neurobiol 18:1–40, 1975

4

Receptor Properties: Receptor Potentials and Coding

Let us begin our discussion of the neurophysiology of sensation by considering what happens in a receptor when a stimulus is applied to it. In later chapters individual sensory receptors for each sense are considered separately, but at this point, it is the general properties of receptors that are of concern. We have already seen that when a suprathreshold stimulus (of strength greater than threshold strength) is applied to a receptor, the nerve fiber associated with that receptor discharges. What we would like to know is how the stimulus energy is transformed into action potentials in the normal operation of the system, that is, what is the nature of the transduction process?

RECEPTOR POTENTIALS

The transduction process appears to be similar in all of the various types of receptors that have been studied. Let us take for our example the **muscle spindle,** a small structure found in skeletal muscle that contains two kinds of receptors both of which can signal the length of the muscle. The anatomy and physiology of the muscle spindle are considered in more detail in Chapter 11. If a recording electrode is placed on the sensory nerve fiber supplying one of the receptors in the muscle spindle (the primary receptor) at a point very near the spindle itself and then the spindle is stretched, recordings like those in Figure 4-1 result. The upper trace of each pair shows the recording from the fiber, whereas the lower trace shows the monitor of the muscle length (longer being indicated by an upward deflection). In Figure 4-1A, the spike discharge is superimposed upon a slow depolarizing potential that develops as the muscle is stretched. If the preparation is bathed in a solution of lidocaine, a local anesthetic agent, or in tetrodotoxin, the action potentials are blocked as in Figure 4-1B, leaving the slow depolarizing potential by itself. This potential, called the **generator potential,** can be shown to originate in part of the spindle receptor, not in the nerve fiber. Nerve fibers are usually not particularly sensitive to the same stimulus that excites their receptors. Some people use the term generator potential synonymously with **receptor potential,** whereas others prefer to reserve the term receptor potential for those cases in which the receptor does not itself generate spikes, as in the receptors of the eye. We use the term receptor potential here in the latter sense.

The generator and receptor potentials are local or nonpropagated events as shown by the degradation of their amplitudes with increasing distance from the receptor. One need only move the recording electrode along the nerve a few millimeters farther away from the spindle before the generator potential disappears. They are graded responses as opposed to the all-or-none character of the action potential; the amplitudes of the generator and receptor potentials increase with increasing stimulus

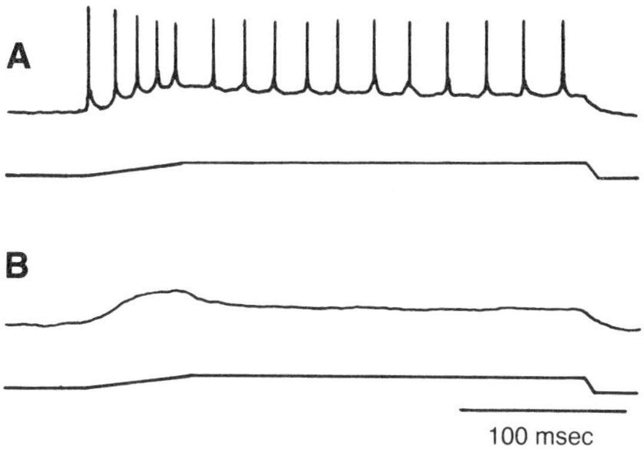

FIG. 4-1. Relation between impulse response and underlying generator potential. A. Response of a muscle spindle receptor to prolonged stretch with nerve recording shown in the upper trace and monitor of the stretch of the muscle in the lower trace. B. The same response after bathing the spindle in 0.2% lidocaine. (Ottoson D, Shepherd GM: Acta Physiol Scand 79:423–430, 1970).

FIG. 4-2. Graded responses of a muscle spindle receptor to stretch. Graded stretches are indicated by the stretch monitor in the lower trace; graded generator potentials are shown in the upper trace. Records are superimposed. (Ottoson D, Shepherd GM: Cold Spring Harbor Symp Quant Biol 30:105–114, 1965).

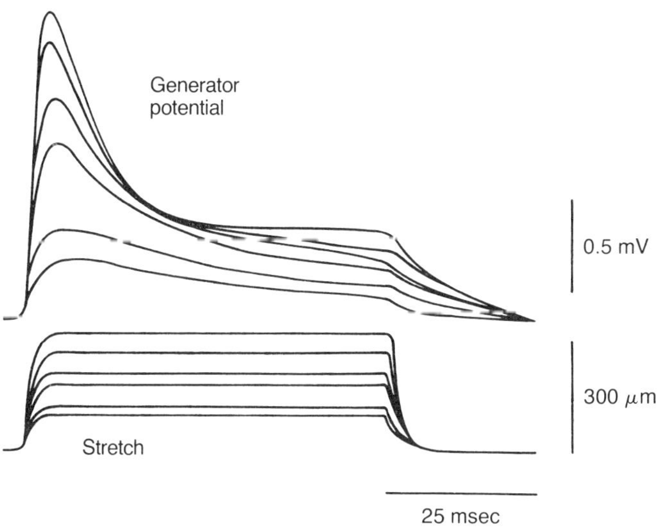

strength. The upper trace of Figure 4-2 shows superimposed generator potentials from a muscle spindle receptor that resulted from the different amounts of muscle stretch, as shown by the heights of the indicators superimposed in the lower trace. For these records, the action potentials have been blocked by application of lidocaine. The graded increases in the generator potential amplitude with graded muscle stretches are clearly illustrated in this figure.

The start of the generator potential results from an increase in the permeability of the membrane of the receptor to sodium ions and an inward sodium current, whereas the potential is terminated by a decrease in sodium ion permeability, an increase in potassium ion permeability, and an outward potassium current. The ionic mecha-

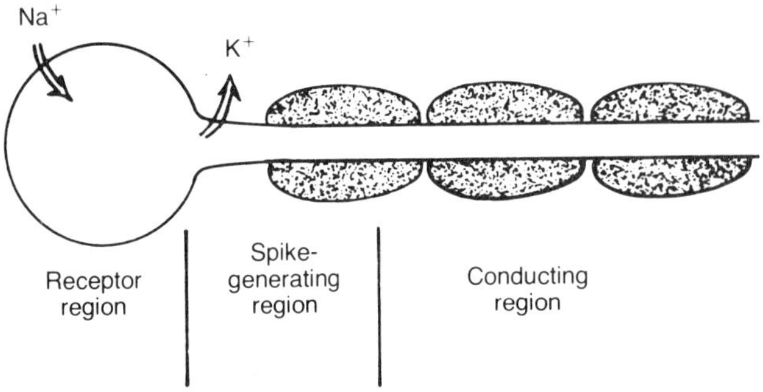

FIG. 4-3. A schematic diagram of a generalized receptor showing the receptor region, the spike-generating region, and the conducting region along with the currents that flow during the generator potential.

FIG. 4-4. Relation between amplitude of the generator potential and frequency of impulse discharge during the dynamic phase of stretch (time when muscle and spindle are actually changing length). (Ottoson D, Shepherd GM: Acta Physiol Scand 79:423–430, 1970)

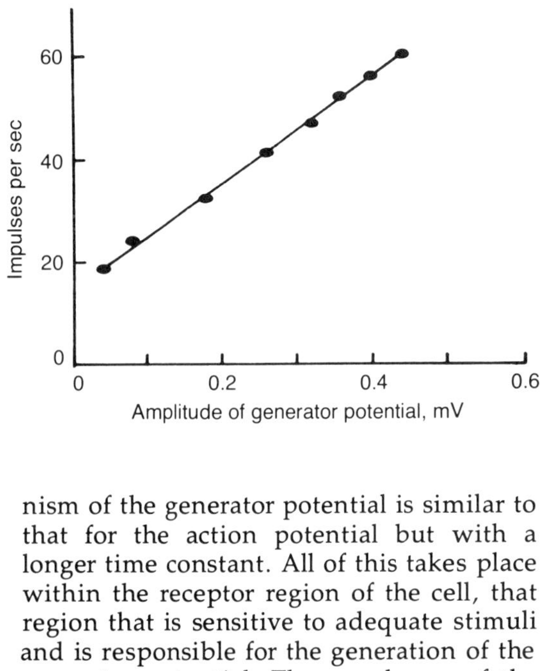

nism of the generator potential is similar to that for the action potential but with a longer time constant. All of this takes place within the receptor region of the cell, that region that is sensitive to adequate stimuli and is responsible for the generation of the generator potential. The membrane of the receptor region is, however, electrically inexcitable; it contains no voltage-gated ionic channels and does not generate spikes. If the receptor region generated action potentials, the graded nature of the generator potential would be destroyed because as soon as the generator potential exceeded the critical firing level an action potential would be initiated, reversing the membrane polarization no matter how large or small the stimulus, that is, the membrane potential would no longer encode the stimulus intensity. The action potentials themselves are usually initiated in a physically separate region of the cell, the pacemaker or spike-generating region. This may be anatomically separate from or continuous with the receptor region or with the axon itself, the conducting region. These parts of a generalized receptor are indicated in Figure 4-3. As illustrated in the figure, the inward sodium current that depolarized the *active* (with changed conductances) receptor region is concomitant with an outward current (probably carried mostly by potassium ions) in the spike-generating region of the cell. That this *must* be true follows from Kirchhoff's current law; current flows only in *complete* circuits. As anywhere in a nerve cell, outward current though an *inactive* (with normal resting conductances) region of membrane causes a depolarization of that membrane. A depolarization, as we already know, leads to the formation of action potentials, provided that the critical firing level is reached or exceeded. Actually, the spike-generating region simply responds to depolarizing current in the same way as any membrane containing voltage-gated Na^+ and K^+ channels. The conducting region of the membrane of the sensory receptor simply "follows" what the spike-generating region does; it simply transmits, without alteration, signals it receives.

In the absence of an anesthetic agent, it is possible to study the relationship between the frequency of discharge in the muscle spindle axon and the amplitude of the generator potential. The relationship obtained for various muscle lengths is linear as plotted in Figure 4-4. Again, recall that the fact that the plot is linear indicates that equal increments in discharge frequency result from equal increments in generator potential amplitude. A linear relationship between the amplitude of the generator potential and the discharge frequency of the nerve has been found for every receptor studied so far. For the muscle spindle, there is also a linear relationship between the amount of stretch applied and the amplitude of the generator potential. The muscle spindle is one of the cases of a receptor in which there is a linear relationship (the exponent of the power function, $k = 1$) between the strength of the stimulus and the response of the cell, that is, the amount of stretch and the frequency of discharge of the associated nerve fiber. If the relationship between stimulus and response is curvilinear for a sensory receptor, as in those cases in which the relationship is a logarithmic or power function (the exponent, $k \neq 1$), then there is a curvilinear relationship between the strength of the stimulus and the amplitude of the generator potential, and, in fact, it is a logarithmic or power function. This must be the case if the relationship between the amplitude of the generator potential and the discharge frequency is always linear.

It is important to bear in mind that the *normal* sequence of events in transduction is (1) stimulus, (2) receptor or generator potential, and (3) action potentials. An adequate stimulus always leads to a receptor or generator potential if it is large enough and applied at the right place. The generator potential normally leads to the formation of action potentials provided that it is large enough to bring the membrane potential of the fiber to critical firing level. In those cases in which a receptor potential results from a stimulus, the receptor potential must somehow give rise to a generator potential before action potentials result. In the retina of the eye, the receptor potential in the receptors, the rods and cones, causes a decreased release of a transmitter substance (a new stimulus, chemical this time) to the bipolar cells that causes them to generate a receptor potential. The second receptor potential causes the release of a transmitter substance (a second new stimulus, again chemical) onto the ganglion cell that sets up a generator potential (an EPSP; see Chap. 13) in the ganglion cell. The generator potential in the ganglion cell finally initiates action potentials in the optic nerve fibers. In the retina, two receptor potentials and a generator potential intervene between the stimulus and the first action potentials, but the sequence of events is still: stimulus, receptor or generator potential, and action potentials.

SUMMATION

In receptors that are suitable for applying two stimuli close together, two other properties of generator potentials can be studied. If a mechanical stimulus is applied to a mechanoreceptor, a generator potential is recorded such that the amplitude of the generator potential is a function of the amount of deformation of the receptor surface. Two identical stimuli applied in rapid succession at the same site result in a generator potential twice the size of that resulting from a single stimulus. In fact, the amplitude of the generator potential that results from any two stimuli applied in close temporal proximity is always equal to the algebraic sum of the generator potentials initiated by each stimulus alone. An example of this behavior is shown in Figures 4-5 and 4-6 for a Pacinian corpuscle, a tiny ellipsoidal body composed of a number of concentric lamellae and with a myelinated fiber running into its center. The corpuscles are found in connective tissue of the mesentery and the popliteal fossa among other places; their function is largely unknown. Their generator potentials have been thoroughly studied. Figure 4-5 shows the way a mechanical stimulator is applied to the isolated corpuscle while recordings are being made from its axon. When the stimulator presses down on the corpuscle, as shown in the lower trace, a depolarizing generator potential is initiated in the receptor. The potential rapidly returns to resting levels, but a new depolarizing generator potential is set up when the corpuscle is released from compression. This behavior is typical of the Pacinian corpuscle. If we were recording from the nerve fiber associated with the corpuscle at a site farther away, we would record an action potential associated with each of the generator potentials, but for now we are concerned about the generator potentials. We can use the first generator potential of the corpuscle to study

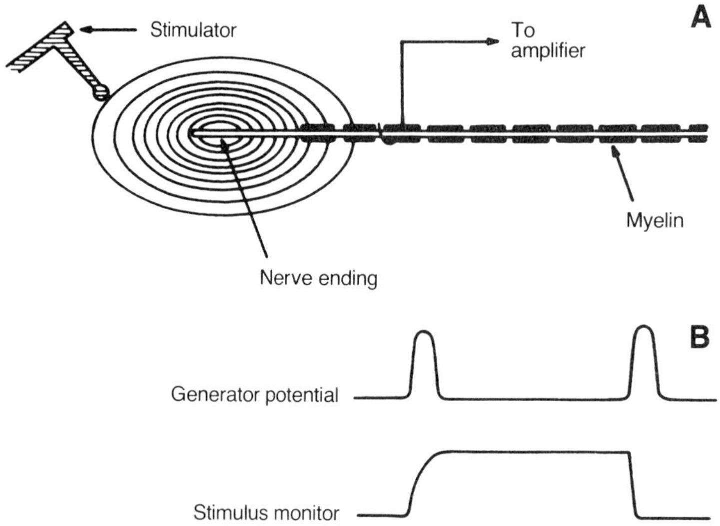

FIG. 4-5. A. The setup for recording generator potentials from Pacinian corpuscles. **B.** The stimulus monitor and an example of a Pacinian generator potential.

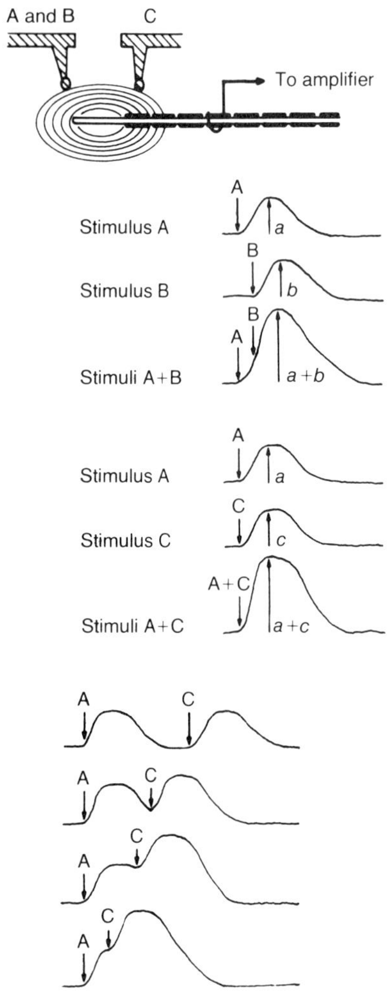

FIG. 4-6. Spatial and temporal summation of generator potentials in a Pacinian corpuscle. Stimuli A and B are applied, with the same stimulator, close together in time. Stimulus C is applied at another place on the receptor at the same time as A in the second set of records. At the bottom of the figure is shown the summation that results from varying the interval between stimuli A and C.

summation. As shown in Figure 4-6, stimulus A results in a generator potential of amplitude a and stimulus B in a potential of amplitude b. When A and B are applied together, the resulting generator potential has amplitude $a + b$. This additive property of generator potentials is called **temporal summation,** because the variable is time. A similar phenomenon results when two stimuli are applied at the same time at two different locations. Again in Figure 4-6, stimulus C results in a generator potential of amplitude c, whereas stimulus A + C results in a generator potential of amplitude $a + c$. In this case, the variable is the spatial distribution of the stimuli instead of time; thus the phenomenon is termed **spatial summation.** Figure 4-6 shows summation of only two generator potentials, but any number of generator potentials can summate in a single cell, limited only by the physical arrangement of the receptor, that is, by how many stimuli can impinge upon it at the same time.

The generator potential rises from the

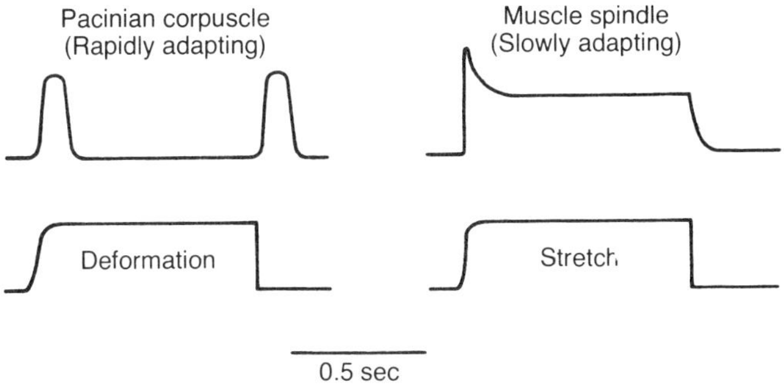

FIG. 4-7. Comparison between rapidly adapting (Pacinian corpuscle) and slowly adapting (muscle spindle) generator potentials.

resting membrane potential, reaches a peak after a given interval, then returns toward the resting membrane potential. If the stimuli are presented so far apart in time that the first generator potential is over before the second stimulus is applied, then there will be no summation. Thus, the amplitude of the summated generator potential depends upon how much the membrane potential of the receptor is altered at the time the second stimulus is applied. At the bottom of Figure 4-6 are shown a number of examples of how summation is affected by varying the time between the two stimuli, A and C; the maximum summed potential occurs when the stimuli are delivered simultaneously and the amplitude falls off as the second stimulus is delayed. The end result of the summation is an increase in the frequency of discharge of the sensory nerve fiber over the frequency that would be obtained for either stimulus alone. Any number of generator potentials can sum in this same manner, each increment in the amplitude resulting in increased discharge frequency, until a maximum frequency, characteristic of that particular fiber, is reached.

ADAPTATION

The time over which summation is obtained depends upon the duration of the individual generator potentials. To a certain extent, the duration of the generator potential depends upon the duration of the stimulus; however, some receptors have generator potentials that last only a short time, no matter how long the stimulus is maintained. Figure 4-7 shows the generator potentials of a Pacinian corpuscle and a muscle spindle for a sustained deformation and stretch, respectively. Notice that the generator potential for the corpuscle increases to a maximum amplitude and then returns to the resting membrane potential in spite of the persistence of the stimulus. On the other hand, the muscle spindle generator potential increases to a maximum and then declines a bit, but is maintained above the resting potential for the duration of the stimulus. We refer to a decrease in the amplitude of the generator potential or the frequency of discharge of the sensory fiber in the face of a persisting, constant stimulus as **adaptation.** Receptors that behave like Pacinian corpuscles are said to be **rapidly adapting;** those that behave like muscle spindles are said to be **slowly adapting.** For some receptors, the rate of adaptation is a function of the physical characteristics of the receptor structure. In the Pacinian corpuscle, which shows an extreme of rapid adaptation, the adaptation is slowed considerably by removal of the lamellae and application of the stimulus directly to the nerve fiber. Membrane accommodation may also play a role in producing adaptation.

The reason for having both slowly and rapidly adapting receptors lies in the different kinds of information they signal. Slowly adapting receptors presumably signal the onset and offset, but most importantly the presence of a long sustained stimulus. They do adapt to some extent as indicated by the gradual waning of the sensation of the chair against your posterior as you read this. (This probably does not represent entirely a receptor process, but involves the central nervous system as well, as is indicated by the fact that the sensation returned to your posterior as soon as mention was made of its absence). On the other hand, rapidly adapting receptors signal the start, velocity, and, in some cases, the stop of a stimulus, but do not signal in between. On the other hand, they give very good responses to repeated stimuli, suggesting that they may play a role in vibration sense. The time over which summation of slowly adapting generator potentials can occur is longer than for rapidly adapting ones for a stimulus of the same duration.

CODING

At one time the nervous system was thought to be a syncytium, a continuous, interconnected, multinucleated mass of protoplasm. The problem of explaining how information was routed from one place to another was most puzzling in such a system, because any stimulus should in theory be able to set the whole mass alive with impulses—all identical. How could any part of the system operate on its own; how could we tell hearing from smelling, high pitches from low? We now know that nervous systems are composed of individual cells strung together and able to communicate with each other in specific patterns. Even with this "simplification," the problem of how the information contained within a stimulus is signaled to distant parts of the nervous system is formidable.

Any stimulus contains within it certain features that are of interest to the organism. Stimuli have *intensities* or strengths; they have *locations* or sites of application; they have *frequencies* of application; they have *rates* of application; and they have *modalities*. We begin our classification of stimulus features with modality, which, broadly speaking, is a class of sensations that are referred to a single type of receptor. Vision, hearing, touch, smell, and taste are all modalities. However, not every sensation can be associated with a single type of receptor, so the term modality becomes somewhat less precise. For example, in the eye there are receptors for three different spectra of light. Is each color we perceive, from mixing these spectra, a modality?

Some physiologists prefer to define modalities of sensation in terms of the stimuli that produce them. They refer to touch, pressure, and pain as modalities or submodalities of somesthesia with particular reference to the way the skin is stimulated. But, do touch, pressure, and pain represent different forms of stimulation or just different strengths of the same stimulus? With your fingers, lightly grip a fold of skin on your forearm, a stimulus you might consider as touch. A stronger grip yields a sensation of pressure, and an even stronger grip a sensation of pain. Yet the manner of stimulation is the same in all three cases. Taking another example, electrical stimulation of a neuron can lead to the same sensation as a more natural stimulation of the skin. Clearly, electrical energy is not of the same form as mechanical energy, still the quality of the sensation is the same. In our discussion, we use the term modality to mean one of the following: **vision, audition, gustation, olfaction,** and **somesthesia** (including skin, muscle, position, and visceral senses). Any part of one of these modalities is called a **submodality.** For example, gustation, or the sense of taste, has only four submodalities—sweet, salty, sour, and bitter—whereas olfaction, the sense of smell, has a very large number.

How do neurons recognize and encode the features of a stimulus? The term **coding** means simply the representation of the facts about the stimulus (information) in terms of neural activity. Most neurons generate action potentials by which they communicate with each other. These action potentials are essentially the same for all neurons. For the neurophysiologist studying coding, the problem is rather like that of a nation that intercepts a secret code sent by a foreign nation—what does the message say? There are quite a few codes possible using neural activity, many or all of which are used somewhere in the nervous system. For the present, the discussion will concentrate on five classes of neural codes, with some specific examples of how they may be used.

CODE OF SPECIFIC NERVE ENERGIES

Typically, sensory receptors are sensitive to many different kinds of stimulus energy. For instance, receptors in the hand respond to touch, heat, or vibration of the skin; the nerve itself can also respond to mechanical stimulation. Anyone who has ever hit his "funny bone" can attest to this fact. However, every receptor has one form of stimulus energy to which it is most sensitive, and this stimulus form is called the **adequate stimulus.** The eye is excitable most easily by light, although it can also be excited by pressure on the eyeball itself; therefore, for the eye, light is the adequate stimulus. The neurophysiologic term, adequate stimulus, does not refer to stimulus strength, only to a form of energy. It is possible to have a subthreshold adequate stimulus.

Complementary to the principle of the adequate stimulus is a notion formulated by Johannes Müller. Müller noticed that, though the eye is excitable by light, by pressure on the eyeball, by electrical stimulation of the optic nerve, and by some irritative pathologic conditions, the sensation experienced is always one of vision—the person "sees light." The **doctrine of specific nerve energies,** as formulated by Müller, says that, although a sense organ may be sensitive to many forms of stimulus energy other than its adequate stimulus, the sensation evoked is always like that associated with the adequate stimulus, no matter what kind of energy was applied. With electrical stimulation of the optic nerve, the sensation evoked is one of seeing light, not one of an electrical shock. The doctrine of specific nerve energies implies that the modality or submodality of a sensation is determined not by the stimulus, but by what specific receptor or nerve fiber is stimulated. The doctrine also implies that the subjective qualities of a modality are determined, not in the receptors themselves, but in the central nervous system.

An extension of the doctrine of specific nerve energies is the concept of **labeled lines.** The concept of labeled lines says that information from a particular receptor travels over particular pathways to particular parts of the nervous system. Thus, the modality of a sensation depends upon which particular cell, pathway, nucleus, or lobe is activated by the stimulus. The concept of labeled lines receives some support from the fact that stimulation of the spinothalamic tract in man causes pain or from the observation that stimulation of the visual cortex leads only to a perception of light in a place within the visual world that depends upon where the visual cortex is stimulated.

The concept of labeled lines implies that between the receptor on the periphery and the place in the central nervous system where the sensation occurs, there is no interaction between the modalities or submodalities. This does not seem to be true. For example, in the cuneate nucleus, a major relay in the somatosensory system, there is interaction between activity arising from hair receptors and activity arising from touch receptors. In addition, there is interaction here between cutaneous, auditory, and visual activity. The nature of this interaction is just beginning to be explored. It is true, however, that some structures within the central nervous system do appear to be associated with particular modalities of sensation.

Even if a specific pathway or labeled line underlies the subjective quality of a sensation, a given neural pathway must use more than one code if other stimulus features are to be signaled. Although any activity in the pathway would evoke an experience of a specific quality or modality, the intensity of the sensation is usually coded within the activity itself.

RATE OR FREQUENCY CODES

One way of coding intensity is in terms of discharge rate. Many mechanoreceptors use modulation of their discharge rates, that is, the number of impulses generated per second, to code the intensity of a mechanical stimulus. Figure 4-8 illustrates a rate code for the amount of displacement of the surface of a Merkel's disc mechanoreceptor found in the hairy skin of cats and on the abdomens of humans. In this experiment, a probe was applied to the dome-shaped surface of the receptor, as shown in A. The probe was pushed down, indenting the surface a certain distance, and held there while recordings were made from the sensory nerve fiber supplying the receptor. A typical recording is shown in B. The upper trace illustrates the movement of the probe, whereas the lower trace is an actual recording of the fiber's discharge. The average frequency of discharge was measured during the time when the displacement was held (the plateau) for a number of different displacement distances, and the results were plotted in the graph of Figure 4-8C. Notice that the fiber codes an increase in displacement by increasing its discharge rate, F, in a linear fashion. The equation defining this relationship is $F = 0.55D +$

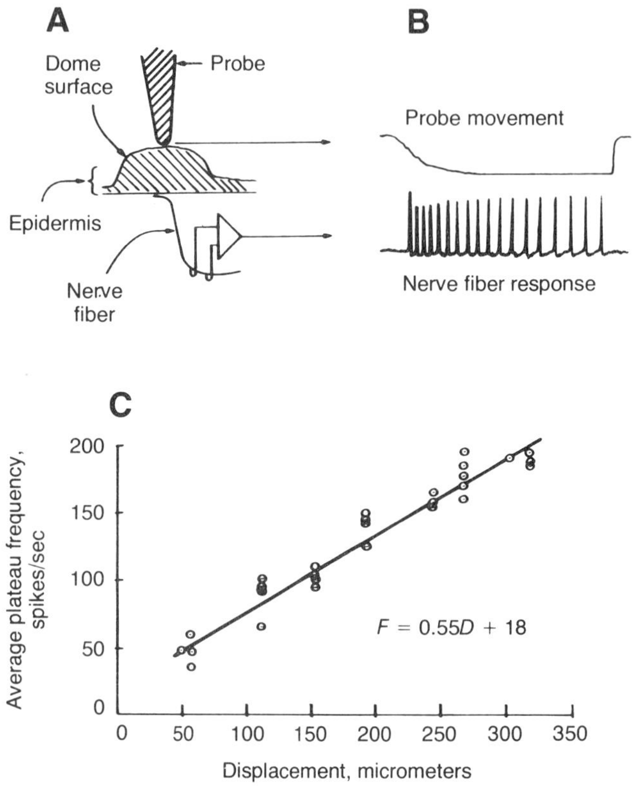

FIG. 4-8. An example of a frequency code. **A.** The physical setup of the experiment illustrates how the probe is positioned over the receptor structure and how the discharges of the nerve fiber are recorded. **B.** A typical response from the fiber (indicated below) to a prolonged displacement (indicated above) of the receptor surface (downward deflection of the trace indicates a downward movement of the probe). Entire record is 40 msec in duration. **C.** A plot of the frequency of discharge of the fiber against the amount of displacement of the receptor. Notice that the amount of displacement is coded as a linear function of the frequency of discharge. (Data from Tapper DN: Trans NY Acad Sci 26:697–701, 1964)

18, where F is the rate of discharge in spikes/sec and D is the displacement in micrometers. Knowing this relationship, we can derive the amount of displacement the receptor must have experienced from the frequency of discharge of its nerve fiber. Presumably the nervous system can do this, too.

INTERVAL CODE

Most neurons generate impulses or action potentials, but they spend most of their time in the resting condition. Even a neuron that is generating impulses at a rate of 50/sec spends most of its time resting. This can be seen in Figure 4-9. If an action potential lasts 0.5 msec, as shown in A (some action potentials are shorter and some are longer), and repeats at a rate of 50/sec, as shown in B, the neuron is silent for 97.5% of the time. Interestingly, one of the possible codes of neural activity is based on this silent time.

For vibrating stimuli, it is possible to encode the frequency of the stimulus in a linear fashion with one impulse for each stimulus, as a frequency code, or with one impulse for every two or more vibrations of the stimulus, as an interval code. Coding of vibratory frequency is perhaps the most trivial example of a possible interval code and, at the same time, the least different from a frequency code. When the stimulus is not periodic, the interval code is more obvious. It is possible that in some cells, such as pyramidal tract cells, a particular short interval between action potentials, in a train where the other intervals are much longer, may signal the start of some move-

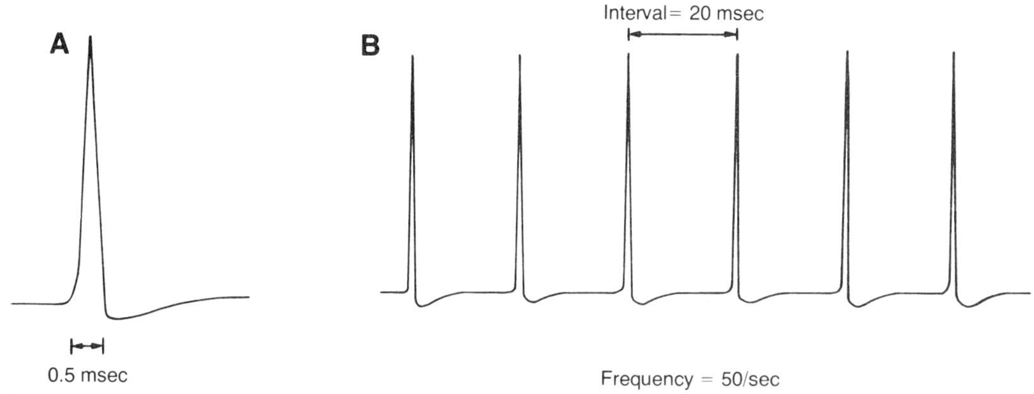

FIG. 4-9. A. The duration of a single nerve impulse. **B.** The interval between impulses in a train of nerve impulses at 50/sec.

FIG. 4-10. An example of a pattern code. Four different taste receptors: Each responds to each of 4 substances of different tastes. None *by itself* signals the substance applied, but by looking at the pattern of discharge in all 4 receptors it is possible to deduce what the substance was.

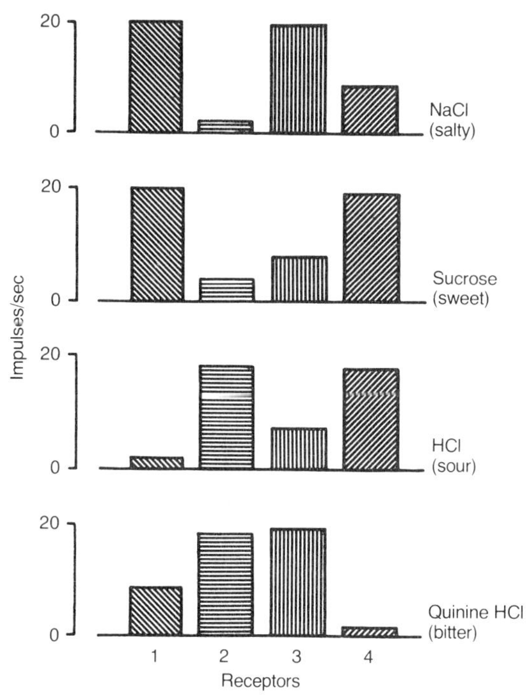

ments. We will examine this in more detail later. Briefly, however, this phenomenon is related to a special event called facilitation that occurs in certain postsynaptic cells only when two presynaptic action potentials arrive at short intervals.

NEURON PATTERN OR ENSEMBLE CODES

In some cases, one neuron may not be capable of signaling all the features of a stimulus that we can sense. In these cases, the stimulus features may be signaled by activity in populations of neurons and decoded by comparison, addition, or subtraction of their activity. It is the ensemble of cells that carries the information about the particular sensation. An example of a possible pattern or ensemble code is the coding of the submodalities of taste: sweet, sour, salty, and bitter. Every gustatory receptor responds to substances of all four qualities. The responses of four such receptors are shown in Figure 4-10.

Each column of the figure represents the responses of a single taste receptor to four different solutions, one from each submodality. The height of the bar indicates the magnitude of the response that particular receptor gave when the particular solution was poured over it. Looking at the response of only one receptor, it is impossible to tell what the stimulus was. For example, receptor 1 responds equally to salty and sweet and thus cannot distinguish between the two. By comparing the responses of the four cells, it is possible to detect which stimulus was presented. Salty corresponds to large discharges from receptors 1 and 3, sweet to large discharges from receptors 1 and 4, and so on. There is a unique pattern of discharge across the group of receptors for each different quality, even though no one receptor can signal a given quality uniquely; obviously, there are more than four taste receptors, but a similar principle could be applied to a much larger set of receptors.

NONIMPULSE CODES

To this point, we have considered codes involving the generation of propagated action potentials. Why do nervous systems use action potentials to communicate information? Would it not be easier to communicate increasing stimulus intensity with increasing amplitude of a voltage? The answer to both of these questions is simple. Voltages are attenuated drastically in a very short distance in volume conductors. Where long distances must be traversed it is imperative to use a brief, self-regenerating potential change that stays the same size all along the fiber. Coding can then be accomplished by modulating the frequency of discharge.

However, some cells in the nervous system do not generate action potentials at all. In these cases, the distances traversed are only fractions of micrometers, and reduction of potential at a distance is no problem. For example, in the eye, information must pass through a minimum of two cells before any action potentials are generated. All of the information in the optic nerve discharges must also be encoded in the depolarizations and hyperpolarizations of the receptor cells and bipolar cells.

Any time the potential across the membrane of a cell changes there is a current flow generated in the extracellular space. These currents are large enough in the cerebral cortex to be recordable on the scalp as the **electroencephalogram** or **EEG.** Small amounts of these extracellular currents can penetrate other nearby cells, altering their membrane potentials and thus their excitabilities. This kind of interaction can sometimes be quite powerful. We presume that this is another manner in which information can be coded and transferred, but as yet there is no proof that this is so.

SUGGESTED READING

Aidley DJ: The Physiology of Excitable Cells. Cambridge, Cambridge Univ. Press, 1971

Loewenstein WR [ed]: Principles of Receptor Physiology. Handbook of Sensory Physiology, Vol. I. Berlin, Springer-Verlag, 1971

Mountcastle VB: Sensory receptors and neural coding: introduction to sensory processes. In Mountcastle VB [ed]: Medical Physiology, 13th ed, Vol. 1. St. Louis, Mosby, 1974

Rushton WAH: Peripheral coding in the nervous system. In Rosenblith WA [ed]: Sensory Communications. Cambridge MA, MIT Press, 1961

Zimmermann, M: Neurophysiology of sensory systems. In Schmidt RF [ed]: Fundamentals of Sensory Physiology. New York, Springer-Verlag, 1978

5

Somesthesia: Peripheral Mechanisms

The broadest definition of somesthesia is the awareness of having a body and the ability to sense the contact it has with its surroundings. Our concerns at this point are about the receptors that serve to make us conscious of our bodies. Receptors are generally put into two broad classes: the **exteroceptors,** which sense stimuli from outside the body and signal what is going on in the outside world, and the **enteroceptors,** which receive stimuli from inside the body and tell us what is going on in the inside world. The broad class of exteroceptors includes, in addition to receptors in the skin, receptors for light in the eye, sound in the ear, and for chemical substances in the nasal mucosa and tongue. These specialized receptors are discussed in future chapters; for now, we will concentrate on the skin.

THE EXTEROCEPTORS

The skin serves many functions: (1) as protection from injury and dehydration, (2) as a radiation surface and regulator in temperature maintenance, (3) in secretion of chemical substances, such as pheromones that function as attractants or repellants, (4) as camouflage due to coloration in some species, and (5) in reception of mechanical, thermal and, to some extent, chemical stimulation. From our present point of view, we may think of the skin as a sheet of sensory receptors held together and supported by a network of connective tissue and blood vessels. Figure 5-1 shows a cross section through a transitional region between glabrous and hairy skin. The outer layer or epidermis is composed of four to five layers of cells and connective tissue and is devoid of blood vessels. The epidermis receives its nutrients from the dermis immediately beneath it. The dermis consists mainly of loose connective tissue. Nerve fibers course into the skin through the dermis, and many of them end at the dermal–epidermal border where many of the sensory receptor structures are located. Figure 5-1 shows several of the types of receptors that are typical of skin. Structure A is a typical hair follicle—note that all hairs are innervated and thus serve as sensory receptors. The nerve fibers associated with a hair enter the follicle and follow a wandering course up and down along the root sheath and also around it. This winding pattern of the nerve fiber may determine how the receptor responds to hair movement, but as yet we do not know how. In addition to hair follicles, there are many encapsulated nerve endings found at the dermal–epidermal border. These are endings surrounded by specialized structures; a few of the types are shown in the figure (B-F). These structures vary somewhat in form so that it is not always clear in which class a particular structure belongs. The largest class of receptors is that with no specialized structure at all, the free nerve endings (G). Near their termination, the nerve fibers simply branch many times, and the many tiny terminal "twigs" lie in the dermis, near the border between the dermis and epidermis, or sometimes penetrate into the epidermis itself.

Many attempts have been made to associate different receptor structures with particular sensations, but there appears to be

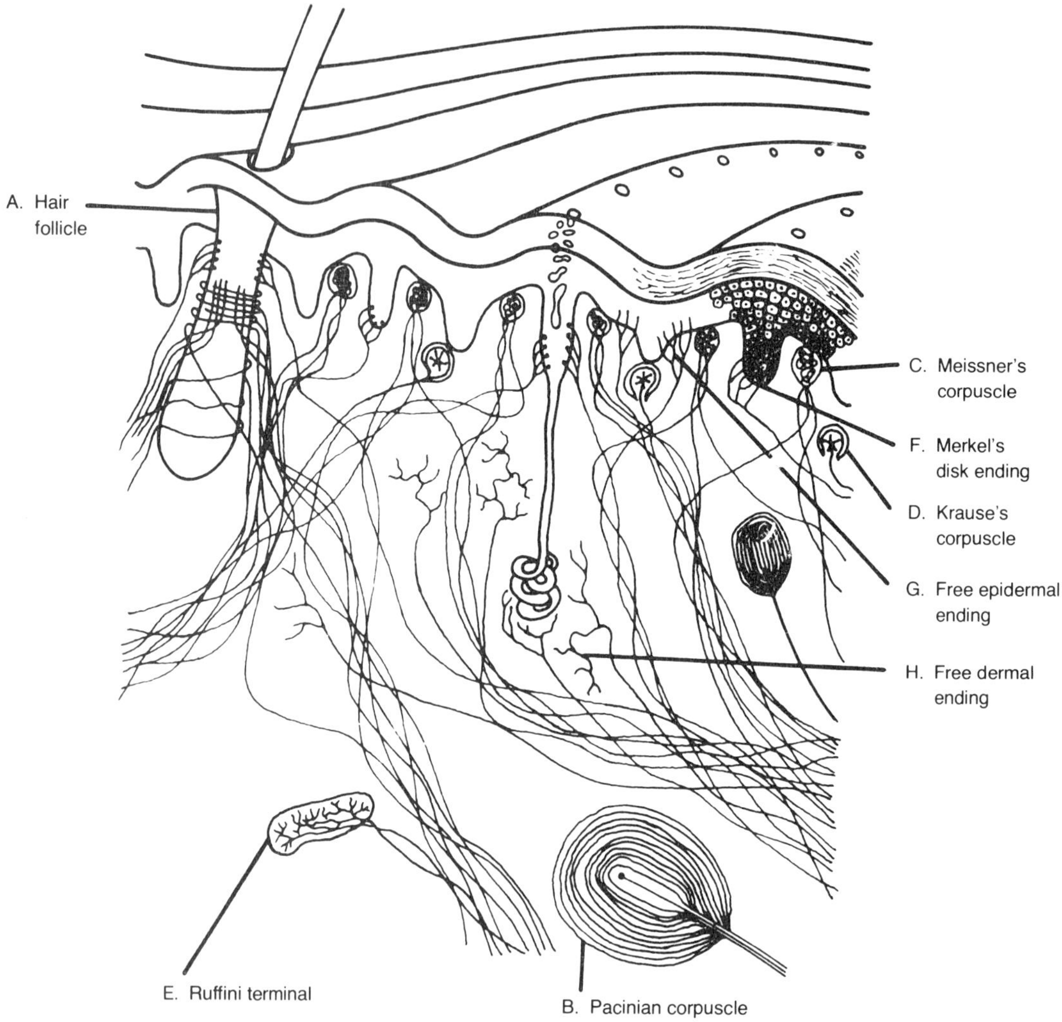

FIG. 5-1. A section through a transitional region between glabrous and hairy skin showing the locations and arrangements of various dermal and epidermal receptors. (Warwick R, Williams PL [ed]: Gray's Anatomy, 35th ed. Philadelphia, WB Saunders, 1973)

no clear relationship between structure and sensation. One problem is that the sensations associated with skin are surprisingly complex. Nearly everyone allows that there are (1) mechanical sensations, (2) thermal sensations, and (3) nociceptive or pain sensations, but only some will divide mechanical sensations into touch, pressure, and pinch, whereas others maintain that the list should also include vibration, tickle, itch, and perhaps even others. Clearly, we may have more describable sensations than we have receptor types to account for them.

The problem is further compounded if we realize that we experience all of the normal skin sensations on the pinna or auricle, the external part of the ear, yet the pinna probably has only free nerve endings. The cornea of the eye can sense temperature and pain, but has only free nerve endings. Although there is not a one-to-one relationship between receptor structure and sensation, that is not to say that there is no relationship at all. Free nerve endings are usually associated with the sensations of pain, temperature, and what many call **crude touch,** a sensation that requires firm pressure to elicit and is difficult to localize. The encapsulated endings are associated with light touch and pressure when they lie

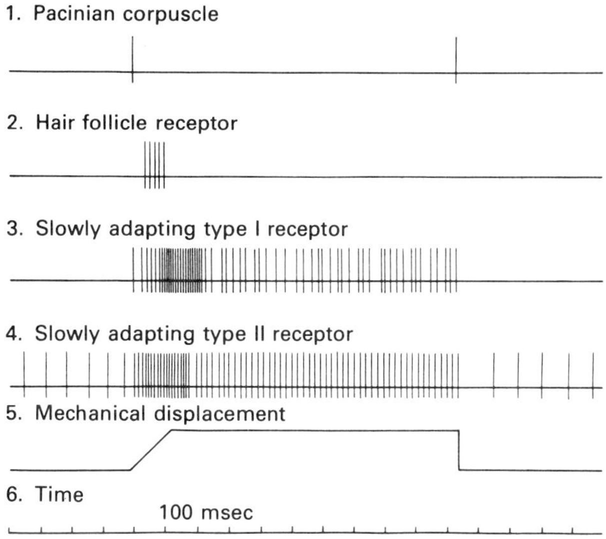

FIG. 5-2. Responses of cutaneous primary afferent fibers. A mechanical indentation or displacement was applied to four different types of receptors, the monitor of the movement being shown in trace **5**. The action potential responses of two rapidly adapting fibers are shown in traces **1** and **2**: They respond only at the onset or offset of the stimulus. Responses of the two slowly adapting fibers are shown in traces **3** and **4**: They discharge throughout the stimulus. A 100-msec time base is shown in trace **6**.

superficially within the skin and with deep pressure and tissue deformation when they lie deep within the tissue. Hair receptors, of course, can be associated with a class of sensations that accompany hair movement; these sensations have no special terminology.

MECHANICAL SENSATIONS

If recordings are made from the sensory nerve fibers innervating particular cutaneous receptors, the stimuli that best excite each type of receptor, the adequate stimuli, can be identified. Examples of recordings from four different fibers serving four different kinds of receptors are shown in Figure 5-2. A monitor of the mechanical displacement of the structure is shown in trace 5—the probe indented the receptors in traces 1, 3, and 4, and pushed the hair laterally in trace 2. Traces 1 to 4 show the spike discharges recorded from the fibers, the **primary afferent fibers.** The bottom trace is a time scale. The discharge pattern of the Pacinian corpuscle should already be familiar. The fiber discharges when the receptor is compressed and again when the receptor is restored to its resting state—the discharge is rapidly adapting or phasic. The same kind of discharge pattern is seen in recordings from hair afferent fibers when the hair (trace 2) is displaced. The hair receptors are all rapidly adapting, that is, they are incapable of signaling sustained stimulation. On the other hand, the slowly adapting receptors, types I and II,* can signal the presence of a sustained stimulus. They begin discharging with the indentation and continue to discharge until the stimulus is removed. The type I receptor is a Merkel's disc receptor, whereas the type II is associated with a Ruffini ending.

There are a number of characteristics of a mechanical stimulus that are distinguished by physiologists, about which the central nervous system might need to be informed. First, there is simple stimulus detection—is there a stimulus present or is there not? All of the receptors just listed are exquisitely sensitive to mechanical stimuli, requiring displacements of only a few to tens of micrometers to excite them. Some require the

* This is an unfortunate terminology, but for the present we are stuck with it. Do not confuse type I and type II cutaneous primary afferent fibers with group I and group II afferent fibers from muscle and skin, to be discussed in Chapter 11.

stimulus actually to contact the skin, for example, type I and type II and Pacinian corpuscles, and some do not, such as hair receptors. The latter class may serve a distance receptor function, allowing stimuli to be detected before they contact the skin.

Every mechanical stimulus causes a displacement of a receptor when it excites one—hairs are moved, skin is indented—and it might be of some value to know by how much the receptor was displaced. A receptor must discharge when the stimulus is stationary, that is, when the receptor is being held at a constant displacement, in order to signal the magnitude of the displacement. Clearly, Pacinian corpuscles and hair receptors cannot signal displacement magnitude because they discharge only when the stimulus is actually moving. That is not to say that the displacement cannot be derived from their discharge. As we shall see, the hair receptors are good detectors of stimulus velocity; all that is required is a relatively accurate internal clock to derive the displacement from the velocity: velocity = displacement/time, or displacement = velocity × time. However, displacement magnitude information is not directly encoded in their discharge. An example of a receptor that does signal displacement is shown in Figure 4-8. The responses shown are for a type I slowly adapting receptor; type II slowly adapting receptors also signal displacement magnitude.

It might also be useful to know the velocity of a mechanical stimulus. To signal velocity, a receptor must either increase or decrease its rate of discharge with increases in stimulus velocity. An example of this behavior is shown for a Meissner's corpuscle in glabrous skin in Figure 5-3 where receptor discharge frequency is plotted on the ordinate against indentation velocity on the abscissa. The relationship between these two variables is clearly nonlinear, although the velocity of the stimulus is encoded in the discharge frequency. Hair receptors also encode the velocity of hair displacement by increasing frequency with increasing velocity. It is normally assumed that a receptor that signals displacement magnitude cannot also signal velocity; however, there is no evidence to support this assumption. Slowly adapting receptors, both types I and II, encode displacement velocity in their discharge frequency, and they must be considered as candidates for velocity receptors.

Another feature of a stimulus that might be detected is its frequency of application. Regular, periodically recurring stimuli induce a sensation of vibration. The Pacinian corpuscle discharges one spike for each displacement over a broad range of displacements and velocities and cannot supply information about either displacement magnitude or velocity. However, it discharges an action potential for each cycle of the vibratory stimulus up to 600 Hz and is normally considered to be a vibration receptor. Again, receptors that encode other features of the stimulus are considered not to be receptors for vibration, but most cutaneous receptors are capable of responding to vibratory stimuli at frequencies of 500 to 600 Hz at least for a short time (Burgess, Petit, Warren, 1968). Human vibration perception is clearly within the ability of these receptors.

Pressure receptors should signal stimulus pressure in their discharge frequency. An example of a receptor that does this is shown in Figure 5-4. This slowly adapting receptor clearly signals increasing force of the stimulus applied to it by increasing its discharge frequency. The increasing force will result in increased displacement as well, and it is not known whether any receptor signals force or displacement independently. Types I and II slowly adapting receptors are capable of signaling pressure as well as the duration of a mechanical stimulus.

In summary, there are obviously candidate receptors to signal stimulus presence, displacement, velocity, force, frequency, and duration. At this point, we can only say that the central nervous system receives this information from particular receptors; we cannot say that the nervous system actually uses the information. There have been a number of attempts to correlate psychophysical measurements in humans with the discharges of particular receptors. Initially, the receptor behavior was studied in animals, but more recently the behavior of human receptors has been observed. Two examples of the results of these experiments are shown in Figure 5-5. In A are shown nerve discharge frequencies and detection thresholds for indentations of the distal phalanx of the thumb. Filled circles indicate

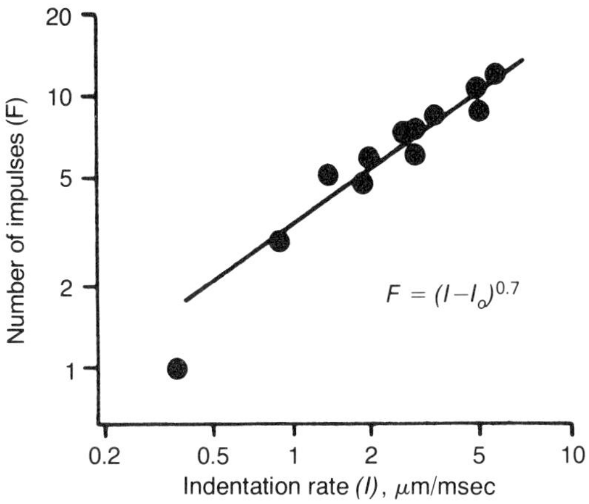

FIG. 5-3. Response of a velocity detector. The relationship between rate of indentation (abscissa) and number of impulses evoked per stimulus (ordinate) in a double logarithmic plot is shown. The threshold stimulus, 1.6 μm/msec, has been subtracted from abscissa values. To find actual stimulus velocity add 1.6 to values on the abscissa. (Schmidt RF: Somatovisceral sensibility. In Schmidt RF [ed]: Fundamentals of Sensory Physiology. New York, Springer-Verlag, 1978)

FIG. 5-4. Response of a pressure receptor to various constant-force stimuli. The relationship between stimulus force (abscissa) and discharge frequency (ordinate) at 1, 5, and 30 sec after the beginning of a 40-sec duration stimulus. Threshold stimulus values at each time during the maintained stimulus were subtracted from applied intensities. Each point is the average of 10 measurements. (Schmidt RF: Somatovisceral sensibility. In Schmidt RF [ed]: Fundamentals of Sensory Physiology. New York, Springer-Verlag, 1978)

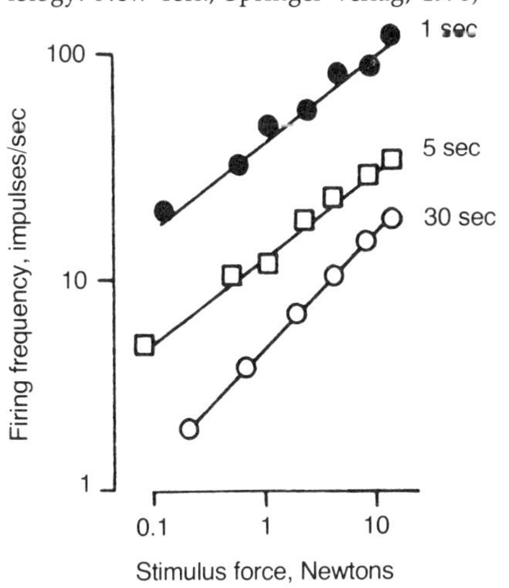

FIG. 5-5. Neural and perceptual thresholds for the same test point on the skin. The stimuli were delivered to a point on the skin that yielded the lowest threshold response from an axon associated with rapidly adapting receptors. The amount of indentation (abscissa) is plotted against the percent of the stimulus presentations in which the stimulus was detected and against the percent of the stimulus presentations in which the axon discharged (ordinate). Data are shown for a stimulus point on the distal phalanx of the thumb (**A**) and a point on the palm of the hand (**B**). Neural data are indicated by **open circles,** perceptual data, by **filled circles.** (Vallbo AB, Johansson R: Skin mechanoreceptors in the human hand: Neural and psychophysical thresholds. In Zotterman Y [ed]: Sensory Functions of the Skin in Primates, with Special Reference to Man. Oxford, Pergamon Press, 1976)

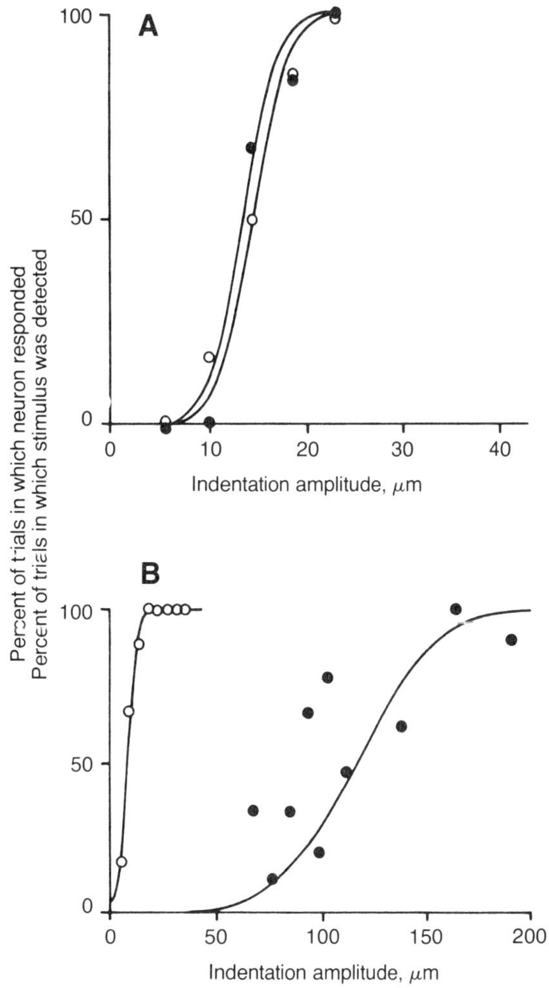

the percentage of the presentations of indentations of a given amplitude in which the stimulus was detected, whereas open circles indicate the percentage of indentations at that amplitude that evoked a discharge from the receptors. There is clearly a close coherence between these two plots, but such a close fit is not always found. The thresholds for similar receptors on the palm of the hand are considerably lower than detection thresholds at the same sites (Fig.

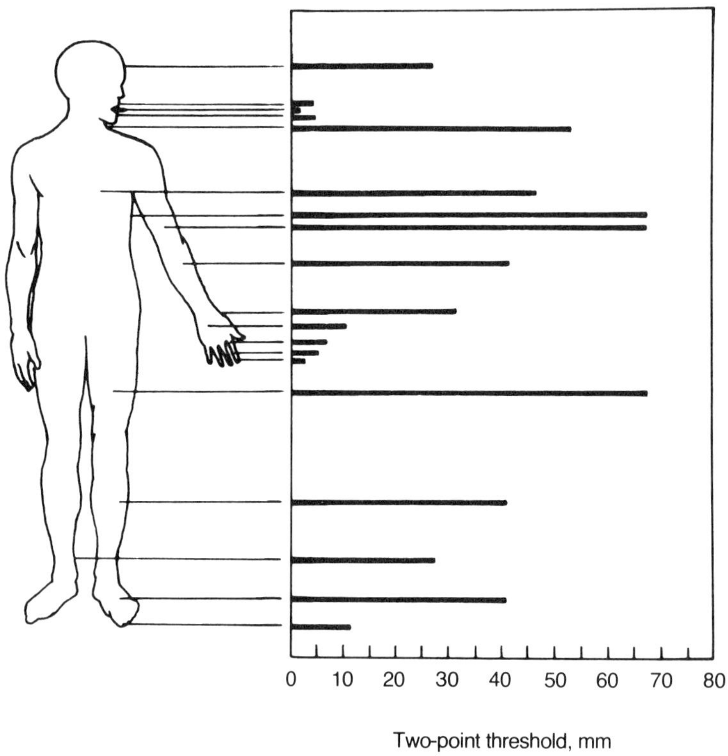

FIG. 5-6. Distribution of two-point thresholds over the surface of the body. The threshold is plotted as the distance between two points that just yields a sensation of two points instead of one. (Ruch TC: Somatic Sensation. In Ruch TC, Patton HD [eds]: Physiology and Biophysics, 19th ed. Philadelphia, WB Saunders, 1965)

5-5B). These data are typical of the results in experiments to date. Sometimes there is a close correlation between psychophysical results and neural results and sometimes there is not. Even when there is a close correlation, we cannot be sure there is a causal relationship, that is, that the neural discharge causes the sensation.

The area of skin over which the application of a stimulus excites a given primary afferent fiber is called the **receptive field** of that fiber. As far as we know, a primary afferent neuron only innervates one particular type of receptor, though it may innervate a number of individual receptors of that type. For example, a hair afferent neuron may innervate anywhere from a few to 100 hairs and a given hair may receive innervation from 2 to 20 different fibers. Thus, there is considerable overlap in the receptive fields of different fibers. The size of a receptive field varies over the body surface, with those located on the extremities being the smallest, of the order of a few square millimeters on the digits, growing in size along the leg or arm, and reaching a maximum size on the trunk. This arrangement might account, in part, for the observed distribution in **two-point thresholds,** a commonly used measure of touch sensitivity. Two-point thresholds can be tested by using an ordinary pair of dividers. When the closed dividers are touched to the skin, the perception is of being touched with only one point. As the dividers are opened more and more on successive applications to the skin, a separation of the points is reached at which the perception is of being touched with two points. The separation at which this first happens is the two-point threshold. Plotted in Figure 5-6 are the two-point thresholds in millimeters on the abscissa against the position on the body on the ordinate. The distribution is very much like the distribution of receptive field sizes described previously. A moment's reflection will show why this should be so. In order for two sensations to be evoked, the stimuli must activate at least two primary afferent fibers. At minimum two-point distances,

TABLE 5-1. SENSITIVE SPOTS PER SQUARE CENTIMETER*

	TOUCH†	PAIN	COLD	WARMTH
Ball of thumb	120	60		
Tip of nose	100	44	13	1.0
Forehead	50	184	8	0.6
Chest	29	196	9	0.3
Volar side of forearm	15	203	6	0.4
Back of hand	14	188	7	0.5

* Data from Woodworth RS, Schlosberg H: Experimental Psychology. New York, Holt, Rinehart and Winston, 1965

† Arranged in descending touch-spot density.

FIG. 5-7. Psychophysical intensity function for the perception of temperature of the palmar surface of the hand, as a function of the actual skin temperature after 30 minutes adaptation. Estimates of temperature **(left ordinate)** and relative intensity estimates **(right ordinate)** are plotted against actual temperature **(abscissa).** Average values for 18 subjects. (Hensel H: Correlations of neural activity and thermal sensation in man. In Zotterman Y [ed]: Sensory Functions of the Skin in Primates, with Special Reference to Man. Oxford, Pergamon Press, 1976)

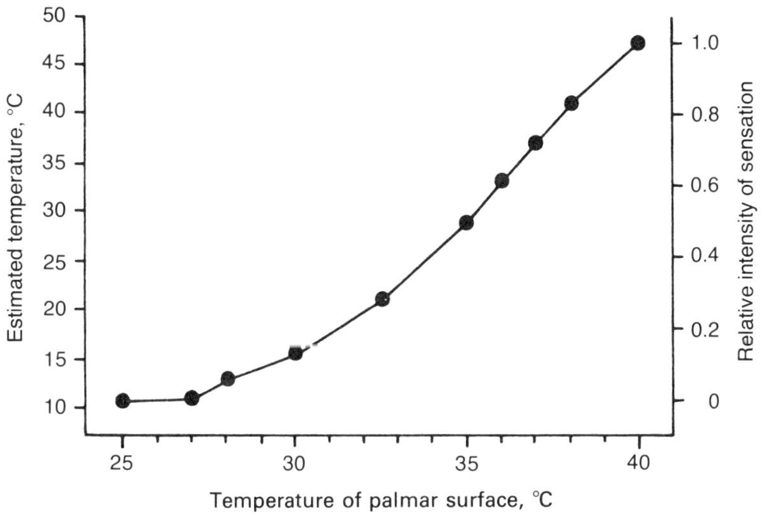

this is more likely in areas of skin with smaller receptive fields than in areas with larger ones.

Receptors are discrete structures embedded in or residing just under the skin. Although in some regions the density of receptors is high, there are always areas in which there are no receptors. Because of their extreme sensitivity to mechanical stimulation and the spread of mechanical disturbances over the skin, receptors may nevertheless appear to be distributed continuously. Table 5-1 shows the density of touch, pain, and temperature spots (presumably these correspond to receptor locations) in various regions of the skin. The data have been arranged in descending order of touch-spot density. On the glabrous surface of the hand and the nose, touch spots are very dense; in hairy skin, the density is much lower.

TEMPERATURE SENSATIONS

Because of the high touch receptor density in some areas, touch sensitivity sometimes appears to be uniformly distributed. In contrast, temperature sensitivity is always

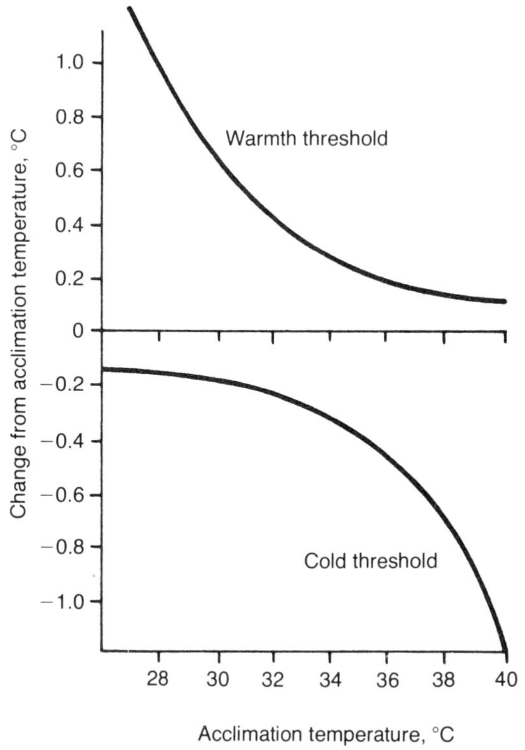

FIG. 5-8. The dependence of thresholds for sensations of warmth and cold upon the initial temperature of the skin. The skin was brought to one of the temperatures on the abscissa and held there for some time. Then the temperature was either raised or lowered until a sensation of warmth or cold was reported, and the threshold value was plotted on the ordinate as either an increase or decrease from the initial temperature expressed in degrees centigrade. Two curves were generated, one for warmth thresholds and one for cold thresholds. Values presented are accurate for temperature changes in excess of 6°C/min. (Kenshalo DR: Correlations of temperature sensitivity in man and monkey: a first approximation. In Zotterman Y [ed]: Sensory Functions of the Skin of Primates, with Special Reference to Man. Oxford, Pergamon Press, 1976)

FIG. 5-9. The response of a single warm fiber to gradual warming of the skin in its receptive field. A monitor of the local temperature of the skin is shown in the lower trace whereas the spike discharge is shown in the upper trace. (Redrawn from Hensel H: Pflugers Arch 313:150–152, 1969)

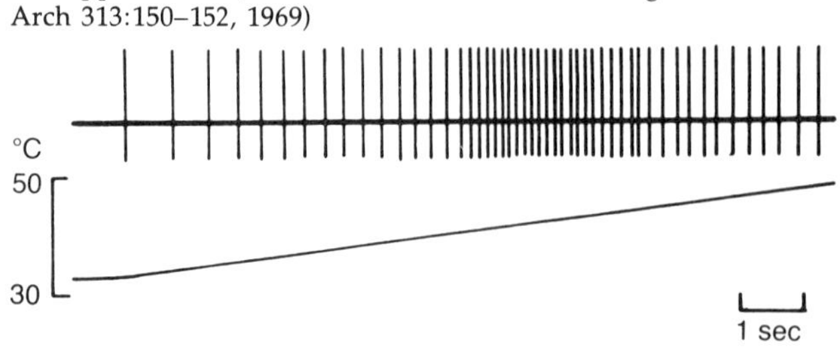

punctate or localized to small spots on the skin. We speak of "warm spots" and "cold spots" on the skin that are areas sensitive to upward and downward changes in skin temperature, surrounded by areas of virtual insensitivity to changes in temperature. The low density of temperature-sensitive spots is indicated in Table 5-1. At no place is the density of temperature spots as high as is the lowest touch-spot density. Note also the low density of warm spots compared to cold spots.

In estimating skin temperature, people are quite accurate in the region of normal body temperature, 37 to 38°C, but they consistently overestimate higher temperatures and underestimate lower temperatures. This can be seen in the graph of Figure 5-7 of estimates of the temperature of the palm of the hand. The inaccuracy is extreme at low temperatures; people estimated the temperature to be 10°C when it was actually 25°C. When the temperature of the skin is changed rapidly, the sensation evoked depends not only on the amount and direction of change, but also upon the temperature from which it is changed, the acclimation temperature. This is illustrated in Figure 5-8 where acclimation temperature is plotted on the abscissa against the change in temperature on the ordinate. Starting at a temperature on the abscissa to which the skin has been adapted for some time, the skin temperature had to be changed by the number of degrees on the ordinate to elicit a sensation of either warmth or cold. Thus, starting at 28°C, the temperature has to be raised by about 1°C (reading upward from 0 to the heavy curve then across to the ordinate) to elicit a sensation of warmth or lowered by 0.15°C to elicit a sensation of cold (reading downward from 0 to the heavy curve then across to the ordinate). On the other hand, if the acclimation temperature is 38°C, the skin must only be warmed by about 0.1°C to elicit a sense of warmth, but it must be cooled by more than 0.6°C to elicit a sense of cold. To convince yourself that these observations are accurate, try the following experiment: Fill three bowls with water: one lukewarm, one cold, and one warm. Put the left hand in cold water, the right in warm water and then place both in the lukewarm water. A clear sensation of warmth will occur in the left hand and a sensation of cold in the right. An important conclusion from Figure 5-8 is that the same temperature can feel either warm or cold depending upon stimulus conditions, that is, the acclimation temperature.

If recordings are made from single primary afferent fibers, it is possible to identify **warm fibers,** which increase their frequency of discharge when the skin is warmed, and **cold fibers,** which increase their discharge frequency when the skin is cooled. The response of a single warm fiber is shown in Figure 5-9. Warm fibers are slowly adapting; they fire continuously at constant temperature. A monitor of the skin temperature at the bottom of the figure shows the temperature gradually increasing from 32°C to 50°C. As the temperature increases from 32°C to 44.5°C, the discharge frequency of the warm receptor increases, but further increases in temperature cause the discharge

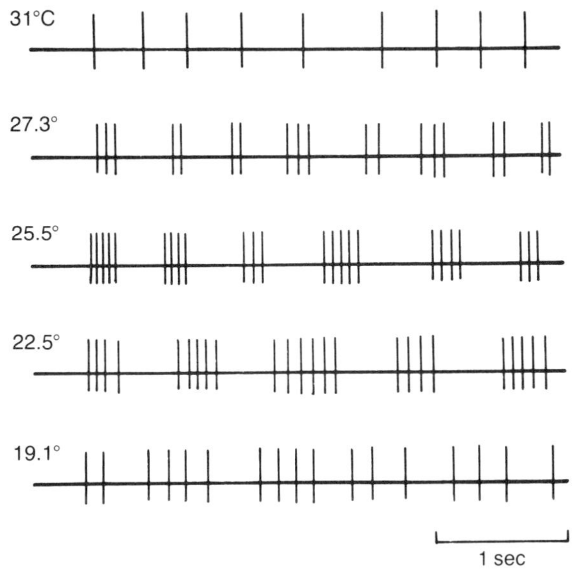

FIG. 5-11. The response of a single cold fiber to 5 different temperatures. At 31°C the fiber fires more or less continuously, fires in bursts in the range from 27.3 to 22.5°C, and then fires more or less continuously at lower temperatures. (Iggo A, Iggo BJ: J Physiol (Paris) 63:287–290, 1971)

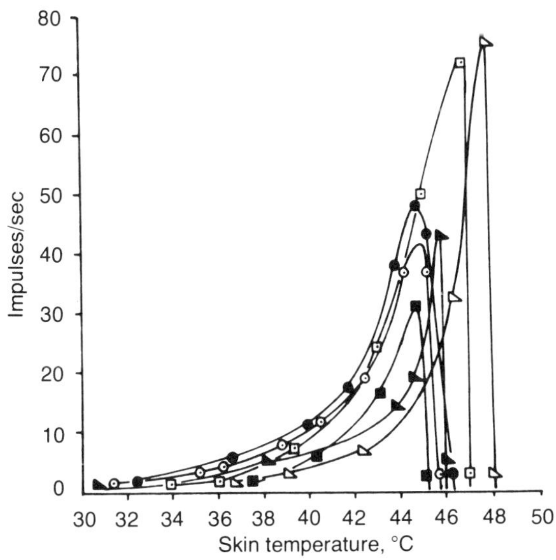

FIG. 5-10. Plots of the responses of six warm fibers. The frequency of discharge of each fiber (to a series of temperatures as in Fig. 5-9) is plotted against the temperature. Note that all curves reach a peak in the region from 44.5°C to 47.5°C. (Hensel H, Kenshalo DR: J Physiol (Lond) 204:99–112, 1969)

frequency to fall. This means that there is only one temperature that is uniquely signaled by the discharge frequency of the fiber, namely, 44.5°C, at which point the discharge frequency is maximum. Two temperatures—one above and one below 44.5°C—are signaled by every lower discharge frequency. Most people are able to detect changes in temperature as small as 0.08°C. The problem for the nervous system is to figure out what the skin temperature is by looking at the discharges of temperature receptors. One possible solution to the problem is to have different fibers, each with its own "best temperature," the temperature that yields the highest rate of discharge, but with best temperatures of the population of fibers distributed across the whole range of temperatures. This would be a pattern or ensemble code. Unfortunately, the system does not seem to be built that way. Figure 5-10 shows the frequency responses of a number of warm fibers. Most of them have about the same "best temperature," namely, 44.5°C. How they signal the changes in temperature to account for our ability to discriminate changes in temperature remains a mystery, but it seems likely that the manner of coding must be in terms

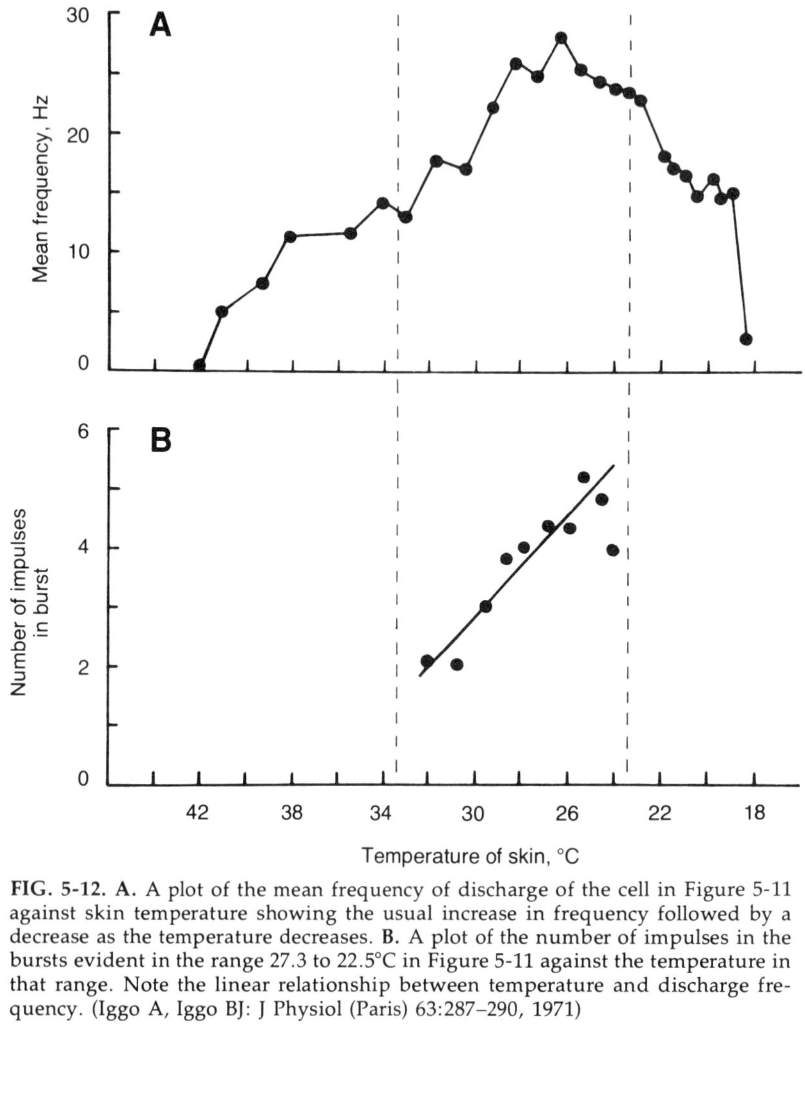

FIG. 5-12. A. A plot of the mean frequency of discharge of the cell in Figure 5-11 against skin temperature showing the usual increase in frequency followed by a decrease as the temperature decreases. **B.** A plot of the number of impulses in the bursts evident in the range 27.3 to 22.5°C in Figure 5-11 against the temperature in that range. Note the linear relationship between temperature and discharge frequency. (Iggo A, Iggo BJ: J Physiol (Paris) 63:287–290, 1971)

of the pattern of activity across a number of fibers. The threshold temperature for pain receptors that are sensitive to noxious heating is about 44 to 46°C. That means they are beginning to discharge (presumably signaling pain) at the temperature at which the response rate of warm receptors is beginning to fall off from its maximum (Fig. 5-10). The temperature range from 38 to 44°C could be distinguished by the central nervous system from that above 44°C by sensing the discharge of thermal pain fibers that would be zero in the former case but not in the latter.

How cold sensations are coded by cold fibers may be easier to understand. Figure 5-11 shows the discharge of a single cold fiber at several temperatures. As the temperature is lowered from 31°C to 27.3°C, the discharge changes from a more-or-less continuous stream of impulses to a series of bursts. Also, as the temperature reaches 19.1°C, the fiber again returns to a more-or-less continuous discharge. If the average frequency of discharge is computed and plotted against temperature, the curve in Figure 5-12A results. It resembles the bell-shaped curve of warm fibers, yielding the same ambiguity for temperature determination. If, on the other hand, the number of impulses in a burst is plotted against temperature, as in Figure 5-12B, an approximately linear relationship results with no ambiguity over the range in which the bursts occur. However, this is only a part of the range over which temperature is sensed and discriminated by humans. It may be that other such cold fibers respond in different parts of the temperature range so that the entire range is covered by the aggregate of cold fibers.

PAIN SENSATIONS

Almost everyone experiences pain: it is hard to ignore and demands our attention. It is the most frequent complaint that the neurologist, in fact, any physician hears. We all know what the word pain means and yet describing pain to someone else is nearly impossible, because it is a highly personal experience. The experience of pain is influenced by prior experience; by the meaning of the situation in which it occurs; by attention, anxiety, and suggestion; and by the sensory adaptation level of the individual.

Prior experience with a stimulus can cause that stimulus to be perceived as either more or less painful, depending upon the nature of the experience. Painful stimulation, repeated in a psychologic trauma-producing situation, may tend to make similar stimulation in the future more painful, whereas painful stimulation, repeated in otherwise pleasant surroundings, may tend to make future stimulation less painful. Parental attitudes about pain and painful stimulation have a big influence on our responses to noxious stimuli. To some extent, these attitudes are determined by our culture; some cultures do not experience pain in certain situations where most others do. In some cultures, women do not experience pain during childbirth; in some cultures, the husbands experience pain during childbirth. There are also many examples of cultures in which people undergo, during religious ceremonies, treatments we would find excruciating, but they do not experience any pain, at least in the ceremonial context.

In some situations, especially emotional ones, a stimulus that would normally be perceived as painful does not evoke pain. For example, football players, during football games, and soldiers, during battle, frequently sustain serious injuries that, if they occurred in another situation, would be extremely painful, but in this situation they are not accompanied by pain.

Similarly, a person anticipating a painful stimulus or anxious about his situation will normally perceive a stimulus as more painful than he would if he did not anticipate the stimulus. For example, a person shown a hot iron, then blindfolded and led to believe he will be touched with the iron, may swear he has been burned when he has been touched with an icicle. Conversely, a painful stimulus may feel less painful if an innocuous stimulus is anticipated instead.

A person's sensitivity to pain also depends upon his immediately preceding sensory experiences. For example, people who live in cold climates are acutely aware that, after spending time outdoors without gloves on cold days, even lukewarm water can "burn" the skin painfully, though no damage is actually being done by the water.

Most people believe that pain is primarily a signal that body tissues are being or have been damaged, and it certainly does have qualities that are consistent with this notion. For example, in many cases, painful sensations are accompanied by a rapid withdrawal of an injured limb from the damaging stimulus. Persons with congenital pain insensitivity frequently injure themselves severely—bad burns, broken bones, appendicitis (unnoticed)—without being aware of it, because they have neither pain sensations nor changes in blood pressure, heart rate, or respiratory rate that accompany them. One of the enigmas of pain is that it can occur without injury and injury can occur without pain. We have already discussed some examples of injury without pain. Spontaneous pain, for example, phantom limb, causalgia or neuralgia pain, can sometimes persist long after damaged tissues have healed and nerves have regenerated.

Most methods of measuring pain treat it as if it were a single unique quality that varies only in intensity—mild versus moderate versus intense. However, pain is a complex category of experiences. Careful observations of pain sensations have shown that all pains are not the same. Pain from the skin is localized accurately, is variable in intensity and duration, but is invariant in quality or tone. No matter how pain is produced in skin, the sensation is always of the same quality, that is, if tests are done properly, the subject cannot say how the pain was produced or whether receptors or nerve fibers were stimulated. Brief stimuli such as hair pull, heating, pin prick, electrical, if applied without associated sensory (but painless) stimuli, all lead to a "pricking" sensation. The sensations only differ if the subject has some other clue, for example, non-noxious movement of nearby hairs, that tells him what the nature of the stimulus was. Prolonged stimuli of sufficient intensity all lead to "burning" sensations even if the stimulus is not heat. Thus, pricking pain is a short-duration pain; burning pain is a cutaneous pain that continues.

Muscle pain, pain from tendon, periosteum and joint, and pain from mucous membranes are all rather diffuse, difficult to locate precisely, continuous, and distinct from cutaneous pain. Muscle pain is indescribable, but disagreeable and inconstant in intensity. Tendon, periosteal, and joint pain are similar in quality to muscle pain, but more constant in intensity. These and muscle pain are often referred to as "aching" pains. The mucous membranes—buccal membranes, conjunctiva, nasal membranes, and glans penis—all are hypersensitive (relative to other tissues) to pain; slight contact or friction can lead to pain of surprising intensity. The quality of this pain also is similar to that of muscle pain.

Some observers have distinguished superficial (cutaneous) from deep (muscle, periosteal, tendon, joint, and mucous membrane) pains. Superficial pain stimuli lead to withdrawal of the limb (for a discussion of the withdrawal reflex, see Chap. 15) or kicking, if applied to the shoulder region. Deep pain stimuli do not. In humans, superficial pain is associated with brisk movements, increased pulse rate, and a sense of invigoration, whereas deep pain is associated with quiessence, decreased pulse rate and blood pressure, sweating, and nausea. Deep pain is sometimes referred to as "sickening," a term never applied to superficial pain. Cutaneous nociceptors are activated by mechanical injury, chemical irritation, ischemia, thermal energy, and certain kinds of electrical stimulation. Deep pain is elicited by ischemia, prolonged muscle contraction, mechanical force, chemical irritation, distension, and spasm.

However, pain is not simply sensation. Some people have even suggested that pain is better classified as a need-state, like hunger, than as a sensation. Clearly, pain has a sensory component and can be induced by noxious stimulation impinging upon receptors. On the other hand, receptors are not required. The existence of **phantom limb pain,** painful sensations referred to an amputated limb, demonstrates this clearly. Peripheral nerves are not required either; central pain mechanisms are clearly able to generate pain after dorsal rhizotomy. Pain also appears to have a memory component that can be triggered by stimulation or triggered spontaneously. In a fascinating experiment, teeth on both sides of a subject's mouth were drilled and filled without local anesthesia. As long as 70 days later, pin pricks of the nasal mucosa led to pain in the filled teeth. This pain was permanently eliminated on one side after recovery from a single injection of novocaine to block the trigeminal nerve on that side, but pain persisted on the unblocked side.

All pain has two psychologic aspects: One is *discriminative,* that is, we can objectively gauge its intensity, location, and quality. The other is *affective* or emotional, that is, pain causes suffering. It is important to distinguish the discriminative aspect from the affective aspect of pain. The importance of this distinction is highlighted by the fact that the two aspects can be dissociated by the proper clinical maneuvers, suggesting that different parts of the nervous system are involved. For example, separation of the prefrontal lobes from the rest of the cerebral cortex in the patient with intractable pain leaves the patient with his pain sensation intact, but the pain no longer bothers him. The suffering is eliminated even though the pain is not. The affective aspect of pain depends upon the integrity of cerebral cortical function; the discriminative aspect does not.

If pain is so complex, can it really be defined at all? Clearly, from what we have discussed so far, the dictionary definition—a more or less localized sensation of discomfort, distress or agony, resulting from stimulation of specialized nerve endings, serving as a protective mechanism insofar as it induces the sufferer to remove or withdraw from the source—is not adequate for clinical pain, where a receptor may not be involved. Another definition—an abstract concept that refers to (1) a personal, private sensation of hurt; (2) a harmful stimulus that signals current or impending tissue damage;

(3) a pattern of responses that operates to protect the organism from harm (Sternbach, 1968)—suggests a bit more of the individual variation, but still links pain inextricably to receptors. Dr. Ronald Melzack has suggested that pain is definable in terms of a multidimensional space that comprises subjective experiences that have both somatosensory and negative-affective components and elicit behavior aimed at stopping the conditions that produce them (Melzack, 1973). This form of definition removes pain from its bond to receptors but still links pain to behaviors that may or may not be directly associated with the sensations. For example, the withdrawal reflex normally occurs with painful stimulation of the foot, but it begins before the pain sensation and, during general anesthesia, occurs in the absence of pain sensation (or in the absence of any pain the patient can later report). In Chapter 15, we shall see that the mechanism of the withdrawal reflex is localized to the spinal cord; higher centers are not required, but the mechanism of pain sensation requires supraspinal structures.

Pain is clearly not a simple phenomenon, and we must keep certain principles in mind in our discussion of it. These principles are as follows:

1. There is *not* a one-to-one relationship between the intensity of noxious stimulation and the intensity of pain it produces.
2. The same injury can produce different pain sensations and responses in different people as a result of cultural variables or prior experience.
3. The same injury can produce different pain sensations and responses in the same person at different times, that is, different times of day (pain sensitivity is lower in the morning than in the afternoon) or different times during the menstrual or other cycle.
4. Psychologic variables can intervene to produce variable pain sensations and responses.
5. Pain perceived varies with the situation in which it occurs and the meaning of the situation for the individual.
6. Pain varies with sensory adaptation levels.
7. Pain refers to a category of complex experiences, not a single one.
8. Clinical pain may not be the same or have the same neurologic mechanism as laboratory or normal pain.

Because pain is so variable, it is not easy to study experimentally, yet some aspects of pain sensation have proved amenable to scientific investigation.

The sensation produced by touching the skin of the hand with a hot iron has three different parts. Shortly after the contact, there are two distinct waves of pain, the first a bright, sharp sensation, then after a short interval of time, a dull, burning sensation. After the second wave, there is a longer interval, up to several seconds in length, during which there is no pain sensation at all. This is followed by a third prolonged period of less intense pain that can be made more severe by warming the skin in the burned area to a degree that would not normally have caused pain. We can account for these waves of pain in terms of the discharges in primary afferent fibers, but first the nature of these fibers should be considered.

The fibers in a peripheral nerve are of different sizes, ranging from less than 1 μm to 22 μm in diameter. A cross section of a nerve is shown in Figure 5-13A, and a distribution of fiber diameters is plotted in Figure 5-13B. The majority of fibers are less than 2 μm in diameter. These fibers are mostly unmyelinated fibers, termed **"C fibers."** There is also a smaller group of fibers with diameters from 1 to 4 μm, termed **A delta** (Aδ) fibers, and another group with diameters of 8 to 22 μm, termed **A alpha** (Aα) and **A beta** (Aβ) fibers. The A-fiber groups consist of myelinated fibers. The threshold of a fiber to externally applied electrical shocks is inversely related to the diameter of that fiber. Accordingly, Aα fibers would have the lowest electrical threshold (require the least current to evoke a discharge), Aδ fibers slightly higher, and C fibers the highest.

It was discovered during stimulation of cutaneous nerves in volunteer medical student subjects that pain was not evoked by shocks to the nerves until the shocks were of sufficient strength to stimulate Aδ fibers. (This strength does not excite C fibers.) It was, therefore, concluded that Aα and Aβ fibers do not signal pain, but that at least some Aδ fibers do. Similarly, stimulation of

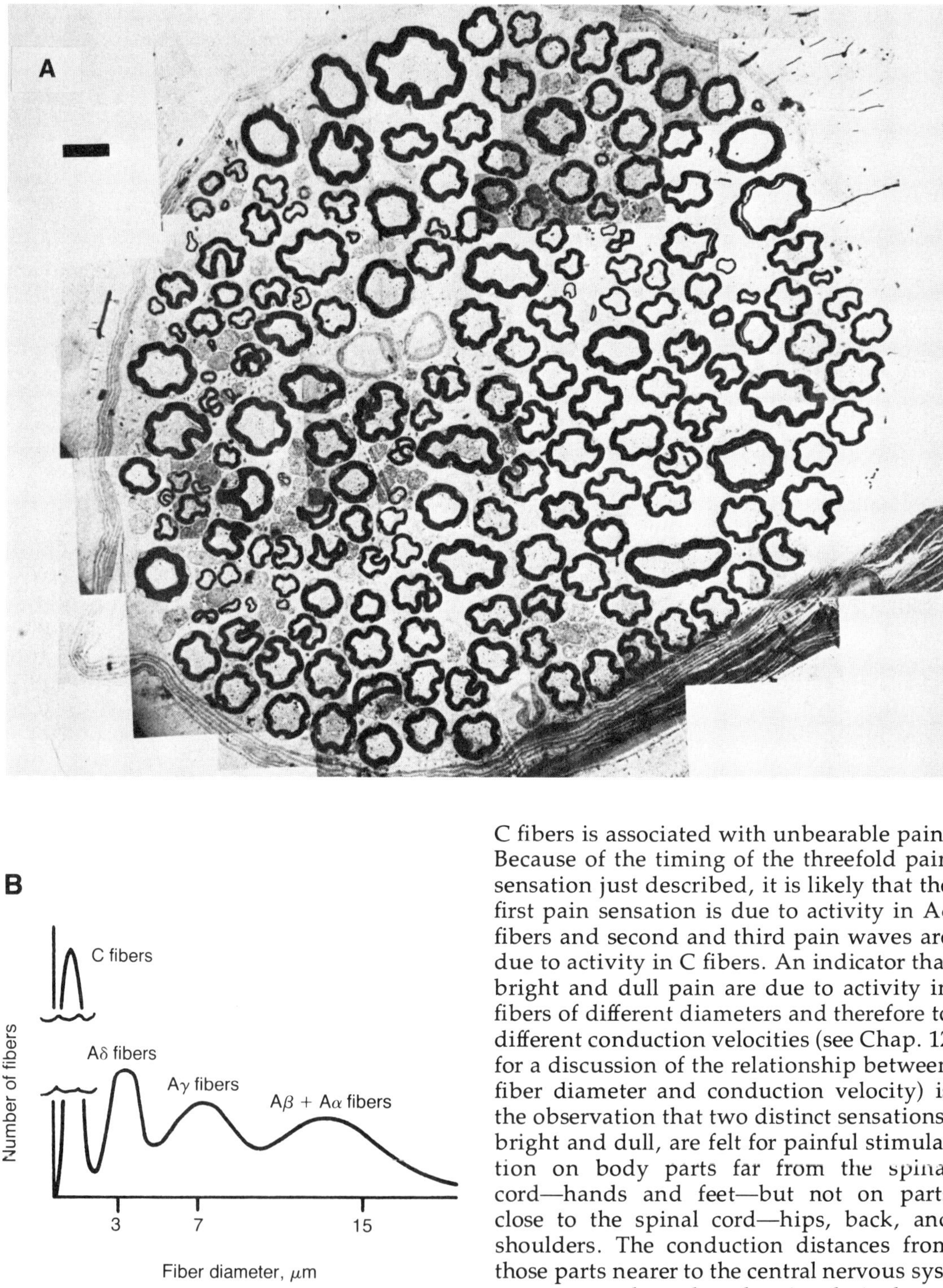

FIG. 5-13. Distribution of fibers within a peripheral nerve. A. A cross section of the posterior articular nerve of the cat showing fibers of different diameters. Calibration: 10 μm. (Courtesy of F. J. Clark). B. A plot of the number of fibers of different diameters in a peripheral nerve. Note the predominance of fibers less than 2 μm in diameter.

C fibers is associated with unbearable pain. Because of the timing of the threefold pain sensation just described, it is likely that the first pain sensation is due to activity in Aδ fibers and second and third pain waves are due to activity in C fibers. An indicator that bright and dull pain are due to activity in fibers of different diameters and therefore to different conduction velocities (see Chap. 12 for a discussion of the relationship between fiber diameter and conduction velocity) is the observation that two distinct sensations, bright and dull, are felt for painful stimulation on body parts far from the spinal cord—hands and feet—but not on parts close to the spinal cord—hips, back, and shoulders. The conduction distances from those parts nearer to the central nervous system are so short that the signals in larger (faster) and smaller (slower) fibers arrive nearly simultaneously, and the sensations therefore fuse into a single one. From farther away, the signals arrive at distinctly different times, and the sensations are separate. When recordings are made from single C fibers during short application of noxious heat, an initial, high-frequency discharge is observed followed by a period of silence. After the period of silence the fibers resume their discharge but at a lower rate than the one observed initially. The rate of discharge in this latter phase is increased by warming the burned area of skin to a temperature that did not influence the cell previous to the burn. It seems that the transmission of pain information is accountable by activity in both Aδ and C fibers.

The study of **nociceptors,** receptors that respond only to stimuli that are strong enough to produce damage and are painful to humans, is a fairly recent development in neurophysiology because these fibers are small and easily damaged during dissection and, as we shall see later, contribute little to whole-nerve recordings, the compound action potentials. These receptors have interesting properties that may have important implications for pain research, but one should be cautious in applying the term "pain receptors" to them. This term implies that activity generated in these nociceptors leads predictably to pain, a fact that is not known. All that is known is that they can detect the existence of a noxious event or environment, that is, that they are nociceptors.

Some nociceptors respond only to painful mechanical stimuli and produce little or no discharge when the skin is damaged by extremes of heat or cold; nor do they respond to acid placed in cuts across the receptive field. The receptive fields of these nociceptors are made up of a number of spots of sensitivity separated by regions of insensitivity. The axons of these nociceptors are small myelinated fibers with diameters in the Aδ range. C fibers with similar properties are rarely found. Another group of Aδ fibers responds to both damaging heat and damaging mechanical stimuli. Among C fibers there are some that respond to damaging stimuli, both mechanical and heat, and others that respond to both damaging mechanical and cold stimuli. The majority of C-fiber nociceptors appear to be of this type, called **polymodal nociceptors** because they respond to more than one type of noxious stimulus.

It is interesting that the topographic distributions of sensitivity to touch–pressure stimuli and pain stimuli are inverse. The thresholds for both pressure and pain are given in Table 5-2. In general, where sensitivity to pain is high, sensitivity to touch is low and *vice versa.* This phenomenon may reflect receptor density to some extent. The rough inverse relationship between touch-spot and pain-spot density is clearly evident in Table 5-1.

TABLE 5-2. PRESSURE AND PAIN THRESHOLDS ON VARIOUS PARTS OF THE BODY*

	PRESSURE† (g/mm^2)	PAIN‡ (g/mm^2)
Tip of finger	3	300
Back of hand	12	100
Calf of leg	16	30
Abdomen	26	15
Back of forearm	33	30

* Data from Woodworth RS, Schlosberg H: Experimental Psychology. New York, Holt, Rinehart and Winston, 1965

† Tested with a human hair.

‡ Tested with a needle.

THE ENTEROCEPTORS

JOINT SENSATIONS

Though joints differ in the range and direction of their movements, most have an enclosed cavity filled with synovial fluid and are surrounded by cartilage. Free nerve endings are abundant in the articular cartilage and nearly everywhere around the joint. In addition, there are spray-like endings in the joint capsule and encapsulated corpuscles both on and in the capsule. Free nerve endings arise from both myelinated and unmyelinated fibers in the articular nerves, whereas spray-like endings and corpuscles arise from myelinated fibers only.

Originally, it was thought that the sense of the position of the joint, that is, the angle between the bones of the joint, was signaled by the myelinated fibers of the articular nerve leaving that joint. However, studies indicate that most of these fibers do not, in fact, signal the static position of the limb. This is because they fail to discharge at any position but the extremes of flexion and extension. In addition, anesthetizing the human knee joint does not diminish position sense for that joint. It appears that the most likely candidate for signaling joint angle would be the muscle spindle receptors or group Ia or II afferent fibers (these are discussed in detail in Chap. 11).

The receptors of the joint may be signaling that the joint is undergoing or about to undergo some undue stress or strain, thus serving a role in protection of the joint itself, not in body orientation. The majority of the fibers serving the joint are small-diameter myelinated and C fibers whose functions are unknown at present, but it is unlikely that they signal joint angle, because their very slow conduction velocities would cause long time delays in our ability to sense changes in joint angle. Such delays do not occur.

OTHER SUBCUTANEOUS RECEPTORS

The Pacinian corpuscle is a rapidly adapting mechanoreceptor. Its distribution in the mesentery, joint capsule, connective tissues, and at pressure points on the palmar and plantar surfaces of the extremities suggests that it may have a number of roles.

In the carotid bodies, aortic bodies, and along the arteries and perhaps veins are receptors that play a role in the control of respiration. These receptors sense the amount of oxygen and CO_2 in the blood and the *p*H of the blood, and trigger reflex changes in respiration volume and rate. In the carotid body, special receptor cells, innervated by the carotid branch of the glossopharyngeal nerve, increase their frequency of discharge in response to a decrease in blood *p*H of 0.1, a decrease in blood O_2 saturation of 4%, and increases in blood CO_2 concentration.

Near the carotid body is a structure called the carotid sinus. In the carotid sinus and also in the aortic arch are mechanoreceptors that sense blood pressure. These receptors increase their discharge rate with increases in blood pressure and decrease their discharge rate in response to decreases in blood pressure. The impulses from these receptors flow into the medullary region of the nervous system and modulate or initiate changes in heart rate and contractility and in the diameter of blood vessels that result in compensatory changes in blood pressure.

There are receptors in the heart that sense the volume of blood in the various chambers, and there are receptors in the lungs to signal the amount of inflation. Evidence exists that there are receptors in the hypothalamus that sense the temperature and osmolality of the blood and perhaps also the concentration of glucose in the blood. There are undoubtedly receptors in various parts of the body, including the brain, that can sense the circulating levels of hormones in the blood. A complete description of these kinds of receptors is beyond the scope of this discussion.

SUGGESTED READING

Burgess PR, Perl ER: Cutaneous mechanoreceptors and nociceptors. In Iggo A [ed]: Handbuch Sensory Physiology II, pp. 25–32. Heidelberg, Springer-Verlag, 1972

Burgess PR, Petit D, Warren RM: Receptor types in cat hairy skin supplied by myelinated fibers. J Neurophysiol 31:833–848, 1968

Clark FJ, Burgess PR: Slowly adapting receptors in cat knee joint: Can they signal joint angle? J Neurophysiol 38:1448–1463, 1975

Iggo A, Young DW: Cutaneous thermoreceptors and thermal nociceptors. In Kornhuber HH [ed]: The Somatosensory System, pp. 1–22. Acton, MA, Publishing Sciences Group, Inc., 1971

Melzack R: The Puzzle of Pain. New York, Basic Books, 1973

Sternbach RA: Pain. A Psychophysiological Analysis. New York, Academic Press, 1968

Wall PD: On the relation of injury to pain. Pain 6:253–264, 1979

Zotterman Y [ed]: Sensory Function of Skin in Primates, with Special Reference to Man. Oxford, Pergamon Press, 1976

6

Somesthesia: Central Mechanisms

In this chapter, we examine the pathways that somatic activity can take in the central nervous system and then consider the mechanisms by which different sensations can occur.

SOMATOSENSORY PATHWAYS

Once the primary afferent fibers leave the skin, they group together into larger and larger bundles in the cutaneous nerves. At some point in their course they are joined by **muscle nerves,** containing sensory and motor fibers of the muscles. Nerves that innervate the skin are termed **cutaneous nerves** and those that contain both skin and muscle fibers are termed mixed nerves. The sciatic is an example of a mixed nerve. Nerve fibers that carry impulses to the CNS are called **afferent;** those that carry them from the CNS are **efferent.** Near the spinal cord, the afferent and efferent fibers separate again; the efferent fibers go to the ventral roots, and the afferent fibers, after passing their cell bodies in the dorsal root ganglia, enter through the dorsal roots. This separation of afferent fibers in the dorsal root and efferent fibers in the ventral root is the so-called **Bell–Magendie law.** Lately, this concept of a rigid separation of dorsal, sensory and ventral, motor fibers has been challenged by findings that, in the cat, up to 30% of the ventral root fibers are sensory. This probably would not have surprised Magendie, who originally stated that *most* fibers in the ventral roots were motor.

The dorsal roots are often divided into two parts, a lateral division consisting mainly of unmyelinated fibers and a medial division consisting mainly of larger, myelinated fibers (Fig. 6-1). Upon entering the spinal cord, some of the afferent fibers bifurcate, with one collateral descending toward the caudal regions of the cord and the other ascending toward the rostral regions. Both myelinated and unmyelinated fibers branch extensively and have terminals near the dorsal root entry zone. The collaterals of the unmyelinated fibers go only a short distance, one or two segments, before terminating in the dorsal horn, but a fiber may put down several collateral branches that terminate in many places in the gray matter. Descending branches of the myelinated fibers generally terminate within one segment from their entry; however, many of the ascending branches can travel uninterrupted for long distances in the dorsal white matter, the dorsal columns, even reaching the lower medullary levels where they terminate in the dorsal column nuclei, the nuclei gracilis (lower limb) and cuneatus (upper limb).

In the dorsal column nuclei, these fibers form connections with cells that live within the nuclei themselves. As illustrated in Figure 6-2, the axons of these second-order neurons immediately cross over to the other side (decussate) of the brain stem, forming a bundle of fibers, called the medial lemniscus. They are soon joined by fibers of the trigeminal system, serving the face, and also by fibers from the spinothalamic tract.

Those fibers that send a branch into the dorsal columns at the segment of entry also send branches down into the gray matter. There they join the branches of other myelinated fibers and unmyelinated fibers to par-

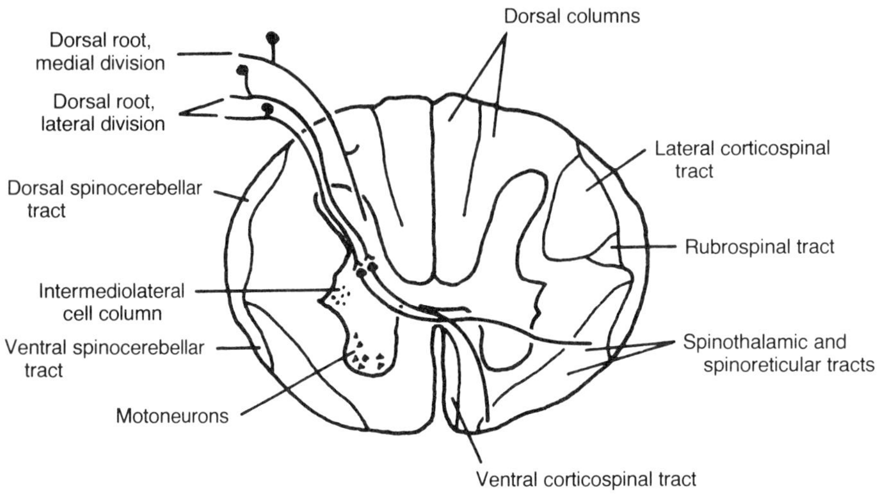

FIG. 6-1. A cross section through the cervical spinal cord showing the entry of the two divisions of the dorsal roots and the routes that fibers take into the major ascending tracts. (Crosby EC, Humphrey T, Lauer EW: Correlative Anatomy of the Nervous System. New York, Macmillan, 1962)

FIG. 6-2. The course and major relay points of the dorsal column system. (Crosby EC, Humphrey T, Lauer EW: Correlative Anatomy of the Nervous System. New York, Macmillan, 1962)

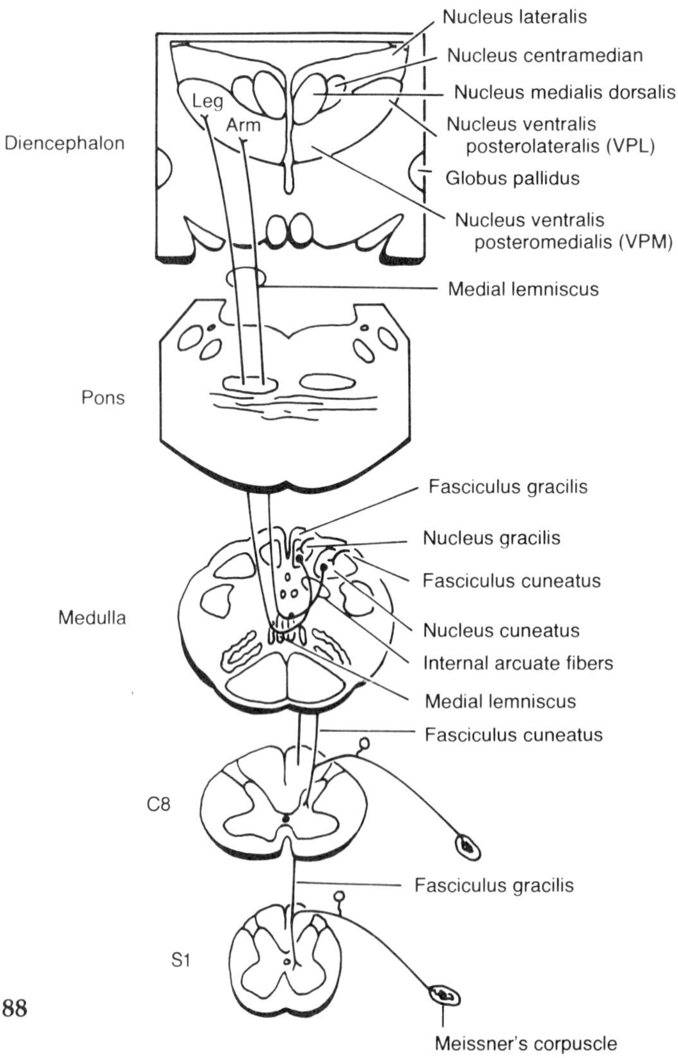

ticipate in reflexes and other spinal cord activities. Some of these fibers cross to the **contralateral** ventral gray columns at or near the segment of entry and establish connections with second-order cells whose axons proceed into the ventrolateral white columns. In this position, they ascend the spinal cord as the spinothalamic tract, until they join the fibers of the already decussated medial lemniscus in the brain stem.

Primary afferent fibers from the region of the face in front of the ears group together into the trigeminal nerve and have their cell bodies in the semilunar ganglion. From the semilunar ganglion the fibers enter the brain stem as a part of the fifth cranial nerve. As in the spinal cord, many of the sensory fibers bifurcate immediately upon entering the brain stem, sending an ascending branch to the main sensory nucleus of the trigeminal and a descending branch to the nucleus of the spinal tract of the trigeminal, a structure analogous to the dorsal aspect of the spinal cord gray matter. Though most of the fibers arising from the second-order neurons of the trigeminal nuclei decussate in the brain stem and soon join the medial lemniscus, a few do not cross, but join the **ipsilateral** medial lemniscus.

The fibers of the medial lemniscus, along with those from the trigeminal nuclei and the spinothalamic tract, proceed directly to the ventral part of the thalamus, contralateral to the primary afferent fibers associated with them. Fibers originating in the main sensory nucleus and the rostral parts of the spinal nucleus of the trigeminal terminate in the nucleus ventralis posteromedialis (VPM) of the thalamus, whereas those of the caudal part of the spinal nucleus terminate in the intralaminar nuclei and the medial geniculate, and a few end in VPM. Fibers originating in the dorsal column nuclei and most fibers of the spinothalamic tract terminate in the nucleus ventralis posterolateralis (VPL) of the thalamus. Some spinothalamic fibers terminate outside of VPL, notably in the medial geniculate body and suprageniculate nucleus.

The third-order fibers arising from the thalamic nuclei can then be traced out through the internal capsule to the somatic cerebral cortex. In man, the primary somesthetic cortex is the region of the postcentral gyrus, the region immediately posterior to the central sulcus, from the Sylvian sulcus to a place within the midsagittal sulcus.

There are other pathways that carry somatic information and other areas of the cortex that receive it, but they play a more subtle and less well understood role in sensation. Consequently, there is less we can say about them.

It has been customary to think of the dorsal column–medial lemniscus pathway as the mediator of touch, pressure, vibratory (**pallesthesia**), and joint position senses. The spinothalamic tract was usually thought to carry information about pain, deep pressure, temperature, and crude touch. The difference between the information in the two pathways was thought to be the sensitivity or threshold (the dorsal columns being more sensitive) and the discriminability of the spatial qualities of the stimulus (the ability to locate the site of stimulus being much greater for the dorsal columns). In the trigeminal system, the caudal part of the spinal nucleus (some people still maintain the whole spinal nucleus) was thought to carry information for pain, temperature, and perhaps also crude touch, whereas the main sensory nucleus was thought to relay information from the face about touch, pressure, and vibration.

There is an increasing body of evidence that has cast doubt on the dichotomy of function of the systems outlined above. Some of the evidence comes from laboratory experiments. When recordings were made of the discharges of single indentified spinothalamic tract cells, it was found that some of them did, in fact, respond to noxious or thermal stimuli, in much the same way as nociceptors or thermoreceptors do (see Chap. 5). In the monkey, these made up 30% of the fibers studied. Other fibers responded to light touch, pressure, or hair movement in much the same manner as do the mechanoreceptive fibers found in the dorsal columns. These made up 40% to 60% of those fibers studied. Most spinothalamic tract fibers (60%) responded to both light tactile stimulation and noxious stimulation (Trevino *et al*, 1974).

Conversely, some dorsal column fibers respond to stimulation that is frankly noxious. These fibers are located primarily deep within the columns and are second-order rather than primary afferent neurons. These second-order neurons make up 10% to 30% of the dorsal column fibers by some estimates and are comprised of fibers that respond to light tactile as well as noxious stimulation (77%), noxious stimulation only (6%), and light tactile stimulation only (17%) (Angaut-Petit, 1975). There appears to be some discrepancy between the responsiveness of single fibers and the roles normally attributed to the tracts that contain them. The same sort of mixture of nociceptive and tactile responses has also been found in the main and spinal trigeminal nuclei. Thus, the supposedly complete segregation of submodalities in the different pathways does not hold up to physiologic testing. Moreover, at least three other major ascending pathways have been shown in animal studies to carry both tactile and nociceptive information.

Finally, cells that could be responsible for signaling the position of a joint, the muscle and perhaps joint receptors, do not form a part of the dorsal column–medial lemniscal system (Clark, 1972). The original data suggesting that the dorsal columns carry joint position information came from patients with tabes dorsalis, a syphilitic infection that causes degeneration of dorsal column fibers, but tabes dorsalis is a dorsal root disease and more than just dorsal column fibers are affected.

Additional evidence that casts doubt on the dorsal column–spinothalamic tract dichotomy comes from the clinical literature. Because the spinothalamic tract and the dorsal columns serving one side of the body are on different sides of the spinal cord and because the dorsal columns are on the dorsal aspect and the spinothalamic tract is on the more ventral aspect of the cord, it is possible to transect one without cutting the other. In some patients with intractable pain, that is, pain that is not diminished by drug treatment or even by cutting the dorsal roots (**dorsal rhizotomy**), the spinothalamic tract was cut (**spinothalamic tractotomy**) at the appropriate level on the side opposite the location of the pain. These patients usually received immediate relief from the pain as predicted, but there were two problems: (1) Pain eventually returned in patients who survived longer than 6 months, and (2) there was a reduction in tactile sensitivity (**hypesthesia**) as well as pain (**hypalgesia**) and temperature sensitivity on the opposite side of the body. These observations, not often made because tractotomies are seldom performed on nonterminal patients, do not exactly fit the dichotomy of function between the two ascending systems. Likewise, surgical lesions of the dorsal columns in animals may result in little or no permanent tactile loss and little analgesic effect. When the dorsolateral columns are included in the lesion, there is a temporary analgesia with gradual recovery of pain sensation. Ventrolateral column lesions (including the spinothalamic tract) are even less effective in producing analgesia. In man, lesions of the dorsal columns produce relief from phantom limb pain, but pain returns in several months. The same is true for various sorts of pain and ventrolateral cordotomy. We will have more to say about this problem later. On the other hand, damage to half of the spinal cord in man leads to ipsilateral paralysis of voluntary (as opposed to reflex) movements, loss or reduction of touch and joint sensation ipsilaterally, and loss of temperature and pain sensation contralaterally, the **Brown-Séquard syndrome.** This is as predicted from the classic notion of dorsal column and spinothalamic tract function, but there are other tracts within half of the spinal cord. At this point, the classic notion of the function of the spinothalamic tract and the dorsal columns is still widely accepted. However, the wise student should expect this notion to be revised before too long and sensory transmission to be attributed to multiple tracts.

DERMATOMES AND SOMATOTOPIC ORGANIZATION

Fibers serving particular areas of skin gather together to form nerves, and the area served by the different cutaneous nerves can actually be mapped. Such a map is shown in lateral parts of Figure 6-3. Each area is the combination of the receptive fields of all the fibers in that nerve, that is, it is the **receptive field** of that nerve. Despite some variation from person to person, the receptive fields of nerves are constant enough in location and extent to be clinically useful.

When a peripheral nerve is cut, the result is an area of complete lack of sensation or anesthesia. The region is called the **autonomous zone** and corresponds to the area in the central part of a nerve's receptive field. Only a part of the total field is anesthetic, as a natural consequence of the overlap of receptive fields of neighboring pe-

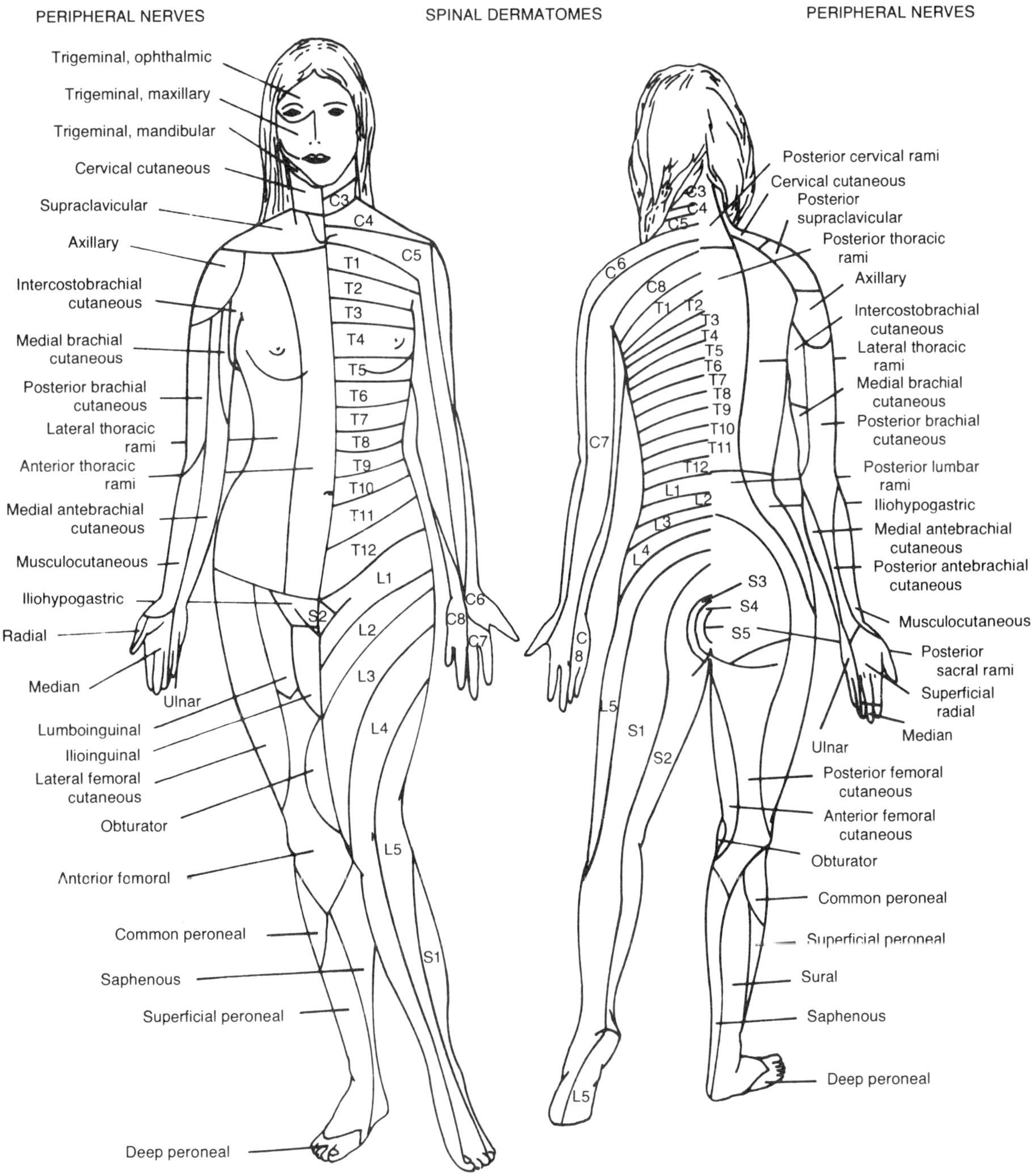

FIG. 6-3. Receptive fields of the peripheral nerves are illustrated on the outside of both views of the figure. Dermatomes of the dorsal roots are illustrated on the inside of both views. Shown are the regions of hypesthesia following nerve or root damage. (Curtis BA, Jacobson S, Marcus EM: An Introduction to the Neurosciences. Philadelphia, WB Saunders, 1972)

ripheral nerves. Surrounding the insentient autonomous zone is an **intermediate zone** in which there is partial sensation. Sometimes the overlap is so extensive that the loss of a small nerve is hardly noticed.

The receptive fields of the fibers in a dorsal root, when combined, also cover a fixed, distinct area, the **dermatome** ("slice of skin"). The dermatome of each dorsal root is illustrated in Figure 6-4. The dermatomal

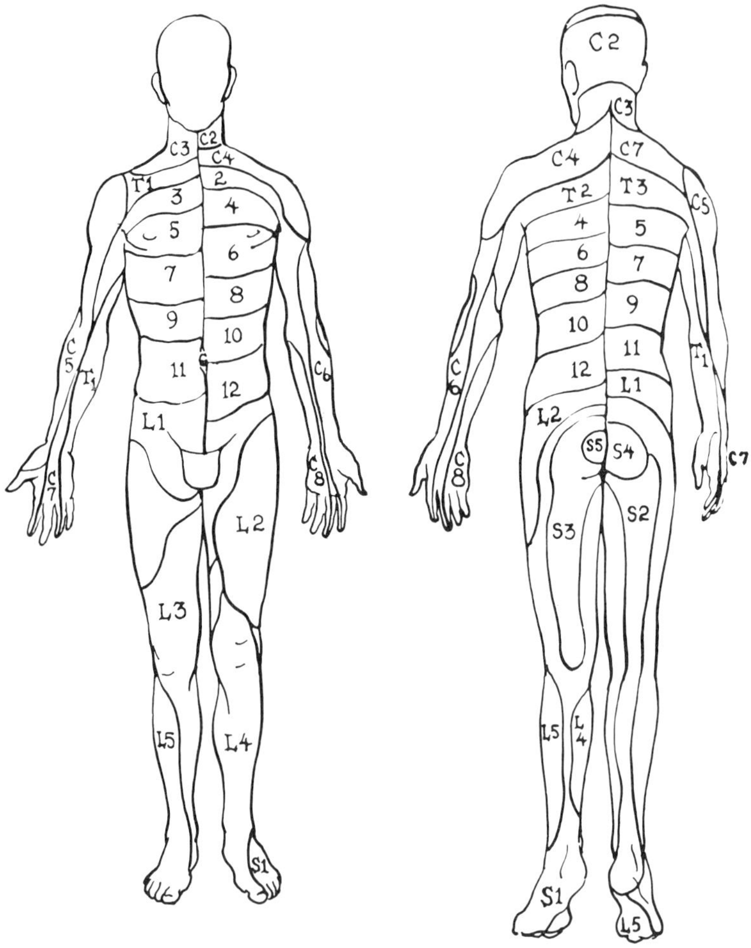

FIG. 6-4. Spinal dermatomes plotted alternately on opposite sides of the body to illustrate the entire extent of the dermatomes. This figure should be compared with Figure 6-3. (Turek SL: Orthopaedics: Principles and Their Application. 3rd ed. Philadelphia, JB Lippincott, 1977)

organization is a constant feature of the nervous system. Dermatomes overlap in the same way that the receptive fields of both nerves and single fibers do. There is, however, a region in each dermatome that is not overlapped by adjacent dermatomes. In the case of a transected root, one should expect to see hypesthesia in the regions indicated in the central part of Figure 6-3. This sort of map is made by tracing areas of hypalgesia following rupture of intervertebral disks. Note that corresponding areas are smaller than the dermatomes of Figure 6-4. Again, the overlap of adjacent dermatomes may be so great that a deficit is hardly noticed unless two or more dermatomes are denervated! This is especially true of thoracic dermatomes for which there is little or no nonoverlapped region.

The nerves serving adjacent areas of skin do not necessarily enter through the same or even adjacent dorsal roots. This is especially true on the limbs and results from the pattern of development of the limb buds. Further information can be found in a textbook of embryology.

Knowledge of the receptive field and dermatomal maps is fundamental in examination of any complaint that involves anesthesia, analgesia, hypesthesia, or hypalgesia over a portion of the body. For example, a patient with anesthesia on the posterior side of the leg, running from over the buttocks down to the most lateral toe probably has a compressed or damaged S1 dorsal root, and a disc problem might be suspected. On the other hand, the patient

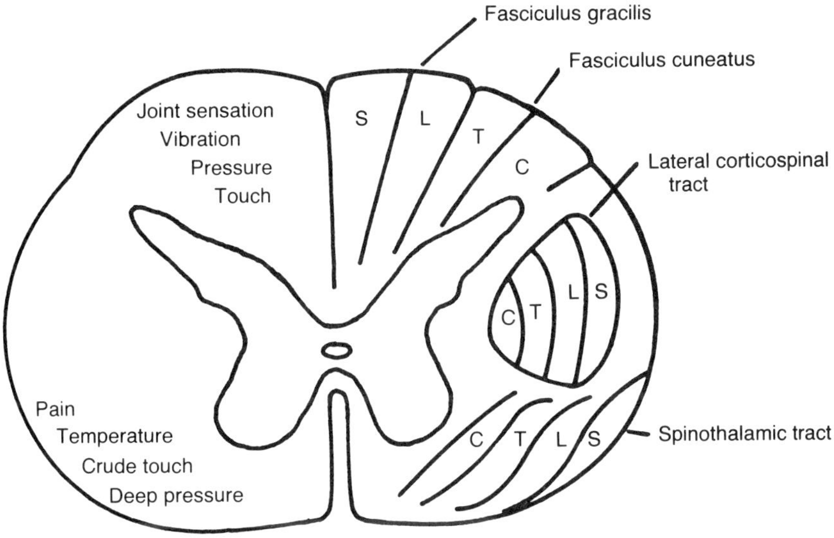

FIG. 6-5. The somatotopic organization of the dorsal columns and the spinothalamic tract and the functions classically attributed to each. (Brodal A: Neurological Anatomy, 2nd ed. New York, Oxford Univ. Press, 1969)

with an analgesia over the middle of the abdomen, in the general region of the rectus abdominis muscle, extending upward to about the region of the clavicle cannot have damaged a dorsal root or even a group of dorsal roots; the damage must be to the anterior thoracic rami. In the first case, you would look for damage somewhere between the dorsal root ganglion and the spinal cord and, in the second case, somewhere peripheral to the ganglion.

Several diseases involving the dorsal root ganglia are conspicuous because of their dermatomal patterns of symptoms. **Tabes dorsalis,** a syphilitic infection of the dorsal root ganglia, often exhibits a dermatomal pattern of hypesthesia because the spirochete shows a preference for larger myelinated fibers. Pain and thermal sensations are normal in the affected area. **Herpes zoster,** a viral infection of the dorsal root ganglia, sometimes called shingles, is characterized by the appearance of a vesicular rash in the dermatome of the affected root.

Knowledge of the dermatomes has other uses besides diagnosing dorsal root damage. In cases of spinal cord transection, the level of section can often be determined by reference to the pattern of sensory loss. The same is true for tumors of the spinal cord that result in a sensory loss. Later we will see that the pattern of motor deficits is equally telling in the neurologic exam. Many times visceral pain is felt to be on the surface of the body (so-called **referred pain**). Often this pain is localized to a dermatome, and knowledge of the dermatomal pattern can lead the alert clinician to the internal organ that is involved.

One of the striking features of the organization of the nervous system is that a picture of the body (though distorted) can be mapped onto the various tracts and nuclei of ascending systems all the way to the cerebral cortex. The tracts are formed so that spatial information from the periphery is preserved in the spatial arrangement of the fibers themselves. This type of organization is called a **somatotopic** representation, referring to the organization by place, "topos," on the body, "soma." The dorsal columns, for example, are formed by the addition of new fibers, at progressively more rostral segments, to the lateral aspect of the columns. This results in an organization such that the dermatomes are laminated, with the sacral segments represented medially and lumbar segments more laterally in the fasciculus gracilis and the thoracic and cervical segments successively more laterally in the fasciculus cuneatus. This organization is illustrated in Figure 6-5.

As a result of this somatotopic organization, it is possible for a spinal cord tumor to disrupt transmission through only the medial fascicles of the dorsal column, producing sensory disturbances in the lower limbs, or through the lateral fascicles, producing sensory disturbances only in the arms. However, it would be extremely unlikely that any lesion of the dorsal columns could produce a sensory disturbance localized to just one dermatome.

The spinothalamic tract likewise appears to be somatotopically organized, but because the fibers are crossed the organization is reversed such that fibers from caudal segments lie laterally, being displaced that way by the progressive addition of fibers to the medial aspect of the tract. (Again, see Figure 6-5.) This is presumably why superficial cuts in spinothalamic tractotomies produce immediate analgesia and **athermesthesia,** that is, the loss of temperature sensation, only in the contralateral lower limb, with graded, more rostral losses resulting from deeper cuts. These deficits are always contralateral to the damage as opposed to the ipsilateral losses due to dorsal column lesions.

It should be mentioned at this point that the somatotopic maps are summary diagrams and should not be taken to indicate that within any marked zone are found only fibers of that type. This is a mistake frequently made. For example, in Figure 6-5, a closed figure surrounds the location of the corticospinal tract; within that figure are found many fibers that are not part of the corticospinal tract. The same warning applies to the somatotopic zones within the dorsal columns or spinothalamic tracts. Within the zone marked for thoracic fibers are found fibers from other levels as well, but the majority appears to be from thoracic segments. This may be one reason why unpredicted effects on sensation are found following controlled tractotomies that do not encroach on the neighboring regions. In any case, these somatotopic maps, whether derived from physiologic or anatomic observations, should be treated as statistical statements only.

The somatotopic arrangement is preserved at higher levels of the nervous system, though the orientation changes. In the dorsal column nuclei, the arrangement found in the dorsal columns is preserved, with lower limbs represented medially and upper limbs laterally. As they course into the medial lemniscus, the fibers of the gracile nucleus take up a ventral position, and those from the cuneate nucleus a dorsal position. Fibers of the spinothalamic tract join the lemniscus, after it decussates, in such a way that they form a cap on the lemniscus, with the leg represented dorsally and the arm ventrally. Addition of fibers from the trigeminal to the most dorsal aspect results in a representation (from top to bottom) of: face, lower limb, upper limb, trunk, and lower limb. In the thalamus, the lower limb fibers terminate laterally and those of the upper limb more medially (the opposite of the spinal cord), with the face represented most medially in VPM. The fibers again cross each other upon leaving the thalamus with the result that the lower limb is represented on the medial aspect of the hemisphere, whereas the representation of the upper limb is more lateral and that of the face most lateral. The resulting organization is illustrated in Figure 6-6. Another representation of the body exists on the cerebral cortex, the so-called somatosensory area II. Its organization is the inverse of that already described for somatosensory area I, namely, face, arm, and leg in that order, going laterally. Area II, however, is not visible on the exposed surface of the human cortex, but is buried in the Sylvian fissure.

This description of the organization of the somatosensory cortex is supported by recordings made directly from the cortex in humans as well as animals. It is possible to open the cranium of an awake human patient under local anesthetics and record from or stimulate the cortex while the patient is awake. This is normally done during surgery to remove a tumor or to treat an epileptic condition. When recordings are made under such conditions, it is usually found that the largest amplitude responses for stimulation of the hand are found on the lateral aspect of the postcentral gyrus, whereas those for stimulation of the leg are on the medial aspects or buried in the midsagittal sulcus. Similarly, if the cortex is stimulated directly, it is possible to elicit sensations *referred to a particular point on the body, not to the cortex itself.* Even though it is the cortex that was stimulated, the feeling is one of being stimulated on the appropriate body part. The particular point of reference depends upon the site of stimulation in the same orderly manner. A detailed map of the human cortex has been made in this way by

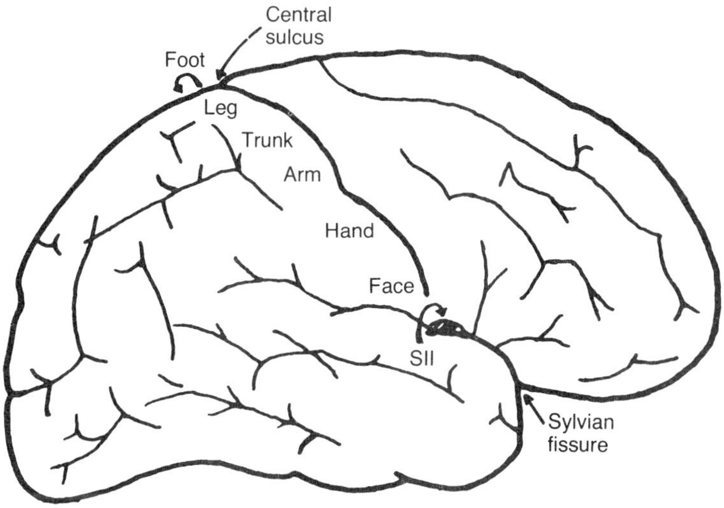

FIG. 6-6. The somatotopic organization of the postcentral gyrus of the cerebral cortex and the position of somatosensory area II.

Dr. Wilder Penfield, the distinguished neurosurgeon. His map is shown in Figure 6-7. It can be seen that the foot is represented on the medial aspect of the hemisphere in the midsagittal sulcus with the leg represented on the medial part of the exposed hemisphere, and the trunk, arm, and hand, more laterally. The face is separate and more lateral yet. The amount of tissue devoted to the hand and face is disproportionately large. This presumably reflects the heightened sensitivity of these parts compared to that of the trunk and legs, as indicated, for example, by the differences in two-point thresholds.

A caution should be introduced in regard to somatotopic maps like that shown in Figure 6-7. In humans, these maps are obtained in two ways. In the first, various sites on the cortical surface are stimulated; where the patient feels a sensation to be is noted; and a mark is made on a photograph of the exposed cortical surface. Not every point on the surface is stimulated in such an experiment; neither is a sensation experienced at every point of the homunculus in every experiment. Rather, it is assumed that if stimulation at two points on the surface of the brain leads to sensations at two points on the body, then stimulation between the points will lead to a sensation localized to the body surface between the two original points. In other words, it is assumed that an intermediate value principle holds for such maps—a fact not known to be true.

The second mapping method involves recording from the cortex while stimulating the skin. Animals cannot indicate the nature or location of any sensations they have, so this is the only method available in animal experiments. It is assumed that the evoked potential (see Chap. 20), recorded from the cortical surface, is an indicator of the occurrence of a sensation (an assumption that is questionable and probably incorrect). Points on the homunculus are then indicated at places where the evoked potential with largest amplitude occurs; the fact that potentials of smaller amplitude are evoked in wide areas of the cortical surface by the same stimulus is ignored. Activity initiated at a point on the body surface converges upon an area of cortex, not upon a point of cortex as the homunculus is usually taken to imply.

That this method of mapping is grossly reliable is indicated by the rough similarity of maps made in different patients and by the similarity of maps made by stimulating the skin and, in different patients, by stimulating the cortex. However, such maps do vary from individual to individual. Some studies (Woolsey, Erickson, Gilson, 1979) clearly show that in some individuals the foot is represented within the midsagittal sulcus whereas in others it is represented laterally on the exposed surface. It is also important to remember that figurine maps are composites from a number of patients,

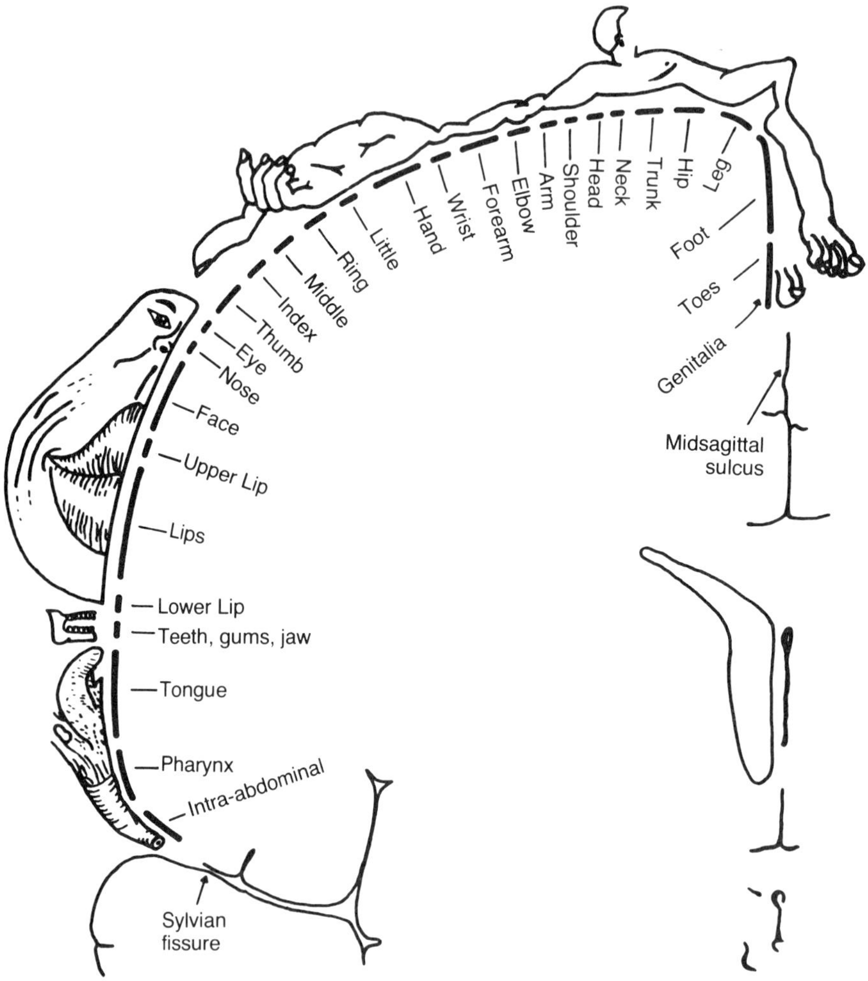

FIG. 6-7. A detailed somatotopic map of the postcentral gyrus. (Penfield W, Rasmussen T: The Cerebral Cortex of Man. New York, Macmillan, 1968)

each of whom was studied only to a limited extent. Thus, the foot may be studied in one patient, the arm in another, and so forth. If there is variability in the position of the representation, then the amount of tissue devoted to a particular area of skin is likely to be overestimated in composite maps.

It should always be kept in mind that these patients are undergoing surgery for an abnormality, tumor, or epileptic focus, in or near the area being studied, and their cortices are not entirely normal. The significance of such maps in understanding cortical organization is also brought into question by the fact that if maps are made using minimum latency of the evoked potential (the time between the stimulus and the beginning of the potential) rather than amplitude as a measure of activity, then a completely different homunculus map is obtained. Who is to say whether latency or amplitude is more important?

CEREBRAL MECHANISMS OF SENSATION

The precise reason for this somatotopic representation in all of the main sensory pathways and nuclei is unknown, though many are of the opinion that it provides the functional and anatomic substrate for coding of spatial localization. Perhaps it does, but perhaps it exists as a mechanical and architectural convenience for a nervous system developing through phylogeny from a simple segmented, metameric pattern.

Many people have the mistaken idea that the cerebral cortex is where the real business of the nervous system is transacted and that the rest of the nervous system is just a conduction pathway to it. This is not the case. For instance, removal of the hand area of the postcentral gyrus does *not* produce anesthesia in the hand. What it does produce is an elevation of the threshold for sensation at the hand, an hypesthesia, and a severe deficit in discriminating the spatial aspects of stimulation, that is, in using sensory information to solve problems. The patient, following such a lesion, has difficulty in pointing to a site on the skin that has been stimulated (**atopognosis**); has difficulty recognizing words written on the skin (**agraphesthesia**); and has difficulty in identifying objects by feeling them (**astereognosis**). The clinical literature contains some studies that indicate that sensory defects following damage to the primary somesthetic cortex are more severe than claimed above and some that indicate that they are less severe. The great variability may be ascribed to a number of factors: (1) Naturally occurring lesions are seldom confined to the primary somesthetic cortex; one would expect the nature of the sensory losses to depend upon the total extent and distribution of damage. (2) The measures of sensory capacity used in different studies vary widely; results may depend upon the test employed. (3) In cases of clinical ablations, the lesions were made in tissue already damaged sufficiently to produce epileptic discharges or already invaded by tumors; the influence of these factors cannot be evaluated. This is especially important when there has been no measure of the sensory capacity of the individual before the surgery. (4) What is usually reported is the location and amount of tissue the surgeon removed, but no information is available about what influence the surgery may have had on surrounding tissues. This influence shows up in cases in which, after unilateral ablation, deficits are seen bilaterally when the patient is compared to normal people (Corkin, Milner, Rasmussen, 1970). Without postmortem examination, there can be no idea how extensive this effect may have been.

The minimum effect of a cortical lesion probably is not a good indicator of the function of the tissue because the minimal lesion probably does not damage the tissue enough. The maximal effect probably represents the function of too many tissues. Therefore, it seems likely that some middle point is at least a good approximation of the deficits caused by removal of this tissue. It really should not surprise us that the cerebral cortex is not required for sensation. Consider how well a frog can sense and act upon stimuli applied to his skin, and he has no cerebral cortex at all.

How can we account for the fact that sensations can be evoked by stimulation of the human somatosensory cortex? Early stimulation experiments resulted in sensations described by the patients as tingling or prickling sensations or a feeling of numbness, and so it was thought not to be possible to evoke "real" sensations, such as touch, by direct stimulation. With improved techniques, such sensations have been evoked, but it is necessary to pass current through the electrodes for about 0.5 sec, a time much longer than that needed simply to excite local neurons. Under these circumstances, identifiable, well-localized sensations have been evoked. Certainly a sensation does not require a cortical neuron to discharge for 500 msec, because for a stimulus to the skin, the stimulus is sensed and a response is executed by a normal person in about 200 msec. One explanation is that the sensation occurs as the result of some event occurring at a distance from the cortical stimulation site and that transmission from the cortex to this element requires the generation of more than one spike in the cortical neuron. Another possible explanation for this discrepancy may lie in the distinction between sensation and perception. It may be that a stimulus can be sensed and acted upon at one level of the nervous system, but only perceived (come into consciousness) if it elicits activity elsewhere. Old ideas about "subliminal perception" would make sense in this context. It is also possible that the somesthetic cortex is not part of the "normal" pathway by which the conscious sensation (perception) is elicited by a stimulus to the skin. The observation that cortical ablations do not eliminate but merely elevate thresholds of sensation begin to make more sense in the light of these considerations.

CENTRAL MECHANISMS OF PAIN SENSATIONS

Stimulation of the surface of the cortex seldom leads to painful sensations. Neither does removal of any portion of the cerebral

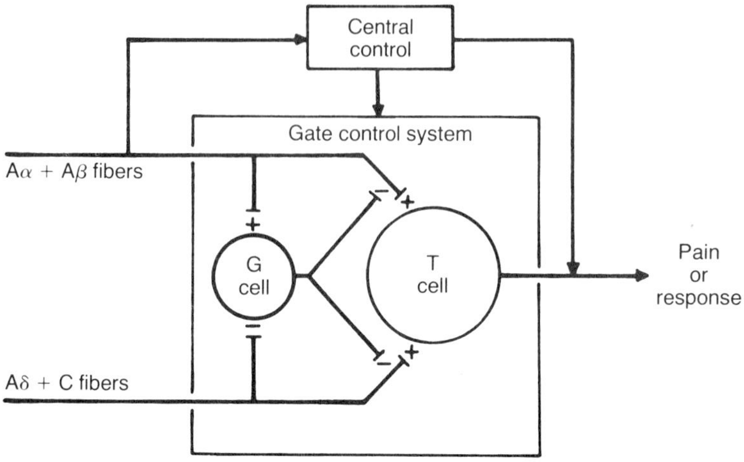

FIG. 6-8. The circuit diagram of the gate-control theory of pain perception as proposed by Melzack and Wall (1965).

cortex eliminate pain sensations; however, this is not to say the cortex plays no role in pain perception. We have already had occasion to point out that removal of the prefrontal lobe, a **prefrontal lobotomy** or **lobectomy,** results in a dissociation between the discriminative and affective aspects of pain. When stuck with a pin, such a patient reports that it hurts, but it does not bother him. There is also the well-known suppression of pain sensations that occurs as an everyday event, but is more prominent during military battles. A person may be wounded seriously and not be aware of it, or he may suppress being aware of it during concentration on some other activity. Whether this sort of suppression is of cerebral cortical origin is unknown, but it could be.

Pain sensations can be elicited by stimulation in some areas of the thalamus. For example, stimulation in the ventral and posterior parts of VPL and VPM in awake patients evokes excruciatingly painful sensations localized to the appropriate area of the body (appropriate according to the thalamic somatotopic organization). Lesions in this area have sometimes proved effective in eliminating, for a short time, certain forms of spontaneous pain such as **causalgias,** burning pain caused by damage of a peripheral nerve, and phantom-limb pain, pain experienced in a limb that has been removed (occurs in 5–10% of amputees, especially those with pain in the limb before amputation). Other areas of the thalamus contain cells that respond to noxious stimulation or when stimulated, lead to pain sensations, or, when removed, temporarily reduce or eliminate pain sensation, but as yet we do not have a thorough understanding of this system. In cases of thalamic lesions, pain is alleviated for a short time, but soon returns, often with even greater severity than before the lesion; this is termed **hyperpathia.** To the patient this may mean an endless series of surgical lesions, he may wish had never begun, just to keep ahead of the advancing pain intensity. It has been customary to think of the experience of pain as occurring in the thalamus simply because it is the "highest" center in which it can be recorded, evoked, or blocked.

GATE THEORY

In most sensory systems there exists a phenomenon known as **masking** that is an increase in the threshold for perception of a given stimulus caused by the presence of another stimulus. In audition, tones of similar frequencies tend to mask each other. There is only a slight increase in the threshold for detection of a 400-Hz tone in the presence of an 800-Hz tone, but there is considerable increase in threshold for a 750-Hz tone in the presence of an 800-Hz tone. In the olfactory system, strong odors tend to mask weaker odors. Similar masking phenomena occur in the somatosensory system. Touching the skin near a hair will block the sensation evoked by flicking the hair with a pencil point. Also, weak cutaneous stimulation and sometimes even strong stimulation can block or reduce cutaneous pain sensations. (All of these masking phenomena probably do not have the same neural mechanisms, but they are similar phenomenologically.)

A number of properties of pain perception (including masking) have led to the proposal of the **gate theory of pain.**

1. Counterirritation, such as lightly rubbing the painful skin, can relieve the pain experienced.
2. Under certain circumstances (*e.g.*, in causalgias), gentle stimulation of an injured area can produce intense pain, though it does not produce pain on normal skin.
3. Intense, spontaneous pain often results from pathologic conditions, such as tabes dorsalis, in which large myelinated fibers (which do not carry pain signals) are affected preferentially.
4. Pain often results in the ten-second period after ischemic pressure-block of a nerve while large fibers fail to conduct.
5. Stimulation of the dorsal columns ipsilateral to the pain often produces relief of pain.

To account for these observations, Melzack and Wall proposed that the perception of pain depends not only upon pain signals in small fibers, but also upon the *balance* of activity in large myelinated *mechanoreceptive* fibers (Aα and Aβ fibers) and small myelinated and unmyelinated *nociceptive* fibers (Aδ and C fibers). It is important to remember that not all small fibers are nociceptive—some are mechano- and thermoreceptive. They proposed that, under normal conditions, anything that increases the activity of the large mechanoreceptive fibers tends to reduce pain, and anything that increases the activity of small nociceptive fibers tends to increase pain by changing the balance. Specifically, they proposed the model illustrated in Figure 6-8. According to the theory, the transmission (T) cells (originally thought to be cells of the spinothalamic tract) activate neural mechanisms that produce pain perception, that is, T-cell activity is interpreted by the central nervous system as pain. A gate cell, or G cell (originally thought to be cells of the substantia gelatinosa), is capable of modulating the activity in afferent pathways (of both large and small fibers) to the T cell, before it gets to the T cell. G-cell activity is, in turn, modulated by activity in both large and small primary afferent fibers. Specifically, volleys in both large and small fibers excite the T cell (drive its membrane voltage toward the critical firing level), whereas the same volleys in large fibers excite the G cell to discharge and the same volleys in small fibers inhibit the G-cell discharge (drive its membrane voltage away from the critical firing level). Activity in the G cell inhibits (reduces or blocks) transmission from both large and small fibers to T cells. Cortical and subcortical influences on the gate control mechanism are indicated in the diagram of Figure 6-8. This diagram is just one module of many; there are many T and G cells and, of course, a million or so afferent fibers.

How does this theory account for the preceding observations? (1) Lightly rubbing the skin increases the discharge of the G cell. This results in decreased transmission through both large and small afferent fibers to the T cell that, of course, is perceived as a reduction in pain sensation, because the severity of pain sensation is proportional to the frequency of firing of the T cell. (2) In causalgias, there can be selective destruction of the large fibers in the affected nerve. This results in diminished G-cell activity caused by reduced excitation from large fibers and the unopposed inhibition from small fibers, thereby opening the gate and letting the T cell receive excitation through the large and small fiber pathways. The result is pain evoked by even the lightest touch. (3) Many C fibers are slightly spontaneously active and, when the gate is open because of large afferent fiber damage, these C fibers are free to excite the T cell. When the excitation builds up enough to bring the T cell to firing level, spontaneous pain is experienced. (4) After an ischemic block of a peripheral nerve, the large fibers recover more slowly than the small fibers. Therefore, there is a period of time when the gate is open due to the absence of the large fiber activity. (5) The dorsal column fibers are branches of the large myelinated fibers of the medial division of the dorsal root. Stimulation of the dorsal columns sends impulses up **(orthodromically)** and down **(antidromically)** the fibers of the columns. When the antidromic impulses reach the point of bifurcation, action potentials are set up in both the dorsal root (antidromic) and in the branch that descends into the spinal gray matter (orthodromic). These orthodromic impulses act just like those from the periphery in closing the gate by activating the G cell; thus, the pain is reduced. Small stimulating devices have been implanted in the dorsal columns of patients with chronic pain. The patient can activate the device himself when the pain recurs. Some success has been reported using this technique.

There was a flurry of excitement when this theory was introduced and with it a great deal of research. The original specifications of the theory assigned to specific cells in the spinal cord the roles of G and T cells. These specific cells do not seem to have all of the properties of G and T cells. In addition, there are some examples of clinical syndromes that do not seem, at first glance, to fit the gate theory. In Friedrich's ataxia, a hereditary disease, the symptoms of which are ataxia, speech impairment, lateral curvature of the spine, swaying, irregular movements, and muscle paralysis, there is a preferential loss of large fibers without pain. Similarly, the polyneuropathy associated with renal failure in adults is not associated with complaints of pain, although there is destruction predominantly of large fibers. Nor do some other neuropathies make any sense in any current theory of peripheral nerve involvement in pain sensation. Fabry's disease, a rare phospholipid storage disease, is associated with both pain and the loss of small myelinated fibers, and one hereditary sensory neuropathy is associated with loss of myelinated fibers, preserved C fibers, and analgesia. One should bear in mind that none of these is a disease of peripheral nerves alone. Friedrich's ataxia also involves sclerosis of dorsal and lateral columns of the spinal cord, including the pyramidal tract, and Fabry's disease involves pathologic conditions of the cardiovascular and renal systems as well as skin and muscle lesions. The effects on pain of these forms of polyneuropathy are not explained by reference to which peripheral nerve fibers are present or absent. Therefore, it may be the involvement of central pain mechanisms that makes these diseases appear not to fit any existing theory.

It should be kept in mind that not all pain is of peripheral origin, that is, some pain does not arise from activity in nociceptors. Causalgias are a class of disorders involving burning pain caused by peripheral nerve damage, not receptor damage. The importance of the separation of "central" and "peripheral" pain is indicated by the observation that patients often obtain relief from spontaneous pain of causalgias when the dorsal columns are stimulated, but the same stimulation does not elevate the threshold for pain induced by pinching the skin in the referral area of the causalgias. The stimulus also does not elevate touch and vibration thresholds. It appears that causalgias may have mechanisms different from those of peripheral pain, but how they differ is as yet unknown.

A further indication of this difference between "normal" and "pathologic" pain is the result of attempts to close the gate by peripheral stimulation. In patients with causalgias, stimulation of large-diameter fibers has been used to attempt to activate the G cells and close the gate. In one-third or more of such patients, partial to complete relief has been obtained, but the same stimulation has no effect on pain due to noxious stimulation of the hand. Pain caused by squeezing the Achilles' tendon can be relieved by large-fiber stimulation, suggesting that all sorts of "normal" pain may not be the same either. Similarly, morphine can decrease postsurgical tonic pain, but has less effect on acute pain of movement or removal of stitches. Nitrous oxide, on the other hand, depresses both.

ENDOGENOUS PAIN SUPPRESSION SYSTEM

It is doubtful that the gate control theory, as it was originally proposed, is adequate to explain all types of pain, but it seems reasonable that some similar gating mechanism(s) are active in pain perception, either in the spinal cord or at some other level of the central nervous system. In fact, there is some evidence for such a mechanism at the brain-stem level. Stimulation of the periaqueductal gray matter of the brain stem (Fig. 6-9) produces analgesia in rats sufficient to do abdominal surgery and equivalent to a dose of 50 mg/kg of morphine, but without the muscular rigidity that accompanies such high doses. It blocks

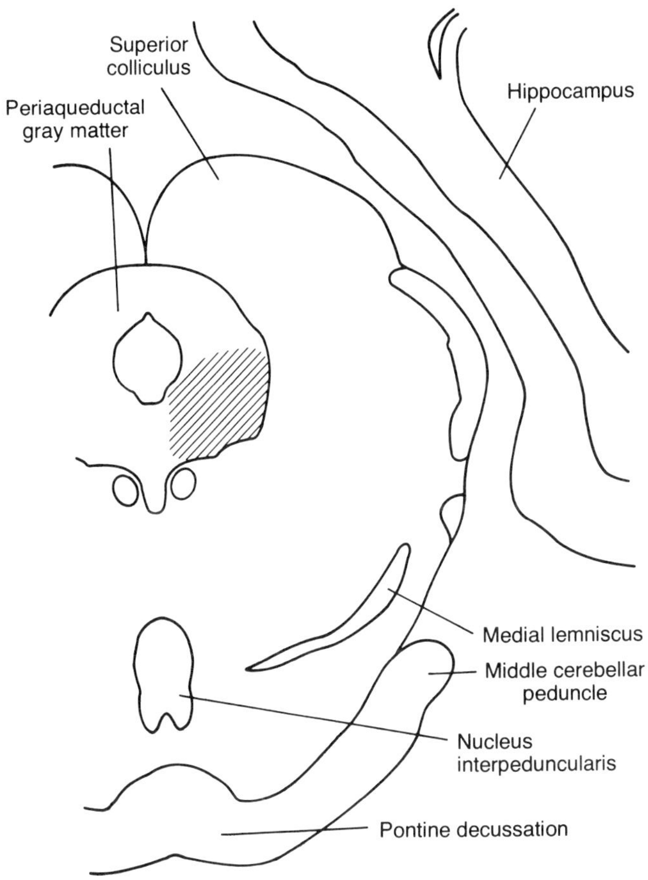

FIG. 6-9. The location of stimulus sites within the periaqueductal gray matter at the level of the superior colliculus (*shaded area*) from which analgesia can be produced in the cat.

withdrawal reflexes caused by skin pinch, noxious heat, tooth pulp stimulation (supposedly evoking pure pain sensations), and chemical irritants. The analgesia induced by a few minutes of high-frequency stimulation lasts minutes, hours, or days, but is not a total analgesia, because some parts of the body are unaffected. Again, pathologic pain is blocked more easily than normal pain.

Injection of minute amounts of opiate drugs into the region of the periaqueductal gray matter induces strong general analgesia similar to that obtained with systemic morphine. The opiate-antagonist drug, naloxone, blocks the analgesic effects of systemic and microinjected morphine and reduces the effects of periaqueductal gray matter stimulation. The effects of morphine and stimulation are also reduced or blocked by depletion, with parachlorophenylalanine, of serotonin (5 hydroxytryptamine, 5HT), a putative excitatory transmitter substance, and blocked by lesions of the ipsilateral dorsolateral funiculus of the spinal cord. These latter observations prompted a search for a pathway descending to the spinal cord in the dorsolateral funiculus from the region of the periaqueductal gray matter and containing serotonin. Such a pathway originates in the nucleus raphe magnus of the medullary reticular formation. Stimulation within this nucleus also produces analgesia similar to that seen with periaqueductal gray matter stimulation. Subsequently, a synaptic link between the periaqueductal gray matter and the nucleus raphe magnus has been demonstrated, and cells in both nuclei have been shown to be responsive to noxious inputs as well as light tactile stimulation.

At about the same time that stimulation-produced analgesia was being discovered, pharmacologic investigations were revealing the presence of receptors in

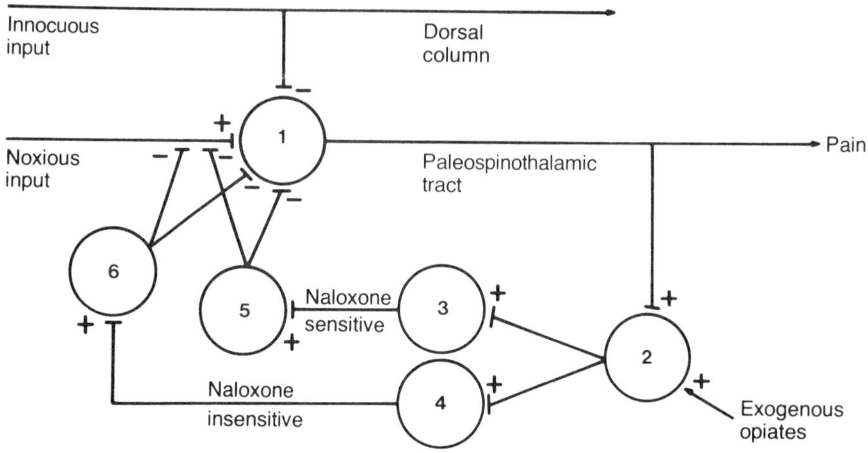

FIG. 6-10. The endogenous pain suppression theory includes a negative feedback system in which spinothalamic tract cells **(1)**, activated by noxious input, activate cells of the periaqueductal gray matter **(2)**, which in turn activate descending pathways from the nucleus raphe magnus **(3)** and the locus ceruleus or nuclei subceruleus and parafascicularis **(4)**. At the segmental spinal cord, interneurons **(5 and 6)** activated by these descending impulses inhibit further activation of spinothalamic tract cells. Also shown are the sites of action of dorsal column influences and morphine. (Basbaum AI, Fields HL: Ann Neurol 4:451–462, 1978)

the brain to which opiates bind specifically. This suggested that there were naturally occurring morphine-like compounds in the brain that could bind to these receptors. Subsequently, two pentapeptides, the enkephalins, and certain other peptides, the endorphins, were isolated from brain tissue and shown to have analgesic effects like that of morphine when injected systemically or into the ventricle. These compounds are found at many places within the central nervous system, but, notably, they occur in the periaqueductal gray matter and the area of the spinal cord from which the spinothalamic tract has been shown to originate. The opiate receptors have also been seen on the terminals of primary afferent neurons in the dorsal horn; some investigators believe these are the terminals of nociceptive axons.

From the preceding observations, Basbaum and Fields (1978) proposed what they call an endogenous pain suppression system. The model, shown in Figure 6-10, proposes that noxious stimulation excites nociceptors, which, in turn, excite cells of the spinothalamic tract, giving rise to pain sensations. Spinothalamic fibers excite cells of the periaqueductal gray matter, which, in turn, excite cells of the nucleus raphe magnus. The latter cells can also be excited by nociceptive inputs through other pathways. Axons of raphe magnus neurons descend in the dorsolateral funiculus and their activity excites interneurons in the spinal cord that contain endorphins as a transmitter substance. The endorphins block the release of transmitter substance (possibly substance P, another peptide compound) onto spinothalamic tract cells, preventing or reducing further nociceptive discharges in them. This is an example of a **negative-feedback loop** in which the output of a group of cells, in this case the spinothalamic tract cells, is used to reduce its input, in this case the amount of nociceptive input. The effect of the system is to reduce subsequent pain sensation. The model suggests that morphine acts by exciting the system at the periaqueductal gray matter.

This model explains the effects of morphine (systemically and locally injected), of periaqueductal gray matter and nucleus raphe magnus stimulation, and of endorphins on pain sensitivity, at least in part. However, naloxone administration and serotonin depletion only partially block the effect of periaqueductal gray matter stimulation, implying that there must be an additional mechanism for this effect.

This model requires that periaqueductal gray matter stimulation and morphine administration actually result in inhibition of nociceptive activity in spinal cord neurons.

Studies have indicated that, in the rat, injection of morphine into the periaqueductal gray matter leads to decreased responsiveness to noxious stimulation in some lumbar spinal cord neurons; others increase their activity or are not influenced. In some of the inhibited cells, naloxone returned the cell discharge to normal despite continued stimulation. Periaqueductal gray matter stimulation does not influence the discharge of most cells that respond to mechanical, non-noxious stimulation. The situation in the monkey and cat is similar, but not as neat. Stimulation of the raphe magnus nucleus inhibits both nociceptive and non-nociceptive, tactile activity in spinothalamic neurons. Thus, it is clear that not all nociceptive activity is inhibited by stimulation in regions that produce analgesia; however, not all nociceptive activity is necessarily associated with pain perception. As we shall see when we discuss synaptic transmission (Chap. 13), it is not necessary to reduce nociceptive inputs to a cell to zero in order to bring the membrane potential below critical firing level, preventing its discharge. Still, the link between the cellular events in the spinal cord and the analgesia observed has yet to be established, so the model is tentative; however, it has already led to new pain treatments.

REFERRED PAIN

Visceral sensations can be classed either as organic sensations or pain sensations. Organic sensations are those that signal a bodily need and that usually lead to an activity designed to satisfy that need. Hunger sensations are an example. All fibers that carry visceral sensation travel the viscera in the company of autonomic efferent fibers and enter the spinal cord through the deep nerve trunks and the ventral ramus of the dorsal root.

Visceral pain is peculiar in that it is often felt to be coming from the surface of the body, not from the organ that contains the pain receptors. We say that the pain is referred to the site on the skin. The area of the referral is always in the dermatome innervated by the same dorsal root(s) as those supplying the irritated structure in the viscera. This is a case in which knowledge of the dermatomes becomes an important diagnostic tool. **Angina pectoris** is a classic example in which pain caused by anoxia of the myocardium is referred to the chest and arm. The pain fibers from the myocardium originate in the dorsal root ganglia T1-T5, which have dermatomes on the chest from below the nipple up to about the level of the clavicle and also down the posterior aspect of the arm. It serves a clinician well to memorize this distribution, because chances are he will see it again.

There are a number of other examples of referred pain. Regurgitation of acid into the esophagus is sensed as burning pain localized to the region of the lower end of the sternum ("heartburn"), whereas referred pain for inflammation of the appendix is experienced in the lower right quadrant. It should be noted that not all visceral pain is referred. Appendicitis is also accompanied by diffuse pain near the midline at the epigastric level, and a myocardial infarction is usually accompanied by deeper aching in the chest in the vicinity of the heart.

Referral of pain is not limited to visceral organs. Pain in some nonvisceral organs such as the peritoneum and the diaphragm is also referred to the appropriate dermatomes. The pain fibers from the central region of the diaphragm travel in the phrenic nerve to enter the spinal cord at C3 and C4. Thus, pain in the diaphragm, for example, caused by subphrenic abscess, is referred to the region of the neck and shoulders. Referral of pain from the diaphragm also occurs following a gynecologic test to determine the patency of the fallopian tubes, Rubin's test. In this test, CO_2 is forced into the uterus and out through the tubes, and if they are patent, the bubble of gas escapes past the fimbria into the peritoneal cavity. It causes no sensation in the horizontal position, but upon rising the patients often report pain in the shoulder because of the localization of the bubble beneath the diaphragm. The pain subsides, of course, as the gas is absorbed.

The mechanism of the referral is undoubtedly the same for visceral and other somatic pain. The visceral pain afferent fibers probably terminate on the same central cells and influence them in the same way as the cutaneous and muscle pain fibers of that dermatome do. Through experience, the discharge of those central cells has become associated with pain of the body surface, visceral pain being an infrequent event. The brain thus interprets activity in those cells as pain at the surface, not deep pain. Whatever the nature and the location of the central pain mechanism, it knows only that the central cell *has* discharged, not what made it discharge.

PAIN TREATMENT

The most common treatment for pain is the administration of so-called analgesic drugs. This is, perhaps, an unfortunate term, because few of these drugs produce analgesia in the sense of insensitivity to pain. In most cases, they produce pain relief—aspirin relieves headaches—but pain sensitivity is not lowered. The patient still responds with the same sensitivity to noxious heat, damaging mechanical or chemical stimulation, or electrical stimulation. As already mentioned, even morphine does not produce analgesia. General anesthetics may produce analgesia, or they may not. We only know that the patient does not report experiencing pain under the influence of a general anesthetic agent, but withdrawal reflexes and reflex changes in blood pressure still occur in response to painful stimulation. Perhaps the patient felt pain, but just did not remember. We cannot say with certainty. We will see that most surgical treatments for pain also produce pain relief, not analgesia, but that is what the patient really wants.

Chronic pain has been treated with a number of destructive surgical interventions. Dorsal rhizotomies have been performed for a chronic pain owing to malignancies, vertebral disc disease, spinal trauma, and other causes, but the success rate (complete pain relief) is less than 30%. There are, of course, fibers other than nociceptive fibers in the dorsal roots, and losses occur in other than pain sensations. The use of this procedure is further complicated by the fact that, even though a nerve block by local anesthetics may alleviate pain totally, subsequent rhizotomy of the same roots may be without effect. A similar treatment for **trigeminal neuralgia** or **tic douloureux** (a severe, unremitting pain in the face associated with large-fiber damage and triggered by gentle but not intense stimulation of the face), involving thermocoagulation of the trigeminal roots or ganglia within the foramen ovale, has achieved a success rate of 90% to 100%, though up to 17% required more than one treatment. This treatment has the advantage of preserving touch sensation in the analgesic field in many cases, but pain still recurs in 22% of cases. The cause of the relief may not be destruction of nociceptive fibers in every case, because a mistaken coagulation of the wrong trigeminal (the one contralateral to the pain) led to pain relief for two years in one patient.

The notion that the spinothalamic tract was the pain pathway provoked a great many anterolateral cordotomies (or spinothalamic tractotomies) for the relief of chronic pain. Initially, these were done surgically, but more recently they have been done percutaneously by inserting metal electrodes into the spinal cord (without a laminectomy) and coagulating a portion of the anterolateral quadrant. As mentioned before, this procedure never produces permanent pain relief. A **dysesthesia,** a persistent, painful sensation produced by gentle stimulation, usually develops sometime after a cordotomy and it worsens with time. For these reasons, cordotomies are seldom done except in terminal disease cases.

It is possible to make small lesions in specific structures within the brain by passing a small amount of current through an electrode placed in that structure. The current produces heat that destroys the nearby cells. Such electrodes can be placed accurately using **stereotaxic coordinates,** a Cartesian coordinate system, read from an atlas and referenced to particular points on the head. The position of the electrode can be checked by using known properties of the cells in the region, for example, the cells of the nucleus ventralis posterolateralis of the thalamus are known to discharge in response to skin stimulation, and by x-ray imaging. Lesions have been made in the various relays for nociceptive information in the thalamus or mesencephalon. However, everyone who has used this type of intervention has found the same result: There is initial relief followed by rapid return of pain. Even large unilateral and bilateral lesions fail to relieve pain and usually lead to exacerbation of preoperative pain or dysesthesia that is worse than the initial complaint. At present, there is little justification for **thalamotomy** in pain treatment.

The causalgias are burning pains associated with peripheral nerve damage, often associated with penetrating wounds, and they are frequently exacerbated or triggered by emotional and thermal stimulation. These pains can also be triggered by light touch or any stimulus that elicits a startle reflex. The involvement of emotion suggests that the sympathetic nervous system may play a role in causalgia; in cases in which pain is exacerbated by such stimuli, **sympathectomy** has produced at least some pain relief. Paravertebral sympathetic nerve blocks are good indicators of the success of sympathectomy. This form of treatment has also been used for pain relief in disease confined to the visceral capsule, for example, angina pectoris, aortic aneurysms, and postcholecystectomy neuralgia, but seldom is effective for pain caused by malignancy. For causalgia with emotional exacerbation, good, long-term pain relief has been obtained in up to 83% of cases where sympathectomies have been performed. The mechanism of the pain relief is not known, but (1) abolition of vasomotor and sudomotor efferent discharge, with relief from ischemia, and (2) interruption of accessory sensory pathways carrying pain discharges from blood vessels have been suggested as explanations.

Pain caused by hormone-dependent tumors is usually not responsive to surgical or nerve-block treatments because the tumors are commonly metastatic and distributed over wide areas or in different organs. Some patients suffering from this sort of chronic pain have been treated by chemical **hypophysectomy.** A small amount of ethanol injected in the region of the pituitary produced complete, immediate, long-lasting relief in 88% of the patients in one study, and some of the remaining patients also received relief when the procedure was repeated. The treatment not only results in pain relief, but there is usually an arrest or regression of the metastasis. Two hypotheses suggest that (1) hormones potentiate transmission through sensory pathways and that removal of hormones reduces pain discharge transmission, and (2) ethanol works not only on the pituitary, but also diffuses to surrounding tissues that are in the pain pathway. Hormones are known to potentiate sensory transmission, but potentiation of nociceptive sensory transmission has not been studied.

Percutaneous stimulation and dorsal column stimulation to activate large-diameter fibers have already been mentioned for pain treatment. Stimulation of a peripheral nerve, central to nerve damage in a patient with causalgia, produces immediate pain relief that outlasts the duration of stimulation. Two minutes of stimulation at 100 Hz has produced relief lasting up to seven hours; eventually pain returned, sometimes with an overshoot (it was worse than before stimulation), but repeated stimulation produced repeated relief. Such stimulation has been effective in 70% to 85% of the patients in different clinics. Percutaneous stimulation has been used to treat headache and pain caused by burns and abrasions; relief is more frequent for this type of new pain than for chronic pain. In a group of patients with chronic low-back pain, 39% obtained complete relief, 28% obtained some relief, but 33% obtained no relief. There are three hypotheses advanced to explain pain relief by percutaneous stimulation. Closure of the pain gate in the gate control theory is one explanation. Blockage of transmission in small fibers as a result of repeated, high-frequency stimulation is another. Masking of pain sensations by evoked **paresthesias** is yet another explanation. This last alternative does not seem to explain all cases, because pain usually fades out gradually during stimulation and gradually reappears, whereas the paresthesias appear abruptly with stimulation and disappear before pain recurs.

Dorsal column stimulation has been used most often in treatment of spinal column disc pain. Some patients experience paresthesias and pain relief during stimulation, but both disappear when stimulation ends. In others, paresthesias may last up to 30 minutes longer than stimulation, and pain relief up to four hours longer. Pin-prick pain, light touch, and vibration sensation, and stereognosis are unaffected by dorsal column stimulation, as they are by dorsal column lesions (Friedman, Nashold, Somjen, 1974). Dorsal column stimulation cannot relieve postoperative pain caused by implan-

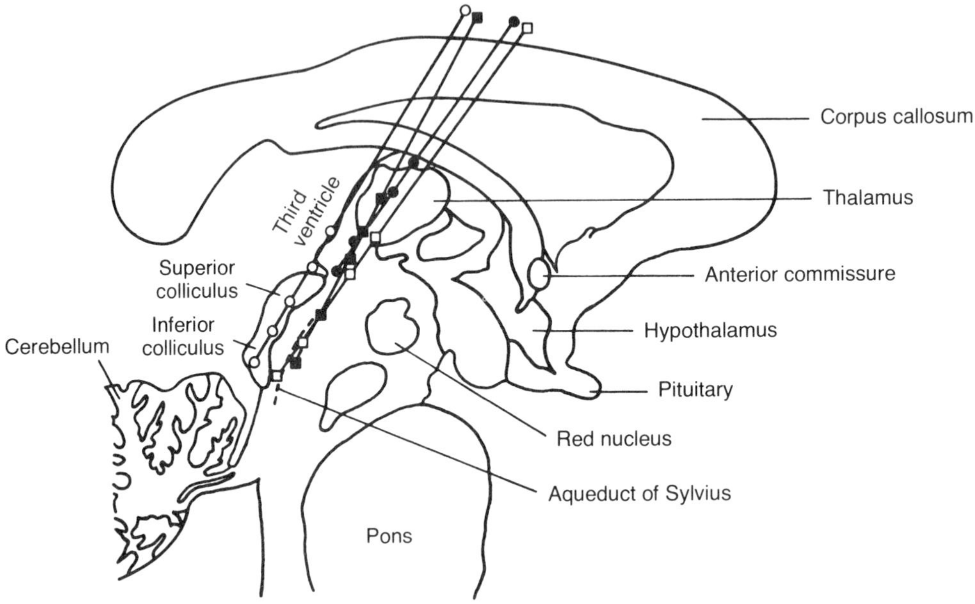

FIG. 6-11. Stimulation sites in human patients from which pain relief has been obtained. Electrode tracks are shown, along which the stimulation sites are marked with different symbols for each patient. These tracts traverse the periventricular gray area along the medial aspect of the nucleus parafascicularis of the thalamus. (Richardson DE, Akil H: J Neurosurg 47:178–183, 1977)

tation of the stimulator or pain due to long-bone fracture, but it has been effective in 81% of the cases of disc pain.

The experimental observations of the effects of stimulation of the periaqueductal gray matter in rats have now been extended to cats and monkeys and, finally, to man. In pain patients, various forms of chronic pain, including disc pain, tumor pain, and phantom-limb pain, have been relieved by such stimulation, without any apparent influence on other sensory modalities (*e.g.*, vision) or submodalities (light touch) or changes in motor or intellectual activity. In some cases, acute experimental pain has also been blocked, but usually with more difficulty and for shorter times. The diencephalic periventricular gray matter, the pretectal nucleus, and some hypothalamic sites have also produced analgesia when stimulated (Fig. 6-11). Medial periventricular thalamic structures are preferred targets for stimulation in humans, because periaqueductal stimulation usually produces unpleasant sensations, including nystagmus and nausea. Chronic pains beginning after implantation of stimulating electrodes may not be influenced by stimulation; electrically induced, radiant heat-induced, and ischemic exercise-induced pains may also be unaffected. When patients are allowed to control stimulation, a tolerance, which generalizes to opiate drugs, may develop in 4 to 5 weeks, but if use is limited, this tolerance does not develop. Bilateral pain relief occurs with unilateral stimulation. About 75% of the patients treated with this kind of stimulation (in one study) received at least some relief from pain; many received complete relief. In 5 of 6 patients, naloxone administration reversed the relief that resulted from stimulation (Richardson and Akil, 1977). In another study, similar stimulation has no effect on pain sensation in any patients (Mazars, Merienne, and Cioloca, 1979). This form of treatment is new and the number of patients treated is too small to form a reliable test.

The treatment of choice for pain is not always clear; nor is it clear that a single treatment is good for all types of pain. Early attempts at treating pain with a new procedure are often more effective than later attempts. One should guard against being overly optimistic about the effectiveness of new treatments. In a review, Shealy (1974) concluded that "traditional destructive procedures—cordotomy, cingulumotomy, rhizotomy—are not only almost useless (except in cancer) but they cause far more harm than good, and they interfere with success of other procedures." In cancer, the patient usually does not survive long enough to suffer the harm of these procedures. The mechanism of action of any pain treatment is not known. Most do not produce true analgesia but only pain relief. Many produce only transient relief and, for no treatment has an appropriate control procedure been done to evaluate the effectiveness of the treatment itself. For example, trigeminal coagulation produces pain relief in most cases of trigeminal neuralgia, but simple manipulations without destruction can also produce relief. Pain is, indeed, a curious phenomenon!

ACUPUNCTURE

The practice of acupuncture in treatment of disorders is very old in China, but interest in it has been stirred in this country in recent years by demonstration that it can be used for analgesia. The technique essentially is to insert metal needles through the skin at certain critical points and then to either manipulate them or stimulate through them using mild electrical currents. Exact sites and number of sites are determined by the position in which the analgesia is desired. The patient usually reports a tingling, pricking, or numbing sensation during stimulation of the needles with a stimulus strength that is great enough to excite $A\alpha$ fibers and perhaps the largest $A\delta$ fibers. Under this intervention, everything from minor dental work to major abdominal and thoracic surgery is performed without anesthetic agents or their side effects. Two advantages of the procedure are a more rapid recovery and the absence of any need for close supervision during recovery.

One is at first tempted to interpret the acupuncture phenomenon in terms of the gate theory. This temptation is brought on by the rather selective excitation of large myelinated fibers by the needles and their stimulation. However, in the gate theory, the large and small myelinated fibers operating the gate supposedly enter the same spinal cord segment. On the other hand, the acupuncture needles are often placed in the hand or ear lobe for procedures in the lower abdomen, a separation of many segments for entry of the appropriate afferent fibers. Indeed, some variation of the gate theory could be invoked to explain the phenomenon, but the pathways involved are not known at this time.

In China, acupuncture is used in about 30% of hospital surgical procedures. If the procedure is so useful, why is it not used in 100%? The most likely answer is that it only works in 30% of the cases. This is about the same proportion of cases that receive relief from placebo treatments or have surgical procedures under hypnosis. It is reasonable to suggest that the monotonous stimulation has a somewhat hypnotic effect upon the patient. On the other hand, acupuncture has been reported to be effective on animals and small children, suggesting that hypnosis is not the only explanation, if it is an explanation at all.

We should recall that some superficial pains can be blocked by intense stimulation or counterirritation. This intense stimulation can be in the form of dry needling, intense cold, or injection of normal saline. Treatment with mustard plasters and blistering agents may also be considered the same form of treatment, sometimes called **hyperstimulation analgesia.** It seems paradoxical that intense stimulation should relieve pain from intense stimulation, but, in some cases, it works. Some investigators have suggested that acupuncture may be just another case of hyperstimulation analgesia. The acupuncture needles apparently have no effect on pain unless they are moved or an electrical current is applied, implying that a significant input to the CNS is required for the analgesia. However, analgesia is usually produced by hyperstimulation near the area of injury; acupuncture needles are effective at a distance.

SUGGESTED READING

Angaut-Petit D: The dorsal column system: II. Functional properties and bulbar relay of the postsynaptic fibres of the cat's fasciculus gracilis. Exp Brain Res 22:471–493, 1975

Basbaum AI, Fields HL: Endogenous pain control mechanisms: review and hypothesis. Ann Neurol 4:451–462, 1978

Clark FJ: Central projections of sensory fibers from the cat knee joint. J Neurobiol 3:101–110, 1972

Corkin S, Milner B, Rasmussen T: Somatosensory thresholds. Contrasting effects of postcentral-gyrus and posterior parietal-lobe excisions. Arch. Neurol 23:41–58, 1970

Dennis SG, Melzack R: Pain-signalling systems in the dorsal and ventral spinal cord. Pain 4:97–132, 1977

Friedman H, Nashold BS Jr, Somjen G: Physiological effects of dorsal column stimulation. In Bonica JJ (ed): Advances in Neurology, Vol. 4, Pain. pp. 769–773. New York, Raven Press, 1974

Iggo A [ed]: Handbook of Sensory Physiology, Vol. II, Somatosensory System. Berlin, Springer-Verlag, 1973

King RB: Principles of pain management. A short review. J. Neurosurg 50:554–559, 1979

Mazars G, Merienne L, Cioloca C: Effets des soi-disant stimulations de la substance grise péri-acqueductale. Neurochirurgie 25:96–100, 1979

Melzack R, Wall PD: Pain mechanism: a new theory. Science 150:971–979, 1965

Nathan PW: The gate-control theory of pain. A critical review. Brain 99:123–158, 1976

Nathan PW, Rudge P: Testing the gate-control theory of pain in man. J Neurol Neurosurg Psychiat 37:1366–1372, 1974

Richardson DE, Akil H: Pain reduction by electrical brain stimulation in man. I. Acute administration in periaqueductal and periventricular sites. J. Neurosurg 47:178–183, 1977

Shealy CN: Six years' experience with electrical stimulation for control of pain. In Bonica JJ [ed]: Advances in Neurology, Vol 4, Pain. pp. 775–782. New York, Raven Press, 1974

Trevino DL, Coulter JD, Maunz RA *et al*: Location and functional properties of spinothalamic cells in the monkey. In Bonica JJ [ed]: Advances in Neurology, Vol. 4, Pain. pp. 167–170. New York, Raven Press, 1974

Woolsey CN: Cortical localization as defined by evoked potential and electrical stimulation studies. In Schaltenbrand G, Woolsey CN [eds]: Cerebral Localization and Organization, pp. 17–26. Madison, WI, Univ. of Wisconsin Press, 1964

Woolsey CN, Erickson TC, Gilson WE: Localization in somatic sensory and motor areas of human cerebral cortex as determined by direct recording of evoked potentials and electrical stimulation. J. Neurosurg 51:476–506, 1979

7

Vision

Photoreception is a particularly important sense for most primates, including man, but it is not unique to primates or even mammals. Even mollusks have photoreceptors, but one may question whether they possess vision in the same sense as we have it. Most objects reflect light, and because light travels at high speed, it is possible almost instantly to assess their shape, size, position, speed, and direction of movement. The light rays emanating from an object are gathered and focused onto an array of photoreceptors. Activities generated in the different photoreceptors by the light interact to produce a two-dimensional representation of the object that is transmitted to the brain. The brain then reconstructs a three-dimensional representation using information received from the two eyes. The end products of the activity of the visual system are sensations that represent the object and its surroundings. These sensations can be used to guide our immediate behavior or they can be stored for future reference. Visual sensations contain a great deal of information, and understanding these complex phenomena is no simple matter. The best place to begin the study of vision is with the eye itself.

Figure 7-1 shows a cross section through the eye. It consists of two fluid-filled chambers separated by a transparent structure, the lens. Nearly the entire eye is covered with a tough, fibrous coating called the sclera that is modified anteriorly to form the transparent cornea. The cornea is made of the same collagenous connective tissue substance as is the sclera, but the fibers of the cornea are oriented in parallel arrays that let light pass through, whereas those of the sclera are random and light cannot penetrate them. Lining the inside of the posterior two-thirds of the sclera are two membranes: (1) the choroid, a pigment layer containing the vascular supply for the eyeball, and (2) the retina, which contains the photoreceptors and other neural elements essential to our visual process. The fine structure of the retina is considered in detail later.

The lens is suspended in place by a circular ligament, the ciliary zonule, that attaches to the choroid anterior to the retina. A set of smooth-muscle fibers, the ciliary muscles, attach to the sclera and insert in the choroid near the attachment of the zonule. Just anterior to the lens is a pigmented structure called the iris, which is like the diaphragm on some cameras in that it has a hole in the center of a variable aperture, the pupil. The pupil is surrounded by two sets of muscles, one that encircles the pupil, the sphincter pupillae, and one that runs radially out from the pupil, the dilator pupillae.

The anterior chamber of the eye is filled with aqueous humor, a watery fluid of low protein content that is formed from plasma. The posterior chamber contains a gelatinous substance, the vitreous or vitreous humor. In many people the vitreous is not completely clear, but contains particulate matter that is not transparent. This material may be stationery or may float around, producing "spots" before the eyes, the floating variety being called floaters.

At this point, we should spend just a moment reviewing the properties of light, a form of electromagnetic radiation. Light is radiant energy emitted by matter when it is at high temperature, when it is electrically excited, and when it is undergoing certain chemical or physical processes. Early on, physicists attempted to account for the properties of light in terms of a stream of particles emitted by a luminous object. Later, they attempted to account for them

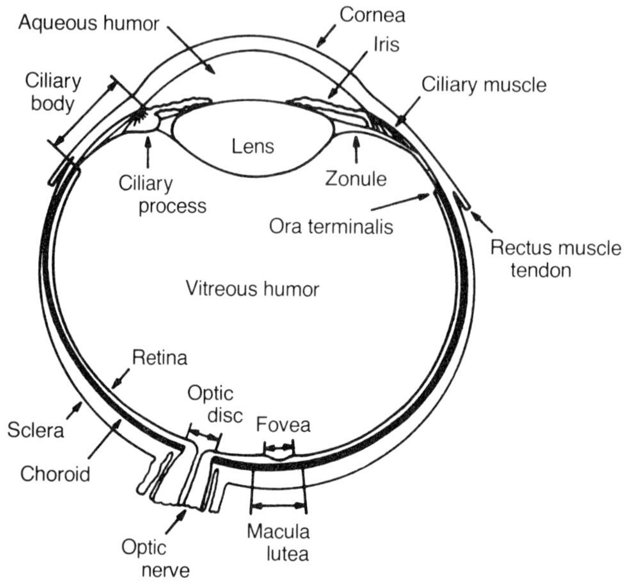

FIG. 7-1. A section through the human eye illustrating the major structures. (Walls GL: The Vertebrate Eye and its Adaptive Radiations. New York, Hafner, 1967)

in terms of waves, but light has properties both of waves and of particles. In any case, light has characteristic wavelengths that are measurable. The total spectrum of wavelengths of electromagnetic radiation is broad, ranging from 1 nanometer (nm) (10^{-9} m) to over 10^4 m, yet we see only a small part of that spectrum (400–700 nm). Some other animals have a broader sensitivity than man, being able to see in the ultraviolet region (less than 400 nm), but not even these animals see the whole light spectrum, 380 to 760 nm.

Light travels in straight lines from its source unless it passes through a high-intensity electromagnetic field or from a medium of one refractive index into a medium of another. In the first case, the light is bent along a curved path. We will not consider this further because it plays no role in normal human vision. When light passes from one medium into another of a different refractive index, the direction of travel of the light beam is changed at the interface. This is the basis for the phenomenon of refraction, which we discuss in detail in the next section.

Psychologically, light has three aspects we need to consider. It has **hue,** a quality correlated with wavelength and analogous to pitch in hearing. It has **saturation,** a quality related to homogeneity or purity of wavelength and comparable to timbre or freedom from noise in audition. The color of a light is a function both of its hue and saturation. Finally it has **brightness,** a quantitative measure of the intensity of the light and somewhat analogous to loudness in hearing. The intensity of light is dependent upon the amplitude of its waves or alternatively upon the number of photons (particles of light).

OPTICAL FUNCTIONS OF THE EYE

The process of light reception and transmission has a number of parts. First, we consider the optical functions of the eye: accommodation,* the process of forming a focused image, and control of the amount of luminous flux at the retina.

ACCOMMODATION

A convex lens like that in the eye has the property of bending rays of light that pass through it toward its axis. This property results from the fact that light travels more

* It is unfortunate that the same term is used for the process of forming a focused image and for changes in critical firing level that occur with small prolonged depolarizations. The only way to distinguish these usages is by the context in which they occur.

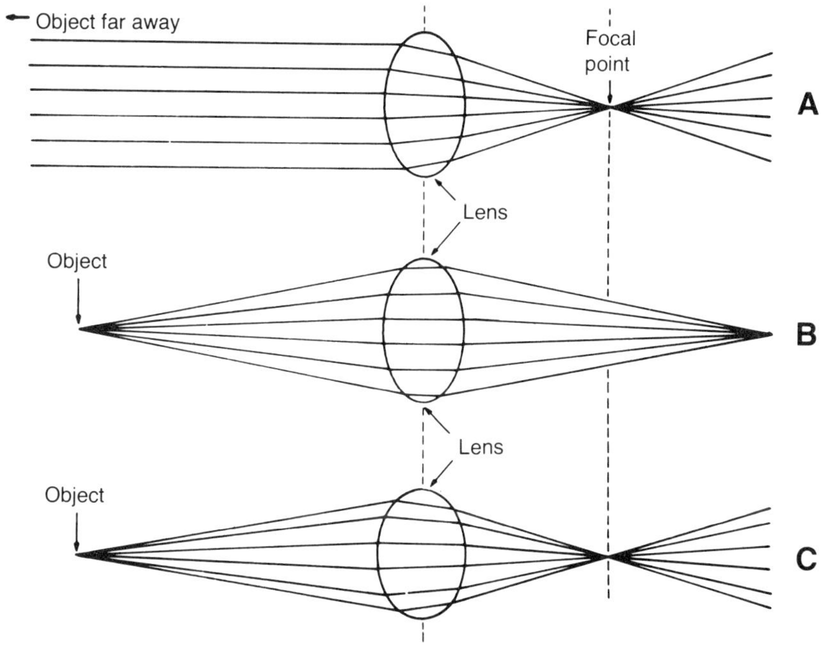

FIG. 7-2. Convergence of light by a convex lens. **A.** Light from an object far away is brought to focus at the focal point of the lens. **B.** Light from a nearer object is brought to focus at a point farther away than the focal point of the lens. **C.** The radius of curvature of the lens must be decreased to bring light to focus at the focal point of the lens in **A.**

slowly in some materials, for example, water and glass, than in air. The amount of slowing in a material is specified by its **refractive index**, which is the ratio of speed of light in a vacuum (the speed of light in air is slightly less, but extremely close) to the speed of light in the material (speed in vacuum/speed in material). If light passes from one medium to another at an angle to the interface between them, the rays are bent as shown in Figure 7-2A, where parallel rays of light emanating from an object far away are bent as they pass through the convex lens in such a way that they converge onto a point in space. Where they converge depends upon the strength of the lens, which is specified by its **focal length.** The focal length of a lens is the distance from the center of the lens to the point of focus of light from a distant object. Focal length is a function of the refractive index of the lens material and the radius of curvature of the lens. The larger the radius of curvature, that is, the less spherical the lens, the longer the focal length is.

A convenient way to specify the focal length or strength of a lens is in terms of the **diopter,** the reciprocal of the focal length of the lens expressed in meters. As you know, there are two kinds of lenses, convex lenses (converging lenses), like that shown in Figure 7-2, and concave lenses (diverging lenses). With a convex lens the image of an object is formed on the side of the lens opposite from the object. With a concave lens no actual image is formed, but physicists identify a virtual image that lies on the same side of the lens as the object. Because the images lie on opposite sides of the lenses in the two cases, convex lenses are assigned positive diopter values (presumably for their real images) and concave lenses are assigned negative diopter values. For example, a convex lens with a focal length of ½ meter is a +2 diopter lens, whereas a concave lens with a focal length of ⅓ meter is a −3 diopter lens. The higher the absolute value of the diopter rating of a lens, the stronger it is, that is, the more it converges or diverges light that enters it.

When objects are close, the distance from the lens to the point of focus varies with the distance to the object. Thus, the light from a source farther away in Figure 7-2A is brought to focus closer to the lens than that from a source nearer the lens in Figure 7-2B. In the eye, the distance from the lens to the

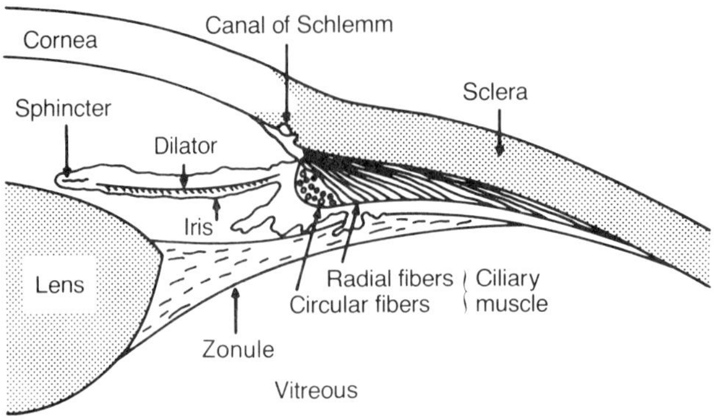

FIG. 7-3. The anterior portion of the eye. The arrangement of the lens, the zonule, and the ciliary muscles is illustrated along with the position of the iris and the arrangement of the muscles associated with it. (Weymouth FW: The eye as an optical instrument. In Ruch TC, Patton HD [ed]: Physiology and Biophysics, 19th ed. Philadelphia, WB Saunders, 1965)

retina is fixed; thus, in order to focus the light from a near source and also light from a far source, the strength of the lens must be alterable (the lens made more spherical), a process called **accommodation** and illustrated in Figure 7-2C. The lens is a flexible structure that, when released from the tension of the zonule, becomes nearly spherical in shape. The lens normally is under considerable tension and thus is flattened, a condition appropriate for focusing objects at a distance. Under these conditions, light from near objects is brought to focus behind the retina but is unfocused on the retina. Because of the way in which the ciliary muscles are attached (see Fig. 7-3), their contraction results in a relaxation of the tension on the lens, causing the lens to become more curved, thereby bringing nearer objects into focus on the retina. By grading the amount of contraction of ciliary muscles and therefore the tension on the lens, the nervous system can focus objects located from about 9 cm from the eye to infinity.

Control of the ciliary muscles is exercised by the autonomic nervous system, which uses information obtained from the retina itself to adjust the focus of an image. Presumably, the pathway for producing accommodation must involve the retina, optic nerve, lateral geniculate nucleus, visual cortex, pretectal nuclei, and finally the oculomotor nucleus, relaying in the ciliary ganglion to reach the ciliary muscles. Participation of visual cortex and pretectal nuclei is inferred from the fact that accommodation is normally accompanied by pupillary constriction and convergent eye movements, in conjunction with the observation that stimulation of visual cortex results in pupillary constriction. This is not a very compelling argument, but it is all we have at present. The nerve fibers supplying the ciliary muscles are parasympathetic postganglionic fibers and cholinergic (they use acetylcholine as a transmitter substance). Transmission through the cholinergic junction is readily blocked by atropine, which produces relaxation of the ciliary muscles so the lens is flattened and focused for distant objects. Ophthalmologists frequently relax the ciliary muscles to test the eye for refractive errors, but they use a shorter-acting parasympathetic blocking agent, such as tropicamide.

Actually, the lens is not strong enough by itself to focus a parallel beam of light on the retina. The cornea also acts as a lens (of fixed strength) and accounts for about 75% of the refractive strength of the optical system. The total refractive power of the eye is about +60 diopters. The cornea accounts for about +45 diopters, the lens only +17 diopters, and the remainder of the +60 is accounted for by the liquid–tissue interfaces. (Note: Some of the interfaces are from regions of higher refractive index, *e.g.*, cornea 1.376, to regions of lower refractive index, *e.g.*, aqueous humor 1.336, and thus act as diverging lenses, in this case with a power of −5.9 diopters.) The lens has a higher refractive index than the cornea (1.386 vs. 1.376), but it is surrounded by fluids with refractive indices much higher than that of the air (1.000) at the anterior boundary of the cornea. It is the ratio of the refractive indices that determines the refractive power of an interface. The greatest ratio occurs at the air–cornea interface. With accommodation, the eye gains another +10 to +12 diopters depending upon age. Loss of the cornea requires a strong convex lens (about +45 diopters) to correct for the loss in refractive power, but a weak lens will correct for loss of lens function. The real problem in loss of lens function is the inability to refocus from near vision to far vision, a fine adjustment that the lens provides.

ERRORS OF REFRACTION

With increasing age, the lens loses some of its plasticity so that even though the ciliary muscles contract and release tension on the zonule, the lens cannot round-up as it should. The result is that near objects cannot be properly focused, calling to mind the image of a man in his 40s or 50s (the age at which this condition becomes apparent) holding a book at arm's length in order to read the small print. The nearest point at which the eye can distinctly perceive an object is referred to as the **near point.** At 10 to 30 years of age, the near point is about 9 cm in front of the eye. It gradually recedes from the eye, being about 28 cm at 45 years and 80 cm at 60 years. There is a gradual loss in ability to see close objects. This condition is called **presbyopia** or old-sightedness. Presbyopia is related to a general condition called **hyperopia** or far-sightedness in which images are formed behind the retina. Hyperopia, shown in Figure 7-4A, results when the length of eye is too short for the refractive power of the lens; this can result from having too short an eyeball or too weak a lens system. When a weak lens system results from age-related changes in the lens itself, the condition is presbyopia. The hyperopic eye sees distant objects clearly only by using the normal accommodative mechanism of the lens. It does this at the expense of constant contraction of the ciliary muscles, which produces eye strain. Further, because part of the accommodative process is used to see even distant objects, less is available for viewing near objects; very near ones are never in focus.

Because the image is focused behind the retina in hyperopia, the correction is accomplished by increasing the stength of the lens system, converging the light beam even more. This involves putting another

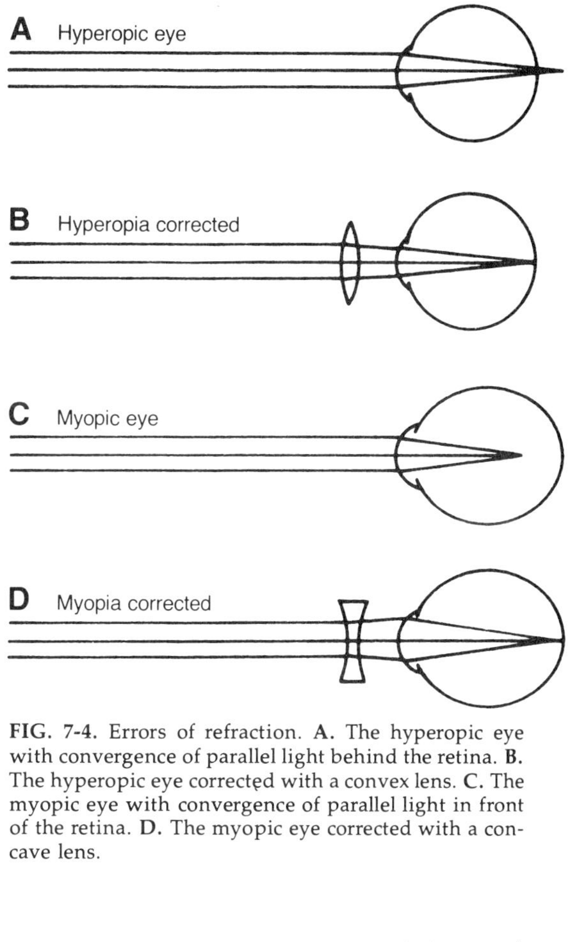

FIG. 7-4. Errors of refraction. **A.** The hyperopic eye with convergence of parallel light behind the retina. **B.** The hyperopic eye corrected with a convex lens. **C.** The myopic eye with convergence of parallel light in front of the retina. **D.** The myopic eye corrected with a concave lens.

convex (or positive, in terms of diopters) lens in front of the eye, as shown in Figure 7-4B.

Another common deviation from the **emmetropic,** or normal eye, occurs when the image comes to focus in front of the retina as illustrated in Figure 7-4C. This condition, called **myopia** or near-sightedness (because near objects are readily focused), results when the eyeball elongates too much for the refractive power of the lens. Most commonly, myopia occurs beginning at puberty. For the myopic eye there are always points sufficiently near, from which light diverges enough to be brought to focus upon the retina, but light from all points at greater distances cannot be focused. Ophthalmologists use the term **far point** to refer to the remotest point at which an object is clearly seen by the unaccommodated eye. In the myopic person, the far point is closer to the eye than normal. The optical correction for this condition is shown in Figure 7-4D. A concave (or nega-

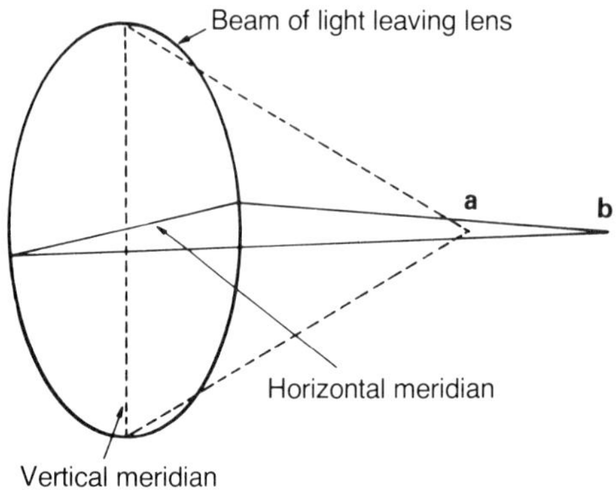

FIG. 7-5. The mechanism of production of astigmatism. Illustrated at left is a beam of light leaving the lens. Because the radius of curvature is greater along the horizontal meridian the light passing through that meridian is focused at point **b** whereas light passing through the vertical meridian of lesser radius of curvature comes to focus nearer, at point **a**.

tive, in terms of diopters) lens of the appropriate power (refractive index and curvature) diverges light rays from more distant objects enough to compensate for the overconvergence of the lens and bring a focused image onto the retina of the lengthened eyeball.

Yet another error of refraction, **astigmatism,** results from asymmetry of the cornea (occasionally also the lens). The ideal refractive surface is symmetric in all meridians such that a line of light would come to focus in the same place no matter how it was oriented. When this is not the case, an astigmatism results. Figure 7-5 shows that in the astigmatic eye a beam of light emerging from the lens is brought to focus along the vertical meridian (the axis of least radius of curvature in our example) at a and along the horizontal meridian (the axis of greatest radius of curvature) at point b. If point a lies on the retina, then a line in the vertical meridian would be focused, a line in the horizontal meridian would be blurred. If point b were on the retina, the situation would be reversed. In the normal eye, points a and b would be the same. Astigmatism usually results from a cornea that is not spherical, but more egg-shaped with the long axis not parallel to the direction light is traveling to the retina. Correction for astigmatism is accomplished by using a combination of a spherical and cylindrical lens, usually ground from a single piece of glass in such a way that (in Fig. 7-5) refraction would be increased in the horizontal or decreased in the vertical meridian or both depending upon the location of the retina with respect to points a and b. An optometrist must determine how the asymmetry is oriented as well as how strong to make the corrective lens.

THE PUPIL

The functions of the pupil are to produce sharp images, especially in close work, to alter the depth of field, and to help regulate the amount of light striking the retina. When the pupil constricts, it prevents light from entering the periphery of the lens. It is on the periphery where **spherical aberrations,** that is, unequal refraction of light by different parts of the lens, and **chromatic aberrations,** unequal refraction of light of different wavelengths, are greatest. Spherical aberrations occur because light passing through the edge of a lens is actually refracted more than light passing through its axis and comes to focus in front of the axial focus. The image formed on the retina of a spot of light in the visual field is a spot surrounded by several rings instead of a single spot. An entire object would appear blurred under these conditions. The pupil partially reduces the influence of this aberration when it constricts, allowing light to enter only through the center of the lens. Light of long wavelengths, like red light, is refracted less than light of shorter wavelengths, like violet light, so the lens tends to separate wavelengths or colors, producing a rainbow effect. This effect (chromatic aberration) would be the worst on the periphery of the lens where spherical aberration is greatest. Exclusion of the periphery of the lens is important in partially reducing the formation of color rings around an image. Constriction of the pupil or **miosis** also helps to reduce the rings around an image that result from light entering the eye from objects too far or too near to the lens to be in focus at a given radius of curvature.

The **depth of field,** that is, the range of distances over which images are in focus for a given strength of the lens, is also a function of pupil diameter. When the eye is focused on objects at a great distance, the depth of field is normally large and pupil size is relatively unimportant. When focused for near objects, however, the depth of field is small and can be increased markedly by closing down the pupil, just as it is by decreasing the aperture in a single-lens reflex camera.

The pupil also changes diameter with changes in light intensity at the retina, an increase causing the pupil to constrict and a decrease causing the pupil to dilate. This response is termed the **light reflex.** Within limits, the light reflex provides an adequate amount of light on the retina, increasing the amount in dim light, decreasing it in bright light. The aperture of the pupil is not a constant function of light intensity because the sensitivity of the retina changes as a result of **adaptation,** which we will consider shortly. Thus, when the light intensity increases moderately, the pupil constricts, but then under constant illumination it gradually dilates again. With larger changes in intensity, the pupil will remain constricted. It is not unusual for the eye to experience a millionfold change in light intensity, but the pupil is only capable of about a fourfold change in diameter that corresponds to about a 16-fold change in light intensity. This is not much compared to the total range the eye can experience; the greater part of the compensation is accomplished through retinal adaptation. However, the pupillary reflex system is extremely fast compared to retinal adaptation that takes minutes.

The light reflex is mediated by the autonomic nervous system. The afferent limb of the reflex involves the retina and the optic nerve. Fibers in the optic nerve give off collaterals to the pretectal nucleus, a structure just rostroventral to the superior colliculus. From this nucleus, fibers run bilaterally to the Edinger-Westphal nucleus, part of the oculomotor nucleus (third cranial nerve), forming connections with fibers of the third cranial nerve that are parasympathetic. These fibers relay again in the ciliary ganglion to innervate the sphincter pupillae. Increasing the amount of light at the retina increases the discharge to the various relays, finally causing contraction of the sphincter, closing down the pupil. At the same time the sympathetic fibers that innervate the dilator pupillae are inhibited by this increased activity, relaxing this antagonistic muscle. Decreasing the amount of light at the retina causes an increase in sympathetic activity and dilation while it reduces the output to the sphincter through the ciliary ganglion. That the pretectal nucleus connects to the Edinger-Westphal nuclei bilaterally accounts for the fact that both pupils normally constrict together even though the light is shown into only one eye. The constriction of the pupil through which the light is shown is called the **direct light reflex;** constriction of the contralateral pupil is called the **consensual light reflex.** The existence of the consensual reflex is a great aid in determining the location of pathology involving this system. A lesion of the **afferent limb** of the reflex (the part conducting toward the brain, including the optic nerve up to the pretectal nucleus) results in abolition of both the consensual and direct responses evoked by shining a light in the eye on the same side as the lesion, whereas a lesion of the **efferent limb** (the part conducting away from the brain) results in abolition of only the direct response evoked from the affected side (though the consensual reflex evoked from the unaffected side is also abolished).

The mechanism of accommodative miosis (pupillary constriction accompanying accommodation) is not identical with miosis of the light reflex, as indicated by their dissociation in certain disease processes. An example is the **Argyll Robertson pupil** that occurs in most syphilitic infections of the central nervous system. The pupil is constricted and is not responsive to light, but does respond normally during accommodation. The only regular pathologic concomitant of syphilitic infections of the central nervous system is gliosis surrounding the aqueduct of Sylvius that has been interpreted to indicate damage to the Edinger-Westphal nucleus. This implies that there are different cells for the two kinds of miosis, one type resistant to the spirochete. However, the cause of the Argyll Robertson pupil is not certain. In **diphtheritic neuritis,** the converse occurs: The pupil responds normally to light, but does not show accommodative miosis.

Dilation of the pupil is a normal concomitant of emotional states such as fright or alarm. The dilator reflex is also elicited by most forms of noxious stimulation. Use has been made of the change in pupil size that occurs with pleasurable sensations in monitoring responses of patients in many clinical situations.

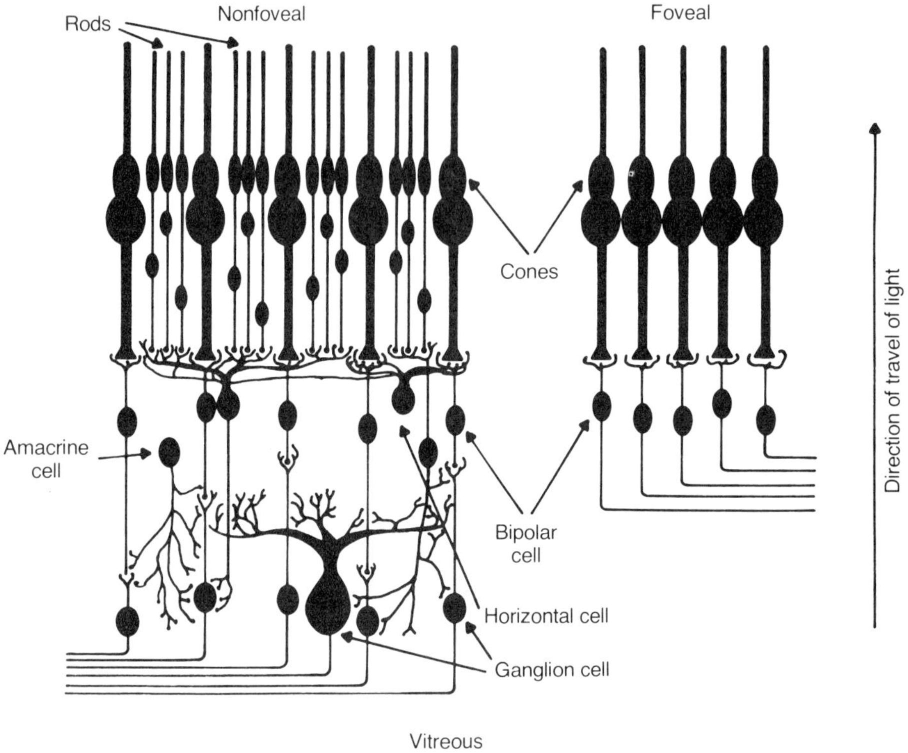

FIG. 7-6. The cellular organization of the foveal **(right)** and nonfoveal **(left)** retina. Notice the higher density of cones, their one-to-one connection with bipolar cells, and the absence of ganglion and other cells in the foveal area. Rods, located only outside the fovea, converge in large numbers onto bipolar cells.

RECEPTIVE FUNCTIONS OF THE EYE

The photoreceptors of the eye are located within a thin sheet of tissue, the retina. The structure of the retina is illustrated in Figure 7-6. Two types of receptors are present in the retina, the **rods** and the **cones,** so named because of their characteristic appearance. The human retina contains about 6.5×10^6 cones and 100×10^6 rods. Both rods and cones are found in the receptor layer of the retina, the outermost layer nearest the choroid. The receptors are connected to cells in the middle layer of the retina, the bipolar cells, which are in turn connected to cells in the innermost layer, the ganglion cells. The axons of the ganglion cells are the fibers that eventually come together to form the optic nerve. Also in the retina are amacrine and horizontal cells that interconnect the bipolar cells and carry activity from receptors to the bipolar cells. These latter two cell types may play a role in sharpening images by surround inhibition. In addition, the retina contains neuroglia and blood vessels that support the tissue. It is important to note that because of the way the retina is oriented, light entering the eye reaches the receptors only after passing through the network of blood vessels, cells, and fibers. The light finally reaches the light-sensitive photopigment in the outer segments of the receptor cells (Fig. 7-6) and what is not absorbed there is absorbed by the pigmented choroid, although a small part may be reflected back to the receptors.

The receptors themselves consist of an inner and outer segment. The outer segment is composed of neatly folded lamellae that contain the photosensitive pigments that change their structure by isomerization when they absorb light. When they do so, they produce a change in the membrane potential of the receptor cell, the receptor potential. The term receptor potential is preferred here because no action potentials are generated in the receptors themselves. In fact, it is in the third-order ganglion cells that action potentials first appear in the visual system. The inner segment is joined to

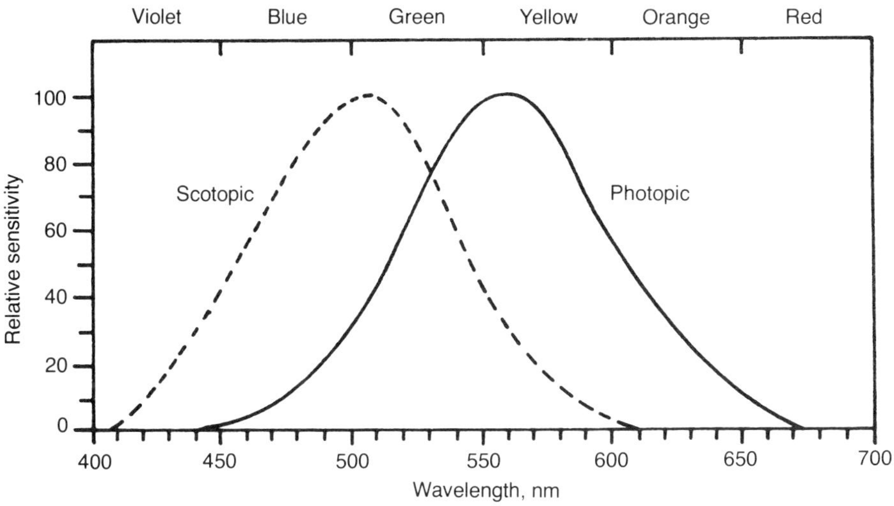

FIG. 7-7. Photopic and scotopic visibility curves. Threshold intensity is plotted against wavelength for the dark-adapted eye **(scotopic curve)** and the light-adapted eye **(photopic curve).** (Winton FR, Bayliss LE: Human Physiology, 5th ed. Boston, Little, Brown, 1962)

the outer segment by a narrow constriction that has characteristics of a true cilium. The inner segment contains mitochondria and endoplasmic reticulum and may be immediately adjoined to the cell body, as in cones, or connected to the cell body by a slender process, as in rods. The axon arises from the soma in both rods and cones.

The retina may be partitioned into several regions that differ somewhat in structure. The central region or **fovea** ("pit") is a small depression of the retina (a concavity on the inner or vitreal side) that is thinner than elsewhere. The fovea is about 1500 μm in diameter in man. Only cones are present in the fovea. The **macula lutea** or "yellow spot" is a region, including and surrounding the fovea, in which yellow pigment is found in the neuron layers of the retina. In the region surrounding the fovea, there is a gradual decrease in the density of cones and a gradual increase in the density of rods until, at the outer margin of the retina, there are almost no cones at all. Finally, there is a region in which there are no receptors, but an accumulation of the ganglion cell axons to form the optic nerve where it leaves the eye. This region, called the **optic disc,** forms a blind spot.

RETINAL SENSITIVITY

Visual systems specialize in the detection of electromagnetic radiation. The human visual system is sensitive to radiation in wave lengths from 400 to 700 nm, that is, the spectrum of visible light from violet through red. Monochromatic sensitivity (sensitivity to one hue) varies continuously through the spectrum; thus thresholds are normally expressed as a curve called the **visibility curve,** relating sensitivity to wavelength. Actually, there are two such curves because the sensitivity varies with the immediate history of the eye. Figure 7-7 shows these curves. If the eye has been in darkness for at least 30 minutes, and the tests are done with brief exposures, the curve on the left results. This is called the **scotopic** visibility curve, and it covers the range from 400 to 625 nm with a maximum sensitivity at about 507 nm, that is, sensitivity is maximum to blue-green light. If, on the other hand, the eye has been in normal daylight, the curve to the right, the **photopic** visibility curve, results. The maximum sensitivity for photopic vision is at 555 nm or in yellow-green light. The values on the ordinate are normalized so that both curves reach a peak at a value of 1.0. If this were not the case, the scotopic curve would be much taller because the eye is much more sensitive after being in the dark than after being in the light. These properties are the result of the characteristics of the receptors that lie in the retina.

Rods and cones not only differ in their appearance, but also in their connections to the bipolar cells and in the kind of visual pigment they contain. Some important dif-

TABLE 7-1. COMPARISON OF RODS AND CONES

	CONES OR "THE CONE SYSTEM"	RODS OR "THE ROD SYSTEM"
Threshold	Relatively high	Exquisitely low
Distribution	Ubiquitous, but concentrated at the fovea	Nonfoveal retina only
Convergence	Limited or none in fovea Probably more elsewhere	Extensive
Illumination	Photopic (day light)	Scotopic (night)
Functions	Central vision Color vision Detail vision	Peripheral vision Achromatic vision Poor detail vision

ferences are summarized in Table 7-1. It is these differences that account for many of the physiological properties of the retina. Cones in the fovea connect in a one-to-one fashion with bipolar cells that connect in a one-to-one fashion with ganglion cells, as illustrated in Figure 7-6. On the other hand, outside the fovea several rods and cones connect to a single bipolar cell, as illustrated at the left in Figure 7-6. Because many rods connect to a single bipolar cell, a given amount of illumination will more strongly excite bipolar cells in the rod system than in the cone system. In addition, the rods themselves are more sensitive to light, showing six times as much change in membrane potential per **quantum** of light as cones. Thus, the sensitivity of the retina is greater where there are more rods and less where there are only cones. This accounts for a phenomenon well known to sailors on watch. A very faint light seen out of the corner of the eye where the image falls on rods disappears when the eyes are turned toward the light, where the image falls on cones in the fovea. The greater sensitivity of the rod-connected system gives it superiority in scotopic or night vision, which lacks color information, whereas the cone system normally functions in photopic or day vision, which is in color. It is not clear why there is such an abrupt shift from rod to cone dominance in the photopic condition, but it appears that rod functioning is somehow suppressed when cones are active.

ACUITY

The measure of **acuity** or detail vision is the minimum distance between two points, which are clearly seen as separate points, at a standard distance from the observer. Humans with normal acuity can distinguish two points separated by an angle of one minute of arc. This is usually expressed clinically as the reciprocal of the angle or 1.0; values less than 1 indicate reduced acuity. Some people can distinguish separations as small as 0.5 to 0.33 minute of arc and therefore have acuities of 2.0 to 3.0. Because the retina is an array of receptors and not a continuous sheet, two point sources of light will only be seen as separate if the light from each one falls on a different receptor and the receptors are connected to separate communication lines to the brain. From what you have already learned about the retina, you should immediately conclude that acuity is greatest in the fovea. This is illustrated in Figure 7-8, where visual acuity has been plotted against position of the test spot on the retina. Acuity is 1.0 in the fovea and falls to 0.1 within 30 degrees. Acuity is, of course, zero in the blind spot where there are no receptors.

The fovea is specialized for detail vision in several ways: (1) The cones are more slender and more closely packed than elsewhere in the retina. (2) There are no rods present. (3) Each cone has its own labeled line in the optic nerve. (4) The blood vessels and extra cells are pushed out to the side of the fovea, reducing their light scattering to a minimum. These factors combine so that the acuity near the edge of the macula is only half that at the fovea, and the acuity at the periphery of the retina is only one-fortieth that at the fovea. The fovea may also act as a lens to magnify the image in that region. Recall that the fovea is concave. Because the retina has a higher refractive index than the vitreous, it could act as a

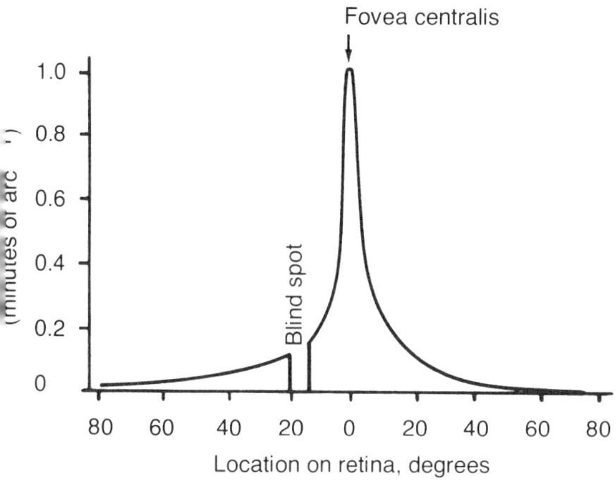

FIG. 7-8. Visual acuity as a function of position on the retina. Note position of blind spot **(abscissa)** and maximum acuity (1.0) at fovea centralis. (Grüsser O-J, Grüsser-Cornehls U: Physiology of Vision. In Schmidt RF [ed]: Fundamentals of Sensory Physiology. New York, Springer-Verlag, 1978)

diverging lens that would magnify the image on the dense array of cones, further increasing acuity in the fovea.

ADAPTATION

Everyone has experienced the changes in visual sensitivity that occur when going from a situation of bright light into one of dim light, such as when entering a darkened theater. At first not much can be seen, but, after a period of time, a considerable sensitivity returns. This is called **dark adaptation.** The reverse condition, a supersensitivity, followed by a decrease in sensitivity on emerging from the dark, is similarly termed **light adaptation.** Figure 7-9 shows the time course of dark adaptation. In the graph, the log of the threshold for vision is plotted against time in the dark on the abscissa. The threshold decreases in two phases, one lasting 7 minutes and the other beginning at about 7 minutes and completed by 30 minutes. During this time, the threshold has decreased by nearly a millionfold.

The two phases probably represent changes first in the cones and then in the rods. There are four pieces of evidence for this conclusion: (1) If colored light is used, the sensation is chromatic to the break point (arrow in Fig. 7-9) and then it becomes achromatic. (2) If red light (rods are insensitive to red light) is used and directed only at the fovea, the second phase is absent (Fig. 7-9, curve a). (3) In persons with severe cases of congenital night-blindness **(nyctalopia),** in whom rod function is apparently completely absent, the second phase is absent (Fig. 7-9, curve a). (4) Individuals lacking cones, that is, completely colorblind persons, show only the second phase of adaptation, but starting at zero time in the dark (Fig. 7-9, curve b).

Dark adaptation results from the fact that vision is a photochemical process. When light strikes the visual pigment, for example, the scotopic pigment, rhodopsin, the pigment is broken down (bleached), but it can be re-formed over a period of time. The sensitivity of the receptor is a direct function of the amount of unbleached pigment. In the light, pigment is bleached faster than it is re-formed and there is a reduction in sensitivity. This is light adaptation. If enough pigment is bleached, a temporary blindness develops. On the other hand, when the light-adapted person goes into the dark, his sensitivity to light is low because most of his pigment is in the bleached condition, but because the pigment is being bleached at a lower rate, the regeneration process can re-form the pigment faster than it is being bleached. The result is a gradu-

FIG. 7-9. The time course of dark adaptation. The threshold in log units for vision is plotted as a function of time in the dark. Adaptation in the normal eye **(solid curve)** occurs in two phases. When colored light is used, sensation is chromatic to the **arrow**, achromatic thereafter. Curve **a** is the adaptation curve for a night-blind person. Curve **b** is the adaptation curve for a completely color-blind person. (Grüsser O-J, Grüsser-Cornehls U: Physiology of Vision. In Schmidt RF [ed]: Fundamentals of Sensory Physiology. New York, Springer-Verlag, 1978)

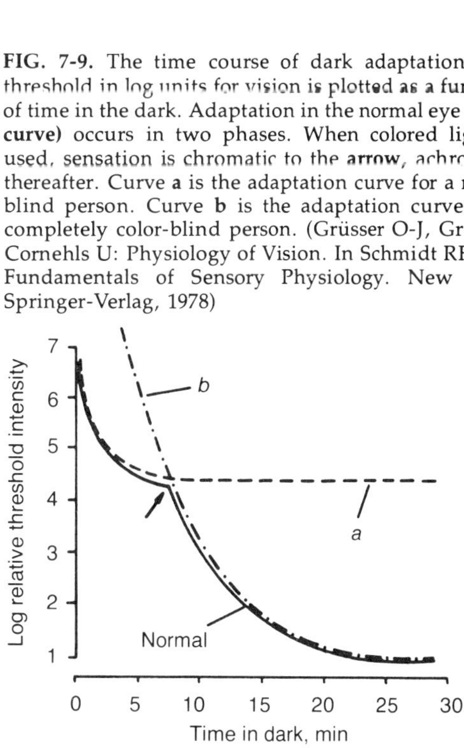

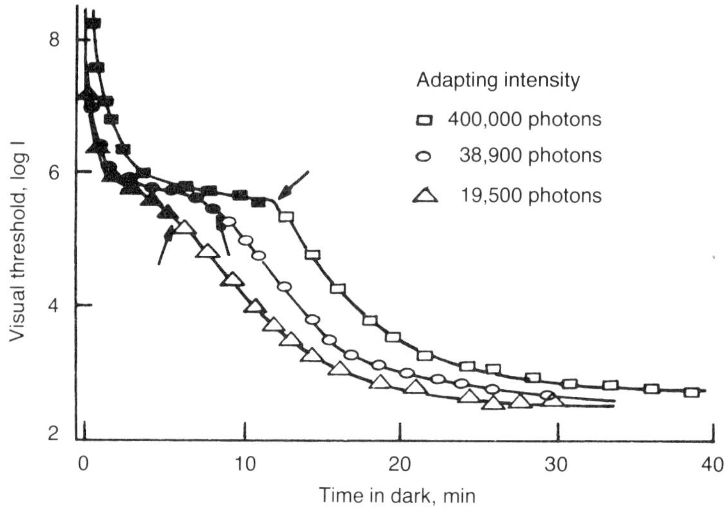

FIG. 7-10. The course of dark adaptation as measured with violet light following different degrees of light adaptation. The **filled-in** symbols indicate that a violet color was apparent at the threshold, whereas the **empty** symbols indicate that the sensation at threshold was colorless. (Hecht S, Haig C, Chase AM: J. Gen Physiol 20:831–850, 1937)

FIG. 7-11. Contributions of the individual color-receptor mechanisms to the total foveal sensitivity of a single human subject. In this particularly blue-sensitive observer, when the total foveal sensitivity is given a maximal height of 1.0, the heights of the B, G, and R curves are 0.053 : 0.575 : 0.542. In the average observer, the blue component is only about one-third as high as that shown here. (Wald G: Science 145:1007–1016, 1964)

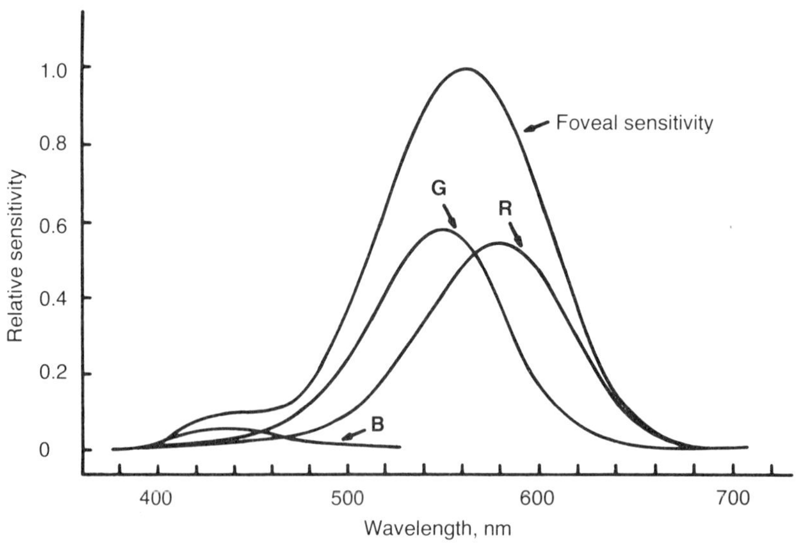

ally increasing quantity of unbleached pigment and thus a gradual increase in sensitivity or dark adaptation.

At first, it may seem puzzling that the rod adaptation curve of Figure 7-9 is delayed. One reason for this is that cone pigments regenerate more rapidly than rod pigments. Also, the cone system seems to exert a suppressive control of the rod system, as mentioned earlier. Clinically, this suppressive effect is manifest in the **photophobia** of the totally color-blind person. The totally color-blind person functions well in dim light but has an abnormally (painfully) high sensitivity in bright light. This presumably reflects the lack of suppression of rods by the cone system.

The break point in the adaptation curve of normal subjects (arrow in Fig. 7-9) comes at a later time in the adaptation period when a brighter light is used in the period before the dark adaptation is measured. This is illustrated in Figure 7-10, where the same data used in Figure 7-9 are plotted (19,500 photons) along with curves for two higher intensities of light during the pre-dark adaptation period. Again, the break points are indicated by arrows. This delay reflects an increase in light adaptation in brighter light that in turn reflects a greater amount of bleaching of the photosensitive pigments.

COLOR VISION

It is the cone receptors that contain the visual pigments that are sensitive to the color of light. In the last century, two physiologists, Thomas Young and Hermann von Helmholtz, proposed that there are three fundamental color (hue) sensations, red, green, and violet (or blue), and that there are three different kinds of color receptors, one for each of these colors. Excitation of a given kind of receptor leads to the sensation of the appropriate color, and all other color sensations result from simultaneous excitation of more than one of these receptors. Thus, equal excitation of all three receptor types leads to the sensation of white light, whereas the appropriate amounts of excitation of red and green receptors yields the sensation of yellow, and so on. This theory, called the **Young-Helmholtz theory** or the **trichromatic theory,** is the generally accepted theory today.

In the early 1960s George Wald (a visual physiologist who later was awarded the Nobel prize) measured the sensitivity of the pigments of the fovea using psychophysical methods. His results are shown in Figure 7-11. The overall spectral sensitivity of the cones was measured by shining lights of various wavelengths on the fovea and determining the threshold strength for each. A plot of these thresholds is seen in the bold (upper) curve in the figure. Then, the fovea was illuminated (adapted) with blue-green light (blue and green), presumably bleaching the green and blue pigments, leaving only the red functioning, and a new spectral sensitivity curve was measured (curve R in the figure). Likewise, the fovea was adapted to purple (blue and red) light and the green pigment curve (curve G) was measured; the fovea was adapted to yellow (red and green) light and the blue pigment curve (curve B) was measured. The blue pigment curve shows peak sensitivity to light of wavelength about 440 nm, the green pigment to light of wavelength about 550 nm, and the red pigment to light of wavelength about 580 nm. It should be noted that only the red pigment is sensitive at all to light of wavelength about 440 nm, the green pigment to rather broad overlap in sensitivity throughout the remainder of the visible spectrum. In addition, the sensitivity of the blue pigment is very much less than that of either of the others.

Spectral sensitivities have also been measured for individual cones. In this case, the absorption of light of various wavelengths by the pigment in a single cone is the variable measured instead of the sensitivity of the person as indicated by his verbal report, as used by Wald. The absorption of light of a given wavelength is determined by shining a light of that wavelength into the eye and measuring how much comes back out. The difference between that amount and the amount that went in is the amount absorbed by the pigments. Plots of absorption spectra for eight cones, including two from human retinae and six from other primates, are shown in Figure 7-12. There are clearly three different kinds of absorption spectra represented in the figure, with peak absorptions at about 445, 535, and 570 nm. These curves are not bad matches for those in Figure 7-11, considering that they were obtained by different methods and that one represents individual receptor responses, whereas the other represents a pigment population response.

Evidence indicates that the three types of cones are not distributed uniformly across the cone portion of the retina. Blue cone density is highest at the edge of the fovea (the human fovea is 1° in diameter) and falls off markedly by 10° from the center. Red and green cones are distributed most densely in the fovea, with the density of green cones being higher than that of red cones. Over the entire retina the green cones are more dense than the red, which are in turn

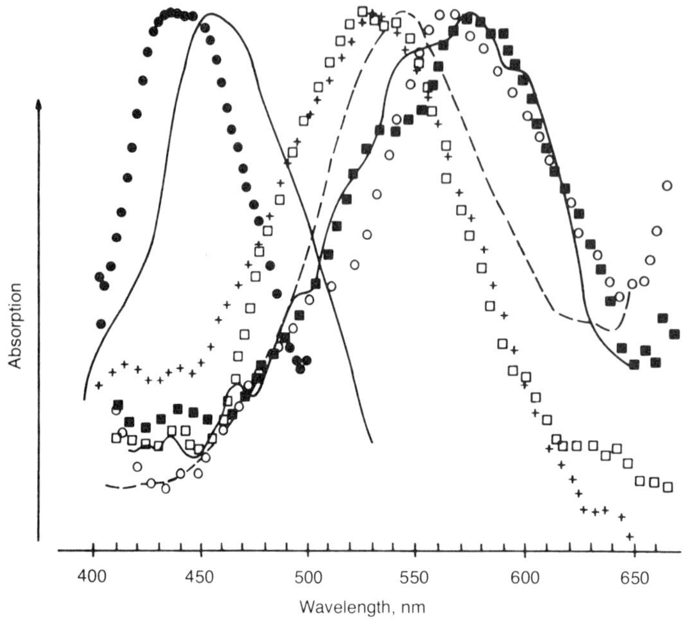

FIG. 7-12. Absorption difference spectra from eight primate cones. Two human cone spectra are indicated by the solid curves. Each symbol represents a different cone. (Wald G: Science 145:1007–1016, 1964)

FIG. 7-13. A. Representation of a color mixture experiment. The top half of the bipartite field is illuminated by the additive combination of red and green light. The bottom half of the field is illuminated with yellow light. **B.** View of the field as seen by the observer.

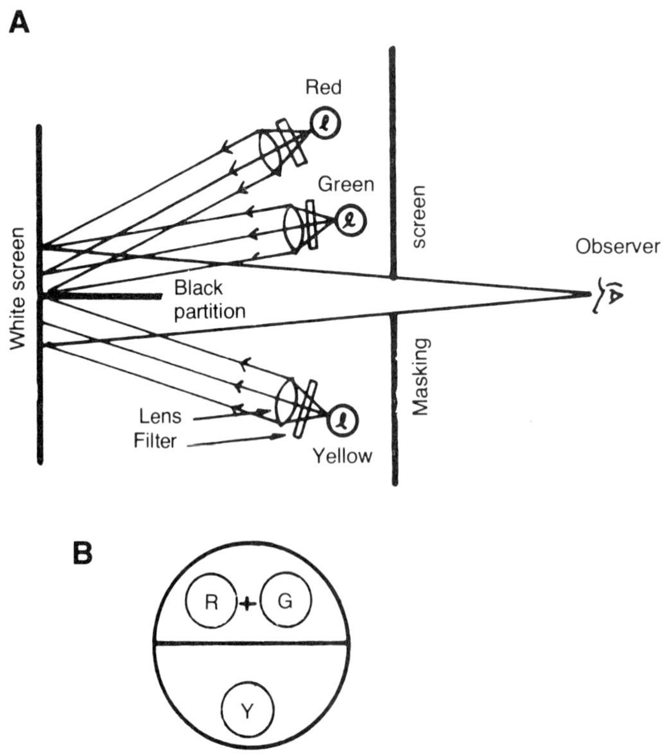

more dense than the blue. Furthermore, blue cones appear in regular arrays, whereas the others appear to be distributed randomly.

There are two ways of producing the various colors of the visible spectrum. One way is to shine a light of the appropriate wavelength in the eye. For example, the sensation of yellow light can be produced by shining a light of wavelength 590 nm in the eye. Alternatively, suitable amounts of light of three other appropriate wavelengths can produce the same sensation when shown into the eye at the same time. The same sensation of yellow light can be produced by mixing light of wavelength 545 nm (green) and 670 nm (red). No blue light is required to produce the sensation of yellow, but for other sensations a certain amount of blue light may be necessary. That this is true is indicated by the following experiment (Fig. 7-13). The observer looks through a hole in a partition at a white surface that is bisected by a black partition. What he sees is shown in Figure 7-13B. A yellow light of 589.3 nm is shown on the lower half of the field, and the observer reports seeing a yellow light. A light of 546 nm is shown on the upper half, and he reports seeing a green light; this is turned off and a light of 670.8 nm is shown on the upper half, which he reports to be red. When both the red and green lights are shown on the upper field at the same time at the appropriate relative intensities, he reports that both the upper and lower fields are the *same* color, namely yellow. This is the basis of function of the **anomaloscope** used to detect color blindness.

Red, green, and blue were taken as the primary hues in this example, because these are the ones used by the human eye. However, from a physical point of view, any three other pure spectral hues could also be used. For the human eye, any color experienced can be produced by a simple additive mixture of the correct proportions of red, green, and blue light.

COLOR BLINDNESS

Color blindness can be partially understood in terms of the mechanisms of color vision discussed above. Essentially, there are three types of individuals with respect to color vision, as follows:

- Trichromats
  - Normal
  - Protanomalous
  - Deuteranomalous
- Dichromats
  - Protanopes
  - Deuteranopes
  - Tritanopes
- Monochromats
  - Totally color blind

There are persons, including normals, who have three visual pigments that they use in their color perception. These are the **trichromats.** Those in a second class, the **dichromats,** match all the colors they see using only two pigments; those in the third class, the monochromats, see everything as a shade of gray, because they only see one color, white.

The **protanomalous** person has all three color pigments, but he has a deficiency in his red responsiveness. In the anamoloscope, he requires at least 1.5 times more red intensity than normal in the upper field to match a yellow in the lower field. The **deuteranomalous** person has reduced green sensitivity and requires at least four times more intense green than normal to match yellow. This is in fact how these abnormalities in color vision are detected, by measuring the amounts, relative to the normal, of red and green that are required to match a standard yellow. As a consequence of this reduced sensitivity, a person with a color anomaly can identify fewer hues than a normal person can. A normal person can distinguish about 150 different hues, whereas a protanomalous or deuteranomalous person distinguishes only 5 to 25 hues depending upon the severity of the deficiency. In addition, there are some interesting contrast phenomena that show up in anomalous individuals. For example, if a yellow light is shown in the lower field of an anomaloscope, the protanomalous individual identifies it as yellow, but if a green light is simultaneously shown in the upper field, he will report that the lower field is red. This does not happen in normal vision; the lower field remains yellow.

The dichromats present a different and more complicated picture. Figure 7-14 shows the luminosity curves for normal subjects, protanopes, and deuteranopes. The

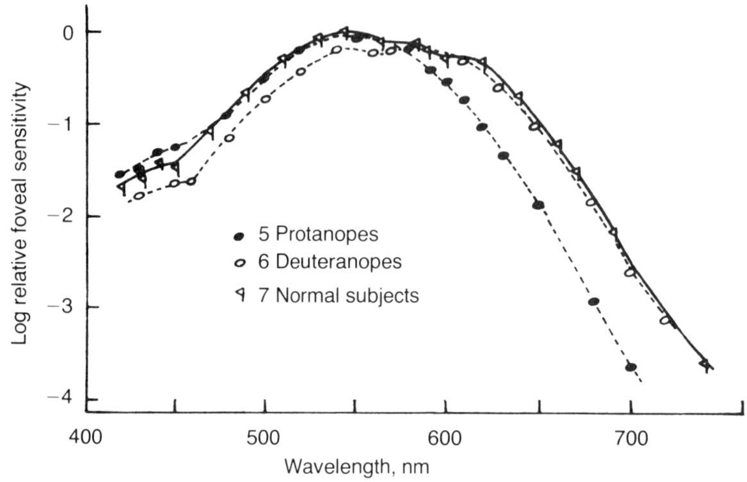

FIG. 7-14. Luminosity curves of color-blind and normal subjects. Downward in the graph represents loss of sensitivity, the log of the reciprocal of threshold energy. (Wald G: Science 145:1007–1016, 1964)

protanope lacks red-sensitive pigment altogether. Notice the more rapid fall of the curve for protanopes at the long end of the spectrum (reds). This is the characteristic that distinguishes protanopes; they are completely insensitive to light beyond about 680 nm. The result is that they see little or no red. They have been known to show up at a black-tie affair with a red tie on. The sensation of black is due to the absence of light and is therefore indistinguishable from red (of wavelength greater than 680 nm) by the protanope.

The **deuteranopes,** on the other hand, are insensitive to green light. There are two types of deuteranopes. There are those who have a reduced sensitivity to light in the middle and shorter wavelengths, which indicates an absence of green pigment (Fig. 7-14), and there are those with normal spectral sensitivity whose problem seems to be that the red and green mechanisms are coupled together to form a single sensory system. This may occur in the retina at the level of the bipolar or ganglion cells, or it may occur in the central nervous system. The **tritanope** is a rare individual who lacks sensitivity to the short end of the spectrum. Some people are of the opinion that tritanopia is not a retinal problem at all, but a disease of the optic nerve. Not enough information is available to say with confidence.

No matter what his deficiency, the dichromat matches all colors he sees with mixtures of only two pure spectral colors. The number of colors remaining chromatic varies with the type of dichromatism, but all of them are interpreted as various saturations of blue and yellow for the protanope and deuteranope, and red and green for the tritanope. For each individual, there is a point between his two basic sensations that he matches with what a normal person sees as white. For the protanope this occurs at about 495 nm; for the deuteranope it occurs at 500 nm; for the tritanope it occurs at 572 nm. One unanswered question is why the protanope (and by analogy, the deuteranope) sees yellow at the middle (long end) of the spectrum and not green (red). It is possible that the pigment present (either red or green) excites both red and green mechanisms in the central nervous system resulting in a sensation of yellow. Kalmus (1965) has reported an interesting individual who was a dichromat in one eye and trichromat in the other.

CASE HISTORY

A healthy young woman had normal color vision in her right eye and was dichromatic in her left. Using her left eye she had only three color sensations: gray, yellow, and blue. When she was shown a spectrum, any light of a wavelength above a neutral zone (wavelength 502 nm) appeared to be yellow whereas any shorter wavelength appeared blue. At 502 nm she described the sensation as gray or neutral using her left eye, but as green using her right. She could match all the longer wavelengths (green to red) seen with her left eye to light of wavelength about 570 nm seen through the right eye and all shorter wavelengths (green to violet) with light of about 470 nm. Altogether in her left eye she lacked any green or red sensations. When using both eyes she perceived the full color range and applied the appropriate names to it.

The cause of **anomalous trichromacy** (protanomaly or deuteranomaly) is usually stated to be an abnormally small amount of the appropriate pigment in the cones. This cannot be the case as evidenced by the following experiment:

A normal observer adjusts red and green intensities to match a yellow in an anomaloscope, as described above. He then looks away from the anomaloscope into an intense red light, bleaching the red pigment. If he looks immediately back into the anomaloscope, he will see green light in both the upper and lower fields, and both are the same green without adjustments of the intensity. If he adapts to green light instead, he will see the same red in both fields. This indicates that the anomaloscope cannot distinguish the color-adapted eye from the non-color-adapted eye. We know that color adaptation results from a simple reduction in nonbleached pigment. It follows that if the anomaly were due to such a simple reduction, the anomaloscope would not detect it, but it does.

What then, is the cause of anomalous trichromacy? A protanope can exactly match green with any red of wavelength less than 680 nm simply by adjusting the intensity of the red. As a result, an experimenter can exchange the matching red with the previously presented green, and the protanope will be none the wiser. The reason for this is that his green-cone pigment catches the light equally and experiences no change when the lights are switched. The same trick cannot be played on a protanomalous individual; he sees the switch. His green pigment cannot detect it; this suggests he may have some anomalous pigment. In fact, such anomalous pigments have been identified by using the preceding trick to measure their sensitivities. The anomalies are probably due to a malfunction in the process for making the pigment. The correct red is replaced by an anomalous one that is less sensitive in the red region in the protanomalous individual, and, in the deuteranomalous individual, the green is replaced by anomalous pigment that is more like the red pigment. The sum of these effects is that the remaining normal pigment (green in the case of protanomaly) and the anomalous pigment sensitivities are much closer together than are the two normal pigments (red and green), and the individual has a harder time distinguishing colors in this region of the spectrum. He thus requires more intensity of red to excite the anomalous pigment than he would to excite a normal red pigment to achieve the proper balance of green and red (anomalous red pigment) excitation.

Protan and deuteran disturbances (terms of protanomaly and protanopia and for deuteranomaly and deuteranopia, respectively) are simple, sex-linked recessive traits. The trait is linked to the X chromosome, so the condition is most common in males. Females show the condition only if they have it present on both X chromosomes. These conditions occur in 1% to 13% of males, depending upon the country (USA about 8%), but only 0.5% females. The normal condition is dominant to the protan or deuteran, and the anomalous condition appears to be dominant to the anopic. The control of green and red pigments seems to be at two separate loci on the chromosome, as indicated by family history data and the existence of women with normal color vision, but with one deuteranope and one protanope son. In the latter case, the women must have carried one defective gene of each type, yet neither was expressed in their phenotype. Deuteranomaly is the most frequently encountered defect, with protanomaly, deuteranopia, and protanopia less but about equally frequent. Tritanopia only occurs in about 0.002% of the male population and thus it is a rare event.

The last color vision defect is monochromatism. This usually shows up in the form of total color blindness in which all colors are perceived as shades of gray. People with this problem are photophobic, as we have mentioned, and show only scotopic luminosity curves. There are cases of subtotal monochromatism in which blue cones are not or only minimally involved or in which mainly macular cones are affected. The result is nearly the same because of the similarity of the blue cone and rod spectral sensitivities and because the macula is the major region used in vision in humans.

PHYSIOLOGY OF SINGLE VISUAL NEURONS

VISUAL NEURONS IN THE RETINA

The receptor cells and the bipolar cells of the retina respond to light with graded, electrotonic responses rather than with all-or-nothing action potentials. The graded responses in the receptors are the result of the photochemical process, but those in the bipolar cells are synaptically driven. Furthermore, it is surprising that the receptors respond to light with a hyperpolarizing receptor potential, which is accompanied by an increase in membrane resistance. Figure 7-15 shows a schematic diagram of a section of the retina with two receptors, one illuminated, the other unilluminated. The responses of the receptors, bipolar, ganglion, horizontal, and amacrine cells are shown in circles representing each cell type. The time when a small spot of light was turned on is indicated by the upward deflection of the lower trace of each pair and the response of the cell by the upper trace. The hyperpolarizing responses of the illuminated receptor and its subjacent bipolar cell are illustrated as are the action potentials generated by the ganglion cell. Apparently, the photochemical process somehow closes membrane channels that are normally open in the dark. It is now known that in the dark there is a constant inward Na^+ current (dark current) flowing through the outer segment membrane and an outward current near the junction with the bipolar cell. This keeps the cell partly depolarized and transmitter substance is continuously released onto the bipolar cell depolarizing it. The light flash decreases the dark current, hyperpolarizing the cell relative to its dark state and decreasing the amount of transmitter released. This accounts for the curious hyperpolarizing receptor potentials. The major line of transmission of information is from receptor to bipolar cell to ganglion cell and then to the brain, but the amacrine and horizontal cells provide lateral transmission lines that can produce the complicated center-surround receptive fields of ganglion cells. The horizontal cells receive their inputs from receptors as do the bipolar cells and, like the bipolar cells, they generate no spikes. Horizontal cell outputs inhibit (reduce transmission at) nearby unilluminated receptor-bipolar cell synaptic junctions. It has been suggested that they may enhance contrast by strongly turning off unstimulated bipolar cells. Amacrine cells produce action potentials and enter into reciprocal synaptic relations with bipolar cells.

The response recorded from ganglion cells following light stimulation of the receptors is more conventional. Depolarizing synaptic potentials initiate trains of action potentials that propagate along the ganglion cell's axon. Ganglion cell responses are of three types: (1) They respond (either discharge or increase their rate of discharge) only when the light is turned on; (2) they respond only when the light is turned off; or (3) they discharge only at the beginning and end of a light period. These are called **on-responses, off-responses,** and **on–off-responses,** respectively. The receptive fields of ganglion cells are usually circular areas of retina, as shown in Figure 7-16. Illumination within the small central area produces an on-response in some cells (a) and an off-response in others (d). In a, the neuron responds when the light goes on, but gives no response when it goes off (on-center); in d, another neuron does not respond when the light goes on, but does respond when it goes off (off-center). Illumination of an annular, fringe area produces an off-response in the first type of ganglion cell (trace b, off-surround) and an on-response in the second (trace e, on-surround). When a ganglion cell fails to discharge at an on- or off-transient of the light, it is not because it is not being excited, but because it is being inhibited, as is indicated by the fact that illumination of both center and surround simultaneously produces both a reduced on-response and a reduced off-response (c and e) compared to those produced by illuminating either center or surround alone. This effect is termed **lateral inhibition** or **surround inhibition.**

A look back at Figure 7-15 may help to understand how responses of ganglion cells are generated. The illuminated receptor cell 1 hyperpolarizes, causing synaptic transmission to be reduced to bipolar cell 1 and

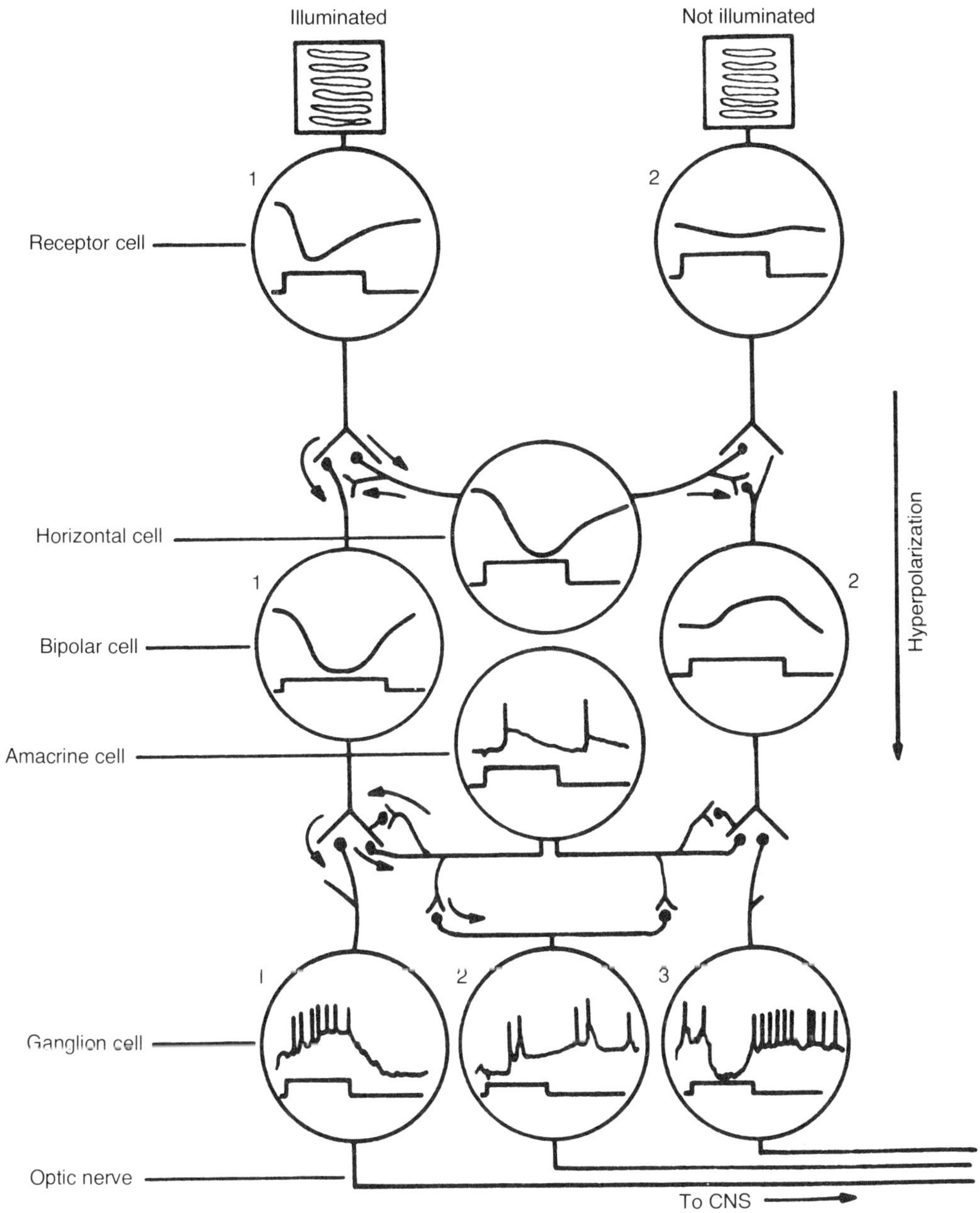

FIG. 7-15. Synaptic organization of the vertebrate retina and responses of retinal neurons. The receptor on the **left** is illuminated, that on the **right** is not. The intracellularly recorded response from each cell is illustrated in the **circle** corresponding to its cell body **(upper trace)** along with a monitor of when the illumination was present over the left receptor. The responses were recorded in the retina of *Necturus.* (Dowling JE, Werblin FS: Vision Res Suppl 3:1–15, 1971)

the horizontal cell. Both of these cells hyperpolarize. Transmission from bipolar cell 1 to ganglion cell 1 causes a depolarization that occurs when the light comes on (on-responses). Transmitter substance is released by bipolar cell terminals in response to hyperpolarization; this is opposite to the situation at most chemical synapses (see Chap. 13). Receptor cell 1 is in the center of the receptive field of ganglion cell 1, but it is in the surround of ganglion cell 3. The hyperpolarization of the horizontal cell by illumination of receptor cell 1 causes bipolar cell 2 to depolarize. This depolarization

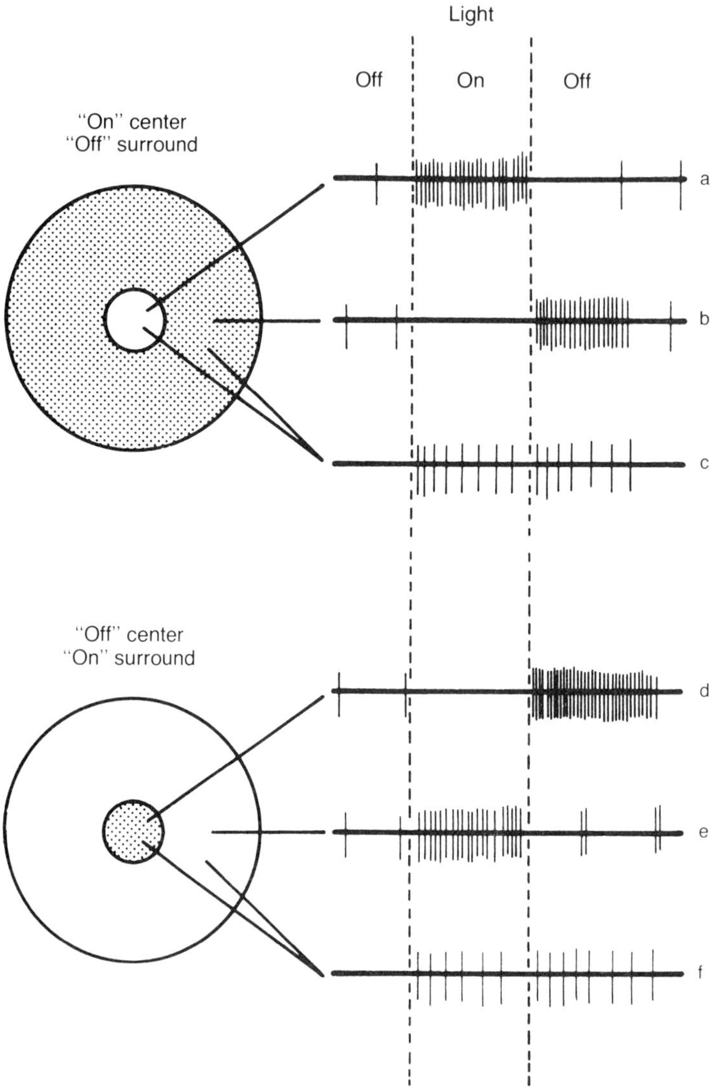

FIG. 7-16. Receptive fields of two retinal ganglion cells. Fields are circular areas of the retina surrounded by an annulus of different properties. The cell in the upper part of the figure responds when the center is illuminated (on-center, **a**) and when the surround is darkened (off-surround, **b**). The cell in the lower part of the figure responds when the center is darkened (off-center, **d**) and when the surround is illuminated (on-surround, **e**). Both cells give on- and off-responses when both center and surround are illuminated (**c** and **f**), but neither response is as strong as when only center or surround is illuminated (Hubel DH: Sci Am 209: 54–62, 1963)

prevents the release of transmitter substance from bipolar cell 2 onto ganglion cell 3 and the ganglion cell does not discharge. Actually, the ganglion cell is also inhibited (prevented from firing by hyperpolarization), perhaps through the amacrine cell. When the illumination of receptor cell 1 is turned off, bipolar cell 2 repolarizes. This repolarization is equivalent, as far as the transmitter release mechanism is concerned, to a hyperpolarization of the bipolar cell; it causes the release of transmitter substance onto the ganglion cell, which discharges (as the light goes off). This mechanism would account for on-center cells; presumably the mechanism for off-center cells would be similar.

The first stage of processing of color information is apparently at the level of the ganglion cell; at least this is the first one studied to date. Color-sensitive ganglion cells are sometimes called **color opponent cells,** because cone mechanisms of different spectral sensitivities (*i.e.,* red, green, and blue) interact in them antagonistically. Most of these cells have concentric receptive fields like other ganglion cells, with either on- or off-centers, and the centers are sensitive to red, blue, or green. The annular surround of an on-center gives an off-response for one of the other cone pigments. Cone mechanisms neighboring each other in the spectrum appear to oppose each other so that red centers have only green surrounds and blue centers have only green surrounds, but green centers can have either red or blue surrounds. Red–blue interactions have not been found. As an example, consider a red on-center, green off-surround cell. This cell discharges when the center of the receptive field is illuminated with red light; it is inhibited when the center is illuminated with green light, but discharges when a green light is extinguished after shining on the periphery; and it is inhibited by illuminating the periphery with red light. The result of these interactions is a rather narrow spectral response of the central portion of the receptive field compared with the absorption curve for the pigments. Thus, some of the very broad overlap in the absorption spectra of the neighboring pigments is eliminated by the nervous system, which forms six fairly narrow spectral channels of information with both on and off information about the image.

VISUAL NEURONS IN THE BRAIN

The axons of the ganglion cells form the optic nerves, which, after leaving the eyeball, proceed toward the brain until they come to the optic chiasm, where the optic nerves divide. Fibers from the nasal half of the retina cross to the opposite side of the brain; fibers from the temporal half go to the same side of the brain (Fig. 7-17). Past the chiasm, crossed fibers from the contralateral eye join the uncrossed fibers from the ipsilateral eye to form the optic tract. Fibers in the optic tract, which are still the axons of retinal ganglion cells, then proceed to the thalamus, where they end on cells of the lateral geniculate nucleus. The fibers of this nucleus project to neurons of the calcarine area of the occipital cortex. This is area 17 as enumerated by Brodmann and is often referred to as striate cortex because of its characteristic striped appearance under the microscope. There are also direct projections to adjacent areas 18 and 19, often referred to as visual association areas.

The receptive fields on the retina of single cells in the lateral geniculate nucleus are similar to those of ganglion cells. Retinal receptive fields of geniculate cells have excitatory centers and inhibitory surrounds or vice versa, but the fields are larger, probably because of convergence of more than one ganglion cell on each geniculate neuron. Despite the presence of both crossed and uncrossed optic tract fibers in the geniculate, each cell there only has a receptive field in one eye.

With respect to spectral sensitivity, geniculate neurons can be put into one of two categories: (1) narrow-band cells and (2) broad-band cells. Narrow-band cells respond with an increase in their discharge rate when their receptive fields are illuminated with light from part of the visible spectrum, and they decrease their discharge rate when their fields are illuminated with light from other parts of the spectrum. The majority of narrow-band cells either increase their response rates when their receptive fields are illuminated with red light and decrease their rates when illuminated with green light, or they increase their rates when illuminated with green light and decrease them when illuminated with red light. The remainder of the cells increase their discharge rates when illuminated with yellow light and decrease them when illuminated with blue light or increase their rates for blue light and decrease them for yellow light. No red–blue cells have been found. In most respects, the narrow-band cells are not very different from color-opponent ganglion cells except for the size of their receptive fields and the width of the spectrum to which they respond. The peak sensitivity in terms of wavelength of the excitatory and inhibitory responses of geniculate cells corresponds nicely to the peak absorption spectra of the three cone pigments. Broad-band cells receive a uniform excitation or inhibition when their receptive

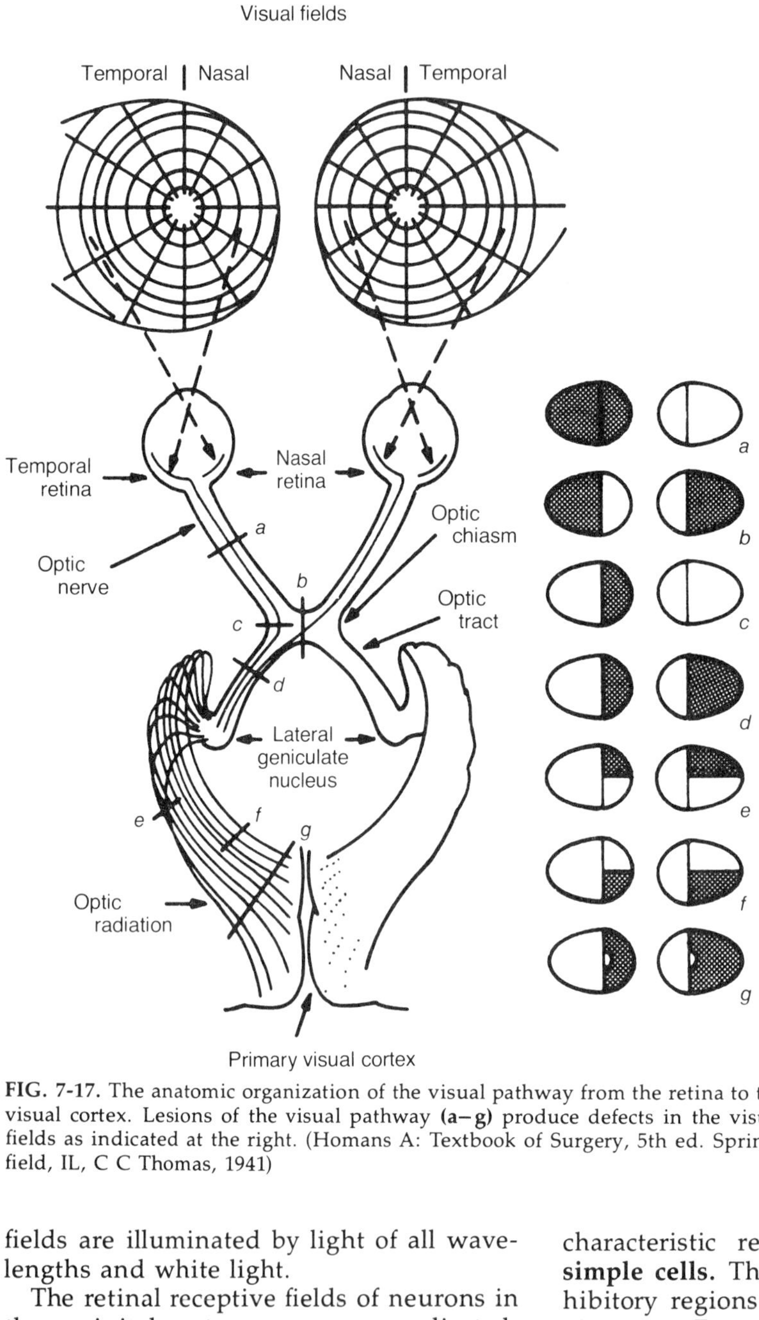

FIG. 7-17. The anatomic organization of the visual pathway from the retina to the visual cortex. Lesions of the visual pathway **(a–g)** produce defects in the visual fields as indicated at the right. (Homans A: Textbook of Surgery, 5th ed. Springfield, IL, C C Thomas, 1941)

fields are illuminated by light of all wavelengths and white light.

The retinal receptive fields of neurons in the occipital cortex are very complicated. Some visual cortical neurons (nonoriented neurons) possess receptive fields not particularly different from those of geniculate neurons; they have circular receptive fields and respond equally to stimuli of all orientations. However, the receptive fields of most cortical neurons are not circular, but are arranged as parallel barlike excitatory and inhibitory areas with straight rather than circular borders. Cortical cells with this characteristic receptive field are termed **simple cells.** These cells can have two inhibitory regions flanking an excitatory region, as in Figure 7-18; the reverse situation can occur; or there can be just two regions side by side, one excitatory, the other inhibitory. As a result, the cells respond best to narrow bars of light oriented in a particular direction across the retina. Rotation of the bar has two effects: (1) It reduces the excitation, because less of the excitatory area is illuminated, and (2) it increases the inhibition, because more of the inhibitory area is illuminated. The result is that the cortical

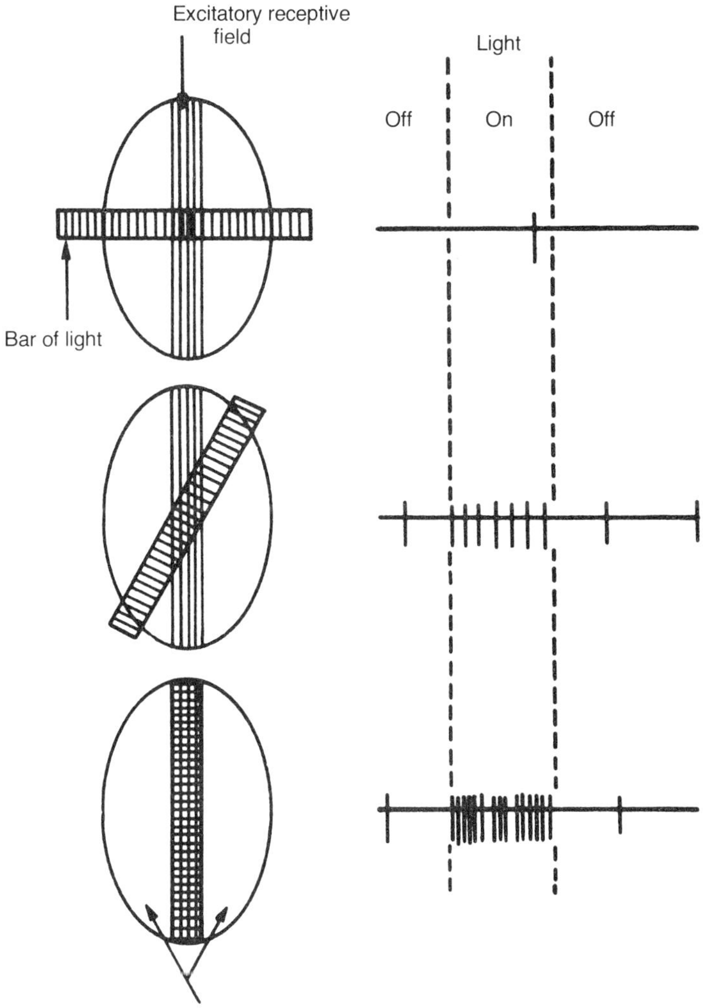

FIG. 7-18. The receptive field on the retina (ellipse) of a simple cell in the visual cortex is shown at the left with a bar of light superimposed on it at various angles. The **vertically striped** portion of the receptive field is the excitatory area (excitatory receptive field), illumination of which excites the cell; the **unhatched** portion is the inhibitory area (inhibitory receptive field), illumination of which inhibits the cell. The bar of light is **striped** across its length. The responses of the cell to the three different orientations of the light are shown at the right. (Hubel DH: Sci Am 209:54–62, 1963)

neuron responds less well when bars are not in their preferred orientation.

Complex cells are similar to simple cells in that they respond to bars or lines of light (or the edges of bright objects) of proper orientation. An example of the response of a complex cell is shown in Figure 7-19. At the right are shown records of discharges of a complex cell made with a patch of light off, then on, then off again, at the position indicated at the left of each record. The contour of the light patch is critical, because this cell responds to vertical lines. The cell responds vigorously when a light with a vertical edge is turned on (A) but hardly at all when the edge is sloping (B). The cell gives an on-response when the left part of the receptive field is illuminated (C and D) and an off-response when the right part is darkened (E and F). However, it gives no response at all if the whole field is illuminated (G). The receptive fields on the retina of complex cells, in general, do not have characteristic excitatory and inhibitory areas, but they may respond with an on-response in part of the receptive field and an off-response in another part. Cells vary widely in which part does which.

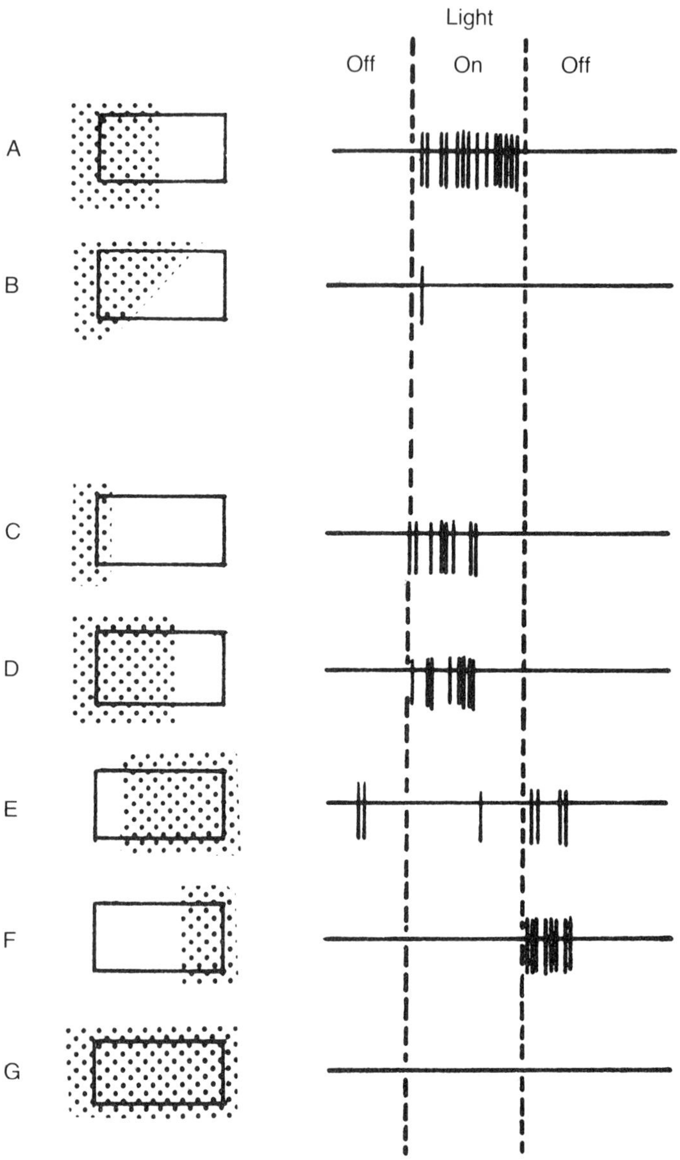

FIG. 7-19. The response of a "complex" cortical cell in the visual field to various illuminations of its large receptive field (8° × 16°) indicated by the rectangle. The **stippled** area is the area illuminated, and the response of the cell to the illumination and its cessation are shown on the **right**. (Hubel DH, Wiesel TN: J Physiol (Lond) 160:106–154, 1962)

In general, complex cells seem to be responsive to lines of sharp contrast. However, unlike simple cells that show only on and off-responses, complex cells respond in a sustained manner to moving lines. They respond better to a line moving in one direction than to the same line moving in the opposite direction across their receptive fields. Figure 7-20 shows the responses of a complex cell to various orientations of a moving bar with respect to the receptive field, as shown on the left. The responses of the cell to movement, first in one direction and then the other (arrows), are indicated at the right. For this cell, the best response occurs when the long axis of the bar is parallel to the long axis of the receptive field and the bar is moving toward the right. Speed of movement of the bar also seems to be an important parameter for some cells.

A third class of visual cortical cells, the **hypercomplex cell,** is much like the com-

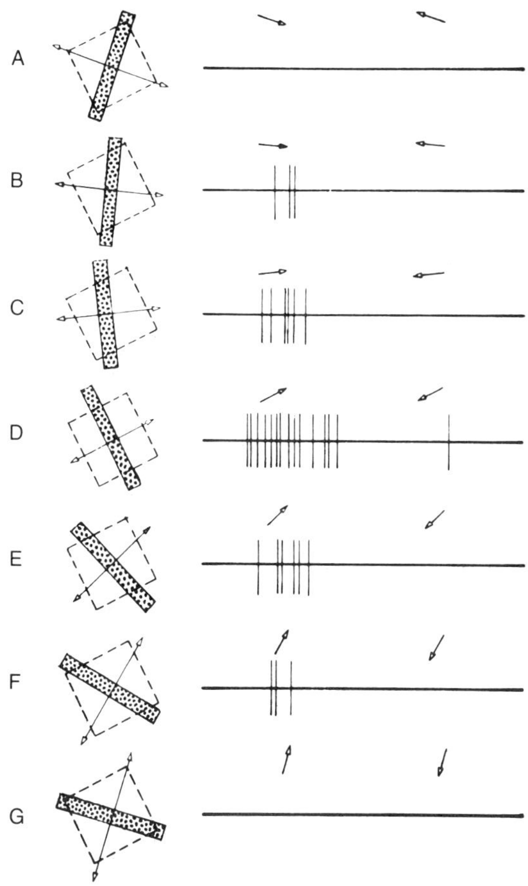

FIG. 7-20. Responses of a complex cell in right striate cortex (layer IV A) of *Macaque* to various orientations of moving black bar. Receptive field in left eye is indicated by interrupted rectangles, approximately 3/8° × 3/8° in size. Duration of each record, 2 sec. **Arrows** indicate direction of stimulus motion. (Hubel DH, Wiesel TN: J Physiol (Lond) 195:215–243, 1968)

plex cell in its response to lines of light or to the edges of bright objects, but with the added complexity that it turns off if the line or edge is too long. This is clearly seen by reference to Figure 7-21. Up to a certain point, increasing the length of the line increases the response, but beyond that point, increasing the length decreases the response. In short, they behave as if the excitatory receptive field is bounded on the ends by an inhibitory field, but no effects (either excitatory or inhibitory) on cell discharge are seen by stimulating these boundary regions alone.

Just how these cells are involved in creating vision is unknown, but some of the features that are abstracted are evident. Contrast, lines, edges, movement, direction of movement and length appear to be relevant variables in whatever these visual cells are doing.

The color sensitivity of visual cortical neurons is much the same as that of geniculate neurons. There are some with broad-band sensitivity and some with narrow-band sensitivity. Most of the narrow-band cells (those presumably signaling color information) are either nonoriented or simple cells. They are excited by light of some wavelengths of the visible spectrum and inhibited by some other wavelengths, much as described earlier for geniculate cells. Other cortical neurons, mainly some complex cells, are excited by illuminating their receptive fields with light from narrow bands at one end or the other of the spec-

FIG. 7-21. Hypercomplex cortical neuron (area 19 of cat). Stimulation of ipsilateral eye. Excitatory portion of retinal receptive field roughly 2° × 2°, represented by interrupted rectangle. **(A** to **G)** response **(right)** to slits 1/8° wide and of various lengths moved downward across receptive field at about 3°/sec **(left).** Note that inhibitory flank on right of excitatory region is weaker than that on left. Sweep duration, 1 sec. (Hubel DH, Wiesel TN: J Neurophysiol 28:229–289, 1965)

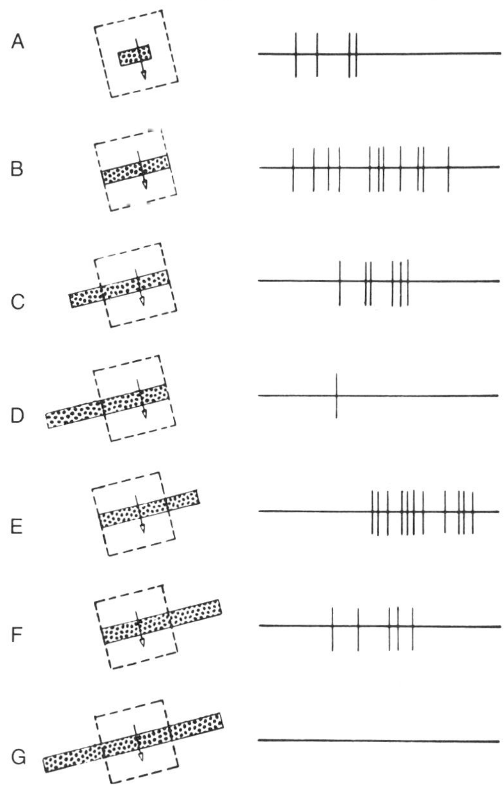

trum. These narrow-band cells make up about 54% of all those cells in samples from the foveal representation in the striate (visual) cortex. The broad-band cells are similar to broad-band cells in the lateral geniculate nucleus.

We have as yet no idea how color is perceived, but its perception seems to involve contrasting excitation and inhibition from the different types of cones or rather cone systems. There is some indication that as a cell's color specificity increases, its spatial selectivity decreases, implying that there are separate mechanisms (cells) for color and form perception.

CLINICAL ASPECTS OF VISUAL FUNCTION

It should be noted, by reference to Figure 7-17, that light striking the nasal retina comes from the temporal **visual field** and that striking the temporal retina comes from the nasal visual field. The monocular visual field is the total extent of the visual world that is seen by one eye at rest. It is customary to describe the defects of vision in terms of losses in the visual field. In the maps of Figure 7-17, the basic reference is a line perpendicular to a tangent to the cornea and passing through the center of the fovea. This is the **visual axis.** The visual axis is marked in the figure as the point in the center of the concentric circles. The vertical diameter of the circles is the same for both eyes so that there is considerable overlap in the visual fields of the two eyes, the basis for stereoscopic vision.

At the right of Figure 7-17 are shown defects of the visual field that would develop from lesions at the levels indicated by the corresponding letters on the diagram to the left. It is possible to work out these defects from knowledge of the anatomy of the visual pathway. Just keep in mind the following points:

1. The retinal image is inverted top to bottom and left to right with respect to the visual field.
2. Fibers from the nasal half of the retina cross over in the optic chiasm.
3. Fibers from the upper part of the retina segregate from those from the lower.
4. Upper retinal fibers from one eye stay with the upper retinal fibers from the other eye; the same is true for the lower retinal fibers.
5. Fibers from the upper part of the retinae are found dorsally in the superior optic radiation passing through the parietal lobe, whereas those from the lower part are ventrally in the inferior radiation passing through the temporal lobe.
6. The macula is represented on both sides of the cortex.

Loss of half of the visual field is called **hemianopsia.** If the visual field is half lost on either the right or the left, as for example in left optic tract section, Figure 7-17d, the loss is called **homonymous hemianopsia,** in this case, right homonymous hemianopsia. If the loss is in both temporal fields, it is called **bitemporal hemianopsia** (Fig. 7-17b). Likewise, the nasal counterpart is **binasal hemianopsia.** A **quadrantanopsia** results from interruption of either the superior or inferior optic radiation (clinically this usually involves a lesion in either parietal or temporal cortex) or alternatively from a partial lesion of the calcarine cortex, lower quadrants in the lingual gyrus, upper in the cuneate gyrus (Fig. 7-17e,f). The representation of the macula on both sides results in **macular sparing** after a complete lesion of one visual cortex. In this condition vision remains in the entire macula, as illustrated by the peculiar picture in Figure 7-17g.

For a long time, it has been generally agreed that complete removal of the visual cortex in man leads to total, permanent blindness in the contralateral visual field. In the last ten years, it has become clear that this is not the case in the monkey. With total striate cortex removal, the monkey is still capable of locating briefly presented stimuli in space and can still discriminate visual patterns. With less than total removal, the impairment is best characterized as a reduction in, not a loss of, sensitivity in part of the contralateral field and, with training, the sensitivity gradually improves. When the lesion involves more than the striate cortex, especially when it includes the posterior parietal and temporal cortices, the animal is reduced only to being able to tell whether the lights in its environment are on or off.

In man, there is seldom a pure striate cortex lesion because the tissue is buried in the calcarine sulcus. However, in a few cases of pure striate lesions, forced-choice discrimination methods have uncovered considerable visual function. The methods involve instructing the patient to guess the identity or point to the location of a stimulus even though he does not see it. Remaining capacities are much like those in monkeys with similar lesions and include the ability to locate stimuli in space, to differentiate the orientation of lines (vertical vs. horizontal vs. diagonal, including white on black and black on white), to discriminate shapes (X vs. O), and discriminate colors (red vs. green). The patients require moderately large stimuli; their performance falls off if the stimuli are too small. For the more difficult discriminations (where the stimuli are more alike, *e.g.*, vertical vs. diagonal lines), a slightly longer duration of exposure may be required.

Even though the human with the striate cortex lesion can perform without errors on such discriminations, he still reports that he saw nothing at all and expresses surprise when he is told of his performance. These observations emphasize the fact that information about stimuli goes to more than one center in the nervous system and show that what are sometimes called "subcortical relays" really do have functions. A person does not have to be able to report verbally the existence of a stimulus to respond appropriately to it. This sort of observation has led some investigators to parcel visual functions as (1) recognizing, identifying, or examining functions, presumably the territory of cortical visual tissues, and (2) detecting or orienting functions, presumably the territory of subcortical visual tissues. Only time will tell if this sort of distinction has meaning, but it does seem to fit the observations described.

There has been a flurry of activity designed to generate a prosthetic device for blindness. Such devices have been of two sorts: The first represents an attempt to use some other modality with pattern recognition capabilities, and the second, more daring effort, actually attempts to produce a visual image. An example of the first type of device is a television camera whose output is transduced into an array of small tactile stimuli that is applied to the skin of the back. The camera is worn on the head and the picture it sees is perceived by the wearer in sufficient detail that he can avoid obstacles while walking around. On the other hand, it can hardly be claimed that the person has vision.

The second type of device uses an array of photocells or a television camera whose output is applied to an array of small electrodes inserted into the retina or into the visual cortex itself. From what we know of the physiology and anatomy of the retina, it should come as no surprise that stimulation there has not reproduced visual experience. After all, the retina consists of about 106 million receptors, each independently sensitive to light. It seems unlikely that the activity of those receptors could be matched by a small array of electrical stimuli.

Electrical stimuli applied to the visual cortex typically produce sensations described as spots or balls of light that are either stationary or in motion. In no case has the sensation been one of perceiving an object, even when an array of stimulating electrodes was used. Although all these devices have proved useful in helping blind people get around, none of them reproduces the lost vision.

SUGGESTED READING

Baylor DA, Fuortes MGF: Electrical responses of single cones in the retina of the turtle. J Physiol (Lond) 207:77–92, 1970

Dowling JE, Werblin FS: Synaptic organization of the vertebrate retina. Vision Res (Suppl) 3:1–15, 1971

Kalmus H: Diagnosis and Genetics of Defective Colour Vision. London, Oxford Univ Press, 1965

Makous W, Boothe R: Cones block signals from rods. Vision Res 14:285–294, 1974

Osterberg G: Topography of the layer of rods and cones in the human retina. Acta Ophthalmol (Suppl) (Copenh) 61:1–102, 1935

Records RE [ed]: Physiology of the Human Eye and Visual System. Hagerstown, MD, Harper and Row, 1979

Weiskrantz L: Some aspects of visual capacity in monkeys and man following striate cortex lesions. Arch Ital Biol 116:318–323, 1978

8

Audition

An object vibrating in air sets up motion of the molecules in the air around it so that when the object moves in the direction of an observer, it compresses the air and when it moves away, it produces a rarefraction. This sequence of compressions and rarefractions is transmitted in a straight line through the air at a characteristic speed. Sound waves, unlike light, cannot travel through a vacuum, but require some medium, gaseous, liquid or solid, each medium with a different speed of conduction. The ear is a structure specialized to receive these vibrations of the air, transduce them into nervous impulses, encoding important features, and transmit the impulses to the central nervous system.

Highly sensitive mechanoreceptors in the ear are capable of sensing amplitudes of vibrations of the air as small as 10^{-8} centimeters (the diameter of a hydrogen ion is 2×10^{-8} cm), yet the ear is structured in such a way that it can withstand sound so intense that it vibrates the whole body (this may come at some cost as we shall see). It transduces sounds of frequencies from 16 Hertz (Hz = cycles/sec) to 20,000 Hz into nervous impulses, allowing the human to distinguish small changes in frequency as changes in **pitch:** The higher the frequency, the higher is the pitch. At the same time, a change in size or amplitude of the vibration is perceived as a change in **loudness.** Perceived loudness is actually a function of both frequency and amplitude because the sensitivity of the ear varies with frequency, being less sensitive at very low and very high frequencies and most sensitive to sounds in the frequency range of the human voice, that is, in the range from 80 Hz to 1.1 kHz.

The clinical procedure in which the sensitivity is tested over the normal range of human hearing is called **audiometry,** and the graphic representation of the sensitivity is an **audiogram.** Normally, clinical audiograms are not done with the precision required to test the absolute sensitivity of the hearing apparatus because it is just too difficult to control extraneous noise. A normal clinical audiogram is shown in Figure 8-1a. This should be compared with the audiogram obtained under ideal conditions (Fig. 8-1b). The human ear, in both types of audiogram, is most sensitive to sound of 1000 to 2000 Hz and that sensitivity is lower for frequencies both above and below this range. The measured thresholds are all higher on the clinical audiogram because it takes more sound intensity to reach the threshold of hearing when the stimulus tone is superimposed on a background of room noise.

The ordinate of Figure 8-1 is plotted in decibels (db), a logarithmic scale, because the useful range of intensity from the minimum audible to the maximum tolerable loudness spans 10^{14}–fold. Specifying intensities over such a range is unwieldly unless they are specified in terms of logarithmic units. The bel system simply designates the ratios between sound intensities in log units (common logarithms, base 10). Thus, 1 bel indicates a 10-fold change, 2 bels a 100-fold change, and so forth. More commonly the **decibel** is used; one bel = 10 decibels. The decibel system compares two intensities or pressures, so to specify a single intensity in decibels we must have a standard reference value. In audiology, the standard value is the threshold for a 1000-Hz tone, which is 2×10^{-4} dynes/cm^2 in terms of pressure. In normal clinical measurement, this standard is used because of its ease of measurement, and it is designated SPL (sound pressure level). To get some idea of sound intensity in terms of decibels, consider the following: Referenced to the threshold of hearing (0 db), a whisper is about +15 db, the average home noise level is about +25 db, conversation is about +60 db, and a jet engine makes noise at about +110 db. Painful sound has an intensity greater than +130 db.

Figure 8-2 illustrates how audiograms are used. In Figure 8-2A are plotted the **threshold of hearing** or **audibility curve** for a patient with a hearing loss (solid line) and a normal curve (dashed line). The patient's threshold is higher for every frequency above 128 Hz. The normal audibility curve is usually converted to a straight line at 0 db loss, and the patient's values are plotted as deviations from the normal values (in this case below, but they can also be above). The result is a **hearing loss curve,** as shown in Figure 8-2B. This particular patient has a high-tone (high-frequency) hearing loss such that there is a 20-db deficiency at 1024 Hz and a 40-db deficiency at 4096 Hz. The threshold of hearing for a 1024-Hz tone is elevated 100 times over normal, that is, 100 times more sound pressure is required for this patient to hear a tone of this frequency than for a normal person. Similarly, the threshold is elevated 10,000 times normal at 4096 Hz. In Figure 8-2B, the patient's loss at 16,384 Hz is about 60 db, which is a 1,000,000-fold increase in threshold in terms of pressure.

The shape of the hearing loss curve is used as an indicator of the type of pathologic condition from which a patient is suffering. Actually, the patient whose audiogram is shown in Figure 8-2 is normal, at least among people his age. Characteristically, advancing age is accompanied by decreased sensitivity to high tones, or **presbycusis.** This loss in sensitivity is the result of degeneration of the receptors in the basal

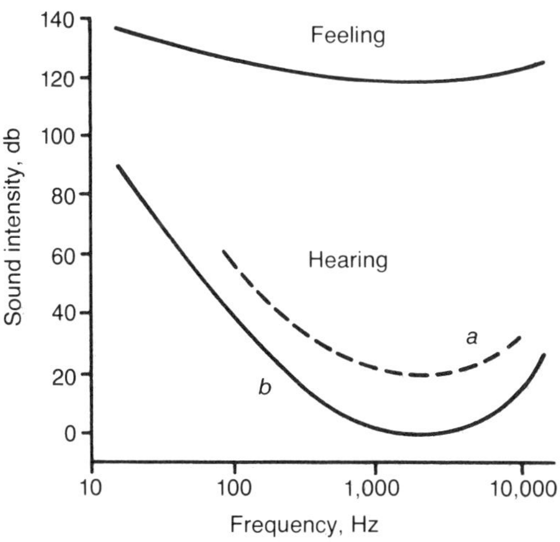

FIG. 8-1. Auditory sensitivity in man. The upper curve shows the threshold of pain for different frequencies. Curve **a** is the "clinical" threshold of hearing curve for a normal human; curve **b,** the laboratory threshold of hearing curve presented to show the effect of room noise on auditory threshold (Licklider JCR: Basic correlates of the auditory stimulus. In Stevens SS [ed]: Handbook of Experimental Psychology. New York, Wiley, 1951)

FIG. 8-2. How the threshold of hearing curve **(A)** is converted to a hearing-loss curve **(B).** The **dashed line** shows data from a normal subject; in the hearing-loss graph, this is converted to 0 db. The **solid line** shows data from a subject with high-tone hearing loss; **arrows** show the magnitude of the hearing loss. (Towe AL: Audition and the auditory pathways. In Ruch TC, Patton HD [eds]: Physiology and Biophysics, 19th ed. Philadelphia, WB Saunders, 1965)

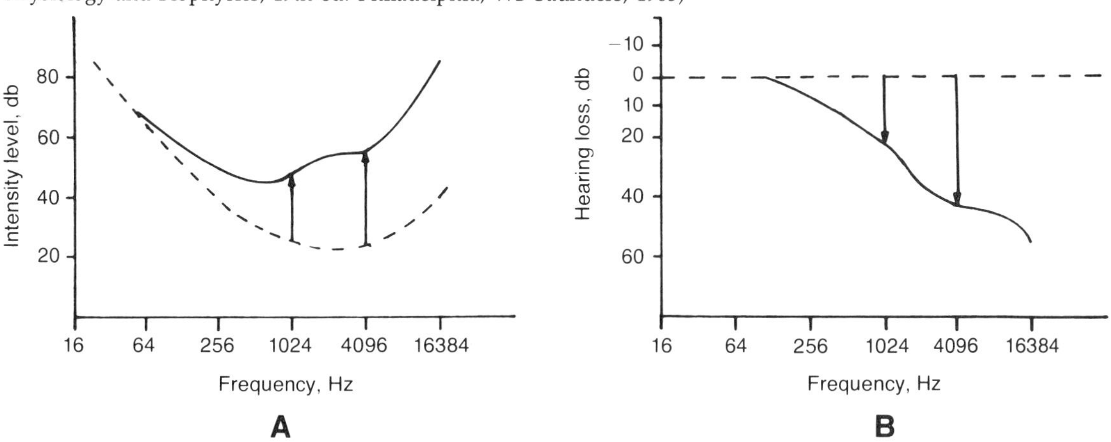

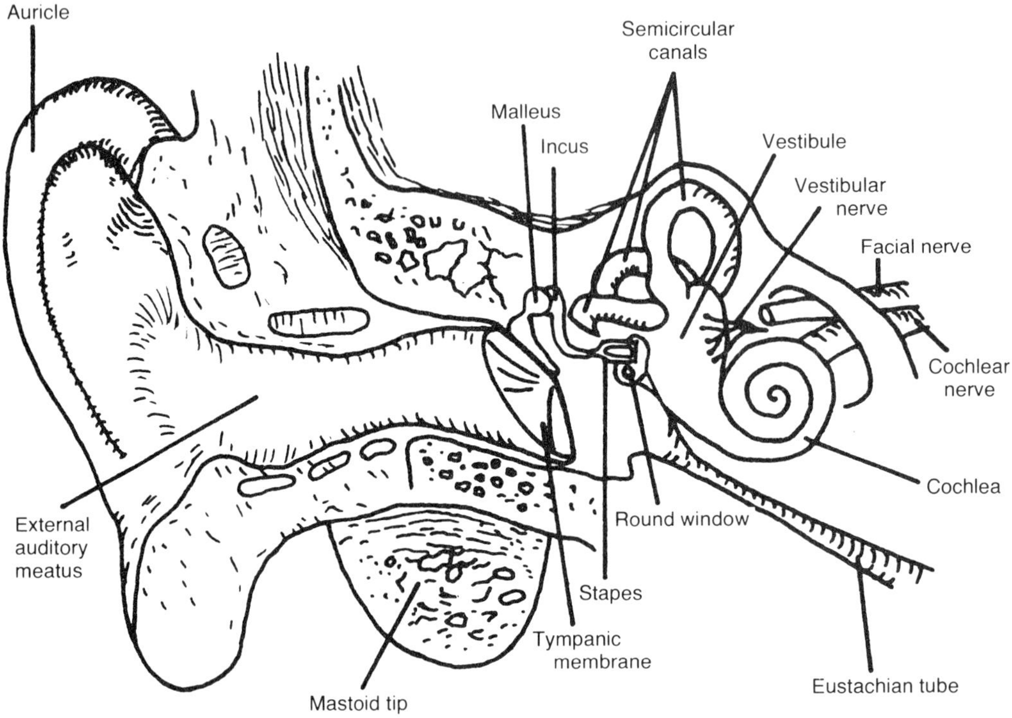

FIG. 8-3. The peripheral auditory apparatus with cochlea rotated slightly to show coils and auditory nerve. (Davis H, Silverman SR: Hearing and Deafness, 3rd ed. New York, Holt, Rinehart, Winston, 1970)

turn of the cochlea. We shall see later that other types of hearing loss also have characteristic audiograms.

ANATOMY AND MECHANICS OF THE EAR

The ear is normally considered to have three parts, an outer ear, a middle ear, and an inner ear, as illustrated in Figure 8-3. The outer ear consists of the auricle or pinna, the part seen on the outside; an elongated tube, the external meatus; and the tympanic membrane. The primary function of the auricle is to capture sound and funnel it into the external meatus, although the human auricle is undoubtedly a lot less efficient than that of many other animals, notably that of the dog. The shape of this structure may be of some help in localizing sounds in space, especially in distinguishing sounds coming from a source in front from those coming from behind the head.

The external meatus certainly acts as a channel for sound to the tympanic membrane, but it also shelters the ear drum and provides a relatively constant environment in terms of temperature and humidity, thus preserving the elasticity of the drum. It also acts as a tubal resonator, amplifying sound pressures particularly in the range of 2000 to 5500 Hz. The pressure amplification in this frequency range can be 5 to 10 db. The tympanic membrane is a cone-shaped piece of elastic tissue whose apex points inward and is the point of attachment of one of the ossicles, the malleus. Normally, the tympanic membrane is kept under tension for better reception of vibrations of high frequency. This tension is somewhat variable and under control of the tensor tympani muscle that attaches to the malleus at its point of contact with the tympanum and to the medial wall of the middle ear dorsal to the opening of the eustachian tube (Fig. 8-4). This muscle is innervated by fibers of the fifth cranial nerve, and its contraction pulls the drum dorsally and medially, tensing it.

Also within the middle ear are three small bones, the malleus, incus, and stapes. These three bones are linked together by hinge-

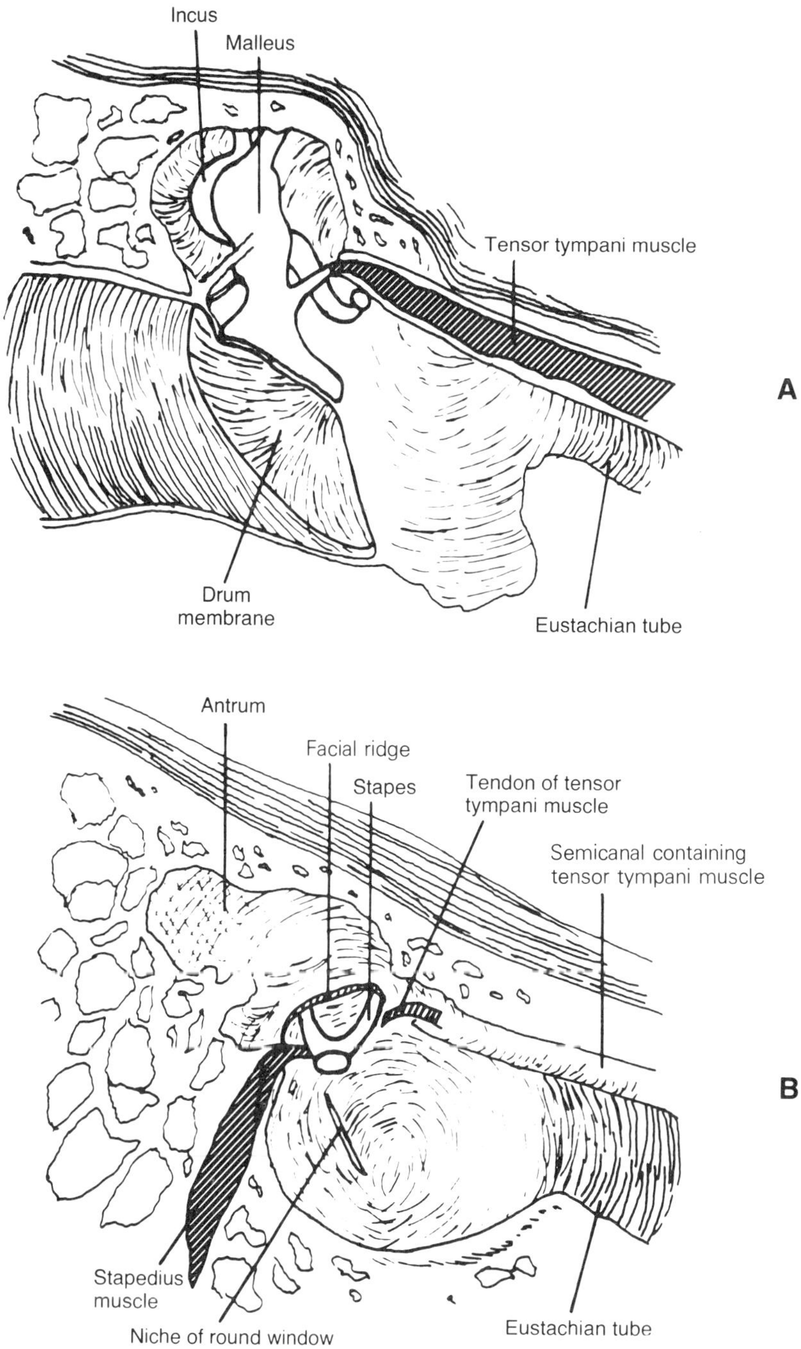

FIG. 8-4. The middle ear and its contents. **A.** Note the connection of the tensor tympani muscle to the malleus and the relationship of the malleus to the tympanum. **B.** A view of the external canal with the ear drum, malleus, and incus removed. Note the attachment of the stapedius muscle to the stapes. (Davis H, Silverman SR: Hearing and Deafness, 3rd ed. New York, Holt, Rinehart, Winston, 1970)

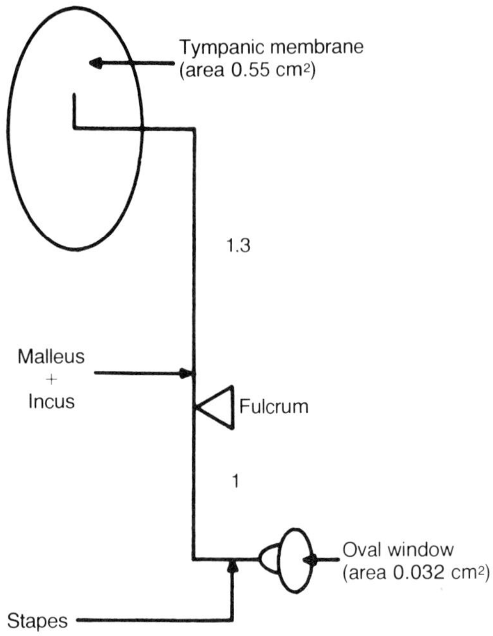

FIG. 8-5. Schematic drawing of ossicle system to illustrate the lever arms and the position of the fulcrum. Relative areas of tympanum and the membrane of the oval window are shown.

like joints and are joined to the tympanum as already described and to the membranous covering of the oval window of the cochlea. Movements of the typanum set the ossicles in motion, the malleus and incus vibrating as a unit and imparting a piston-like motion to the stapes, which pushes against the membranous covering of the oval window. The ossicular chain functions as an **impedance-matching device,** to compensate for the difference in impedance between air and the fluids of the inner ear. Acoustic impedance is the property of a material, roughly speaking, that relates the pressures produced to the amplitudes of vibrations when sound energy passes through a medium. If the impedances of two materials are drastically different, sound will not easily pass from one to the other. The impedance of the fluid in the cochlea is about 30 times higher than that of air, and if the sound were applied directly to the oval window, most of it (~97%) would be reflected, leaving only 3% transmission. It is necessary somehow to compensate for this difference, to match the characteristics of one material to those of the other. The ossicular chain converts the large-displacement, low-pressure signal in air to the small-displacement, high-pressure signal needed for transmission through the cochlear fluid. It does this by acting as a lever system and by exerting all the force at the tympanum on a smaller surface.

The lever formed by the malleus and incus is illustrated in Figure 8-5. The pivot point or fulcrum is located farther from the tympanum than from the stapes, and the ratio of the lengths of the lever arms is 1.3 : 1. This means that the displacement at the oval window is less than at the tympanum by a factor of 1/1.3, but the force at the oval window is amplified by a factor of 1.3. The area of the tympanic membrane is 0.55 cm^2, whereas that of the oval window is only 0.032 cm^2. If the same force exerted on the tympanic membrane were exerted on the membrane covering the oval window, which is only $^1/_{16}$ the area, then the force per unit area at the oval window would be 16 times that at the tympanum. However, the lever arm itself exerts an amplification of 1.3, yielding a total pressure amplification of about 21-fold (about 13 db). With this matching alone, 60% of the signal is transmitted, much improved over the 3% that would be obtained using direct coupling. A further matching effect, almost to the point of 100% transmission, is provided by variations in the mode of vibration of the ear drum.

One last structure of the middle ear is the stapedius muscle. This muscle receives its innervation from a branch of the seventh cranial nerve, and it has its origin in the posterior wall of the middle ear and its insertion in the head of the stapes. Its contraction rocks the stapes out of the oval window (Fig. 8-4). The action of the stapedius, coupled with that of the tensor tympani, is to stiffen the ossicular chain and reduce transmission by as much as 40 db, particularly at low frequencies. Reflex contraction is elicited by intense sound (>70 db above threshold) to protect the delicate inner ear, but the latency of the contraction is so long (40–160 msec) that it can hardly offer much protection against brief, loud sounds. Military cannons frequently incorporate a clicker that activates these muscles in the operator's ears shortly before the large charge is detonated.

The oval window opens into the inner ear, a structure called the bony labyrinth,

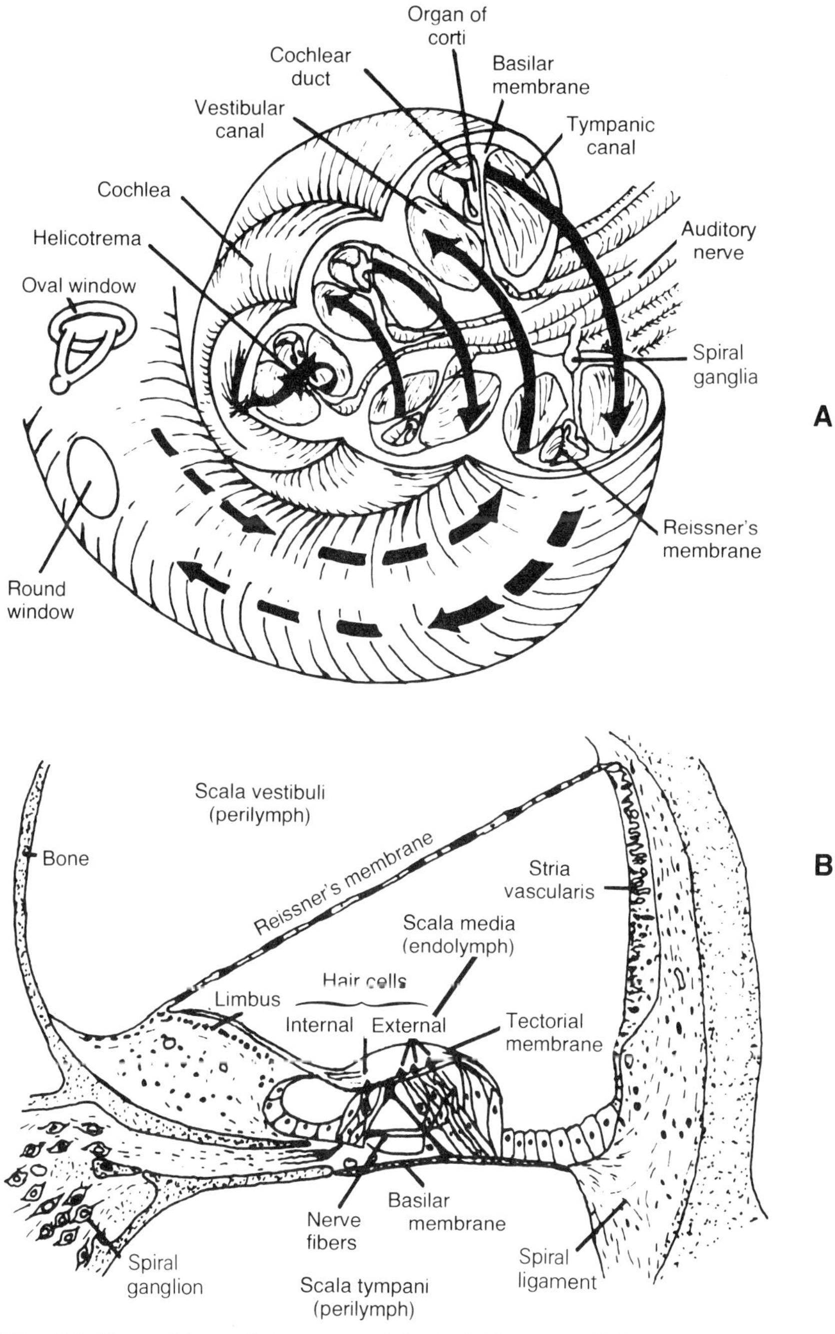

FIG. 8-6. The cochlea and the organ of Corti. **A.** Diagram of the cochlea cut through along the modiolus to show the partition of the cavity by the basilar and Reissner's membranes. **Arrows** indicate the pathway of pressure waves originating in the oval window. **B.** The cochlear partition and the organ of Corti. (**A.** Curtis BA, Jacobson S, Marcus EM: An Introduction to the Neurosciences. Philadelphia, Saunders, 1972. **B.** Davis H, Silverman SR: Hearing and Deafness, 3rd ed. New York, Holt, Rinehart, Winston, 1970)

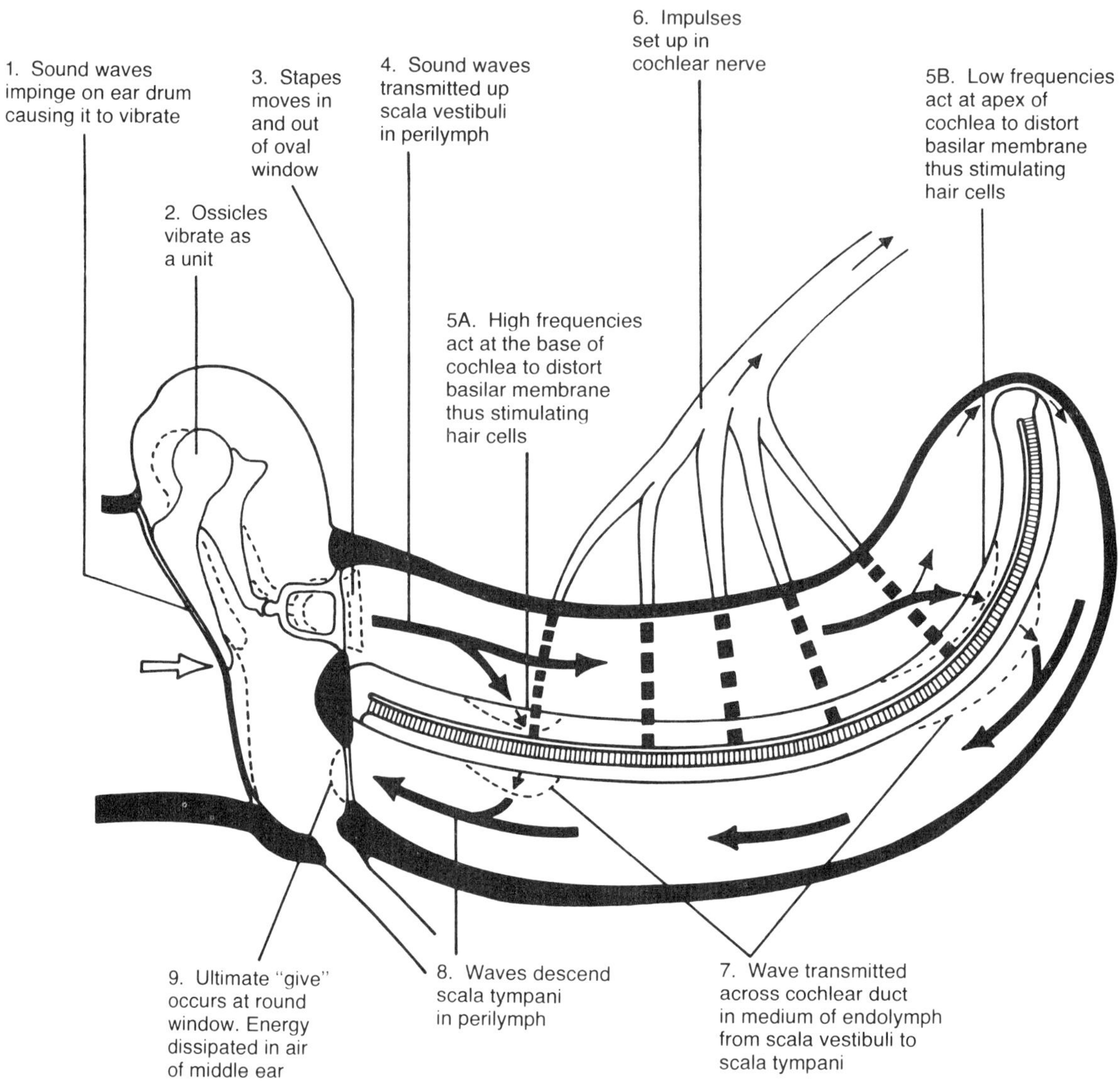

FIG. 8-7. Movement of pressure waves through the cochlea.

which is composed of the semicircular canals, the vestibule, and the cochlea. The bony labyrinth is filled with a fluid, called perilymph. In the perilymph is a membranous structure, the membranous labyrinth, filled with endolymph. The cochlea is a spiral structure whose corresponding membranous structure extends into the spiral as a blind tube. The cochlea, spiraled like a snail shell, contains two and one-half turns from its base at the oval window to its apex. A vertical section of the cochlea, taken along the central pillar or modiolus, is shown in Figure 8-6A. A close look at one section is shown in Figure 8-6B. A bony shelf, an extension of the modiolus, extends part way into the canal. Attached to this shelf and to the lateral wall by the spiral ligament is a delicate membrane, the basilar membrane, which supports the receptor elements of the ear. The basilar membrane, which is about one inch long in humans, divides the canal approximately in half, and the upper half is further divided by Reissner's membrane. Between Reissner's and the basilar membrane (the cochlear duct) is endolymph; outside is perilymph. The cochlear duct is sometimes called the scala media, whereas the portion of the canal above Reissner's membrane is the scala vestibuli, and the portion below the basilar membrane is the scala tympani. At the apex of the cochlea, the scala vestibuli and scala tympani communicate through a tiny opening, the helicotrema.

When the stapes moves inward at the oval window (Fig. 8-7), pressure waves are transmitted to the perilymph of the scala vestibuli and thence through Reissner's membrane and the basilar membrane to the scala tympani. In the scala tympani, the vibrations pass again through perilymph to the round window at the base of the cochlea. The membranous covering of the round window bulges into the middle ear cavity and forms the ultimate "give" in the system, because the helicotrema is so small that little fluid moves through it. This means that the displacement in the cochlea caused by movement of the stapes is almost all *across* the basilar membrane.

On the basilar membrane sits the sensory structure of the ear, the organ of Corti, composed of a complex of supporting cells and sensory or hair cells. The hair cells are arranged in two groups, the inner and outer hair cells. Each hair cell (there are about 15,000) is approximately goblet shaped, with up to 80 tiny hairs or stereocilia projecting out of it into the endolymph. The stereocilia grade in length from inside (toward the modiolus) to outside (toward the stria vascularis). Overlying the hair cells is a gelatinous structure, the tectorial membrane, in which the longest stereocilia are imbedded. When the basilar membrane moves up and down, the tectorial membrane does not move quite with it because their centers of rotation are different, as shown in Figure 8-8, the result being that the stereocilia are subjected to a shearing force that bends them over. Apparently, it is this movement of the stereocilia that gives rise to the receptor potential in the hair cell.

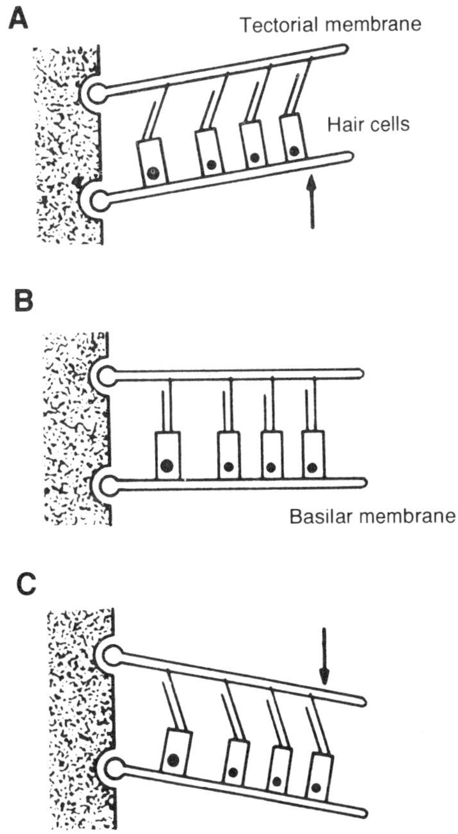

FIG. 8-8. Movements of the basilar membrane and the bending of the stereocilia. The basilar membrane at rest is shown in **B. A.** Upward movement of the basilar membrane **(arrow)** bends hairs away from the modiolus. **C.** Downward movement **(arrow)** bends hairs toward the modiolus. (Klinke R: Physiology of hearing. In Schmidt RF [ed]: Fundamentals of Sensory Physiology. New York, Springer-Verlag, 1978)

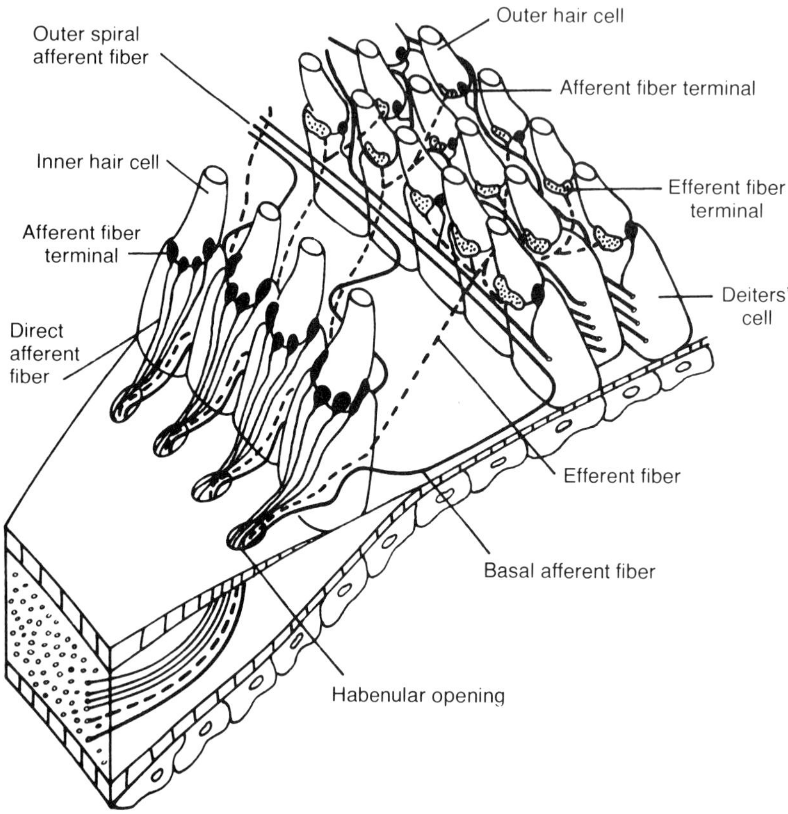

FIG. 8-9. Distribution of the afferent fibers to inner and outer hair cells. Direct afferent fibers innervate inner hair cells; outer spiral afferent fibers run between Deiters' cells before innervating outer hair cells. (Spoendlin H: The innervation of the cochlear receptor. In Møller A [ed]: Basic Mechanisms in Hearing. New York, Academic Press, 1973)

Only the longest (outer) of the stereocilia of each hair cell are buried in the tectorial membrane, yet when these outer stereocilia are bent, the other, shorter stereocilia move with them. Electron micrographs show that the stereocilia are connected together by fine fibrils that serve to interlock them. Some investigators have reported that the stereocilia appear to be rather flexible, whereas others have shown them to be rather stiff. They may, in fact, be able to vary their stiffness and therefore the ease with which they are bent. This may provide a mechanism for adjusting the threshold for hearing. Tiny filaments within the stereocilia contain a substance that behaves much like actin, the protein of muscle that confers upon it contractility. In the stereocilia, the actin-like filaments could be bound together and to the cell membrane or change into a more crystalline conformation to bring about increased rigidity.

Movement of the stereocilia in a direction toward the largest of them excites auditory nerve fibers; movement of the stereocilia in the opposite direction silences the fibers. An upward movement of the basilar membrane bends the stereocilia toward the outside (as shown in Fig. 8-8), toward the larger stereocilia, and thus excites the associated nerve fibers. A downward movement of the basilar membrane has the reverse effect.

As shown in Figure 8-9, the base of each hair cell receives the endings of 10 to 20 nerve cells that reach the hair cell through the modiolus. The modiolus houses the spiral ganglion, composed of the somata of these primary afferent auditory neurons. It is in these nerve endings that impulses are initiated by the receptor potential, and it is the axons of these cells that form the auditory nerve. Most of the 35,000 axons in the auditory nerve (about 95%) innervate inner

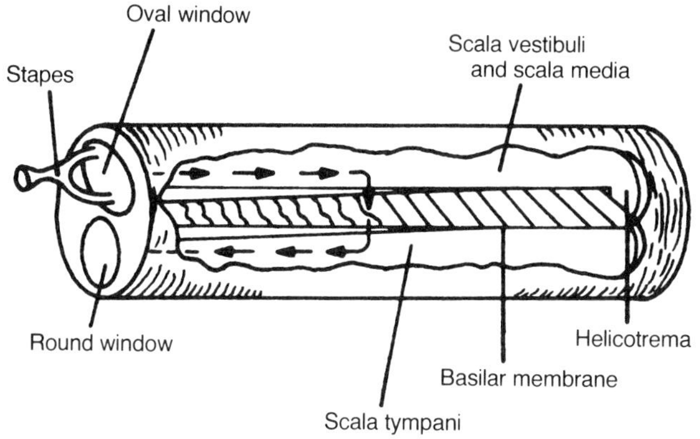

FIG. 8-10. The cochlea uncoiled to show the thinning and widening of the basilar membrane at the apex. (Guyton A: Textbook of Medical Physiology. Philadelphia, WB Saunders, 1976)

FIG. 8-11. Traveling wave in the basilar membrane. **A,B.** Surfaces represent the same wave at two instants in time. **C.** The envelope of the traveling wave indicating the maximum displacement at 28 mm from the stapes for a 200-Hz tone.

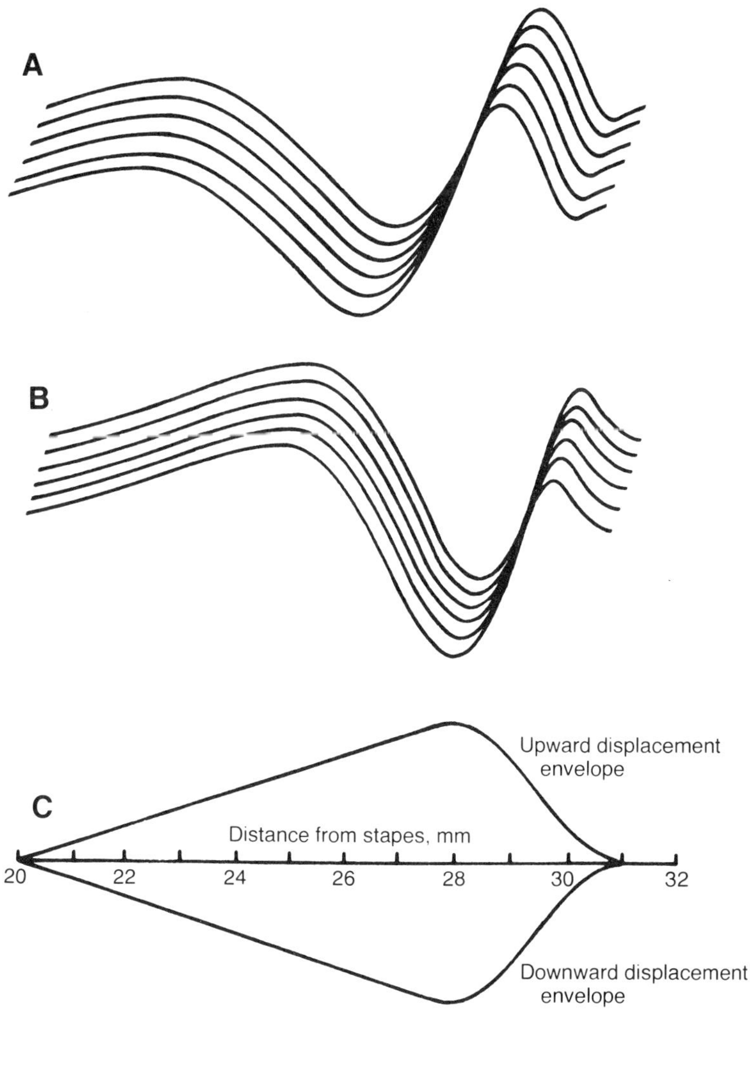

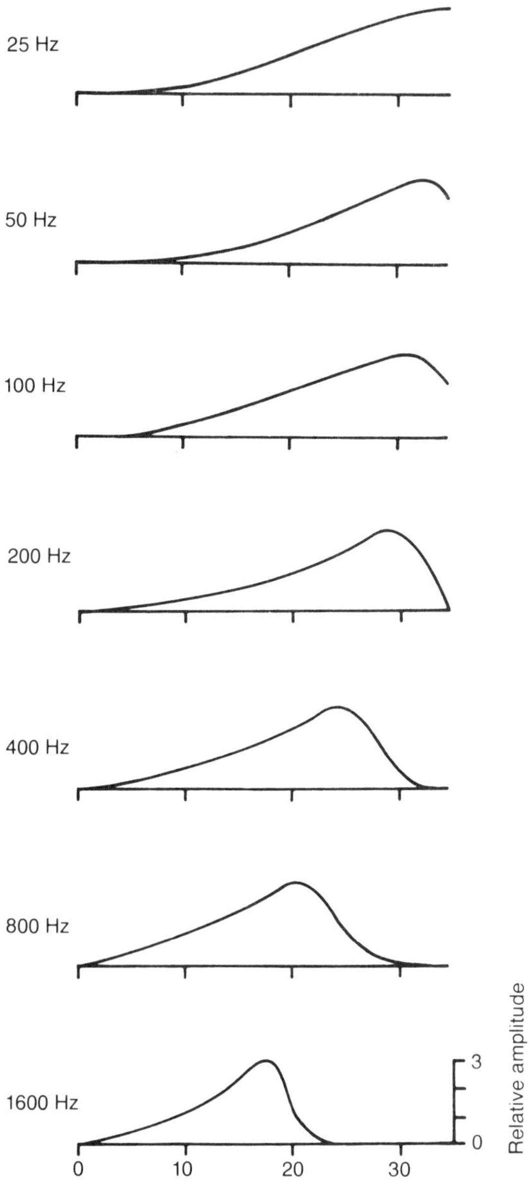

FIG. 8-12. Magnitudes of the upper half of the envelopes of traveling waves elicited in the basilar membrane by pressure oscillations of different frequencies. Note maxima for high frequencies near the base, low frequencies near the apex. (von Békésy G, Rosenblith WA: The mechanical properties of the ear. In Stevens SS [ed]: Handbook of Experimental Psychology. New York, Wiley, 1951)

hair cells, but about 5% innervate outer hair cells. There are three rows of outer hair cells, but there is only one row of inner hair cells. Why most of the fibers end on the minority of hair cells is not known.

PITCH PERCEPTION

There are two theories to explain how pitch, or the frequency of vibration, is encoded by the auditory system. The first theory, the **frequency theory,** says that the pitch is encoded by the frequency of discharge in the primary auditory fiber. If the code consists of one action potential for each cycle of the stimulus, then the code would obviously be limited by the refractory period of the axon. An upper frequency limit of 1000 Hz, of course, falls short of the 20,000-Hz upper limit of pitch perception by the human ear. Actually, auditory nerve fibers can signal frequencies up to about 4000 Hz in their discharge by discharging 1 spike/cycle up to their maximal discharge frequency and then, above that level, discharging 1 spike every so many cycles, locked to a particular phase of sound vibration.

The other theory, the **place theory,** suggested by von Helmholtz, says that specific parts of the basilar membrane vibrate in response to different frequencies. This would make pitch perception a matter of *which* fibers were active (determined by where their hair cells were located along the length of the basilar membrane), rather than how much total activity they generated. If the cochlea were straightened out, it might look like the illustration in Figure 8-10. Notice that the basilar membrane is thicker, narrower, and stiffer at the base and thinner, wider, and more flexible at the apex. This suggested to von Helmholtz, by analogy to piano strings, that the base of the basilar membrane might vibrate in response to high frequencies, whereas the apex would vibrate in response to low frequencies. In its modern form, the place theory claims that, in response to vibration of the oval window, traveling waves are set up and move from base toward the apex in the basilar membrane, just like those set up in a string, one end of which is vibrated. Figure 8-11 shows a traveling wave at two instants in time (A,B) along with the envelope of the displacements (C). The maximum excursion of the envelope occurs in this case at 28 mm from the stapes. As shown in Figure 8-12, the place where this maximum occurs varies with frequency, being nearer the stapes with higher and nearer the apex with lower frequencies. Systematic investigations by von Békésy have shown that each frequency

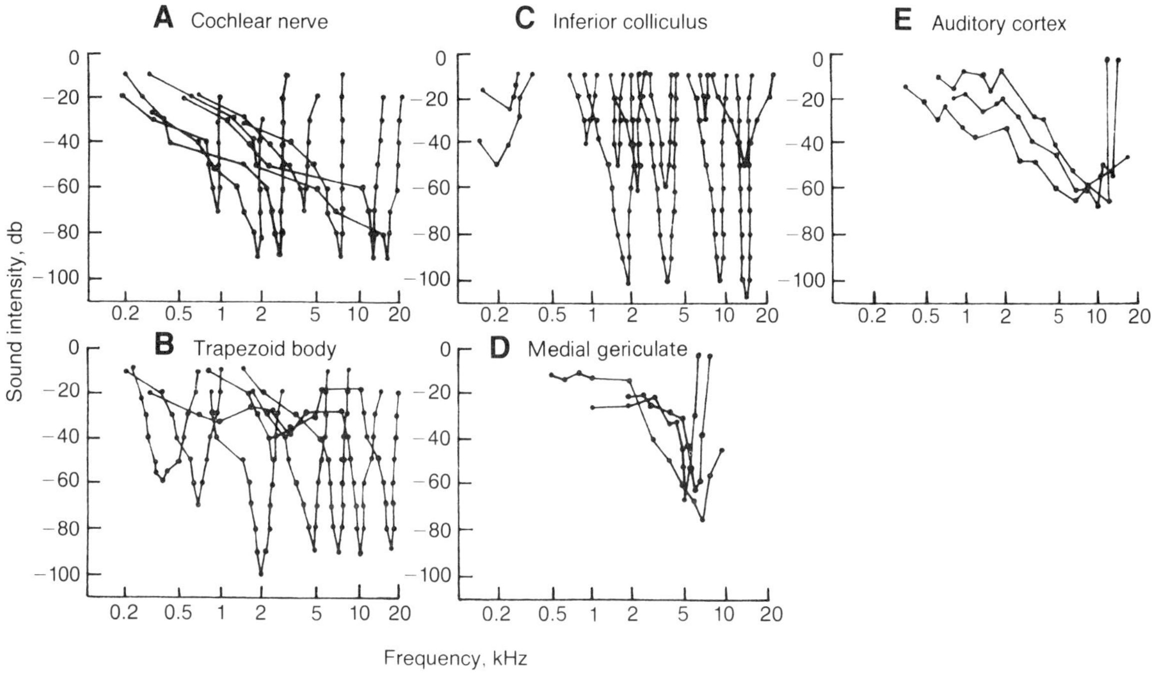

FIG. 8-13. Tuning curves of auditory nerve fibers in a cat (A). All tones within the curves increased the firing of the cell, but the intensity required to increase the firing varied with frequency. The nadirs represent "best frequencies" of the cells. Also shown are tuning curves for neurons in the trapezoid body (B), inferior colliculus (C), medial geniculate nucleus (D), and auditory cortex (E). (Katsuki Y: Neural mechanisms of auditory sensation in cats. In Rosenblith WA [ed]: Sensory Communication. Cambridge, MA, MIT Press, 1961)

through the audible range has its place of maximal displacement on the basilar membrane, just as shown in the figure, but at low frequencies the entire basilar membrane moves up and down. Actually, because the base is stiffer than the rest of the membrane, traveling waves always begin at the base and progress toward the apex regardless of how they are initiated. This is true for waves induced by oval window movement, by bone-conducted vibration, or by pressure waves induced directly in the cochlear fluid (Wever and Lawrence, 1952).

It would appear that perhaps the frequency code is used for lower frequencies and the place code for higher frequencies, or, alternatively, both kinds of codes are used for some or all frequencies. The existence of traveling waves is given some credence by the discharge pattern of fibers in the auditory nerve. Figure 8-13A is a plot of the threshold intensity curves or **tuning curves** for several auditory fibers. The threshold for discharge of a cell varies with the frequency of the sound, but there is a single frequency for which each cell has the lowest threshold. This frequency is called the **best frequency** for that cell. It is this sort of discharge pattern that one would expect to see if traveling waves, such as those in Figure 8-12, are set up in the basilar membrane; cells should respond over a range of frequencies with a best one, and the tuning curves of cells with low best frequencies should be broader than those with higher best frequencies.

The problem for the place theory is how to encode sound intensity. At first, it would appear that a simple frequency code would suffice, but pitch coding cannot be completely independent of discharge frequency, compromising a simple frequency code for intensity. This occurs because of the existence of traveling waves. For example, a tone of 250 Hz sets up a traveling wave in the basilar membrane with maximum excursion near the apex. At slightly greater intensity, the maximum excursion is greater, but still occurs at the same point. A point adjacent to the 250-Hz maximum that corresponds to say the 300-Hz maximum

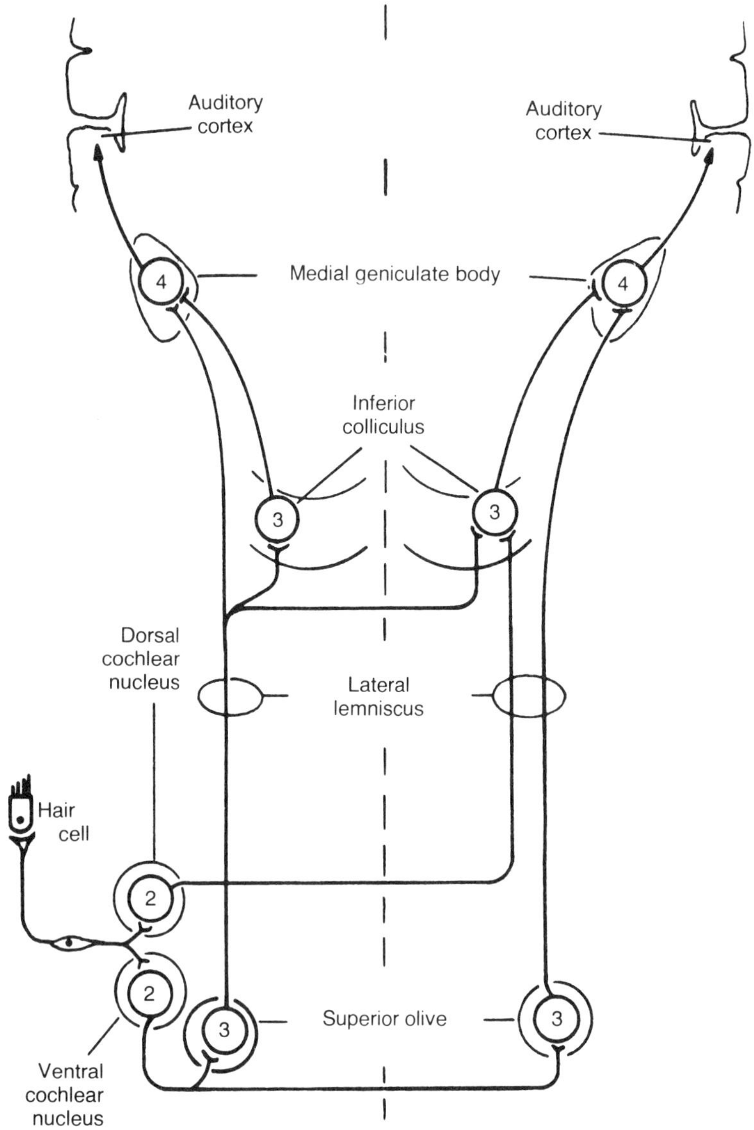

FIG. 8-14. Central auditory pathways. First, second, third, and fourth-order fibers are indicated by the numerals.

point is also caused to vibrate by the more intense 250-Hz tone at amplitude "x." Now the frequency of the tone is increased to 300 Hz. At some lesser intensity of the 300-Hz tone, the 300-Hz maximum point will also be moved by an amount "x." The problem for the place theory is to distinguish the louder 250-Hz tone from the softer 300-Hz tone. The rather wide tuning curves of auditory nerve fibers suggest that single neurons cannot in fact distinguish them, but we know the nervous system can and does. How is yet a mystery. Perhaps some kind of ensemble code is used to encode intensity, which is likely if a frequency code is used for pitch.

CENTRAL AUDITORY PATHWAYS

Primary auditory fibers enter the brain stem and immediately make connections with secondary neurons in the cochlear nucleus, as illustrated in Figure 8-14. From here, the auditory information goes to a remarkable number of places in the central nervous system. Fibers arising from the cochlear nuclei

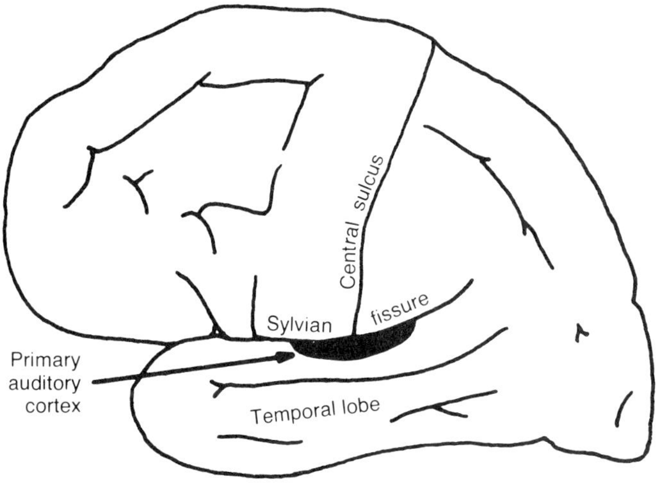

FIG. 8-15. Diagram to indicate the location of the primary auditory cortex on the superior lip of the temporal lobe. (Guyton A: Textbook of Physiology. Philadelphia, WB Saunders, 1976)

ascend in both a crossed and an uncrossed projection, which either enters the lateral lemniscus directly or first relays in the nucleus of the trapezoid body or the superior olive before joining the lateral lemniscus.

The lateral lemniscus contains both second and third-order neurons that project either directly or indirectly to the inferior colliculus, which is an obligatory relay for all auditory fibers. Cells of the inferior colliculus project to the medial geniculate nucleus bilaterally, and the medial geniculate nucleus projects to the primary auditory cerebral cortex, located on the superior and medial aspect of the temporal lobe, as indicated in Figure 8-15.

The responses of neurons in the various nuclei of the central auditory system resemble those of primary auditory neurons in many ways, but they also differ in important ways. As shown in Figure 8-13, the cells of the trapezoid body (B), inferior colliculus (C), medial geniculate nucleus (D), and primary auditory cortex (E) respond to a wide range of sound frequencies and exhibit tuning curves reminiscent of those for auditory nerve fibers (Fig. 8-13A). The curves are narrower (*i.e.*, the range of frequencies that cause the cell to discharge is smaller) for higher order neurons (indicated by numbers in Fig. 8-14) up to the level of the medial geniculate nucleus, and then they get wider again. This narrowing represents a sharpening of the cells' frequency discrimination abilities and probably results from a process like lateral inhibition, in which cells with close best frequencies inhibit each other. Some investigators have concluded on the basis of this observation that frequency and intensity discriminations are accomplished at or before the medial geniculate level, because cortical neurons simply do not have fine discriminative behavior (*i.e.*, they have wide tuning curves). As we shall see, this is probably true at least in animals.

Neurons in the auditory nerve change their frequency of discharge with changes in sound intensity. Sample intensity functions for these and other cells of the auditory system are illustrated in Figure 8-16. The relationship between intensity and discharge frequency is sigmoid for auditory nerve fibers and for cells of the trapezoid body and the superior olive. They increase their frequency of discharge with increasing sound intensity, slowly at first and then more rapidly, to a certain intensity, at which the frequency reaches a maximum. At even higher intensities, there is no further increase in frequency. Cells of the medial geniculate nucleus and the auditory cortex do not increase their frequency of discharge with increasing intensity of sound. (This is the reason for claiming that intensity discriminations occur below this level.) Neurons at successively higher levels of the auditory system discharge fewer spikes in response to a standard tone. Below the level of the inferior colliculus, neurons give repetitive responses to maintained tone stimuli, but at and above the

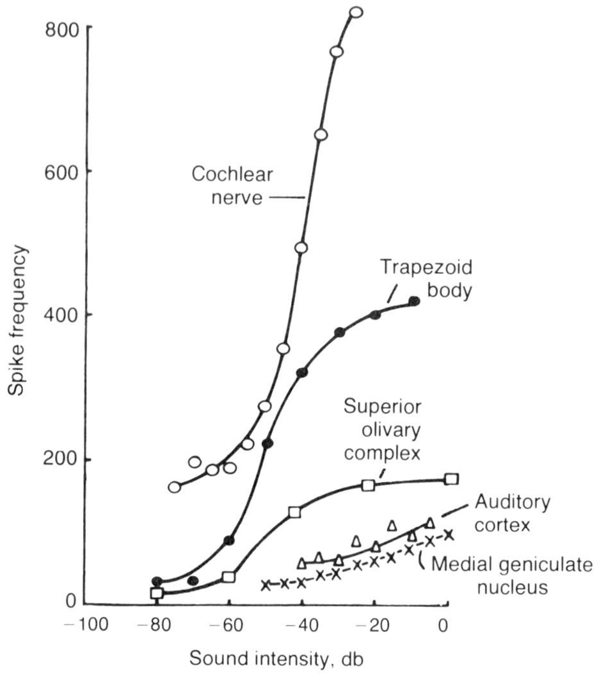

FIG. 8-16. Intensity functions for neurons in the cochlear nerve, trapezoid body, superior olivary complex, auditory cortex, and medial geniculate nucleus of the cat. Frequency of discharge of the neurons is plotted on the ordinate against sound intensity on the abscissa. (Katsuki Y: Neural mechanism of auditory sensation in cats. In Rosenblith WA [ed]: Sensory Communication. Cambridge, MA, MIT Press, 1961)

level of the colliculus, they more often give on-, off-, or on-off responses (these terms are used here in the same manner as for visual cells). In the auditory cortex, there are seldom continuous responses to sustained tones; most cells signal sound onset or offset or both.

However, sounds that we hear are seldom pure tones (*i.e.*, tones of a single frequency) as were those employed in the preceding experiments. More often, they are composites of sine waves of different frequencies and amplitudes. We know little about how the nervous system deals with such complex sounds, but a beginning has been made. In the cochlear and medial geniculate nuclei, the response to a tone is unaffected by a second tone (of different frequency) presented simultaneously at weak intensity. As the second tone is increased in intensity, the response to the first tone is gradually suppressed until it finally fails completely. At this intensity, only responses to the second tone are seen if its frequency lies within the response range of the neuron. In the cerebral cortex, the same maneuver performed on a cell with high best frequency results in enhancement of the cell's response if the tones are harmonically related (*i.e.*, if the ratio of their frequencies is 1 : 2, 1 : 3, 1 : 4) or if the difference in frequency is such that it results in 50 to 200 beats/sec. The greater the frequency of beats, the larger the discharge up to 100 beats/sec. Above 100, the response falls off again. It is tempting to speculate that cortical neurons are playing some role in decoding complex sounds or tone patterns, somehow using beats and harmonics.

The auditory system appears to be arranged topographically, much like the somatosensory system. It is possible to map the cochlea onto the various structures of the auditory system by mapping best frequencies. The auditory nerve has a predominance of fibers with high best frequencies on the outside of the bundle; fibers with low best frequencies lie in the center. The cochlear nucleus is arranged such that cells with high best frequencies are dorsal, and succeedingly more ventral cells have lower best frequencies. This is often called a **tonotopic representation** (or a receptotopic or cochleotopic representation, if the particular author is a strong adherent to the place theory). Unlike the somatic system, the auditory system has a plethora of such representations at each level. Thus, there are three in the cochlear nucleus and two in the superior olivary complex, the inferior colliculus, and the medial geniculate nucleus. At the cortex, the sublime becomes ridiculous, with five tonotopic representations having been defined. These representations are either strict or loose depending upon whether anesthetized or unanesthetized preparations are used. In unanesthetized animals, a good many "ringers" (apparently inappropriately placed) appear in an otherwise orderly arrangement of neurons based upon best frequencies. As in the somatic system, we do not know if the spatial arrangement of neurons has some functional significance or if it is an "accident" of the developmental process.

Removal of all cortical areas dealing with audition bilaterally is a rare event in humans, but the surgery can be performed in experimental animals, although the testing of the auditory capacities is not an easy matter. Unilateral removal of the auditory cortex produces only slight changes in auditory threshold, but bilateral removal produces a significant elevation of auditory threshold (70–75 db in dogs), profound deficits in frequency discrimination ability (perhaps related more to performance than sensation), inability to discriminate simple tone patterns, and severe deficits in ability to localize the source of a sound in space.

The human with normal hearing in both ears uses differences in the time of onset and in the phase of the signals at each ear to localize the source of low-frequency sound, whereas differences in intensity are used to localize the source of high-frequency sound. Binaural phase differences are useful in localizing sound below 1.2 to 1.5 kHz, and interaural intensity differences appear to be useful for judging the source of sound up to about 15 feet. Resolving power of the human auditory apparatus is greatest in the median plane where changes in position of a sound source as small as 1° can be detected. At 90° from the median plane, a change in position by as much as 40° may be undetected. Localization of sound sources also depends upon frequency, with best performance for sounds of 2 to 8 kHz. Because sound localization depends upon comparison of signals from the two ears, a lesion of the auditory system at sites that receive convergence from both ears should produce impairment in this ability. Transection of the trapezoid body, lesion of the superior olive, lesion of the inferior colliculus, and transection of the lateral lemniscus all produce impairments of this ability in animals just as severe as lesions of the auditory cerebral cortex.

EFFERENT CONTROL OF COCHLEAR SENSITIVITY

In addition to the primary afferent connections to hair cells already described, there are efferent (with respect to the central nervous system) connections from fibers originating in both the contralateral and ipsilateral superior olive and running in the eighth nerve. These fibers terminate on the bases of the inner hair cells and on the primary afferent neurons near their points of contact with the outer hair cells (see Fig. 8-9). Together these 500 fibers form what has been called the **olivocochlear bundle.** They discharge in response to sound stimulation of either ear with thresholds of about 40 db (SPL) and show typical auditory tuning curves. Each fiber appears to have a best frequency that corresponds to the best frequency of the afferent fibers arising from the same hair cells it innervates. Thus, axons going to the basal turns of the cochlea have high best frequencies, whereas those going to apical turns have low best frequencies.

The effect of stimulation of the olivocochlear bundle upon the intensity functions of auditory primary afferent neurons is illustrated in Figure 8-17. Without stimulation of the bundle (solid curve), the auditory neuron shows a typical sigmoid intensity function. With stimulation of the bundle (dashed curve), the same kind of response curve is generated, but it is shifted about 10 db to the right, toward higher thresholds. The amount of this shift varies from 1 to 25 db, and it is greatest for cells with best frequencies in the range of 6 to 10 kHz.

It has been suggested that the function of the olivocochlear bundle is to raise the threshold of auditory nerve fibers in order to make them insensitive to noise, yet still sensitive to moderate to loud sounds. With activity in the bundle, the organism can be

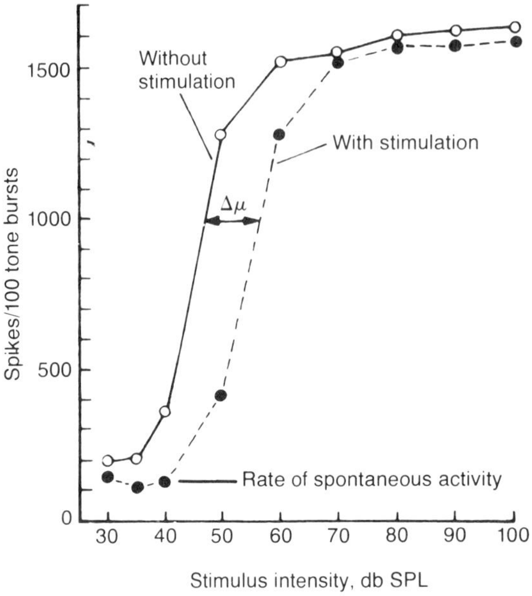

FIG. 8-17. Intensity function for primary auditory neurons with and without efferent stimulation. **Solid curve** shows responses to 40-msec tones at the best frequency (16.5 kHz) at various intensities. **Dashed curve** shows the responses to the same tones preceded by 10 msec by 32 shocks to the crossed olivocochlear bundle at 400/sec. $\Delta\mu$ is the shift in the function due to efferent activity; the average shift is 10 db. (Wiederhold ML: J Acoust Soc Am 48:966–977, 1970)

insensitive to environmental noise, yet still be responsive to other important signals. This hypothesis receives some support from observations that responses of the auditory nerve to moderately intense clicks were almost completely masked by simultaneous low-intensity clicks delivered at high rates. Stimulation of the bundle unmasked the responses to the intense clicks by reducing the responses to the low intensity ones. In addition, discrimination by monkeys of vowel sounds presented against a background noise was impaired by sectioning the bundle.

ALTERNATE ROUTES OF CONDUCTION AND HEARING LOSS

It is clear that the primary or dominant pathway by which vibratory energy reaches the cochlea is through the ossicular chain, but this is not the only route. Vibrations may be conducted through the air of the middle ear directly to the cochlea, mainly through the round window. In addition, the perilymph can be caused to vibrate by oscillations conducted through the bones of the skull and the bony labyrinth. Bone conduction is responsible for the different sound of your voice when you listen to it as you speak, which involves both bone and air conduction, and when you listen to a tape recording of it, which involves air conduction alone. It is bone conduction that lets you hear the loud crunch as you bite a piece of something hard. The existence of these alternate routes to the auditory receptors offers the clinician some easy tests of the origin of many hearing losses.

Audiologists normally distinguish two types of deafness, **conduction deafness** and **nerve deafness.** Conduction deafness can be the result of obstruction of the external meatus, some damage to the tympanic membrane, or some disease of the middle ear. The most common form of middle ear disease is an infection (otitis media), which, if prolonged, can lead to the formation of scars that reduce the mobility of the tympanum or the ossicles. Otosclerosis is a condition in which there is abnormal growth of bone that may cement the stapes in the oval window or reduce its ability to move. Nerve deafness may result from some damage to the cochlea, the hair cells, the auditory nerve, or some auditory structure of the central nervous system.

These two forms of deafness are easily distinguished using a simple tuning fork (preferably one of frequency 500 Hz, because it is easily heard above room noise). In **Weber's test,** the fork is struck and placed in the middle of the patient's forehead. If he has normal hearing or equal deafness on both sides, he will report that the sound comes from the middle of his head. If he has nerve deafness that is worse in one ear, he will report the tone to be heard better in the better ear. Alternatively, the tone will be heard better in the poorer ear if he has an asymmetric conduction deafness.

It is commonly said that Weber's test works because the signal of the tuning fork is masked in the good ear by room noise that cannot reach the ear with conduction deafness. This cannot be the case because the test works even in extremely quiet rooms or if the sound is not allowed to reach either ear by conduction through the air. The most reasonable explanation for the result is in terms of the conduction system

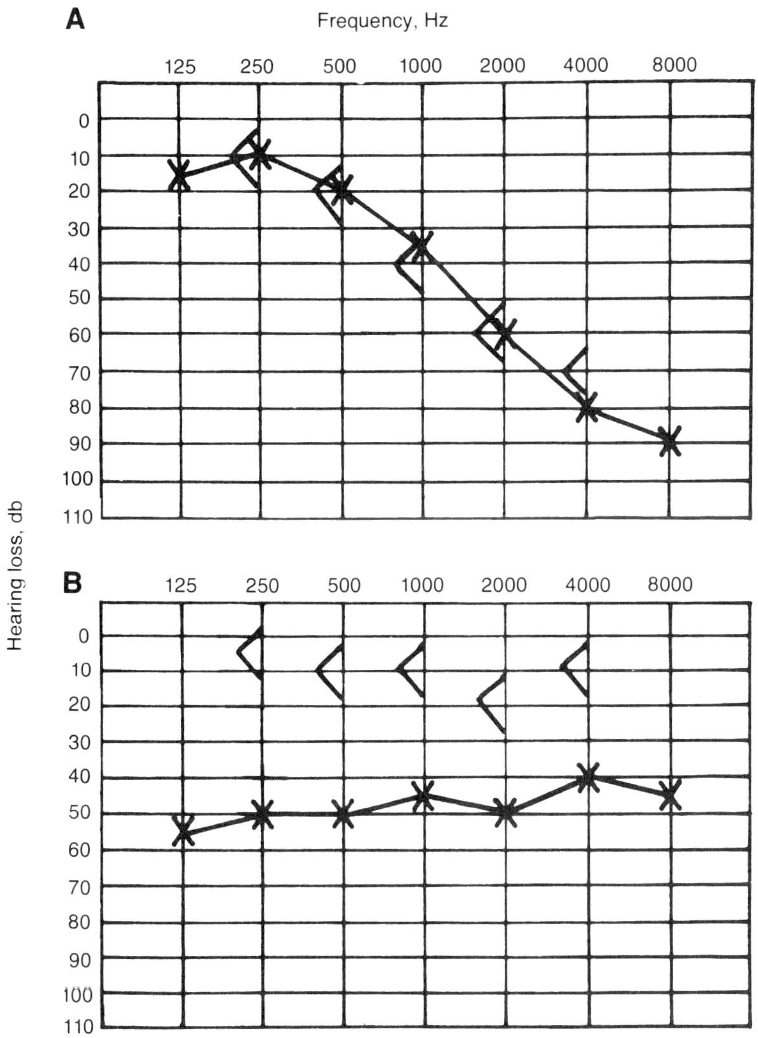

FIG. 8-18. A. Audiogram or hearing loss curve for a patient with neural deafness. *X*s indicate hearing losses for air conduction whereas **arrows** indicate hearing loss by bone conduction. In neural deafness both curves tend to show similar losses. **B.** Audiogram of patient with pure conduction deafness. Note that bone conduction is unimpaired at all frequencies. (Myer D, Schlosser WD, Winchester RA [eds]: Otologic Diagnosis and the Treatment of Deafness. Summit, NJ, Ciba, 1970)

itself. Bone-conducted sound sets the fluids of the cochlea in motion, vibrating the basilar membrane and also vibrating the membrane of the oval window. The ossicles and tympanum are set in motion by these vibrations at the oval window, shunting off some of the vibratory energy in the cochlea. If the ossicles cannot move, say because of otosclerosis, then this shunting is reduced and more of the energy is transmitted to the basilar membrane, increasing the apparent loudness of the sound. The same effect can be achieved in a normal individual. To demonstrate this, try the following maneuver. Say something out loud, and while you say it, stick your finger in your ear. The sound will become louder in that ear because you have prevented the tympanum from pushing air out of the external meatus. The tympanum cannot move as readily under these conditions so less energy is lost through the ossicular chain and the sound becomes louder.

So far, using Weber's test, only a comparison of the two ears has been made. However, following this procedure with **Rinne's test** will tell whether the deficit is in conduction or not. After being struck, the fork is placed on the mastoid process or bulla until its vibration can no longer be

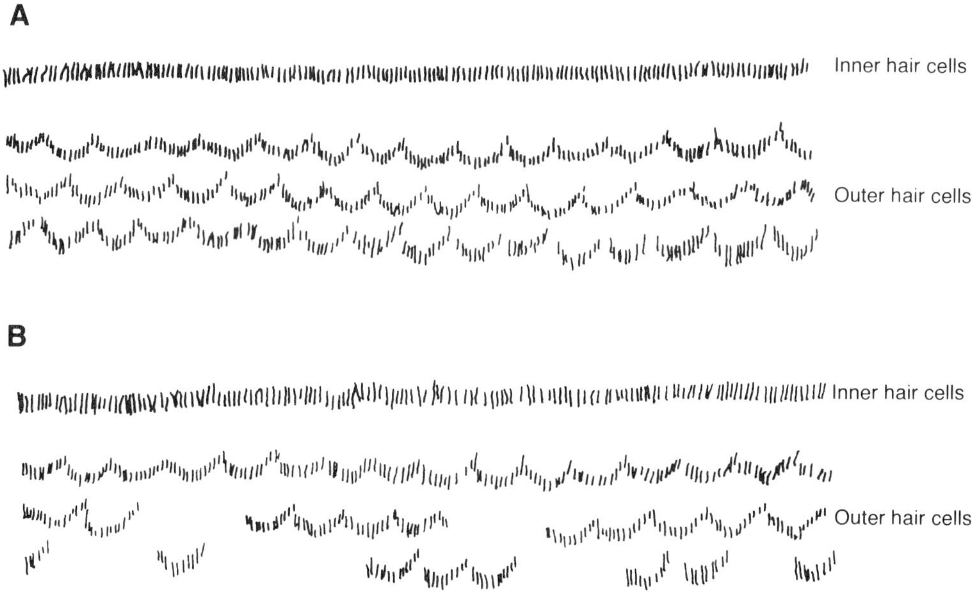

FIG. 8-19. Drawing from a scanning electron micrograph of the dorsal surface of the organ of Corti showing stereocilia of inner hair cells **(top)** and three rows of outer hair cells **(bottom)**. **A.** Normal organ in a guinea pig. **B.** Organ of a guinea pig exposed repeatedly to the noise of a starter's pistol. (Angelborg C, Engström H: The normal organ of Corti. In Møller A [ed]: Basic Mechanisms in Hearing. New York, Academic Press, 1973)

heard. Then the fork is held next to the auricle while it is still vibrating. It is normal to hear the vibration in air after none can be heard through bone conduction, but if it is known that there is some impairment, this result indicates a mixture of both conduction and neural deafness. Conduction deafness alone is indicated by the inability to hear the sound by air conduction in Rinne's test.

If deafness of either origin is indicated, a quantitative indication of the deafness is obtained from an audiogram. Figure 8-18A shows the audiogram of a patient with neural deafness. The *x*s in the audiogram indicate the hearing loss as measured by air conduction, whereas the arrows indicate the hearing loss as measured by bone conduction. Typically, in neural deafness, both measures show the same pattern of loss. Surgery is not indicated for this form of deafness because the neural tissue probably cannot be repaired, but some improvement in hearing is possible with a hearing aid, depending upon the nature of the damage. Figure 8-18B shows the audiogram of a person with pure conduction deafness. In this case, bone conduction is near normal, that is, near 0 db loss, but air conduction is impaired. The air audiogram is nearly flat with conduction deafness (Fig. 8-18B), but there is a differential loss, depending upon frequency, in nerve deafness (Fig. 8-18A). This is a typical result. Surgery may be helpful in many cases of conduction deafness, because removal of the obstruction to normal movement in the middle ear may be possible. In some cases, the stapes may be removed entirely and a prosthetic stapes put in its place.

THE EFFECT OF LOUD NOISE ON THE COCHLEA

Earlier, it was indicated that the intrinsic muscles of the middle ear cannot completely protect the delicate apparatus of the inner ear. With the advent of the scanning electron microscope, it is possible to see the damage done by extremely loud sounds. Figure 8-19A shows a drawing made from a scanning electron micrograph of an organ of Corti from a normal guinea pig. Figure 8-19B shows the same kind of drawing of the organ of Corti of a guinea pig exposed repeatedly to gunshot noise. Some of the outer hair cells are missing in the exposed animal. With more severe exposure to loud sounds, there can be more severe degeneration and even complete obliteration of the organ of Corti or even of the basilar membrane itself. This sort of damage (primarily to outer hair cells), which can be mimicked by the drug kanamycin, results in increases in the displacement threshold of auditory nerve fibers and broadening of their tuning curves. Obviously, this kind of damage is not repairable. It is interesting that in cases of high-frequency overstimulation, the damage is found near the base of the cochlea; when lower frequencies are used the damage is found closer to the apex.

SUGGESTED READING

Dallos P: The Auditory Periphery: Biophysics and Physiology. New York, Academic Press, 1973

Engström H, Ades HW, Hawkins JE II: Structure and functions of the sensory hairs of the inner ear. J Acoust Soc Am 34:1356–1363, 1962

Kiang NY-S, Watanabe T, Thomas EC, Clark LF: Discharge Patterns in the Cat's Auditory Nerve. Cambridge, MA, MIT Press, 1965

Møller AR [ed]: Basic Mechanisms in Hearing. New York, Academic Press, 1973

Nomoto M, Suga N, Katsuki Y: Discharge pattern and inhibition of primary auditory nerve fibers in the monkey. J Neurophysiol 27:768–787, 1964

Sachs MB: Stimulus–response relation for auditory nerve fibers: two-tone stimuli. J Acoust Soc Am 45:1025–1036, 1969

Sataloff J, Sataloff RT, Vassallo LA: Hearing Loss, 2nd ed. Philadelphia, JB Lippincott, 1980

Spoendlin H: The Organization of the Cochlear Receptor. Basel, S. Karger, 1966

Webster WR, Atkin LM: Central auditory processing. In Gazzaniga MS, Blakemore C [eds]: Handbook of Psychobiology. New York, Academic Press, 1975

Wever EG, Lawrence M: Sound conduction in the cochlea. Ann Otol Rhinol Laryngol 61:824–835, 1952

Wiederhold ML: Variation in the effects of electric stimulation of the crossed olivocochlear bundle on cat single auditory-nerve fiber responses to tone bursts. J Acoust Soc Am 48:966–977, 1970

von Békésy G: Experiments in Hearing. Huntington, NY, Kreiger, 1978

9

The Vestibular System

The vestibular apparatus is the nonauditory portion of the inner ear. It serves three primary purposes in man: (1) It plays the dominant role in the subjective sensation of motion and spatial orientation of the head. (2) It adjusts muscular activity and body position to maintain posture. (3) It stabilizes the fixation point in space of the eyes when the head moves, providing a stable image upon the retina. It is important to keep in mind that the vestibular apparatus provides to the senses and to these other control systems information about the position of the *head* in space. Because it provides this information only with respect to the head, it cannot accomplish postural adjustments on its own. Sensors in the neck and perhaps other postural muscles are extremely important in signaling changes in the relationship between the head and the body to the central nervous system. These two systems function in conjunction with the eyes to form a remarkable control system that maintains us in an erect position in a wide variety of unstable postures.

This control system can function adequately without the vestibular input. People with labyrinthine disease or damage to the vestibular nerve, as sometimes occurs with inappropriate streptomycin therapy, can still orient in space, provided that they keep their eyes open or maintain a very rigid relationship between head and body. It is a difficult activity, requiring considerable concentration, and is not the automatic activity that the vestibular apparatus provides.

VESTIBULAR ANATOMY

The basic design of the labyrintine organs was discussed in Chapter 8 with respect to the auditory structures. The vestibular apparatus consists of the same tube (membranous labyrinth) within a tube (bony labyrinth) construction. Both tubes are fluid-filled: endolymph in the membranous and perilymph in the bony labyrinth. The vestibular apparatus contains two sack-like structures, the utricle and saccule, and three semicircular canals that are joined together in the same fluid environments. The utricle and saccule are termed **otolith organs** because they contain some crystals of calcium carbonate that play a major role in their excitation. Both otolith organs are dilatations of the labyrinth that contain sensory epithelia, specialized to sense static position and linear acceleration.

The utricle is an oval tube, whereas the saccule is flattened and irregular; otherwise, their structures are similar. Their positions within the inner ear are shown in the drawing of Figure 9-1. The sensory epithelium of the utricle, the utricular macula, is situated so that it is approximately parallel to the ground when the head is upright. The saccular macula is oriented vertically in the upright human. Both macular organs, in fact the entire vestibular epithelium, contain two types of sensory hair cells, positioned only on the superficial aspect of the epithelium, as shown in Figure 9-2. The type I cell is goblet-shaped and reminiscent of the sensory cells of the basilar membrane. The type II cell is essentially cylindrical. Projecting from the free surface of each type is one kinocilium flanking a group of stereocilia. This arrangement makes the cells polarized, and it has important functional implications.

The sensory epithelia are overlaid by a gelatinous substance that contains the calcium carbonate crystals and in which the cilia are embedded. These crystals are called the **otoliths** ("stones in the ear") or **statoconia,** and the gelatinous membrane

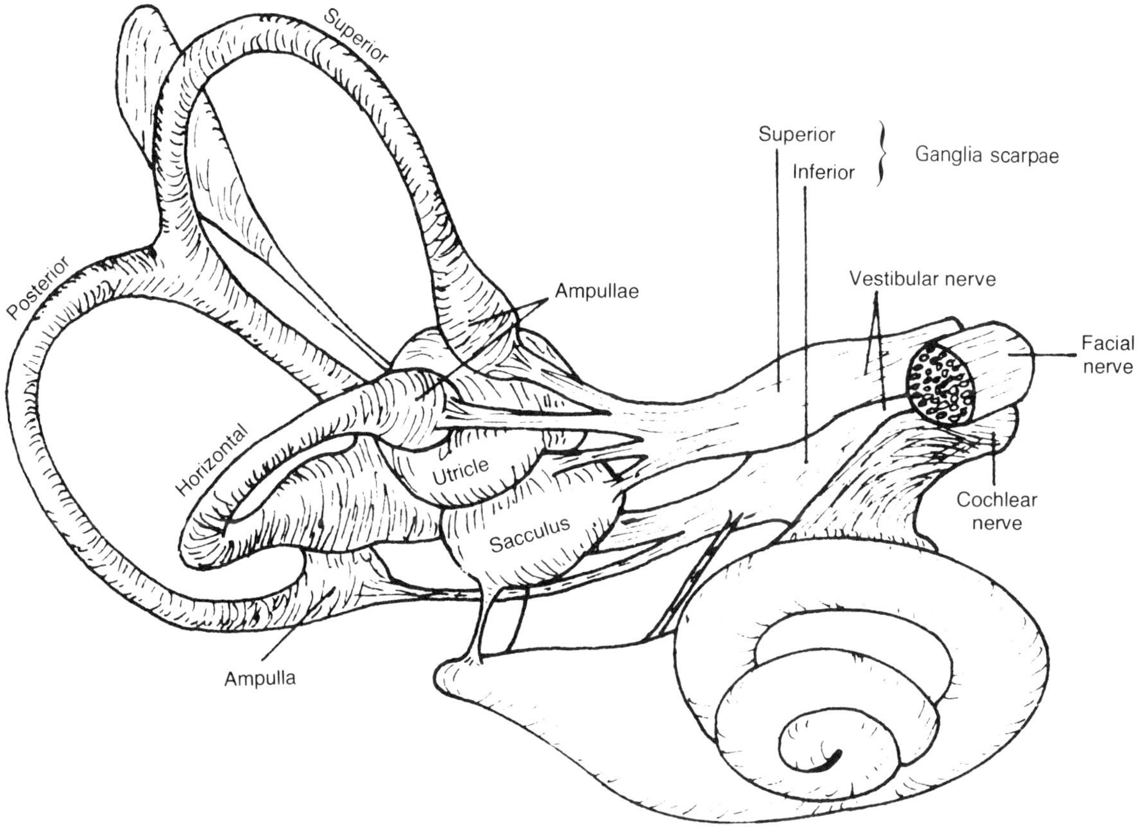

FIG. 9-1. A nearly lateral view of the right human labyrinth. (Hardy M: Anat Rec 59:403–418, 1935)

that contains them is the otolithic membrane. A schematic diagram of the relationship between the hair cells and the otolithic membrane is shown in Figure 9-3.

There are both afferent and efferent fibers to the maculae. Both lose their myelin as they pass through the basement membrane, and the larger afferent fibers contact a small group of type I sensory cells all with the same polarity, that is, they all have the kinocilium on the same side of the cell. They form synapses on the sensory cells that nearly completely engulf the basal end of the cell. The smaller afferent fibers contact both types of sensory cells, with different polarities, forming the same type of synapses on type I cells as larger fibers and ordinary boutons on type II cells.

In each ear there are three semicircular canals oriented approximately at right angles to each other, as shown in Figure 9-1. One canal (the horizontal) is located in a plane that is about 30° from horizontal; it can be brought into the horizontal plane by tilting the head forward by 30°. The other two canals (the posterior and superior) are in vertical planes. It is important to remember that they occur on both sides of the head, that is, there are two horizontal, two posterior, and two superior canals. The posterior canal on one side of the head is in a plane parallel to that containing the superior canal on the other side.

The lumina of the semicircular canals are connected with the utricle. The superior and posterior canals join each other before entering the utricle; thus, there are five openings into the utricle. Near the junction of one arm of each canal with the utricle, there is a dilatation of the canal, called the ampulla. Inside the ampulla and running at right angles across it is the sensory epithelium of the semicircular canal, the crista ampullaris or crista acustica. The hair cells of the crista are similar to those in the maculae except they are all polarized in the same direction. In Figure 9-4, it can be seen that the crista is a folded structure with the

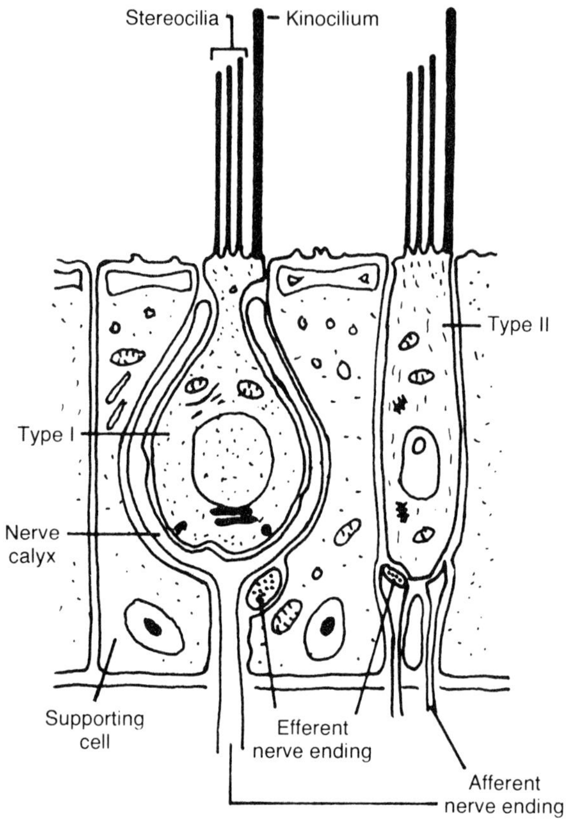

FIG. 9-2. Schematic drawing of the vestibular epithelium showing the two cell types and the nerve connections made on each. (Brodal A: Neurological Anatomy in Relation to Clinical Medicine, 2nd ed. New York, Oxford Univ. Press, 1969)

FIG. 9-3. The effects of different positions of the head upon the otolith organs. A. Upside down, C. right-side up, and B. in between. The **arrows** indicate the direction of gravitational force. (Eyzaguirre C, Fidone SJ: Physiology of the Nervous System. Chicago, Year Book Medical Publishers, 1975)

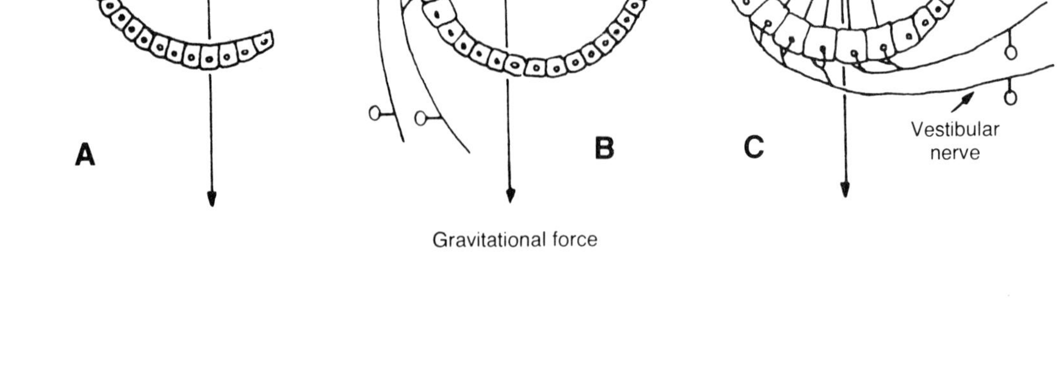

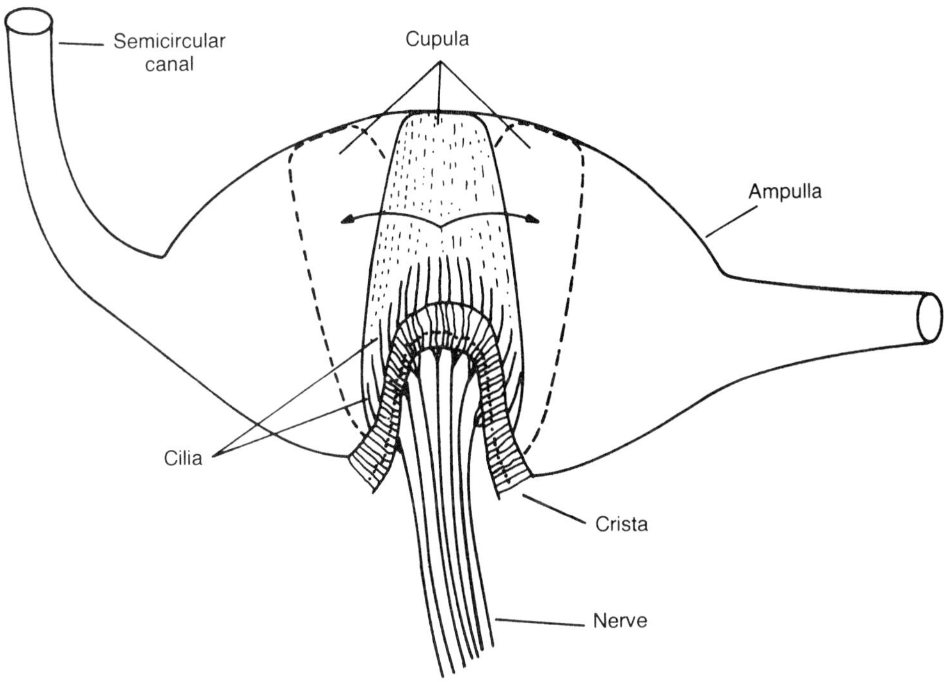

FIG. 9-4. The position of the crista ampullaris and cupula within a cross section of the ampulla of one semicircular canal. Also shown is the movement of the cupula and its embedded cilia during rotation first in one direction and then in the opposite direction. (Eyzaguirre C, Fidone SJ: Physiology of the Nervous System. Chicago, Year Book Medical Publishers, 1975)

cilia of the hair cells projecting out into a gelatinous substance, the cupula. The cupula extends from the crista across the ampulla, dividing it completely and not allowing fluid to pass by it. The result is that if there is relative movement of the fluid with respect to the canal, the cupula and thus the cilia will be bent to the side.

VESTIBULAR PHYSIOLOGY

Presumably, the sequence of events in the excitation of vestibular nerve fibers is similar to that for auditory nerve fibers. Movement of the cilia to one side results in a depolarization of the hair cell, a receptor potential that in turn depolarizes (the generator potential) the afferent fibers that contact it. Thus, when the head tilts forward the gravitational force on the otolithic membrane of the otolith organs changes and the hairs are subjected to a new force that displaces cilia to the side (Fig. 9-3B); pulls them down, away from the epithelium in the inverted position (Fig. 9-3A); or pushes them back against the cell in the upright position (Fig. 9-3C). Maximal discharge of the nerve occurs when the cilia are bent to one side (B); minimal discharge occurs when they are bent to the other side. An intermediate response occurs in any intermediate position (A and C). Because the hair cells are polarized in different directions in various regions of the macula, some hair cells are excited by movement of the head in any direction. The fibers innervating the utricular macula are slowly adapting and therefore can signal position of the head. They also signal linear acceleration because the forces exerted on the otolithic membrane by such acceleration also cause bending of the cilia, much as a wire coat hanger (straightened out) with a weight on the end is bent when you begin to run with it. The function of the saccule is not known.

The semicircular canals are positioned and structured to sense angular rotation. Forces that bend the cilia of hair cells in the cristae are generated by relative movements of the endolymph and the labyrinth. The principle is the same as that which operates in a glass of fluid containing ice cubes. Did you ever try to get a particular ice cube out

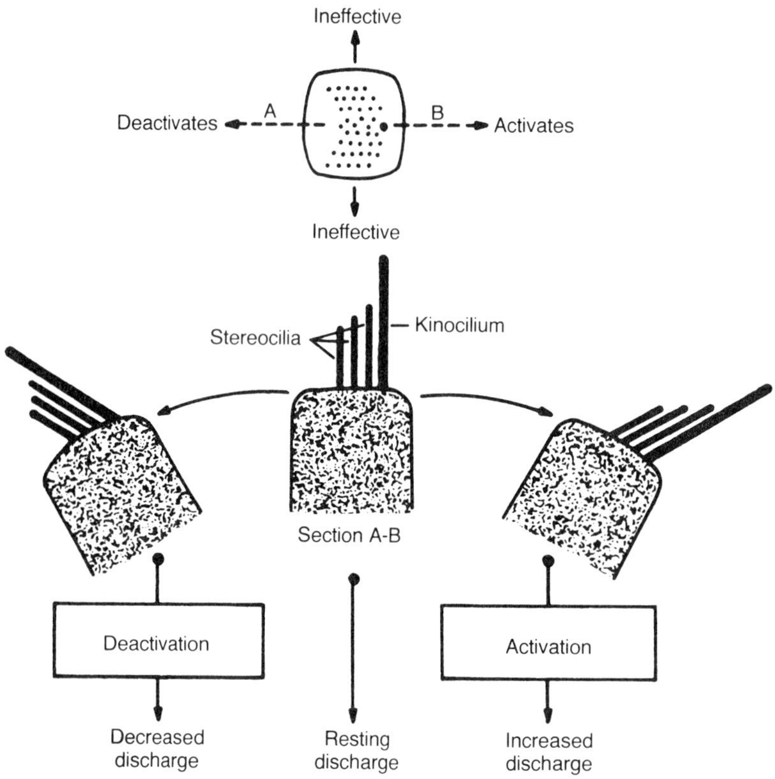

FIG. 9-5. Shearing force in vestibular organs. **Upper diagram** shows arrangement of cilia on a hair cell as seen from above; position of kinocilium indicated by **larger dot. Dotted line** indicates direction of effective shearing forces; forces at right angles are ineffective. **Lower diagram** shows section through hair cell along **dotted line** with cilia at rest **(center)** and tilted right and left. Tilt toward kinocilium excites, tilt away decreases excitation. (Klinke R: Physiology of hearing. In Schmidt RF [ed]: Fundamentals of Sensory Physiology. New York, Springer-Verlag, 1978)

of such a container? You rotate the glass, but the ice cube stays in the same place with respect to you! The inertia of the fluid makes it lag behind the glass in rotation. However, if you continue to rotate the glass at constant velocity, the fluid and the ice cubes will soon be rotating at the same speed as the glass. Now, if you suddenly stop the rotation, the fluid and the ice will continue to rotate until they gradually slow down and stop. If the ice stops on your side of the glass you get it, if not try again.

When the head is rotated the canals move with it, but the inertia of the endolymph causes it to lag behind. This results in a bending of the cupula in the direction opposite that of the rotation (Fig. 9-4) and in either an increase or a decrease in the discharge rate of the nerve cells innervating the crista, depending upon the direction of movement. If the rotation continues, the endolymph catches up with the movement of the canal; the cupula is returned to the upright position; and the discharge of the nerve fibers returns to its former rate (it adapts). If the rotation is suddenly stopped, the canals immediately stop their rotation, but the endolymph does not, so the cupula is bent in the other direction. This has the opposite effect on discharge in the vestibular nerve fibers.

Because of the nearly orthogonal orientations of the semicircular canals, rotation in any direction is sensed by one or more of the cristae. As in any three-coordinate system, any direction of rotation can be signaled uniquely by the combined discharges from the three canals. In the horizontal canal, the kinocilium is polarized toward the utricle. Figure 9-5 shows that when the cilia are bent in the direction of the kinocilium, the vestibular nerve fibers are excited and when they are bent the other way, the discharge is reduced. This means that in the horizontal canals, the vestibular

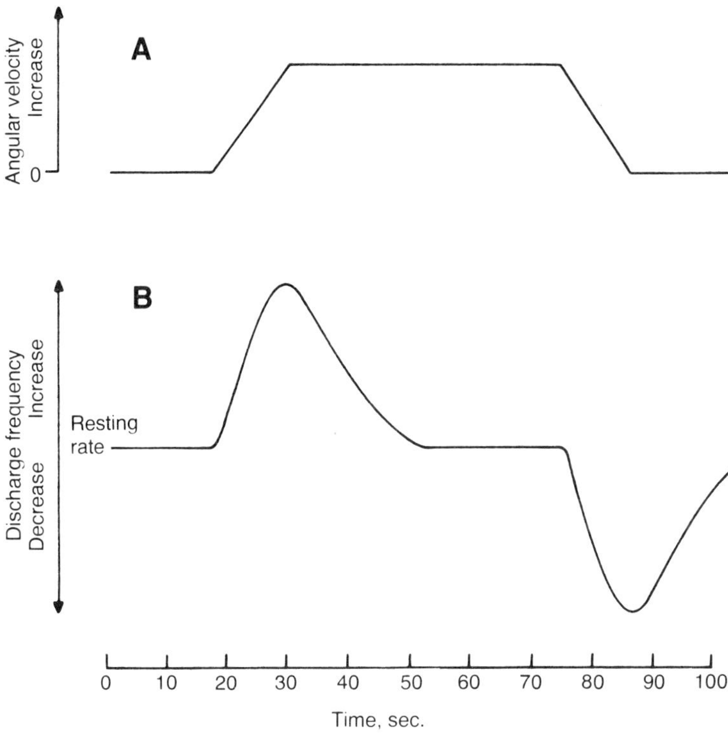

FIG. 9-6. Response of semicircular canals to angular rotation. **A.** The velocity of an angular rotation of the body (ordinate) plotted against time (abscissa). **B.** The change in frequency of discharge of a receptor innervating one of the semicircular canals during periods of constant acceleration, of constant velocity, and of constant deceleration of the head.

nerve activity increases when the endolymph moves (relatively) in the direction of the ampulla. Thus, when the head rotates to the *left*, the fluid in the *right* horizontal canal moves away from the ampulla (reduced excitation), and the fluid in the *left* one moves toward it (more excitation). The reverse movement or a deceleration has the opposite effects. In the vertical canals, the hair cells are polarized away from the utricle. Thus, the activity originating in the right superior canal is increased and that from the left posterior canal is reduced by moving the head forward and to the right, whereas the reverse effects are seen when the head is rotated backward and to the left. The horizontal canals are activated almost exclusively by movement around the vertical axis (the movement is like a "no" gesture with the head); the posterior canal on one side and the superior canal in the other labyrinth are activated by movement of the head in the anterolateral or posterolateral direction (like a "yes" gesture but at a bit of an angle). Note that effects are always bilateral and reciprocal.

ELECTROPHYSIOLOGY OF THE VESTIBULAR NERVE

Recordings made from single axons innervating the monkey's semicircular canals indicate that they have a high resting discharge rate and increase their discharge rate with angular acceleration; however, the receptors adapt rapidly to constant angular velocity, adapting completely to resting rates in less than one minute. The neurons decrease their discharge rates with angular deceleration, and adaptation also occurs with constant (decreased) angular velocity. This is indicated by the records in Figure 9-6. The upper record shows the angular velocity of the head, starting at zero, increasing at a constant acceleration to some higher value, remaining constant at that value for a time before returning at constant deceleration to zero velocity. The discharge rate of the neuron, shown in the lower record, increases from resting rate during constant acceleration, adapts with a time constant of 6.7 sec back to resting discharge rate, although velocity remains constant at the new value. Discharge frequency decreases during constant deceleration and adapts (this time increasing frequency) to the resting rate with a time constant of 4.9 sec. Figure 9-7 shows a simultaneous plot of responses to constant accelerations (open circles) and decelerations (filled circles) to illustrate the longer time constant of adaptation to accelerations. All receptors in the same ampulla have the same polarization so all are excited or inhibited by acceleration in the same direction.

In contrast, receptor cells in the utricle are not all polarized in the same direction so not all the neurons respond to the same sort of movement. For example, 70% of the neurons in one study were most sensitive to ipsilateral sideways roll of the head, whereas contralateral roll was most effective in exciting 30% of the neurons. About half of the neurons were most sensitive to nose-up pitch and half to nose-down pitch. An example of the discharge characteristics of a

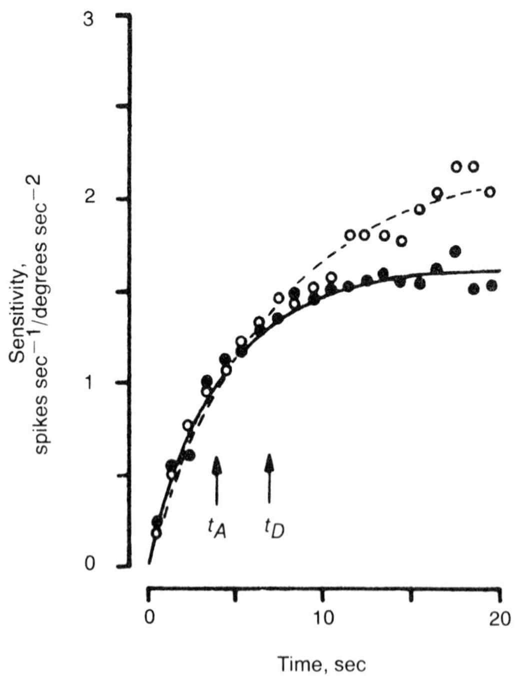

FIG. 9-7. Time course of responses to constant acceleration **(open circles)** and deceleration **(filled circles).** Sensitivity to acceleration in spikes/sec/degree/sec^2 (ordinate) is plotted against time (abscissa). The vertical **arrows** indicate the acceleration and deceleration time constants, t_A and t_D, for a slightly adapting neuron from the horizontal semicircular canal. (Goldberg JM, Fernandez C: J Neurophysiol 34:635–660, 1971)

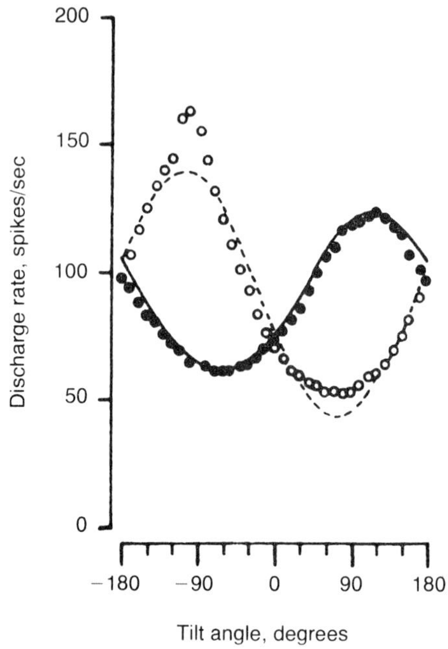

FIG. 9-8. Response curves for a utricular receptor to various pitches and rolls. Discharge rate (ordinate) is plotted against tilt angle (abscissa). Positive angles correspond to forward pitch and ipsilateral roll. **Open circles** are for pitch, **filled circles** for roll. (Fernandez C, Goldberg JM, Abend K: J Neurophysiol 35:978–997, 1972)

utricular receptor to pitches (open circles) and rolls (filled circles) is shown in Figure 9-8. This particular receptor increased its discharge rate with nose-up (backward) pitch until the angle of pitch reached about 90°; thereafter the discharge decreased. The discharge rate decreased with nose-down (forward) pitch to about 60° and increased with larger forward pitches. The response of the neuron to an ipsilateral roll was an increased discharge up to about 120°, then a decrease, whereas the response to a contralateral roll was a decrease, then an increase.

VESTIBULO-OCULAR REFLEX

The vestibular nerve fibers project to the vestibular nuclei and to the flocculonodular lobe of the cerebellum. The vestibular nuclei give rise both to the vestibulospinal tracts, which play a role in movement and posture, to be discussed in Chapter 16, and to connections with cranial nerve nuclei III, IV, and VI and motoneurons of the neck by

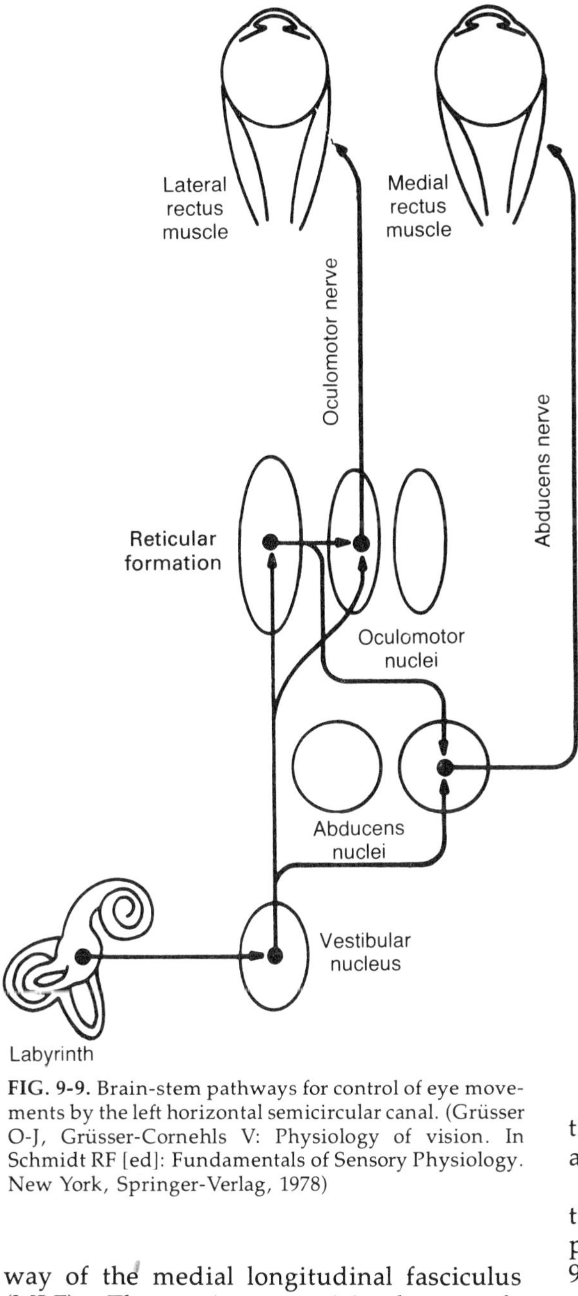

FIG. 9-9. Brain-stem pathways for control of eye movements by the left horizontal semicircular canal. (Grüsser O-J, Grüsser-Cornehls V: Physiology of vision. In Schmidt RF [ed]: Fundamentals of Sensory Physiology. New York, Springer-Verlag, 1978)

way of the medial longitudinal fasciculus (MLF). The various semicircular canals make preferred connections with motoneurons in the cranial nerve nuclei that control particular eye muscles. Horizontal canals drive motoneurons of the abducens nucleus (sixth cranial nerve) that innervate the contralateral lateral rectus muscle and of the oculomotor nucleus (third cranial nerve) that innervate the ipsilateral medial rectus muscle, while producing appropriate inhibition in the antagonist muscles. The vertical canals drive motoneurons that innervate the superior and inferior recti and oblique muscles.

One result of these connections is termed the **vestibulo-ocular reflex.** The neural pathways of the reflex are shown in Figure 9-9. If the head is moved to the left, the eyes are moved **conjugately** to the right, in order to maintain the gaze fixed on an object as the head moves. The mechanism for this reflex has been worked out in some detail. As the head is rotated to the left, the discharge of the vestibular fibers supplying the left horizontal canal is increased; concurrently, the discharge on the right is decreased. This results in an excitation of the right abducens nerve fibers innervating the right lateral rectus muscle and the left oculomotor nerve fibers innervating the left medial rectus muscle. The ensuing muscle contractions deviate the eye to the right. The reflex, of course, also occurs when the head is rotated in the other direction, but the eye movement is in the reverse direction as well.

The vestibulo-ocular reflex has an important clinical use. As a result of the reflex, when the head is moved from side to side, the eyes remain fixed on an object. This is called the **doll's-eye maneuver** by analogy to old-fashioned dolls with counterweighted eyes. It is a normal response to head rotation. Its absence in cases of head injury is usually taken to indicate involvement of the MLF and, therefore, a lesion of the brain stem. There are also reflex rotations of the eyes in compensation for rotation of the head toward the shoulder that involve the vertical canals; these too are normal responses.

NYSTAGMUS AND THE CALORIC TEST

The vestibular system, because of its bilaterality, is a balanced system. Effects of activity from one vestibular organ are balanced by effects from the other. A vestibular imbalance causes overstimulation on one side and slow tonic deviation of the eyes away from that side. Cortical mechanisms rapidly return the eyes to their former position. The tonic nature of the vestibular-induced movement causes this slow movement followed by a rapid or **saccadic** return to be repeated over and over. The complex movements are called **nystagmus.** By convention, the direction of the nystagmus is taken to be the direction of the quicker and more easily observed saccadic movement. It must be remembered that this is opposite to the vestibular-induced movement. Overstimulation can result in several ways. An irritative lesion can produce overstimulation ipsilaterally; natural stimulation by rotation can produce overstimulation ipsilaterally, but a destructive lesion will produce overstimulation contralaterally.

The presence of nystagmus in a patient usually indicates some problem with the labyrinth, vestibular nerve, or vestibular nuclei, but it also occurs as a part of the cerebellar dysfunction following overconsumption of alcohol. Nystagmus apparently also results from certain viral infections involving the vestibular system. In labyrinthine disease, the nystagmus is usually independent of gaze, but with more central lesions it usually occurs in the direction of gaze. Vertical nystagmus is nearly always evidence of a central nervous system lesion.

The functioning of the vestibular system is often checked clinically by means of the **caloric test.** For this test, the head is tilted backward by about 60° to bring the horizontal canal into a vertical position. Then either warm or cold water is introduced into the external auditory meatus on one side. The immediate results are usually vertigo (sensations of spinning), nausea, and twisting of the head and body. Nystagmus also results. When warm water is introduced into the meatus, it may set up convection currents in the nearby horizontal canal. The warm endolymph rises toward the ampulla and stimulates the vestibular nerve fibers there. This increase in activity however it comes about results in nystagmus toward that side of the head (the vestibular activity deviates the eyes in the other direction). Cold water induces nystagmus toward the opposite side of the head, apparently by reducing activity in the vestibular nerve (remember: a balanced system). With diseases involving the cerebral cortex, the saccadic phase of nystagmus is often absent, and the eyes merely deviate to a side appropriate for the temperature of the water.

RESPONSES TO ANGULAR ROTATION

The responses of individuals to rotation have been studied thoroughly because understanding them is important to controlling performance in high-speed aircraft or in spacecraft. When a person, with eyes closed, is submitted to angular rotation, for example in a Bárány chair, he accurately signals the direction of rotation when he first begins to move; however, after a period of rotation at constant velocity, he reports that he has ceased to rotate. This is precisely what is predicted from the rapid adaptation of receptors in the semicircular canals at constant velocity (Figs. 9-6 and 9-7). During the period of acceleration at the beginning of the rotation, the person also experiences a nystagmus in the direction of rotation, the eyes apparently attempting to stay fixated on some target. When the sensation of rotation fades at constant velocity, the nystagmus also disappears.

If the chair is abruptly stopped at this point, the person has a sensation of rotation in the direction opposite to that he previously experienced and that too fades with time. In addition, there is a **postrotatory nystagmus** also in the direction opposite that of the previous rotation. Again, these are phenomena consistent with the discharge properties of receptors in the semicircular canals. When a rotation stops, the discharge frequency of the canal receptors falls below resting levels, just as it would if there were actually a rotation in the opposite direction. Although rotation has ceased, the central nervous system cannot distinguish this signal from the signal that would occur for an opposite rotation and, therefore, it is interpreted as an opposite rotation. This sensation fades with time because of receptor adaptation. Another consequence of rotation in the postrotatory period is **past-pointing.** If a person is asked to point at a target immediately upon being stopped from a period of constant velocity rotation, he will consistently point inaccurately, with the deviation always in the direction of the previous rotation. Thus, if the previous rotation was clockwise, he will consistently point to the right of the target.

People who must undergo this kind of rotation frequently learn to ignore what their vestibular senses tell them. Figure skaters, for example, can spin for long periods without showing past-pointing or postrotatory nystagmus. Obviously, they must be able to do this if they are to continue skating after the spin. Airplane pilots can suffer what is called a Coriolis effect, a false sense of spinning. A pilot who has put his airplane into a spin, either intentionally or accidentally, may be unaware of it after a while if he relies upon his vestibular sense because of the adaptation of the receptors. When he stops the spin (usually because someone tells him to), he experiences a sensation of spinning in the opposite direction, the Coriolis effect. Were he then to attempt to correct for this illusory spin, he would set himself in a spin again. Many aircraft have been sent spinning to earth by pilots who failed to read their instruments and relied on the Coriolis effect to navigate.

DISTURBANCES OF VESTIBULAR FUNCTION

The most common disturbance related to vestibular function is motion sickness. This condition is characterized by vertigo, nausea, and vomiting and is apparently primarily precipitated by repeated vertical movements. Most people adapt readily to such movements, but particularly sensitive people become ill when traveling in a car, boat, or airplane. Motion sickness often can be avoided by eating sparing, fat-free meals or by taking antihistamines such as meclizine or dimenhydrinate (Dramamine) *before* traveling.

Vertigo, the *false* sensation that either the person or his world is rotating, is associated with vestibular malfunction. Clinicians, but not the man on the street, distinguish vertigo from dizziness, which is a disturbed sense of relationship to space or a sensation of unsteadiness with a feeling of movement within the head. Paroxysmal attacks of vertigo may cause the patient to fall down because of his postural responses to the false sensations of movement. Vertigo may occur acutely, as a result of labyrinthitis, or chronically, as a result of damage to the eighth cranial nerve. The symptoms of **Meniere's disease,** resulting from an accumulation of endolymph within the inner ear, can involve deafness or **tinnitus,** ringing or humming in the ears, because of the involvement of the cochlea and also vertigo because of labyrinthine involvement. The cause of Meniere's disease is unknown. The vertigo component of the disease can be treated surgically by labyrinthectomy or partial section of the eighth nerve, though the latter procedure is now seldom used. Meniere's disease is also treated pharmacologically with low-salt diets and diuretics as well as with antihistamines or histamine (a desensitizing procedure) or with large doses of thiamine. Vertigo can also be caused by eighth nerve tumors or ill-advised, prolonged treatment with streptomycin.

Rapid destruction, as opposed to slow destruction by disease, of a labyrinth leads to short-term disturbances of equilibrium, vertigo, and nystagmus. These are symptoms of a disbalance of the vestibular inputs; recall that the vestibular system compares the signals from the two labyrinths. With time, most of these symptoms weaken and disappear. For example, in cats a unilateral labyrinthectomy produces contralateral nystagmus (overstimulation opposite the lesion), head tilt toward that side, and a tendency for the body to roll toward the lesion. After three days, only the head tilt remains. Bilateral destruction of the labyrinths causes only a transient (lasting months) disturbance in equilibrium, but even this can be compensated by the positional information supplied by the eyes. In the cat again, bilateral lesions do not lead to nystagmus or tilt; however, walking is broad-based and swaying, and there is no righting reflex if the eyes are covered. After two weeks there is considerable improvement. In man, compensation for labyrinth destruction is complete; as long as the eyes are open, no chronic effects are obvious. The importance of the neck reflexes to movement and posture are emphasized by the observation that a bilateral block of the C1 to C3 dorsal roots produces the same kind of effect on an animal as bilateral labyrinthectomy (see Cohen, 1961).

SUGGESTED READING

Brodal A, Pompeiano O [ed]: Basic Aspects of Central Vestibular Mechanisms. Amsterdam, Elsevier, 1972

Cohen LA: Role of eye and neck proprioceptive mechanisms in body orientation and motor coordination. J. Neurophysiol 24:1–11, 1961

Flock Å: Sensory transduction in hair cells. In Loewenstein WR [ed]: Handbook of Sensory Physiology, Vol. I. Principles of Receptor Physiology. Berlin, Springer-Verlag, 1971

Hallpike CS: The caloric test: a review of its principles and practice with especial reference to the phenomenon of directional preponderance. In Wolfson R [ed]: The Vestibular System and its Diseases. Philadelphia, Univ Pennsylvania Press, 1966

Kornhuber HH [ed]: Handbook of Sensory Physiology, Vol. VI. Vestibular System, Part 1. Basic Mechanisms. Berlin, Springer-Verlag, 1974

Wersäll J, Flock Å: Physiological aspects of the structure of vestibular end organs. Acta Otolaryngol (Suppl) (Stockh) 192:85–89, 1964

Wilson VJ, Melvill Jones G: Mammalian Vestibular Physiology. New York, Academic Press, 1979

Young LR: Role of the vestibular system in posture and movement. In Mountcastle VB [ed]: Medical Physiology, 13th ed, Vol. I. St. Louis, C.V. Mosby, 1974

10

Gustatory and Olfactory Senses

GUSTATION AND OLFACTION

It is appropriate to consider taste and smell together because they are so intertwined in our experience that most people are unaware that most of what they call taste is really an olfactory experience. The sensations evoked by a substance put into the mouth are complicated and involve much more than taste. For example, a mouthful of orange soda pop gives one a taste that is a combination of sour and sweet; it is cold; it may sting or tingle a bit if it is carbonated; it evokes a complex touch sensation in the mouth, and it smells fruity or fragrant. The only part of this complex of sensations that is taste in origin, that is, resulting from receptors on the tongue, palate, or pharynx is the sensation of sweetness or sourness. Anyone who has ever had a head cold can attest to the flatness or blandness of his diet during that time. This is due to the fact that access of odorants to olfactory receptors is blocked by the copious secretions of mucus.

TASTE

The gustatory system is much simpler than the olfactory system. Four primary taste submodalities are generally recognized: sweet, sour, salty, and bitter. Different regions on the tongue exhibit different maximal sensitivities to the four taste submodalities (Fig. 10-1). The tip of the tongue is most sensitive to sweetness and saltiness. The sensation of sourness is experienced best on the lateral aspects of the tongue, and bitterness is experienced best and perhaps only on the back of the tongue. Next time you put some bitter substance such as tonic water (quinine) into your mouth, you can verify this for yourself.

The chemical senses are difficult to study experimentally because the stimuli that lead to gustatory and olfactory sensations are not well understood. Sour tastes are evoked by all acids in dilute solutions. Apparently, it is the hydrogen ion that activates taste receptors and leads to a sensation of sourness. Accounting for salty tastes is more difficult. Sodium chloride is the only substance known to evoke a purely salty taste in any concentration that is suprathreshold. With other compounds, having one of the cations, Na^+, K^+, Li^+, Ca^{2+}, and one of the anions, Cl^-, Br^-, I^-, SO_4^{2-}, NO_3^{2-}, CO_3^{2-}, the saltiness varies with concentration. For example, a very dilute solution of KCl tastes sweet and, as the concentration increases, it becomes first bitter, then both bitter and salty, and finally purely salty. Both the anion and the cation are apparently involved in evoking the salty sensation.

The basis for sweet and bitter tastes is not known. Sucrose is a carbohydrate, a disaccharide formed from one molecule each of fructose (a fruit sugar) and glucose. Glucose, fructose, and starch are also carbohydrates. Fructose (grape sugar) is the sweetest; glucose is less sweet than sucrose or fructose; and starch is not sweet at all. Some alcohols are sweet. For example, xylitol is used as a sweetener in Europe and in some chewing gum in the United States. Saccharin is also sweet (and bitter), but chemically it bears little similarity to either the sugars or the alcohols. The only known commonality for

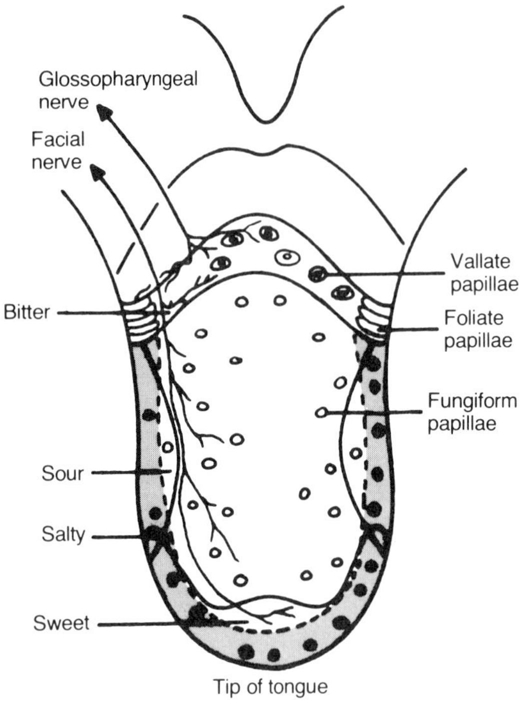

FIG. 10-1. The distribution of gustatory papillae, their innervation, and the regions of maximum sensitivity to different submodalities of taste on the human tongue. (Altner H: Physiology of taste. In Schmidt RF [ed]: Fundamentals of Sensory Physiology. New York, Springer-Verlag, 1978)

all these substances is that they excite gustatory receptors leading to sensations of sweetness.

The sensation of bitterness is evoked by many vegetable alkaloids, such as quinine, and by some metallic salts. Some people think that our sensitivity to bitterness may be a protective mechanism because many plant poisons are alkaloids and are bitter. However, the sense of bitterness may not be a real deterrent to ingesting bitter substances. Many of the favored foods of gorillas are found to taste bitter to humans. Either gorillas do not taste them as bitter or they are attracted to bitter substances. Interestingly, the substance phenylthiocarbamide tastes bitter to some people, but for others it is nearly tasteless, indicating that the characteristics of some receptors vary across individuals.

There are also interactions between taste stimuli or sensations. Sucrose tastes sweeter after caffeine than after water; tartaric acid is more sour after KCl than after water; and caffeine is more bitter after sucrose than after water. After eating miracle fruit (a tropical fruit), even substances that are normally very sour taste sweet. You experience this sort of interaction any morning you eat grapefruit (it tastes very sour) after drinking a glass of sweet pineapple juice.

Taste sensitivity varies widely depending upon the submodality and the substance being tasted. For example, the absolute threshold for detection of sucrose (sweet) is a concentration of 0.02 M, whereas the threshold for sodium chloride is 0.035 M, for hydrochloric acid (sour) is 0.002 M, and for quinine sulfate (bitter) is 0.0000004 M. These absolute thresholds cover five orders of magnitude of concentration difference. Another substance that is sweet, saccharin, has a threshold of 0.00002 M, three orders of magnitude lower than that for sucrose. Taste thresholds for different submodalities are also influenced differentially by changes in temperature. Thus, the sensitivity to NaCl and quinine sulfate decreases with increasing temperature in the range from 17 to 42°C; sensitivity to HCl is unaffected over the same range; and sensitivity to sweet substances increases. With the exception of sweet substances, none of the submodalities behaves as if it involved a chemical reaction, the rates of which are usually speeded by increasing temperature.

TASTE ANATOMY

Gustatory receptor cells are found in the taste buds of fungiform, foliate, and circumvallate papillae located mainly on the tongue. The distribution of the different papillae on the tongue is shown in Figure 10-1. In the intact **papilla,** about all that can be seen from the surface, even with a scanning electron microscope, is a small hole, the taste pore, through which the sapid substance must pass. Inside is the taste bud, which is composed of elongated sensory cells arranged with other nonsensory cells like the segments of an orange, as shown in Figure 10-2, which is a drawing of a cross section through a taste bud. The apical portions of the sensory cells have microvilli that project into the region of the taste pore. These microvilli are 2 to 5 μm long and 0.05 to 0.2 μm wide, and function perhaps to increase the surface area of the cell membrane. There are 40 to 60 densely packed and interdigitated taste cells per bud. It is

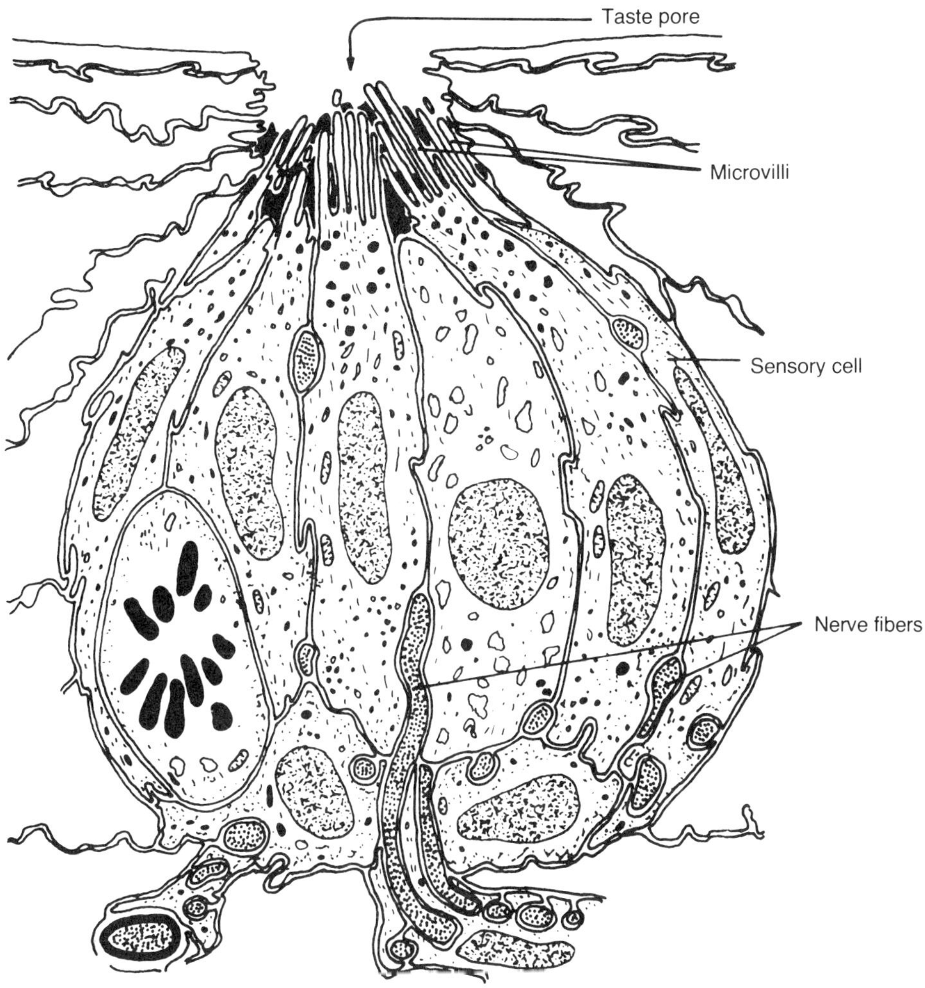

FIG. 10-2. Drawing of a cross section through a taste bud from a foliate papilla of a rabbit indicating the arrangement of receptor cells and the locations of the taste pore, microvilli, and nerve fibers. (Andres KH: Discussion of paper by Murray RG, Murray A: The anatomy and ultrastructure of taste endings. In Welstenholme GEW, Knight J [eds]: Taste and Smell in Vertebrates. London, Churchill, 1970)

unlikely that substances can get between the densely packed cells down to the sensory nerve fibers, so it must be the cells themselves that respond to chemicals. Diffusion in this direction is also impeded by a substance found between the sensory cells at their apical ends. The location of this substance is shown by the blackened areas in Figure 10-2. Even if a taste substance could get between the cells, it could not get to the nerve fibers that are buried, sometimes completely, in invaginations of the sensory cells. It is unlikely that sapid substances excite the sensory nerves directly, but more likely indirectly through the sensory cells.

It is known that taste sensory cells are among the shortest-lived cells in the body. It has been estimated that taste cells live only 250 ± 50 hours. The cells are formed from undifferentiated epithelial cells, and their formation is presumably under neural control. (The initimate relationship between taste buds and the nerve fibers that innervate them is discussed in Chapter 18.) The taste sensory cells begin on the periphery of the bud and move toward the center in a matter of a few days; then they die. This means there is a constant, rapid turnover in taste cells, implying that the specific sensitivity of the sensory cell is determined by the nerve fibers that innervate it. If it were otherwise, our sense of taste would be constantly changing, whereas taste is relatively stable over time.

Beneath the taste bud there is a plexus of myelinated nerve fibers of 1 to 6 μm diameter that enter the bud. The smaller diameter fibers associate with only one sensory cell, but the larger fibers associate with two or more cells. A given sensory cell may receive contacts from up to 30 nerve fibers. In addition, a given nerve fiber can innervate up to nine separate taste papillae.

Afferent fibers carry impulses from the tongue to the brain stem in the chorda tympani branch of the seventh cranial nerve, the lingual branch of the ninth nerve, and the pharyngeal branches of the tenth nerve. The chorda tympani innervates the anterior two-thirds of the tongue, whereas the lingual innervates the posterior one-third. The vagus innervates mainly the pharyngeal and laryngeal areas (see Fig. 10-1). In addition to taste signals, these nerves also carry temperature and tactile information from their receptive fields. Taste fibers in these nerves tend to be Aδ fibers with conduction velocities of 2 to 18 m/sec. There may be pathways for taste fibers other than the three nerves previously mentioned, but this is debatable (sometimes hotly).

In the brain stem, taste nerves relay in the nucleus tractus solitarius where they contact secondary cells that are organized in a roughly topographic manner. These secondary cells then project fibers to the medial part of the ventral thalamus near the somatic face projection from the trigeminal nerve and also to a pontine taste area. The cortical projection sites appear to be in the pre- and postcentral gyri near the face representation and in the insular region.

TASTE PHYSIOLOGY

Taste neurons normally respond to several different kinds of chemicals so that chorda tympani taste fibers typically respond to substances that are salty, bitter, sweet, and sour. That is, they appear to respond to stimuli of two or three or even four different taste submodalities. An example of the discharges evoked in a single taste fiber in the chorda tympani nerve by substances flowing over the tongue is shown in Figure 10-3. This particular nerve cell gives a brisk discharge when NaCl and saccharin flow over the tongue, but it is only minimally, if at all, excited by sucrose, HCl, or quinine. It is also not especially sensitive to changes in the temperature of the fluid bathing the tongue. The question then is; How can we distinguish sweet from sour when our taste receptors respond nonspecifically to taste stimuli?

It appears that most taste receptors do not signal single submodalities uniquely, but the submodality, that is, the quality of the taste, must be determined by the central nervous system from the discharge pattern across the ensemble of sensory nerve fibers. To see this, examine the histograms of Figure 10-4, which are plots of the number of spikes discharged by 28 different chorda tympani nerve fibers in the first 5 seconds after various solutions were allowed to flow over the tongue of a hamster. This figure should be reminiscent of Figure 4-10, which was "invented" to illustrate an ensemble code. In Figure 10-4, the data plotted are from actual experiments, and they illustrate that taste nerve fibers respond better to one or two of the taste submodalities than to others. Few receptors signal a single submodality uniquely; therefore, submodality must be signaled in the form of the ensemble code.

Taste intensity, on the other hand, seems to be signaled in terms of the total number of impulses discharged per second (*i.e.*, the frequency) in the ensemble of primary taste fibers. Single cells increase their discharge frequencies with increasing concentration of taste substances, as illustrated in Figure 10-5. The graphs indicate the responses of three different chorda tympani fibers to increasing concentrations of taste stimuli. The number of impulses evoked in 5 seconds is plotted against the concentration of the solution (on the abscissa). Fiber #1 was quite sensitive to NaCl, less so to sucrose. However, the discharge of the cell increased steadily as the concentration of either NaCl or sucrose was increased. Fiber #2 was more sensitive to sucrose than NaCl, but it still increased its discharge frequency when either substance was in higher concentration. Fiber #3 was sensitive to NaCl, quinine, and HCl, and it showed the same sort of increased response to increasing concentration of any of the three substances. The

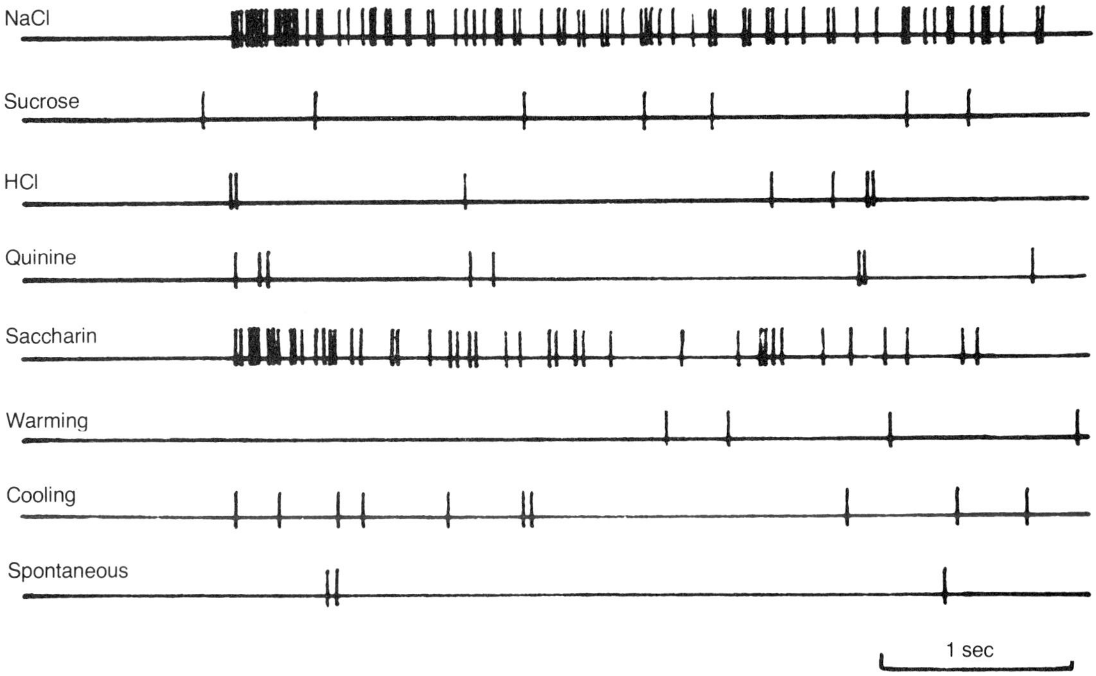

FIG. 10-3. Impulse discharges in a single chorda tympani nerve fiber of a rat. Responses elicited by application to the tongue of 0.1 M NaCl, 0.5 M sucrose, 0.01 N HCl, 0.02 M quinine hydrochloride, 0.02 M sodium saccharin, 40°C water and 20°C water. Spontaneous discharges are shown in the bottom trace. Between traces the tongue was rinsed with 25°C water. (Ogawa H, Sato M, Yamashita S: J Physiol (Lond) 199:223–240, 1968)

total number of impulses per second increased in all the fibers, but their relative discharge for each substance was the same.

In an attempt to correlate psychophysical data for taste intensity with neuron responses to changing stimulus concentration, subjective intensities for citric acid and sucrose were estimated by two human subjects for six different concentrations of each substance. Responses of chorda tympani nerve fibers were recorded at the same six concentrations. The results of these two experiments are plotted together on the same log–log plot in Figure 10-6. There is remarkable agreement between the psychophysical and neural data, both showing a power function relation between stimulus intensity and response magnitude.

However, the problem of intensity coding is not always a simple one. It should be recalled that there is an interaction between quality and intensity for some substances, for example, KCl. For those substances, the response of the cell ensemble to a given concentration should be like the response to another substance that yields the same sensation. That this does occur is shown in Figure 10-7. In this graph are plotted the responses of 12 cells, six in the chorda tympani nerve (lower three curves) and six in the nucleus tractus solitarius (upper three curves). Three solutions were allowed to flow over the tongue. Quinine hydrochloride, QHCl, tastes bitter at any concentration above 4×10^{-7} M. Potassium chloride is bitter at 0.03 M, but it is salty at 0.3 M concentration. The two curves for QHCl and 0.03 M KCl for the chorda tympani nerve are nearly identical as predicted (the substances taste the same), and they are noticeably different from the curve for 0.3 M KCl (that tastes different). This means that this ensemble of six neurons signals the same thing to the CNS about both bitter solutions, but it signals something different to the CNS about the salty solution. The same thing happens in the nucleus tractus solitarius. In fact, the discharges of the second-order neurons are not greatly different from those of first-order neurons except

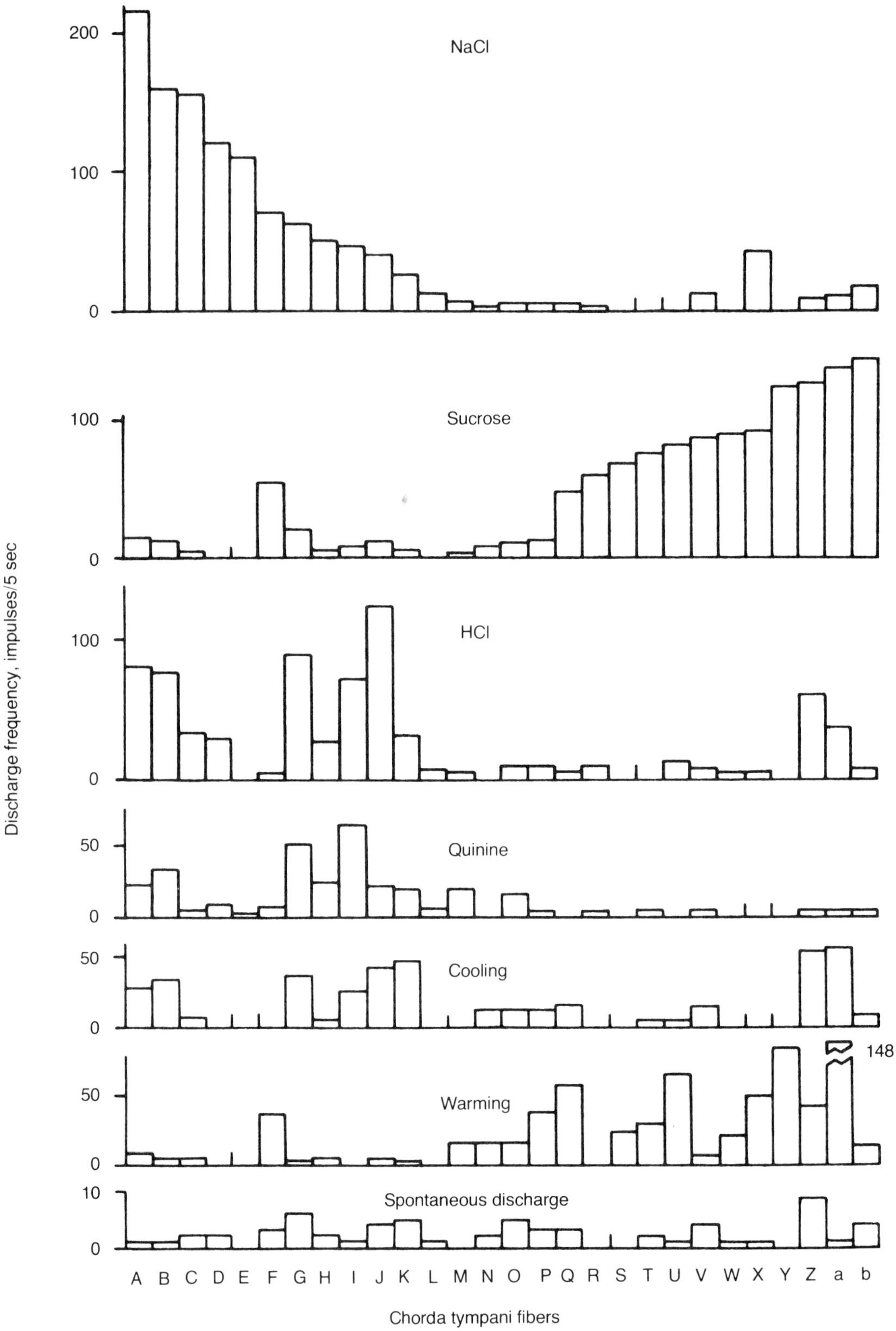

FIG. 10-4. Response profiles of 28 hamster chorda tympani fibers. Stimuli were 0.1 M NaCl, 0.5 M sucrose, 0.01 N HCl, 0.02 M quinine hydrochloride, 20°C water and 40°C water. The response of a single fiber to each stimulus is found by reading up columns indicated by the letters on the abscissa (Ogawa H, Sato M, Yamashita S: J Physiol (Lond) 199:223–240, 1968)

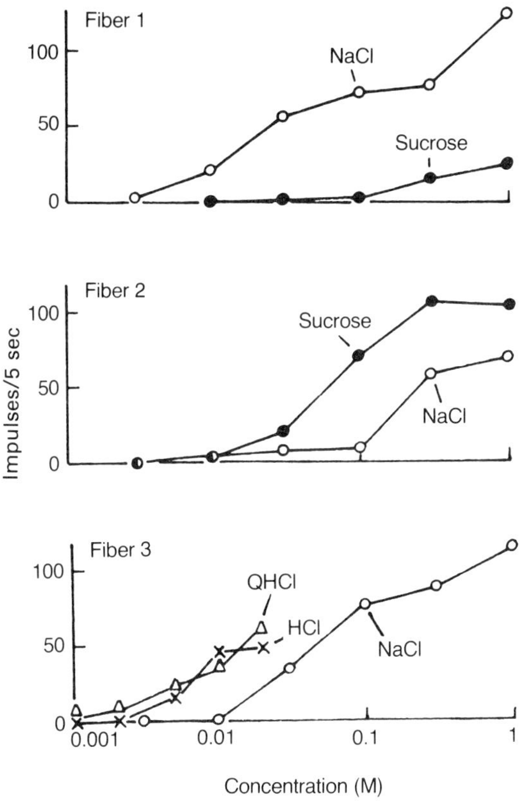

FIG. 10-5. Concentration–response magnitude relationships in three typical chorda tympani fibers of rats. Ordinate indicates the number of impulses discharged by the fiber in the first 5 sec after the substance was applied. Fiber #1 was predominantly sensitive to NaCl, fiber #2 was more sensitive to sucrose than NaCl, and fiber #3 was sensitive to NaCl, quinine, and HCl. (Ogawa H, Sato M, Yamashita S. J Physiol (Lond) 199:223–240, 1968)

that the discharge frequencies are higher. The same is true of discharges in thalamic third-order neurons. To date, only a few cortical taste neurons have been recorded from, so their response characteristics remain a mystery. This is not for lack of attempts to record taste-related activity in the cortex. It appears that the cortex may not play a major role in gustatory sensation.

SMELL

The identification of primary olfactory submodalities has been attempted many times. The first serious effort at identification was made by Linnaeus, the Swedish botanist, in 1756. Over the years a large number of other classifications of odors have been made, but there is not a general agreement about primary odors in the sense of the primary tastes: sweet, sour, salty, and bitter. The human can distinguish the odors of a vast number of different molecules and describes them as aromatic, fragrant, repulsive, ethereal, resinous, spicy, burned, putrid, and so forth. Whether any of these can be considered primary is a point of debate.

Odorous substances have in common that they are either gases or volatile liquids that can evaporate. This is the form in which the odorant reaches the sensory epithelium, either through the nostrils with inspired air or by the backdoor through the mouth and throat. The receptor structures for olfaction

FIG. 10-6. Dependence of subjective intensity of taste sensations **(open circles)** and of the frequency of discharge in fibers of the chorda tympani nerve **(filled circles)** upon the concentration of citric acid and sucrose solutions. Log–log plot. The slopes of the lines correspond to the exponents, k, of power functions with $k = 0.85$ and 1.1. (Borg G, Diamant H, Ström L et al: J Physiol (Lond) 192:13–20, 1967)

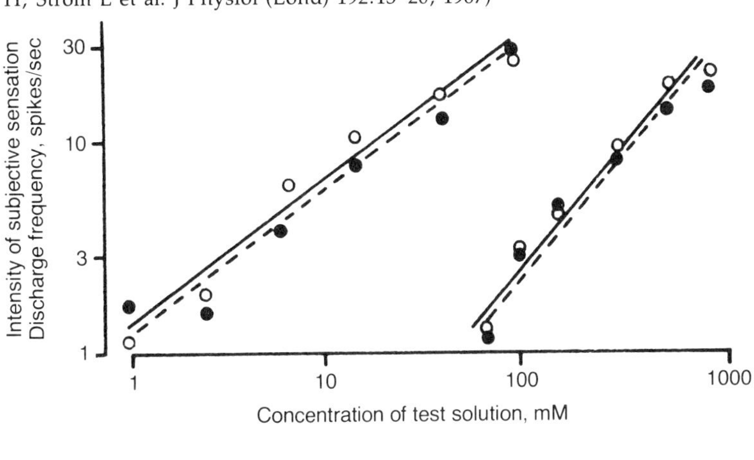

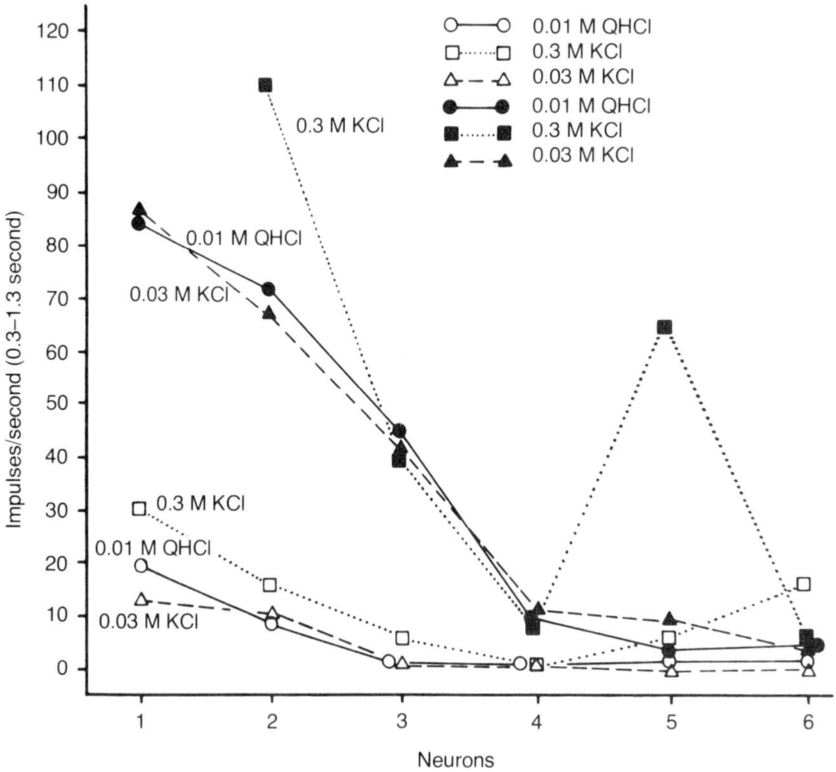

FIG. 10-7. Neural representation of a change in taste quality with a change in the concentration of KCl. Six chorda tympani neurons and six neurons of the nucleus tractus solitarius are indicated by the numerals on the abscissa. The responses of these chorda tympani fibers **(open symbols)** and nucleus tractus solitarius neurons **(filled symbols)** to two different concentrations of KCl and one of quinine hydrochloride are shown by the six sets of curves. To a human, 0.3 M KCl is salty, 0.03 M KCl is bitter, and 0.01 M QHCl is bitter. (Doetsch GS, Ganchow JJ, Nelson LM et al: Information processing in the taste system of the rat. In Pfaffmann C [ed]: Olfaction and Taste, III. New York, Rockefeller Univ Press, 1969)

are covered with mucus so that aqueous solubility is an asset to an odorant.

Of all the chemical elements, only 16 seem to play any role in the production of odor sensation. These are hydrogen, carbon, silicon, nitrogen, phosphorus, arsenic, antimony, bismuth, oxygen, sulfur, selenium, tellurium, fluorine, chlorine, bromine, and iodine. Only the halogens and ozone, O_3, are odorous as elements. There have been many attempts to group odorants in terms of chemical structure, with some success. The gross profile of the molecule, that is, its size and shape, seems to be important. Many people have also emphasized the importance of other physicochemical features, especially the characteristics of functional groups.

The olfactory system is extremely sensitive. For example, ethyl mercaptan can be detected at a concentration of 4×10^{-8} mg per liter of air. However, even at this low concentration, there would be millions of molecules in a single sniff. On the other hand, for certain odorants, a single molecule may be sufficient to excite a single olfactory receptor cell, at least in some animals. Sensitivity is no more constant in the olfactory system than in any other sensory system. It diminishes upon continuous exposure to an odor. This kind of adaptation is familiar to everyone. The smell of fried fish is not even noticed by the cook unless he leaves the kitchen and returns after some time. Odors also interact in rather specific ways. For example, adaptation to the odor of camphor results in a simultaneous increase in the threshold concentration of eucalyptus (eucalyptol) and cloves (eugenol) but not to bitter almonds (benzaldehyde). When two odorants are presented together, they can blend (violets and H_2S together yield a blend smell); they can be sensed successively; one odor can mask the other (especially if one is much stronger); or the combination can give no odor at all. The perfume industry is based on these principles.

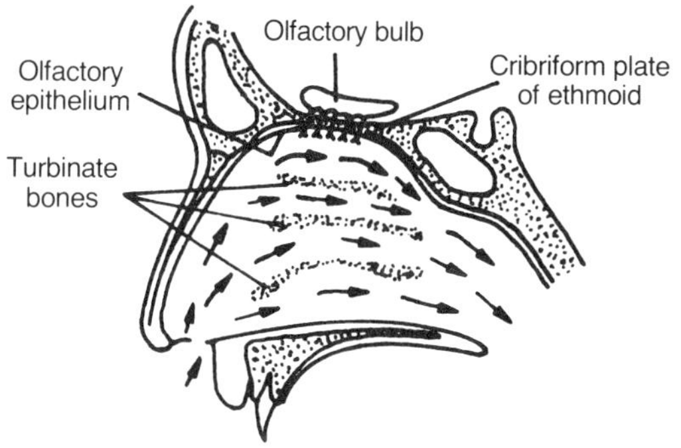

FIG. 10-8. Sagittal section of the human nasal passages, showing the nasal fossae, the location of the olfactory epithelium and olfactory bulb, and the direction of travel of inspired air **(small arrows).** (Douek E: The Sense of Smell and Its Abnormalities. Edinburgh, Livingstone, 1974)

FIG. 10-9. The olfactory mucosa showing arrangement of olfactory receptor cells in interconnected rings, one of which is illustrated. Receptor cells are connected together by gap junctions both between spines and less frequently at their apical expansions (two shown). The centers of the rings are apparently filled with supporting cells. (Graziadei PPC: Z Zellforsch 118:449–466, 1971)

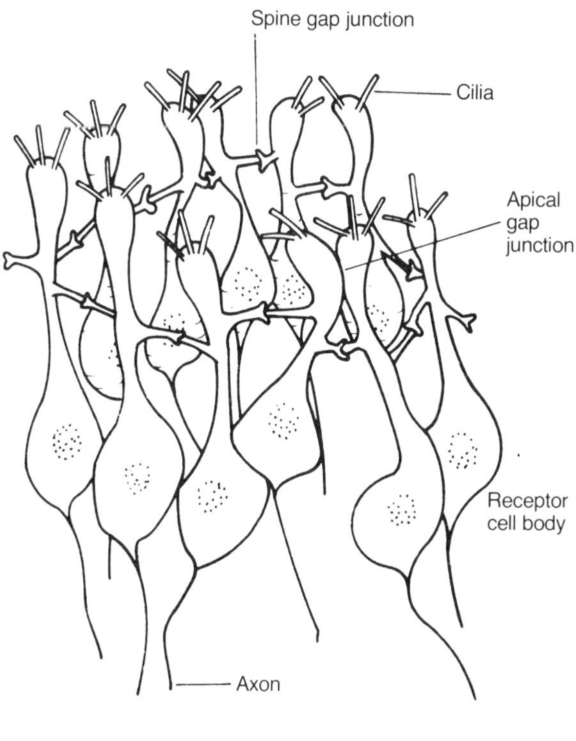

SMELL ANATOMY

The olfactory receptors are located in the posterior portion of the nasal cavity in a mucosal area that measures about 5 cm^2. The location is shown in Figure 10-8. The sensory epithelium sits at the top of the nasal cavity above the superior turbinate bones. It is yellow in color and has no synchronously beating cilia and therefore is distinguishable from the surrounding respiratory epithelia. Within this sensory region are found Bowman's glands that contain most of the yellow pigment and secrete much of the mucus that covers the sensory epithelium in a 10- to 40-μm layer. The odorant must dissolve in this mucus layer in order to reach the olfactory receptors.

The olfactory epithelium contains the receptor cells, as shown in the diagram of Figure 10-9, as well as sustentacular and basal cells. The receptor cells are really bipolar nerve cells and therefore unlike the receptor cells of the eye, ear, and tongue, which are specialized epithelial cells. The olfactory re-

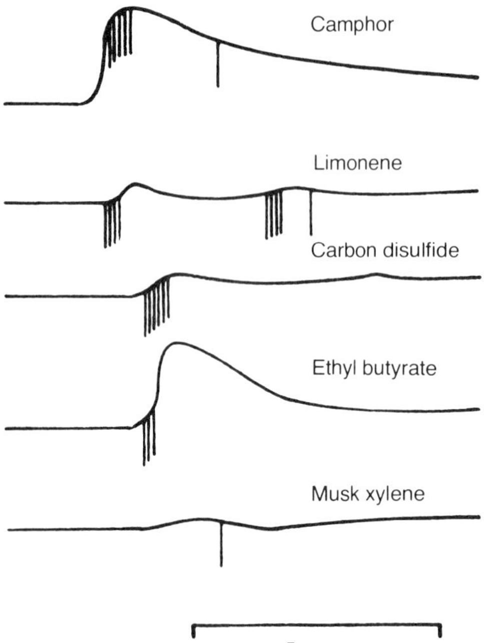

FIG. 10-10. Responses of a single cell in the olfactory epithelium to stimulation with camphor, limonene, carbon disulfide, ethyl butyrate, and musk xylene. (Gesteland RC, Lettvin JY, Pitts WH et al: Odor specificities of frog's olfactory receptors. In Zotterman Y [ed]: Olfaction and Taste. New York, Macmillan, 1963)

ceptor cells have their nuclei in the lower two-thirds of the epithelium, but their apical ends project to the surface. The apical ends are slightly enlarged, and they possess numerous cilia that project 50 to 150 μm out into the mucus. The location of the receptor sites on the receptor cell is unknown. Many people believe they are on the cilia, but the existence of olfactory cells without cilia and the persistence of olfactory sensation after the cilia have been removed argue against this idea.

At its basal end, each receptor cell gives rise to an axon that forms a part of the olfactory nerve. Olfactory nerve fibers are unmyelinated and average about 0.2 μm in diameter. In the rabbit, the olfactory epithelium contains about 100 million receptor cells, and thus there are about the same number of fibers in the olfactory nerve. In man, the olfactory nerve is short, merely perforating the cribriform plate into the brain cavity and terminating in the olfactory bulb. Olfactory nerve fibers converge onto mitral cells in the bulb, which send their axons (about 100,000 of them) in the olfactory tract to the piriform cortex, the periamygdaloid area, and the olfactory tubercle. The olfactory bulb contains interneurons, the granule cells that mediate a form of lateral inhibition between mitral cells; an active mitral cell inhibits (reduces) activity in its neighbors. There are also centrifugal fibers to the olfactory bulb that primarily mediate inhibition of mitral cell activity. The functions of this connection and of the lateral inhibition are not known.

Unlike other sensory pathways to the cerebral cortex, the olfactory pathway does not relay in the thalamus as we have just seen. However, fibers do leave the olfactory cortical areas and relay in the thalamus on their way to the hypothalamus or other areas where they perhaps play a role in the regulation of the intake of food and other behaviors that depend upon olfactory information.

SMELL PHYSIOLOGY

The coding mechanism for olfactory quality (submodality) has been just as elusive as the identification of the qualities themselves. Microelectrode recordings from the olfactory epithelium yield two sorts of responses to olfactory stimulation. Both can be seen in Figure 10-10. First, there is a slow-wave potential reminiscent of the generator potentials of mechanoreceptors (see Chap. 4). However, this potential is much larger than generator potentials recorded extracellularly from single receptors elsewhere. It also does not have a fixed relationship to the time of spike initiation, as can be seen in the figure. This potential probably is the summation of the generator potentials of a number of nearby receptor cells and perhaps potentials generated by supporting cells.

Second, there are the familiar spike discharges in the receptor cell axons or somata. It can be seen from this typical example that receptors are not highly specific in their responses to odorants. This particular cell responds to camphor, limonene, carbon disulfide, ethyl butyrate, and musk xylene, but it was insensitive to nitrobenzene, benzaldehyde, n-butanol, and pyridine. In general, each olfactory receptor responds to a variety of odorants, suggesting a complex ensemble code.

The same sort of behavior has also been

seen in mitral cells of the olfactory bulb. Perhaps, like the gustatory system, the olfactory system signals smell quality by the pattern of activity in the ensemble of olfactory receptors. The larger number of odorants compared to taste stimuli makes this hypothesis difficult to test. Studies have shown that odors may be encoded in terms of the position in the epithelium of responding receptors and the relative timing of discharges across the sheet of receptors. Spatial–temporal patterning is the basis of chromatographic separation of molecules; a similar process might be used by the olfactory epithelium in odor discrimination. Compounds with similar smells have been shown to be similar in terms of these two parameters. As yet, the evidence favoring this hypothesis must be viewed as preliminary.

SUGGESTED READING

Amoore JE: Stereochemical theory of olfaction. In Schultz HW, Day EA, Libbey LM [eds]: Chemistry and Physiology of Flavors. Westport, CT, Avi Publishing Co, 1967

Beidler LM [ed]: Handbook of Sensory Physiology. IV. Chemical Senses. 1. Olfaction. New York, Springer-Verlag, 1971

Beidler LM [ed]: Handbook of Sensory Physiology. IV. Chemical Senses. 2. Taste. New York, Springer-Verlag, 1971

Mozell MM: The spatiotemporal analysis of odorants at the level of the olfactory receptor sheet. J Gen Physiol 50:25–41, 1966

Shepherd GM: Synaptic organization of the mammalian olfactory bulb. Physiol Rev 52:864–917, 1972

Shibuya T, Tucker D: Single unit response of the olfactory receptors in vultures. In Hayashi I [ed]: Olfaction and Taste. II. Oxford, Pergamon Press, 1967

11

Muscle Receptors

So far, our discussion of receptors has dealt only with exteroceptors. Now we will deal briefly with three kinds of enteroceptors, all found in muscle. These are sometimes termed proprioceptors, because they sense what goes on in the body itself. The term proprioceptor is usually reserved for receptors in muscle, tendon, and joint, but the term is sometimes used more loosely as a synonym for enteroceptor. Primary and secondary muscle spindle receptors and Golgi tendon organs all send information about the state of the muscle to the central nervous system. All muscles, with the exception of extraocular and facial musculature, contain all three types of receptors.

MUSCLE SPINDLE AFFERENT FIBERS

The primary and secondary muscle spindle afferent fibers both arise from a specialized structure within the muscle, the **muscle spindle,** a fusiform structure 4 to 7 mm long and 80 to 200 μm in diameter. The spindles are located deep within the muscle mass, scattered widely through the muscle body, and attached to the tendon, the endomysium, or the perimysium, so as to be in parallel with the **extrafusal** or regular **muscle fibers.** Although spindles are scattered widely in muscles, they are not found throughout. Figure 11-1 shows the distribution of spindles in the medial gastrocnemius muscle of the cat, in dorsal and midsagittal projections. It can be seen that nearly 40% of the muscle is devoid of spindles, especially marginal areas. A drawing of a muscle spindle is shown in Figure 11-2. It contains two types of **intrafusal muscle fibers** (intrafusal = inside the fusiform spindle): the **nuclear bag fibers** and the **nuclear chain fibers.** The nuclear bag fibers are thicker and longer than the nuclear chain fibers, and they receive their name from the accumulation of their nuclei in the expanded bag-like equatorial region—the nuclear bag. The nuclear chain fibers have no equatorial bulge; rather their nuclei are lined up in the equatorial region—the nuclear chain. This distinction is illustrated in Figure 11-3. A typical spindle contains two nuclear bag fibers and four to five nuclear chain fibers.

The sensory innervation of the muscle spindle arises from both group Ia and group II afferent fibers. As shown in Figure 11-3, a single, large group Ia fiber coils around the equatorial regions of both nuclear bag and nuclear chain fibers, forming the **annulospiral endings** or **primary muscle spindle receptors.** Current thought is that all group Ia afferent fibers form annulospiral endings; therefore, the terms primary muscle spindle afferent fiber and group Ia afferent fiber are used interchangeably. The smaller group II fibers terminate at either end of the nuclear region primarily on the nuclear chain fibers (there is apparently some innervation of bag fibers by secondary muscle spindle afferent fibers, but there is disagreement as to how much); they form **flower-spray endings** or **secondary muscle spindle receptors.** Not all group II fibers form such endings, so these terms are not synonymous.

The intrafusal fibers are striated muscle fibers that receive innervation from the **fusimotor neurons** or **γ motoneurons.** Activity in fusimotor neurons produces a contraction of the muscular, polar regions of the spindle, putting stretch on the equatorial region (where the receptor regions are) that has few myofibrils and therefore little contractility. It is apparently the stretching of this central region, regardless of how it is accomplished, that is the adequate stimulus

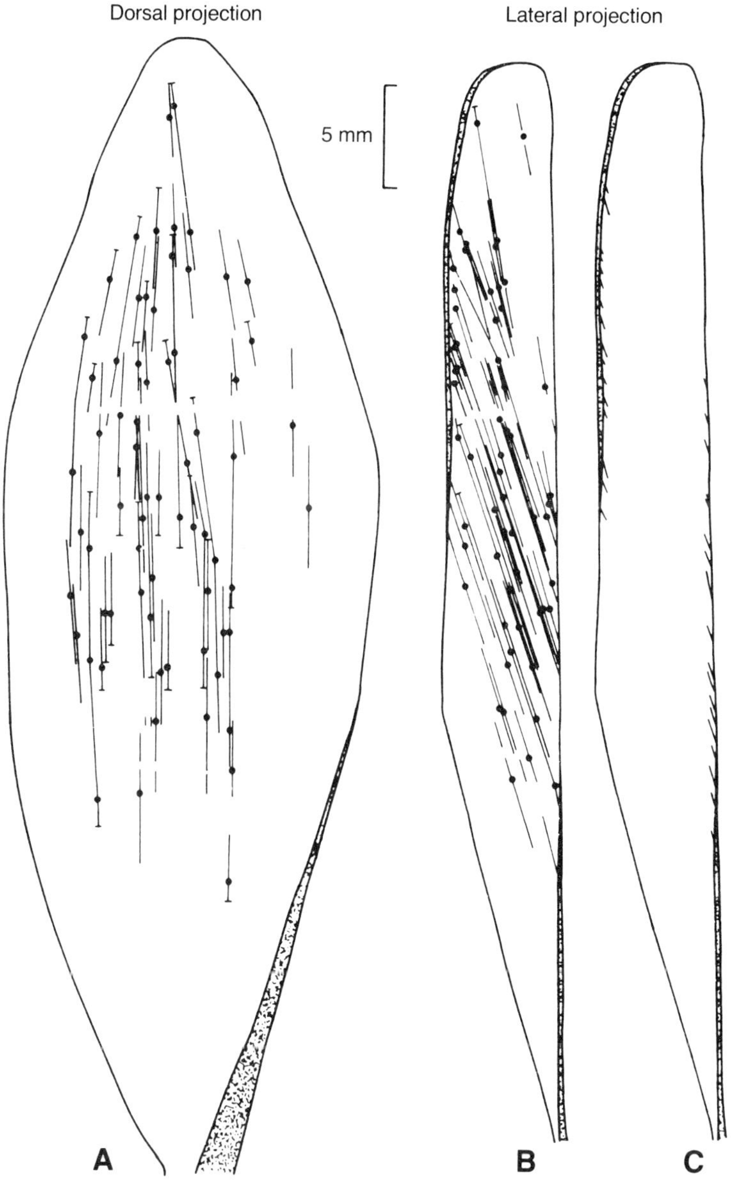

FIG. 11-1. The distribution of muscle receptors in the medial gastrocnemius muscle of the cat. The locations and orientations of spindles are shown in dorsal **(A)** and midsagittal **(B)** views. The locations of Golgi tendon organs are shown in a midsagittal view only **(C)**. The aponeuroses of the muscle are indicated by *shaded* areas. (Swett JE, Eldred E: Anat Rec 137:453–460, 1960)

for both primary and secondary spindle receptors. The fusimotor neurons or γ motoneurons should not be confused with the larger **skeletomotor neurons** or **α motoneurons,** whose activity produces contraction of the extrafusal fibers that do the work of the muscle. The difference in diameter of fusimotor (γ motoneurons) and skeletomotor fibers (α motoneurons) is illustrated in Figure 11-4. The former average about 5 μm in diameter, the latter 13 μm. Contraction of all the intrafusal fibers at once does not produce any measurable tension in the muscle. The intrafusal fibers are much smaller than the extrafusal fibers, 4 to 7 *millimeters* compared with 3 to 50 *centimet-*

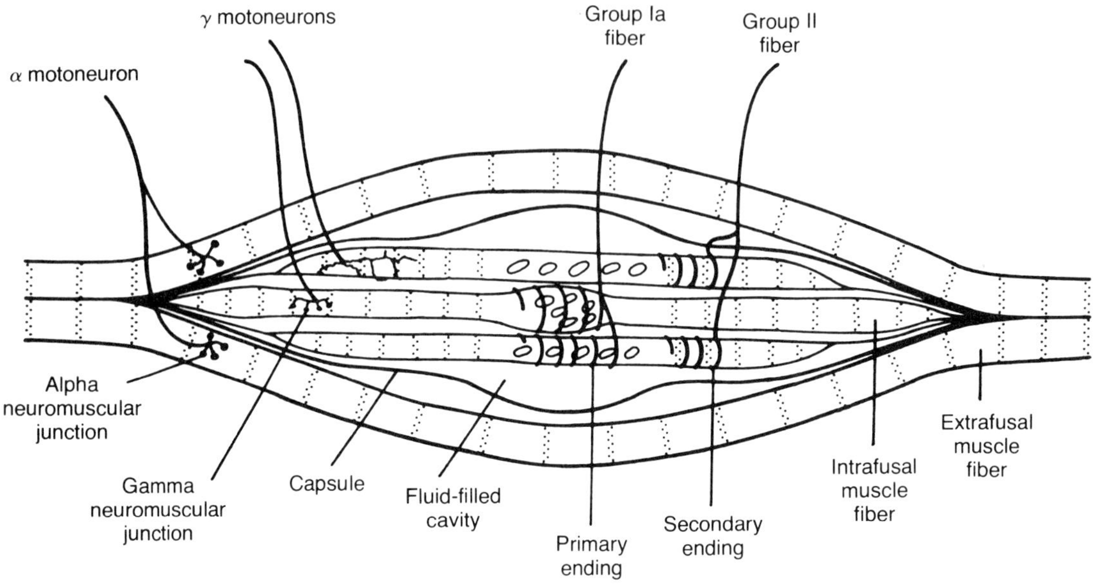

FIG. 11-2. Drawing of a muscle spindle to show the points of attachment, the arrangement of the intrafusal fibers, and how the afferent and efferent fibers enter the spindle.

FIG. 11-3. A nuclear bag and a nuclear chain fiber showing their innervation by group Ia and group II afferent fibers and γ motoneurons. (Matthews PBC: Physiol Rev 44:219–288, 1964)

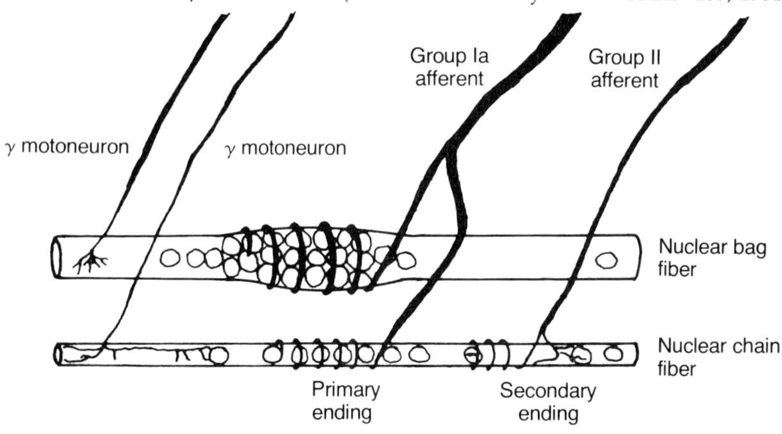

ers in length. Extrafusal muscle fibers can shorten by as much as 40% of their resting length, which for a 20-cm muscle would be 8 cm. The largest intrafusal fiber, shortening by the same percentage, would only change length by 2.8 mm. The extrafusal fiber is therefore capable of a 30-fold greater change in length. The average human striated muscle fiber has a diameter of about 60 μm; the intrafusal fiber averages about 10 μm. Because the force produced by a skeletal muscle is proportional to its cross-sectional area, the extrafusal fiber is capable of producing at least 36 times more force than the intrafusal fiber.

Another way to stretch the equatorial region of the spindle is to stretch the muscle and thereby stretch the entire spindle, because it is attached *in parallel* with extrafusal muscle fibers. Muscle spindle receptors respond to stretch of the muscle and signal *muscle length* and *rate of change of length* to the central nervous system. Both primary and secondary spindle afferent fibers give

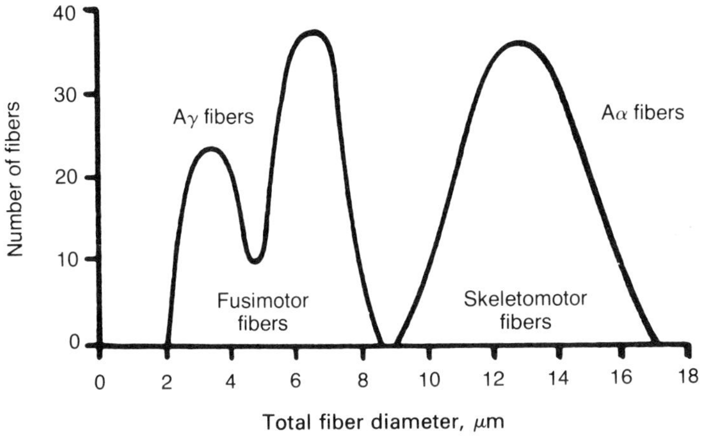

FIG. 11-4. Fiber spectrum of efferent portion of a muscle nerve. Indicated are Aα and Aγ fibers, fusimotor and skeletomotor fibers. (Boyd IA, Davey MR: Composition of Peripheral Nerves. Edinburgh, Livingstone, 1968)

FIG. 11-5. Responses of spindle afferent fibers to muscle stretch. A monitor of the stretch (lengthening, upward deflection) is shown in the upper trace. The response of a primary spindle afferent fiber is shown in the second trace, that of a secondary spindle afferent fiber in the third. (Matthews PBC: Physiol Rev 44:219–288, 1964)

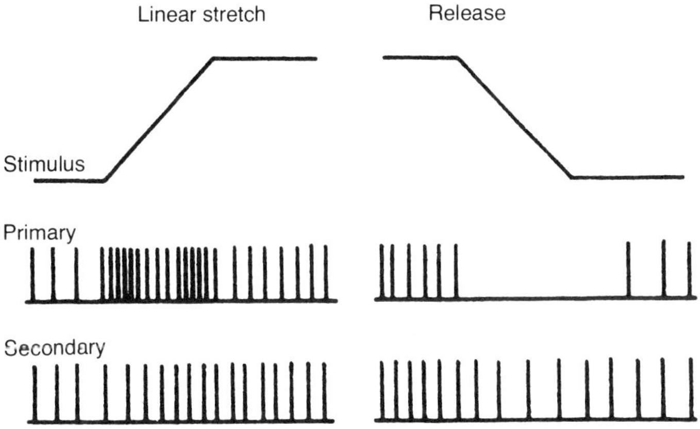

static or length-sensitive responses to stretch, that is, they respond to maintained stretch in a sustained (tonic) fashion at a frequency proportional to the length of the muscle (Fig. 11-5). Both types of fibers usually discharge tonically when the muscle is at its resting length. When the muscle is stretched and held at some new length, both types increase their discharge rates and maintain a discharge for as long as the new muscle length is maintained (an example of a slowly adapting response). When the muscle is returned to its resting length, the primary spindle afferent fiber is observed to stop discharging briefly and then begin again at a frequency appropriate for its new resting length, whereas the secondary spindle fiber discharge does not stop, but just slows to the appropriate rate. This is illustrated in Figure 11-5, where the monitor of the muscle length is shown in the top trace (upward displacement is an increase in length) and the responses of a primary and secondary spindle afferent fiber are shown in the second and third traces. The greater the muscle length, the greater is the stretch on the spindle and the greater is the static discharge of either type of spindle afferent fiber.

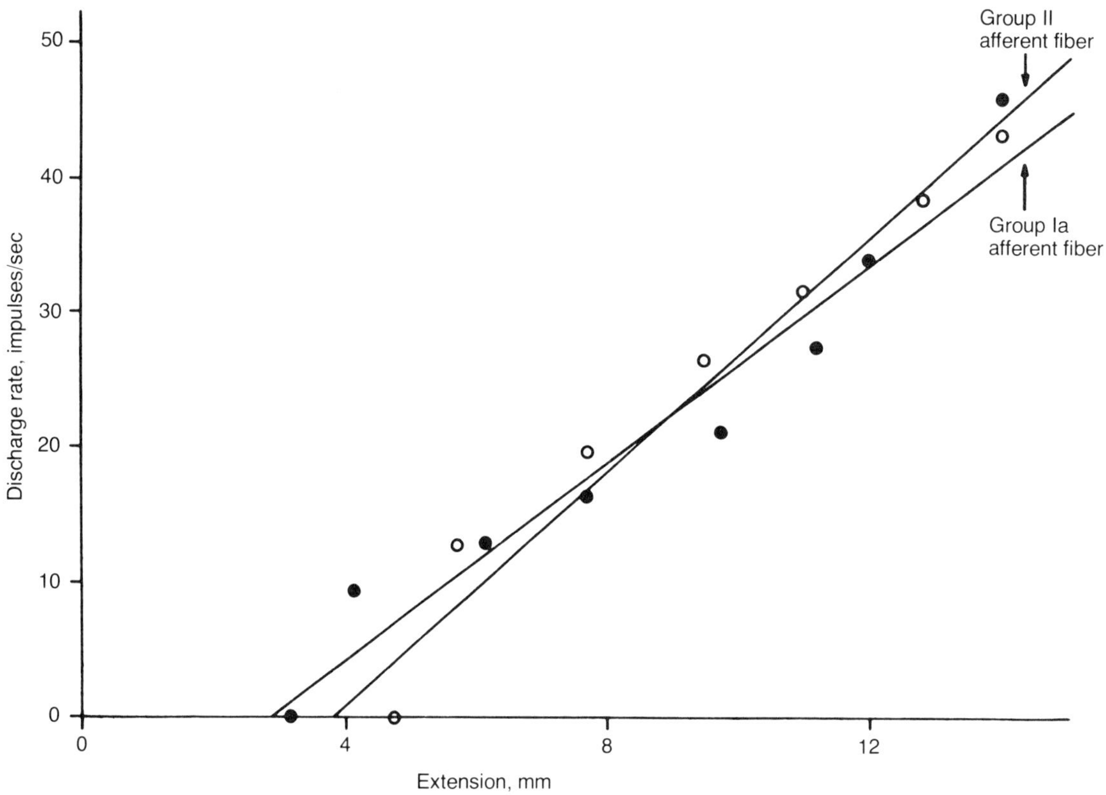

FIG. 11-6. A plot of the frequency of static discharge of a primary and secondary muscle spindle against the length of the muscle. Recordings were made with ventral roots cut. Primary responses are plotted with **filled circles.** (Jansen JKS, Matthews PBC: Acta Physiol Scand 55:376–386, 1962)

FIG. 11-7. The dynamic response. The monitor of the stretch at two different rates **(A** and **B)** is shown in the upper traces. Note that both stretches start and end at the same muscle length. The responses of a primary ending are shown in the second traces; those of a secondary ending are shown in the third traces. Note the higher frequency of discharge of the primary ending at the higher rate of stretch **(B).** Note that the length of the muscle is changing in phase 2, but is constant in phases 1 and 3 of these records.

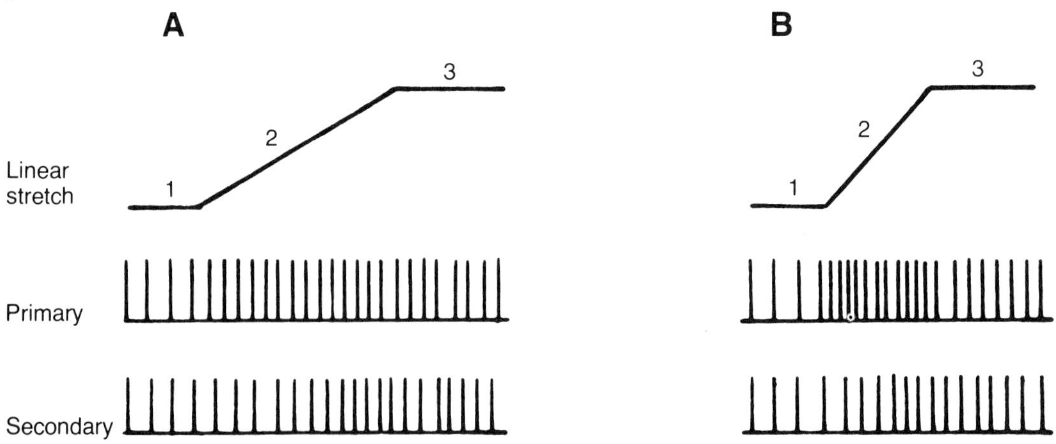

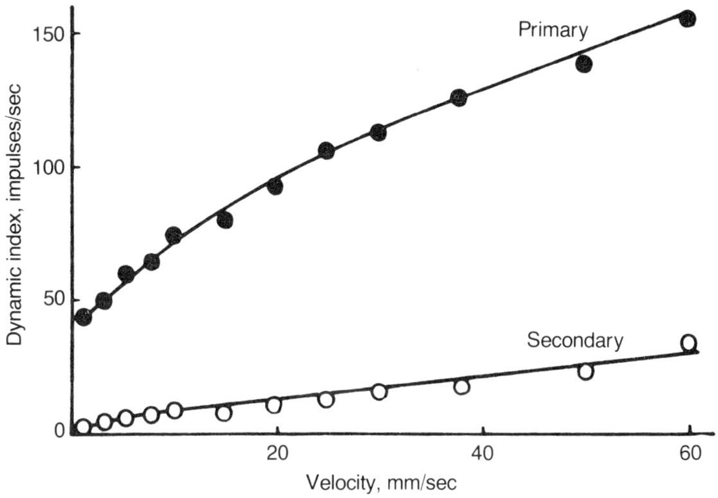

FIG. 11-8. A plot of the dynamic index versus the rate of stretch for a primary and a secondary muscle spindle afferent fiber. Note the flatness of the secondary curve. (Matthews PBC: J Physiol (Lond) 168:660–678, 1963)

In fact, for static conditions, there is an approximately linear relationship between the rate of discharge of the afferent fibers and the length of the muscle. This is illustrated in Figure 11-6, which is a plot of discharge frequency versus length of the muscle, for a primary and a secondary spindle afferent fiber. The frequency of discharge increases monotonically and linearly with increases in muscle length. The slope of these relations is called the position-sensitivity and is usually about the same for primary and secondary spindle receptors.

Only the primary muscle spindle afferent fiber gives a **dynamic** or velocity-sensitive response to muscle stretch. As the muscle length is being changed, the primary ending signals the rate at which it is being changed. The faster the muscle is stretched, the higher is the rate of discharge of the ending. Figure 11-7 shows the responses of both primary and secondary spindle endings to two stretches of the muscle at different rates. A monitor of the muscle length is shown in the upper traces, and the response of the primary ending is shown in the second traces. Notice that the primary ending responds with a higher frequency during the faster stretch in B, even though the initial and final lengths are the same in each case. Also, note that the rate of discharge decreases from its peak after the final length has been reached. This decrease defines the **dynamic index,** which is the difference between the dynamic response frequency for that rate of stretch and the static response frequency for that final length and serves as an indicator of rate sensitivity. When the velocity of stretch is zero, that is, when the muscle length is constant (phases 1 and 3 of Fig. 11-7), the discharge of the cell will be signaling only the length of the muscle. The primary spindle codes zero velocity with zero "velocity" discharge, but with an appropriate "length" discharge. When the muscle is changing length, that is, when the velocity is not zero, there will be a velocity discharge as well as a length discharge that is appropriate for the length of the muscle at each given instant of time. Near the end of phase 2 in Figure 11-7, the muscle has nearly reached its final length as in phase 3, but it is still changing length. Because its length is nearly that in phase 3, they can be taken as equal for a first approximation. This gives the following conditions:

$$\begin{array}{rl} \text{Discharge end phase 2} = & \text{Velocity discharge} + \text{Length discharge} \\ -\text{Discharge start phase 3} = & \text{Length discharge} \\ \hline \text{Dynamic index} = & \text{Velocity discharge.} \end{array}$$

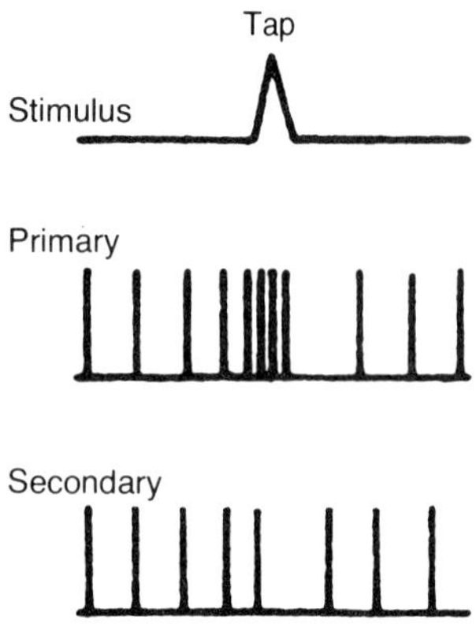

FIG. 11-9. Responses of primary and secondary muscle spindle afferent fibers to tapping the tendon of the muscle that they innervate. Monitor of change in length caused by tap is shown in upper trace; upward is an increase. (Matthews PBC: Physiol Rev 44:219–288, 1964)

Thus, the dynamic index can be used as an indicator of the velocity discharge. Figure 11-8 is a plot of the dynamic index versus velocity (or rate) of stretch for both primary and secondary endings. The curve for secondary endings is flat compared with that for primary endings.

It is the dynamic response capacity of the primary muscle spindle ending that provides for the vigorous response to tapping the muscle tendon as the physician does in reflex testing (Fig. 11-9). The tap rapidly stretches the spindles, and the primary endings respond to this rapid rate of stretching. The secondary endings, because of their lack of dynamic sensitivity, respond little (if at all) to the tap, which produces only a small change in the length of the muscle. After a brief stretch, the spindle is returned to its original length, and the discharge of the primary ending stops; it then returns to its prestretch rate of discharge. This behavior is important in our consideration of the tendon-tap reflex (Chap. 15).

FUSIMOTOR EFFECTS ON SPINDLE AFFERENT FIBER DISCHARGES

Fusimotor neurons are physiologically separable into two groups, based on their effects on the dynamic and static responses of the spindle afferent fibers. Activity in **static fusimotor fibers** increases the static responses of both primary and secondary spindle afferent fibers, whereas activity in **dynamic fusimotor fibers** increases the dynamic response in primary spindle receptors. These effects are illustrated in Figure 11-10. Trace A is again the monitor of muscle length and trace B is the response of a single primary spindle afferent fiber to the stretch. The effect is similar to that illustrated in Figure 11-5. During trace C, a single static fusimotor fiber was stimulated at 70/sec. The effect on the static discharge was so marked that the cell discharged at the initial length when it had not before; it discharged more vigorously at its final length (but still signaled both lengths in its discharge); and the dynamic response was masked by the increase in the static response, resulting in a decrease in the dynamic index, the indicator of the velocity response. The same procedure, this time while stimulating a dynamic fusimotor fiber, produced a marked change in the dynamic discharge but had much less effect on the static response, although there was some increase (Fig. 11-10D). Such changes in the discharge properties show up more clearly perhaps when the muscle is stretched and relaxed in a sinusoidal fashion rather than a linear fashion. Records made of the discharge of a primary muscle spindle afferent fiber are shown in Figure 11-11. The first and fourth traces show the action potentials discharged by the fiber. The second and fifth traces are a monitor of the stretch (upward deflection) and relaxation (downward deflection) of the muscle. This sinusoidal stimulus was applied to the muscle so that the zero position was approximately at the resting length, the muscle being stretched and relaxed equally around it. The two remaining traces show the period during the record when a dynamic fusimotor neuron (third trace) and a static fusimotor neuron (sixth trace) were stimulated. At the beginning of each record there is a period of time when there was no fusimotor stimulation. The group Ia fiber discharges during the stretch of the muscle and ceases its discharge when the muscle is relaxed. The average length of the muscle was not sufficiently great in this experiment to provoke a continuous discharge from the fiber. The effect of dynamic fusimotor activity was to increase the rate of discharge during the stretch portion of the stimulus, but it did not induce the cell to discharge during the relaxation phase of the sine wave

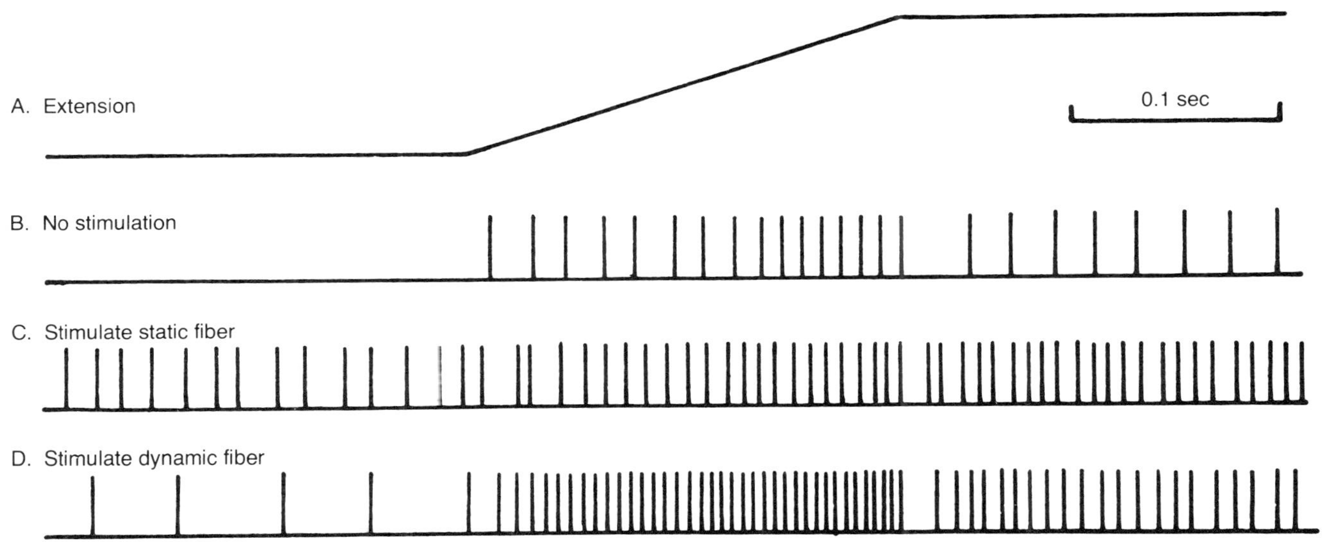

FIG. 11-10. Effect of γ motoneuron discharges on spindle sensitivity. **A.** Monitor of the muscle length during a stretch. **B.** Response of a primary spindle ending to the stretch. **C.** Response of the ending to the stretch during continuous stimulation of a single *static* fusimotor neuron at 70/sec. **D.** Response of the ending to the stretch during continuous stimulation of a single *dynamic* fusimotor neuron at 70/sec. (Crowe A, Matthews PBC: J Physiol (Lond) 174:109–131, 1964)

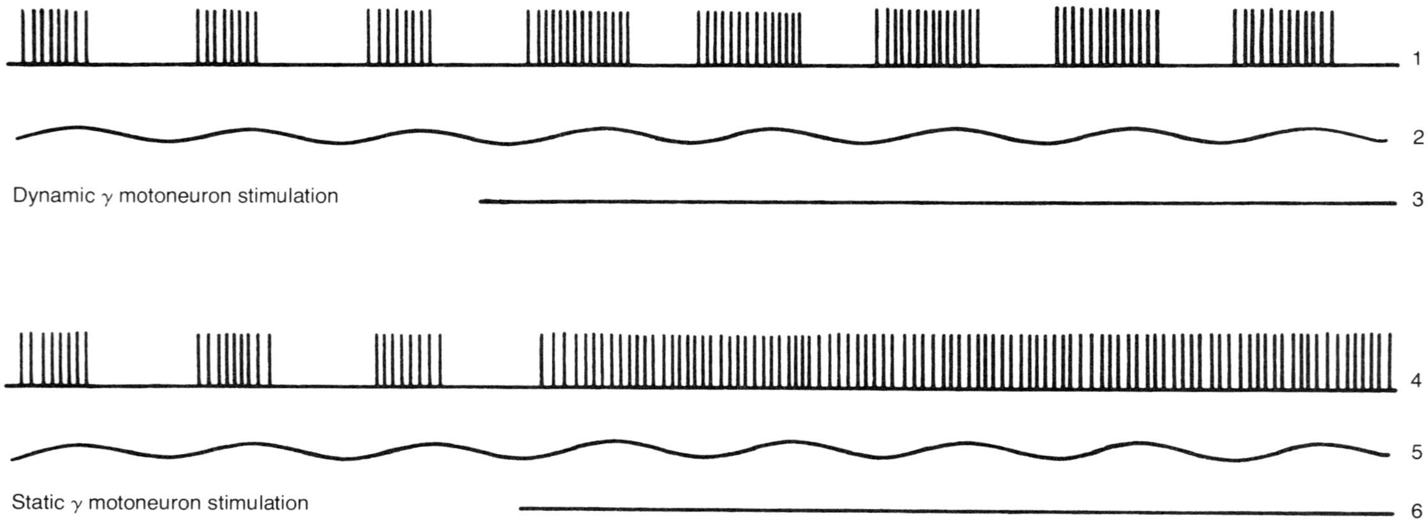

FIG. 11-11. The effect of fusimotor stimulation on the responsiveness of the mammalian primary ending to a sinusoidal stretching of medium extent (1 mm peak-to-peak movement at 3 Hz). (Crowe A, Matthews PBC: J Physiol (Lond) 174:132–151, 1964)

TABLE 11-1. COMPARISON OF ACTIONS OF STATIC AND DYNAMIC FUSIMOTOR NEURONS

PHENOMENON OBSERVED	DYNAMIC NEURON STIMULATION	STATIC NEURON STIMULATION
Static response of the primary ending	Increase	Slightly larger increase
Static response of the secondary ending	No effect	Increase
Dynamic response of the primary ending	Increase	Decrease in dynamic index, though rate may increase
Dynamic response of the secondary ending	No effect	Remains small
Frequency of occurrence	One-fourth of γ fibers	Three-fourths of γ fibers
Intrafusal fiber type affected	Nuclear bag	Nuclear chain

FIG. 11-12. Effects of fusimotor neuron activity on the sensitivity of the primary or secondary muscle spindle afferent fibers to length of the muscle **(A)** and of primary muscle afferent fibers to rate of change of length of the muscle **(B)**.

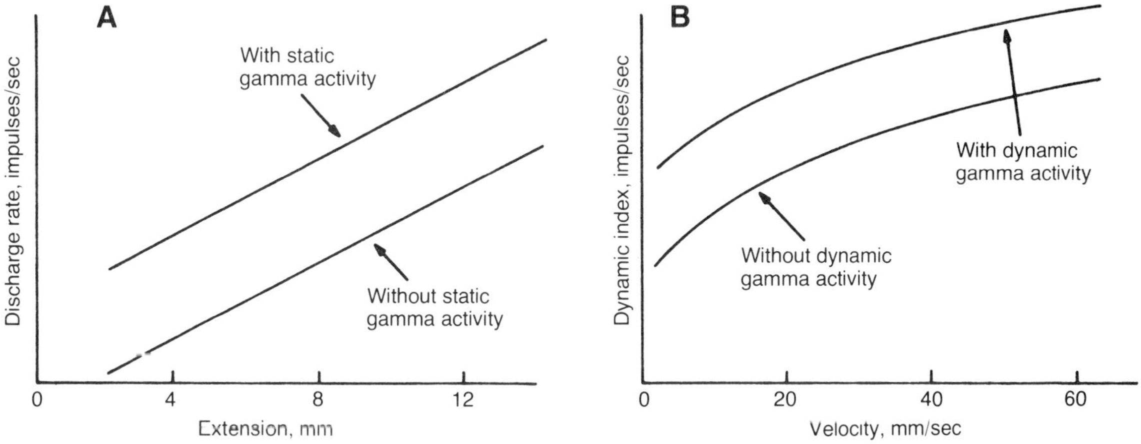

stimulus. The static fusimotor activity, on the other hand, converted the bursting response into a continuous response that occurred at a frequency appropriate for the average length of the muscle during the stimulus. A similar effect could have been achieved by increasing the length of the muscle before the sinusoidal stimulus was applied, that is, by setting the zero position of the sinusoid at some length longer than the resting length. The effects of fusimotor activity on spindle receptors are summarized in Table 11-1. From the distribution of the primary and secondary spindle afferent fibers and the nature of the fusimotor effects on them, it is possible to deduce that dynamic fusimotor fibers innervate primarily nuclear bag fibers, whereas static fusimotor neurons innervate primarily nuclear chain fibers. In a study of single chain and bag fibers, it was found that stimulation of a single dynamic γ motoneuron caused contraction of only bag fibers; chain fibers were not affected. Static γ motoneurons caused contraction of bag fibers only, chain fibers only, or both depending upon the static γ motoneuron.

The important physiologic effect of the fusimotor innervation of the spindles seems to be to alter the sensitivity of the spindle afferent endings. Stimulation of a static fusimotor neuron increases the length discharge of both primary and secondary muscle spindle afferent fibers for any muscle length. This is shown in Figure 11-12A. The discharge rate without the fusimotor activ-

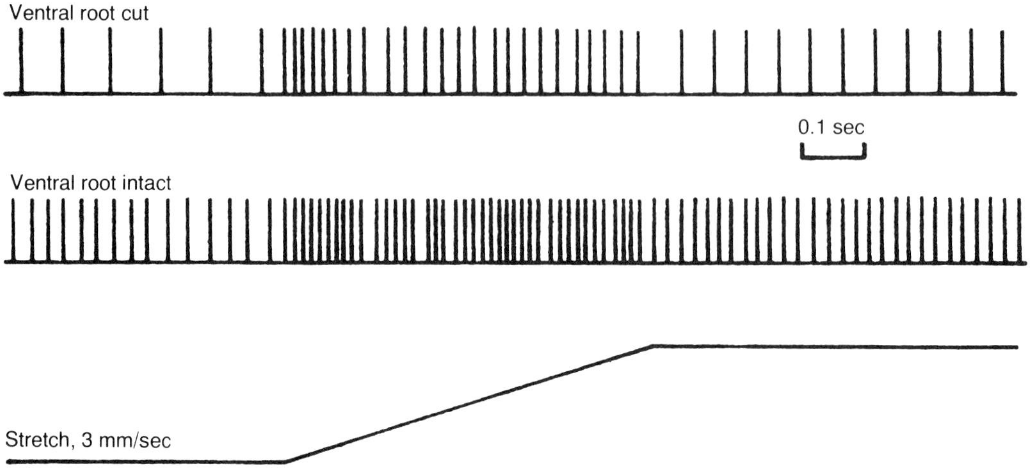

FIG. 11-13. Response of a primary spindle ending to stretching the muscle. **Lower trace** is a monitor of the muscle length. **Middle trace** shows the response to the same stretch with ventral roots intact; **upper trace,** with ventral roots cut. (Jansen JKS, Matthews PBC: J Physiol (Lond) 161:357–378, 1962)

FIG. 11-14. The location of the Golgi tendon organ at the muscle–tendon junction.

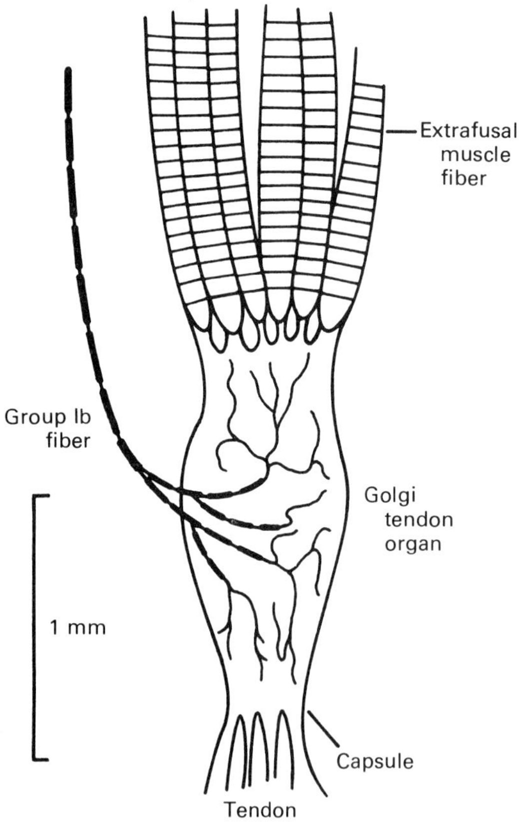

ity is plotted against muscle length as the lower line, as in Figure 11-6. With fusimotor activity a new relationship is generated roughly parallel to but slightly above the lower line. Actually, a family of such roughly parallel lines would be generated by different rates of discharge in the γ motoneuron. For any muscle length, the rate of discharge is higher with γ activity than without, and it is higher by a constant amount.

Likewise, dynamic fusimotor neuron stimulation increases the velocity discharge of a primary muscle spindle afferent fiber for any velocity of stretch. Figure 11-12B shows two parallel curves relating velocity of stretch to the velocity discharge rate, expressed as the dynamic index. The upper curve is the sensitivity of the spindle under the influence of a γ discharge; the lower is without such influence. Again, there would be a family of such parallel curves for different rates of γ-motoneuron discharge. The velocity discharge rate is higher for any velocity with γ-motoneuron stimulation, and it is higher by a constant amount. The effect of both static and dynamic fusimotor neurons on the muscle spindle receptors is to increase their sensitivity, in the one case, their sensitivity to the length of the muscle (static fusimotor neurons on both primary and secondary spindle afferent fibers) and in the other case, their sensitivity to rates of change of the length of the muscle (dynamic fusimotor neurons on the primary spindle afferent fiber).

It appears that there is ongoing fusimotor activity **(gamma tone** or **gamma bias).** Figure 11-13 shows that the sensitivity of the primary spindle ending, both dynamic and static, is reduced by cutting the ventral root, suggesting that this fusimotor modulation is an ongoing thing, and that both dynamic and static fusimotor fibers are active in the absence of movement or stimulation. Position-sensitivity (the slope of the lines in Fig. 11-12A) can fall from as high as 10 impulses/sec/mm to four impulses/sec/mm when the ventral roots are cut. In addition, spindle receptors become silent at minimum lengths (see Fig. 11-6), a condition never obtained with ventral roots intact. Except during rapid shortening, primary endings discharge some spikes even at shortest muscle lengths.

GOLGI TENDON ORGANS

The third muscle receptor of concern to us is the **Golgi tendon organ.** This receptor lies near the muscle–tendon junction (Fig. 11-14) or buried deep within the tendon itself. The receptor consists of specializations of the terminals of the group Ib afferent fiber itself, with a delicate capsule that surrounds the nerve that, in turn, surrounds several fascicles of tendon. Group Ib seems to be composed entirely of Golgi tendon organ afferent fibers, so these terms are used interchangeably.

The Golgi tendon organ signals to the central nervous system the tension developed by the muscle during contraction or exerted on it during a stretch. For many years, it was thought that these receptors had high thresholds to muscle tension and participated in controlling muscle activity only at extremes of tension, functioning as a protective device. Actually, the tendon organs are relatively insensitive to tension applied to the muscle by stretching it, but they are extremely sensitive to tension *developed by the muscle* when it contracts. The reason for this is that the tension on tendon organs is different under passive and active conditions. A muscle like the cat's soleus muscle has many extrafusal muscle fibers in it (about 25,000), but only a few Golgi tendon organs (about 45). Each tendon organ is arranged *in series* with a few muscle fibers (average 7). When the muscle is stretched, the tension applied is distributed across all 25,000 muscle fibers, but the seven fibers associated with each tendon organ only experience 7/25,000 of it—quite a small amount. In addition, the tension caused by stretching the muscle is exerted on the tendons at an angle to the Golgi tendon organs, so that only the component of the force parallel to the muscle fibers actually stretches the tendon organ. This can be small, especially in pennate muscles. On the other hand, if the muscle contracts, the

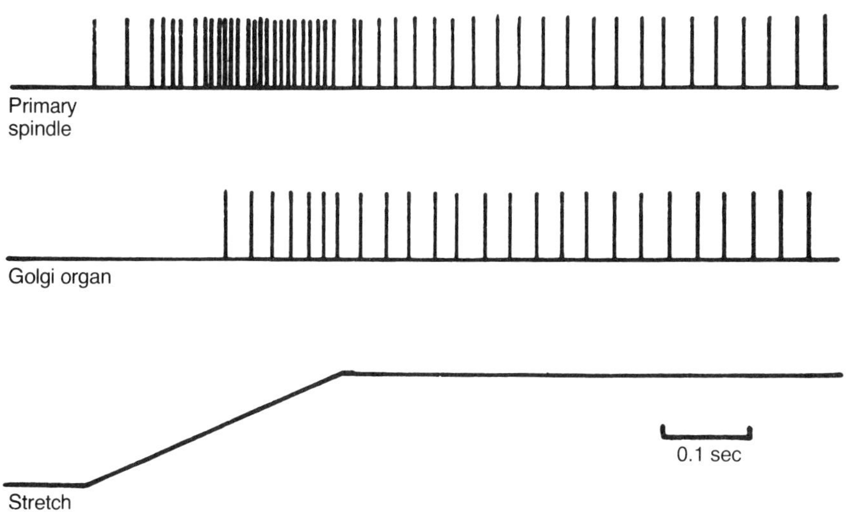

FIG. 11-15. Comparison of the responses of a primary spindle ending and a tendon organ. A monitor of the muscle stretch is shown in the lower trace and the response of the spindle ending in the upper trace. The response of the tendon organ is shown in the middle trace. Note the later start in the discharge of the tendon organ and the less vigorous response. (Matthews BHC: J Physiol (Lond) 78:1–53, 1933)

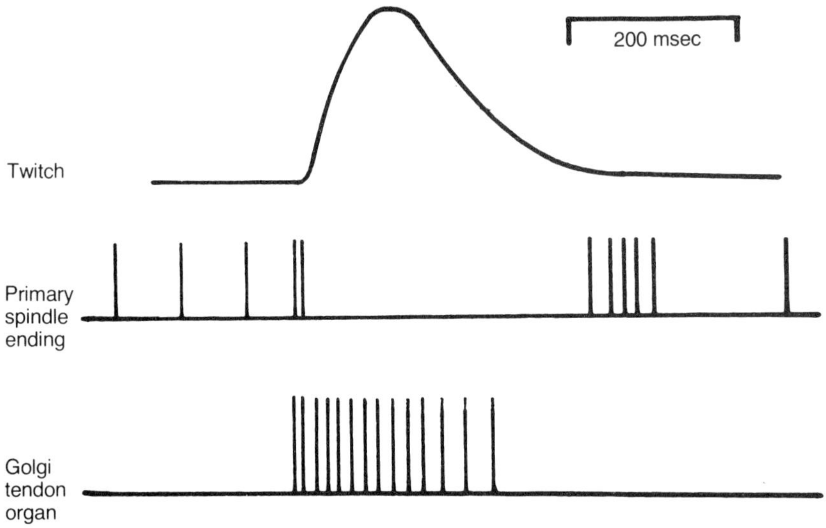

FIG. 11-16. Response of a tendon organ **(lower trace)** and a primary spindle ending **(middle trace)** during a twitch contraction of the muscle containing them. A monitor of the muscle tension is shown in the **upper trace;** an upward deflection is an increase in tension. (Matthews PBC: Mammalian Muscle Receptors and Their Central Actions. Baltimore, Williams and Wilkins, 1972)

TABLE 11-2. COMPARISON OF PROPERTIES OF RECEPTORS IN MUSCLE

PROPERTY	PRIMARY ENDING	SECONDARY ENDING	GOLGI TENDON ORGAN
Location	Midequatorial region of bag and chain fibers in spindles	Juxtaequatorial region of chain fibers in spindles	Muscle–tendon junction
Afferent fiber	Large, group Ia	Small, group II	Large, group Ib
Efferent control	Both static and dynamic fusimotor	Static fusimotor	None known
Response to ramp stretch with plateau	Dynamic and static	Static	Dynamic and static
Response to release of stretch	Abrupt silence	Progressive decrease	Abrupt silence
Response to tendon tap	Low threshold, vigorous	High threshold, little	High threshold, vigorous if threshold is exceeded
Sensitivity to small stretches	High, especially if rapid	Low	Low
Response to twitch contractions	Abrupt silence	Abrupt silence	Vigorous discharge
Signals	Muscle length and rate of change of length	Muscle length	Muscle tension and rate of change of tension

tension developed by the extrafusal fibers is transferred directly to the tendon organ associated with them. Not every tendon is innervated by a Golgi tendon organ. It appears that the system of tendon organs "samples" the average tension in various parts of the muscle in the same way spindle afferent fibers sample its length.

The response to muscle stretch of a Golgi tendon organ is compared with that of a primary spindle ending in Figure 11-15. The tendon organ has both a dynamic and a static response, but it, of course, is signaling tension and rate of change of tension rather than the length or rate of change of length that the primary muscle spindle signals. Because of the series elastic properties of the muscle, the tendon organ does not begin to discharge until long after the spindle ending has already begun to discharge. The real distinction between the responses of the two receptors is seen when an isometric twitch contraction is elicited in the muscle (Fig. 11-16). When the extrafusal fibers shorten, the spindle is unloaded because it is attached in parallel, and the equatorial region relaxes. The result is that the primary spindle ending stops discharging. On the other hand, when the muscle contracts isometrically, it develops tension, and the in-series-attached Golgi tendon organ increases its discharge.

The differences between the three types of muscle receptors are summarized in Table 11-2. Although differences in location and sensitivity to different forms of stimulation exist, these receptors work together in controlling the activity of the muscles with which they are associated, as we shall see in another chapter. Anatomic evidence suggests that among muscle fascicles that contain muscle spindles, Golgi tendon organs are usually present at the muscle–tendon junction. This is shown in Figure 11-1B and C. This relationship suggests an even closer cooperation than was previously expected.

SUGGESTED READING

Barker D [ed]: Symposium on Muscle Receptors. Hong Kong, Hong Kong Univ. Press, 1962

Bessou P, Pagès B: Cinematographic analysis of contractile events produced in intrafusal muscle fibres by stimulation of static and dynamic fusimotor axons. J Physiol (Lond) 252:397–427, 1975

Bourne GH [ed]: The Structure and Function of Muscle, 2nd ed, Vols. I-III. New York, Academic Press, 1972

Matthews PBC: Muscle spindles and their motor control. Physiol Rev 44:219–288, 1964

Matthews PBC: Mammalian Muscle Receptors and Their Central Actions. Baltimore, Williams and Wilkins, 1972

Olkowski Z, Moncha SL: Muscle spindle. In Bourne GH [ed]: The Structure and Function of Muscle, 2nd ed, Vol. II, Part 2. New York, Academic Press, 1973

12

Peripheral Nerves

THE COMPOUND ACTION POTENTIAL

If we took a 10-mm length of mixed peripheral nerve, for example, the sciatic nerve, and recorded changes in electrical potential from one end of it while electrically stimulating the other end, as illustrated in Figure 12-1A, we could make some interesting observations that tell us a great deal about peripheral nerves. Sample records from such an experiment are shown in Figure 12-1B. In the uppermost trace, the strength of the stimulus is low, and we see no response from the nerve. This stimulus strength is **subthreshold.** If the strength is raised, a tiny response appears in the record and, as the strength is increased even more, the response grows to a maximum value (next to bottom trace); further increases in shock strength do not further augment the response. The stimulus strength that just gives a response is termed a **threshold stimulus;** any stimulus of greater strength is **suprathreshold.** The strength that just gives the **maximal response** is a **maximal stimulus;** any strength greater is **supramaximal.** The response of the nerve is called the **compound action potential.** The compound action potential is graded in nature, in striking contrast to the all-or-none response of single axons.

There is a simple explanation for why the response of a nerve is graded, whereas that of a single fiber is all-or-none. The nerve is composed of many fibers of different diameters, with these different diameters seemingly distributed at random throughout the nerve. It turns out that the threshold of an axon to externally applied current is *inversely related to the diameter* of the axon, so that for a large and small axon equidistant from the stimulating electrode, the large axon will have the lower threshold. Furthermore, if two axons of the same size are at different distances from the stimulating electrode (that is, one is buried deeper in the nerve or on the other side of the nerve from the electrode), the one closer to the electrode will pick up more current and therefore reach threshold at a lower stimulus strength than the one farther away. Thus, as the stimulus strength was increased in Figure 12-1B, the largest axons closest to the electrode began responding at lowest stimulus strengths. Then, at higher strengths, smaller axons close to the electrode and large axons farther away from the electrode responded, and their individual action potentials were added to the compound action potential. Finally, at maximal stimulus strength, every axon in the nerve was contributing its own all-or-none action potential, whence no further increase in the response was possible. It should be kept in mind that at all strengths, the recorded response is the sum over time of the action potentials of all of the discharging cells.

The shape of the compound action potential in Figure 12-1 may look like a temporally expanded action potential followed by an after-hyperpolarization; however, the positive potential of the compound action potential does not represent a membrane hyperpolarization. After-hyperpolarizations are really too small to contribute much to the compound action potential. Rather, the biphasic nature of the potential results from the bipolar extracellular recording setup. Note that two electrodes were used for recording, one closer to the stimulus, one farther away, and the voltage was recorded at one electrode with respect to the other, that is, the difference in potential was recorded, but neither electrode was over inactive tissue. Figure 12-2

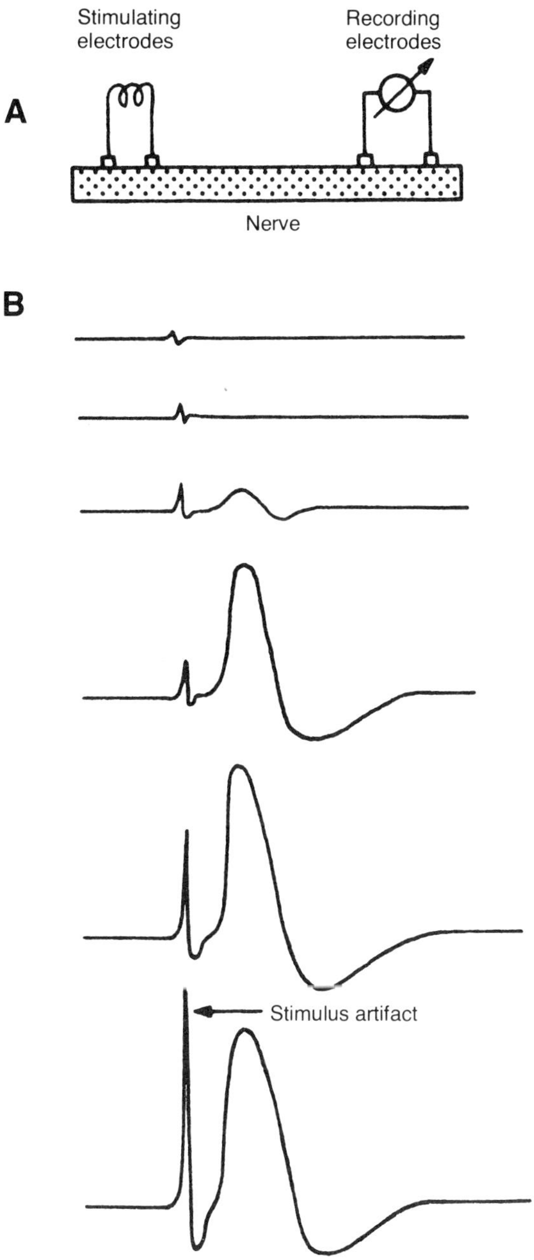

FIG. 12-1. A. Setup for recording the compound action potential from the sciatic nerve. **B.** Sample records taken at stimulus strengths increasing from top to bottom. Trace deflects upward when left recording electrode is negative with respect to the right one. Note the graded nature of the compound action potential. (Katz B: Nerve, Muscle and Synapse. New York, McGraw-Hill, 1966)

shows the events that occur as the compound action potentials are propagating under the electrodes. In A, the action potentials have not yet reached the recording site; the membrane potential of most cells is at rest. (**Note:** Some cells discharge spontaneously.) Both electrodes are at the same potential; the difference is zero as shown. The advancing spikes have reached the first electrode in B; many cells have reversed their membrane polarity, and the potential at the first electrode has become negative with respect to the second. In C, the action potentials have begun to invade the membranes under the second electrode; the potential at the first electrode is still more negative than at the second but less so than in B. The membranes under the first electrode are al-

FIG. 12-2. Axon membrane polarization at various times during conduction of an action potential. Shown are polarizations when the spike is approaching the segment **(A)**, under one electrode **(B, D)**, under both electrodes **(C)**, and retreating from the segment **(E)**. The meter, connected to two external electrodes, shows the polarity of the recorded voltage.

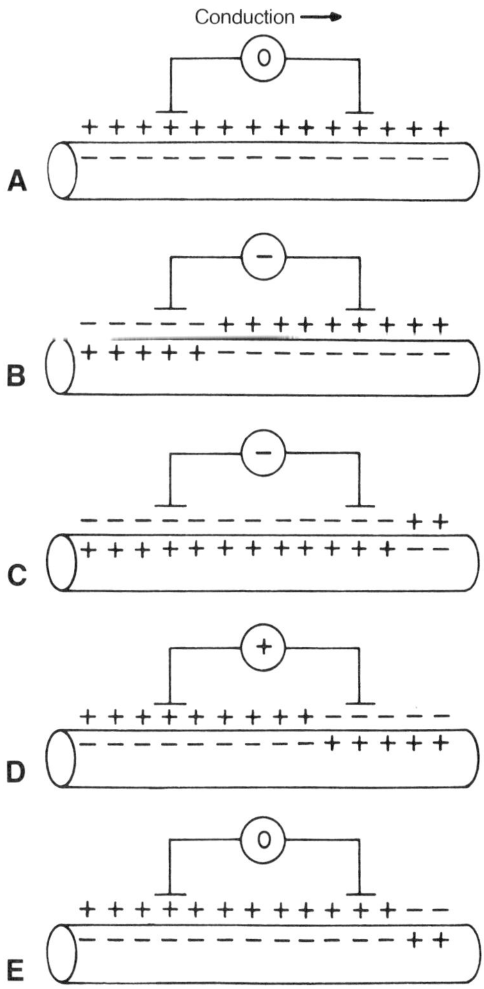

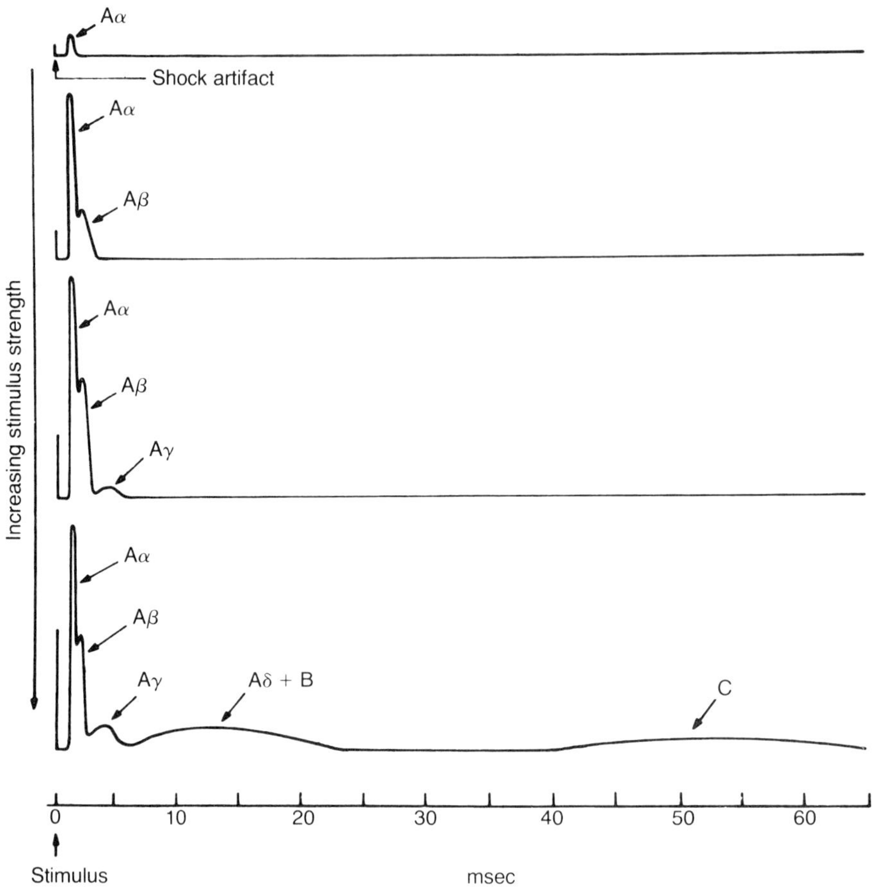

FIG. 12-3. Sample records from the sciatic nerve of responses elicited by electrical stimuli applied to the nerve 80 mm away. The various components of the compound action potential are labeled where they appear. Shock strengths increase from top to bottom.

ready repolarized as the action potentials have passed, but they are still depolarized under the second electrode in D. The potential at the first electrode is now positive with respect to the second. In E, the spikes have passed both electrodes; the electrodes are at the same potential again and the difference is again zero. The recorded configuration is therefore a result of the recording setup.

The compound action potential is an artifact of the manner in which the nerve was stimulated. It is doubtful that such a potential is often elicited in nerves under normal conditions of sensation or movement, but they may occur in some special circumstances. For example, in muscle nerves, when a person jumps off an object and lands on the ground, a relatively synchronous volley of action potentials is set up in the group Ia afferent fibers from the quadriceps muscles, and this in turn results in a relatively synchronous volley in the alpha motoneurons of the quadriceps muscles, as we will see in Chapter 15. Usually, however, there is a constant, asynchronous trickle of action potentials coming into the central nervous system and also leaving it. However, the study of the compound action potential has given us a lot of information about conduction in peripheral nerves.

TYPES OF FIBERS IN PERIPHERAL NERVES

If, now, a greater length of sciatic nerve is used in the same experiment (say 80 mm of nerve), a new phenomenon appears in the recording. Figure 12-3 shows an intensity series recorded under these conditions. At just suprathreshold strength, a response (the Aα response) appears in the record at about 2 msec after the shock artifact. At higher shock strengths, this response grows in size, and a new response (the Aβ response) appears in the record about 4 msec after the artifact. Further increases in shock strength result in further increases in both the α and β responses and the addition successively of the new responses: Aγ, Aδ and B, and C. Based on the discussion of the previous paragraphs, it is appropriate to assume that the components added to the response at higher stimulus strengths represent the responses of successively smaller fibers, and this is indeed the case. Also, the responses of successively smaller fibers occur later and later in time after the artifact. This is because the conduction velocity of an axon is a *direct function of its diameter*, and it requires a longer time for the action potentials in more slowly conducting axons (smaller ones) to travel the 80 mm than for action potentials in more rapidly conducting axons (larger ones).

These different responses were not seen in the experiment in Figure 12-1 because the short conduction distance in that experiment caused the action potentials in all sizes of fibers to arrive at the recording electrode at nearly the same time; there was not sufficient time for differences in conduction velocity to show up. The individual responses were all bunched up together and were thus superimposed in the record. Nevertheless, the same fibers were discharging at the same shock strengths in both experiments.

Take a moment at this point to note in Figure 5-13 that the smallest fibers are the most numerous by far, whereas the largest are least numerous. In cutaneous nerves, measurements have indicated that there are about twice as many Aδ fibers as Aα fibers and about 4.6 times as many C fibers as A fibers.* Though this is the case, the maximal response (Fig. 12-3) recorded from the largest fibers, the Aα fibers, is many times larger than that recorded from the smallest fibers, the C fibers. This is because fibers contribute voltage to the recording *in proportion to the square of their diameters.* The result is that a fiber 2 times as large as another contributes 4 times as much voltage to the recording. In our case, the largest Aα fiber is 22 μm in diameter, the largest C fiber, only 1 μm in diameter; they differ by a factor of 22, and they contribute voltage to the recording in the ratio of $(22)^2:(1)^2$ or 484 : 1.

We find that fibers of particular receptor systems are often separable to some extent on the basis of their conduction velocities. Table 12-1 summarizes the two different classification schemes for peripheral neurons based upon their conduction velocity or diameter. The Roman numeral scheme refers to afferent fibers only, whereas the letter scheme includes both afferent and efferent fibers. It may help to note that Aα, Ia and Ib fibers are mostly of muscle origin or destination, and C and group IV fibers are all unmyelinated. Normally, we use the letter classification scheme to designate cutaneous afferent fiber types and the Roman numeral scheme to designate muscle afferent fiber types, but unfortunately this is not always the case, so care must be exercised. The fiber diameter spectra of a muscle nerve and a cutaneous nerve are indicated in Figure 12-4 for comparison with the classifications in Table 12-1. The sum of the two fiber spectra in Figure 12-4 is approximately equivalent in shape to that in Figure 5 13. Be careful not to confuse the fiber spectra of Figure 12-4 with the compound action potential of Figure 12-3.

PROPERTIES OF DIFFERENT TYPES OF NERVE FIBERS

Nerve fiber types differ in their response to local anesthetics, in their susceptibility to anoxia, and in their susceptibility to pressure block. Using the letter classification, these differences are summarized in Table 12-2. B fibers are most influenced by anoxia, A fibers are most susceptible to pressure block, and C fibers are most readily blocked by local anesthetics. You may be acutely aware that hypoxia blocks A fibers before C fibers if you are in the habit of sleeping with your arm under your head. Upon waking, you may commonly observe that your sense of touch is dulled (you may have a tingling sensation), but your pain

* The precise ratios vary with position on the body. The lingual nerve, which supplies the tongue, contains few unmyelinated fibers, and the nerves supplying the extremities, especially glabrous skin, contain fewer unmyelinated fibers than those supplying proximal skin. Larger animals also have relatively fewer unmyelinated fibers than smaller ones.

TABLE 12-1. TWO SYSTEMS FOR CLASSIFYING AXONS IN PERIPHERAL NERVE BY DIAMETER

LETTER SYSTEM (BOTH AFFERENT AND EFFERENT)				ROMAN NUMERAL SYSTEM (AFFERENT FIBERS ONLY)		
Type of Fiber	**Diameter (μm)**	**Conduction Velocity (m/sec)**	**General Function**	**Conduction Velocity (m/sec)**	**Diameter (μm)**	**Type of Fiber**
Aα	13–22	70–120	α Motoneurons			
			Muscle spindle primary endings	70–120	12–20	Ia
			Golgi tendon organs	66–114	11–19	Ib
			Touch			
Aβ	8–13	40–70	Touch Kinesthesia Muscle spindle secondary endings	20–50	5–12	II
Aγ	4–8	15–40	Touch Pressure γ Motoneurons			
Aδ	1–4	5–15	Pain Crude touch Pressure Temperature	4–20	1–5	III
B	1–3	3–14	Preganglionic autonomic			
C	0.1–1	0.2–2	Unmyelinated fibers			
			Pain Touch Pressure Temperature	0.2–3	0.1–2	IV
			Postganglionic autonomic			

FIG. 12-4. Fiber diameter spectra for a cutaneous **(A)** and a muscle nerve **(B)** to indicate the types of fibers in each and the use of the naming systems of Table 12-1. (Boyd IA, Davey MR: Composition of Peripheral Nerve. Edinburgh, Livingstone, 1968)

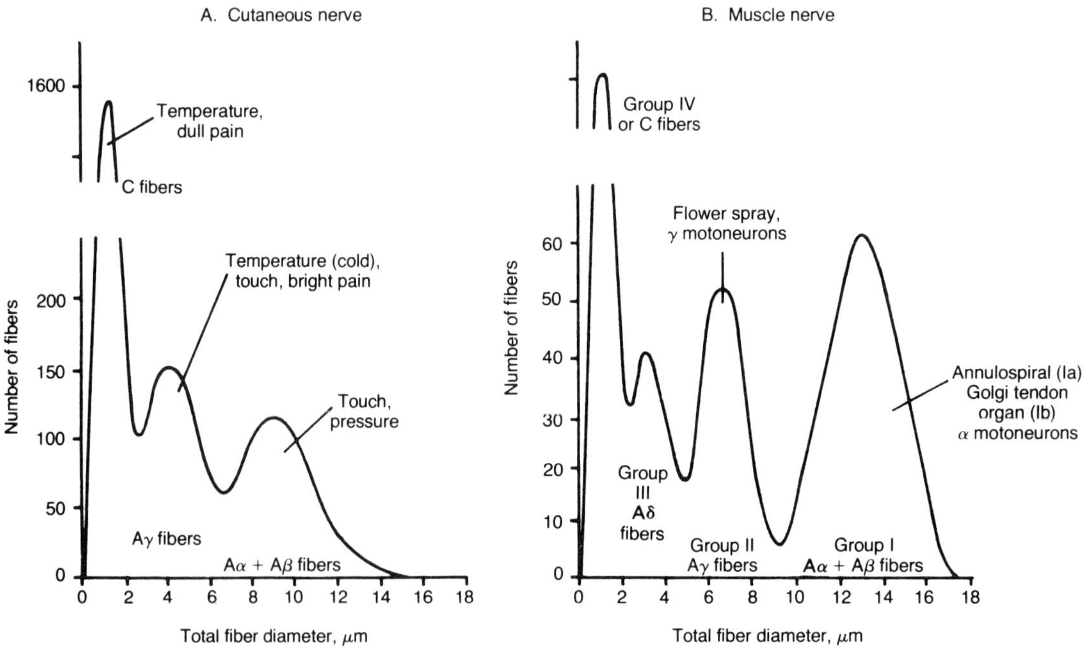

TABLE 12-2. SUSCEPTIBILITY OF DIFFERENT TYPES OF FIBERS TO CONDUCTION BLOCK BY VARIOUS AGENTS

EFFECT	MOST SUSCEPTIBLE	INTERMEDIATE	LEAST SUSCEPTIBLE
Block by hypoxia	B	A	C
Block by pressure	A	B	C
Block by local anesthetics	C	B	A

sensitivity is either normal or perhaps even slightly higher than normal.

THE MEASUREMENT OF CONDUCTION VELOCITIES

It is common in peripheral nerve damage that the conduction velocity is slowed drastically in the damaged portion. For example, in carpal tunnel syndrome, where the bones of the wrist are broken in such a way that the fragments put pressure on the median nerve, partially blocking conduction, it is possible to assess the extent of the damage by measuring the conduction velocity of the nerve and comparing it with that on the normal side.

Measurement of the velocity is straightforward. First, two sets of stimulating electrodes are placed on the skin over the median nerve, one near the top of the forearm and one 10 cm closer to the wrist. It is important that this distance is measured accurately or, at least, that it is the same on both arms if they are to be compared. Next, a pair of surface electrodes or needle electrodes, pushed through the skin into the belly of the abductor policis brevis muscle, is used to record the muscle activity. Recordings are made from muscle because recordings from nerves are more difficult. The position of the stimulating electrodes can be checked by stimulating and looking for abduction and flexion of the thumb, the action of the abductor policis brevis. Electrode position is adjusted to obtain the lowest threshold for contraction with both pairs of stimulating electrodes. The nerve is then stimulated with each set of electrodes while looking at the electromyogram (EMG) from the muscle, and conduction time between the shock artifact and the beginning of the EMG response is measured. Ten centimeters divided by the difference between the conduction times for the two electrodes is the maximum conduction velocity for axons in the nerve. Two pairs of electrodes are used instead of just one because this procedure eliminates the need to estimate and compensate for the utilization time in the nerve, that is, the time it takes for the membrane potential to reach the critical firing level and discharge a spike, and the delay in transmission at the neuromuscular junction, that is, the time it takes for chemical transmission (see Chap. on synapses). In the normal individual the velocity should be nearly the same in both arms.

FIG. 12-5. Recordings of compound action potentials **(arrows)** in the medial and lateral plantar nerves in a normal person **(A)** and in a patient with tarsal tunnel syndrome **(B)**. Note that tarsal tunnel syndrome is accompanied by slowing of conduction and reduction in amplitude of the compound action potential. (Oh SJ, Sarala PK, Elmore RS: Ann Neurol 5:327–330, 1979)

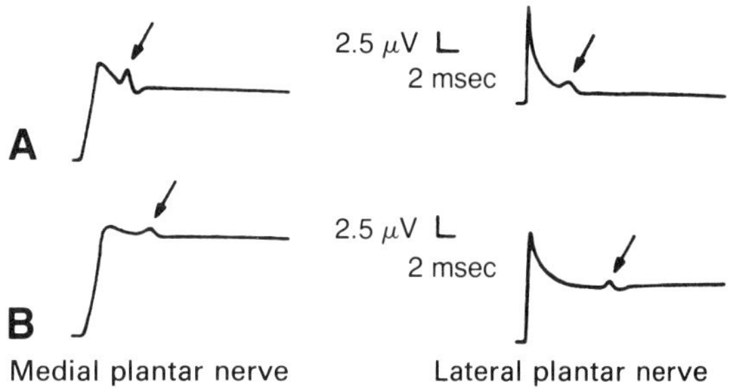

Tarsal tunnel syndrome is the lower limb equivalent of carpal tunnel syndrome, but rarer. In tarsal syndrome, there is compression neuropathy of the posterior tibial nerve associated with burning pain and paresthesia in the toes and on the sole of the foot. Figure 12-5 shows recordings from the medial and lateral plantar nerves of a normal person (A) and a patient with tarsal tunnel syndrome (B). Note that the compound action potentials are smaller and later in the patient than in the normal person, because of the slowing of conduction in some fibers and block of conduction in others. Conduction velocities measured in normal records are 41.25 and 34.80 m/sec respectively, whereas those in the patient are 26.10 and 17.78 m/sec, a slowing of 37% and 49%, respectively.

SUGGESTED READING

Hodgkin AL: Evidence for electrical transmission in nerve. Part I. J Physiol (Lond) 90:183–210, 1937

Hodgkin AL: Evidence for electrical transmission in nerve. Part II. J Physiol (Lond) 90:211–232, 1937

Junge D: Nerve and Muscle Excitation. Sunderland MA, Sinauer, 1976

Katz B: Nerve, Muscle, and Synapse. New York, McGraw-Hill, 1966

Lloyd DPC: Neuron patterns controlling transmission of ipsilateral hind limb reflexes in cat. J Neurophysiol 6:293–315, 1943

Patton HD: Special properties of nerve trunks and tracts. In Ruch TC, Patton HD [eds]: Physiology and Biophysics, 19th ed. Philadelphia, WB Saunders, 1965

13

Synapses

The nervous system consists of billions of neurons, each one an individual cell, receiving signals from some other cells and generating signals of its own to be sent to other cells. We consider here how these signals are transferred from one neuron to another. In most cases, there is a gap between neurons that must be bridged in order for transmission to continue throughout the nervous system. How this is accomplished is the subject of this chapter.

ANATOMY OF A SYNAPSE

If we follow a primary afferent fiber to its termination, we find that the fiber may branch many times, becoming smaller each time. If the fiber is myelinated, then near its termination the myelin disappears and there is a swelling of the axon, called the **bouton terminaux, end bulb, terminal, synaptic knob,** or just **bouton;** with this swelling, the fiber simply ends. Unmyelinated fibers also possess a swelling at their ends. The boutons, whether from myelinated or unmyelinated fibers, are always found in proximity to a soma, axon, or dendrite of another cell.

At the site of the termination of a fiber, the specializations of the terminal and the cell it contacts are called collectively a **synapse.** Synapses on somas are termed **axosomatic synapses;** those on dendrites are termed **axodendritic;** and those on other axons are **axoaxonic.** The fiber's bouton is called the **presynaptic element** and the structure it contacts is the **postsynaptic element.** A schematic diagram of a synapse is shown in Figure 13-1. The pre- and postsynaptic elements are separated by a space 15 to 100 nm wide, known as the **synaptic cleft.** At the synapse, the membrane of the postsynaptic element is slightly thickened, and there is often an accumulation of some densely staining substance near the thickened membrane. On the presynaptic side, there is normally an accumulation of mitochondria in the bouton and, in electron micrographs, a large number of spherical or irregularly shaped structures are seen near the synaptic region. These are called **synaptic vesicles.**

It is believed that transmission from one cell to another at a synapse like the one just described (a chemical synapse, as opposed to an electrical synapse) is accomplished by release of a substance, the **transmitter substance,** from the synaptic vesicle into the synaptic cleft by the process of exocytosis. The identity of the transmitter substance is unknown for most synapses. Many candidate transmitter substances have been suggested; however, we can be certain a substance is a transmitter substance only if it meets all of the following criteria:

1. The substance must occur naturally in presynaptic terminals, and either the precursors and enzymes for its formation or an adequate, specific transport system for its uptake into the terminal must exist.
2. The substance must be released from the terminals by nerve stimulation.
3. A mechanism must exist for *rapid* inactivation of the released transmitter substance, that is, it must be degraded or taken up again by the terminal.
4. A synaptic action must be identified for the substance, and local application must produce effects "exactly" like those of the synaptically released transmitter substance.
5. Drugs must produce similar effects upon actions of the substance and natural transmitter substance.

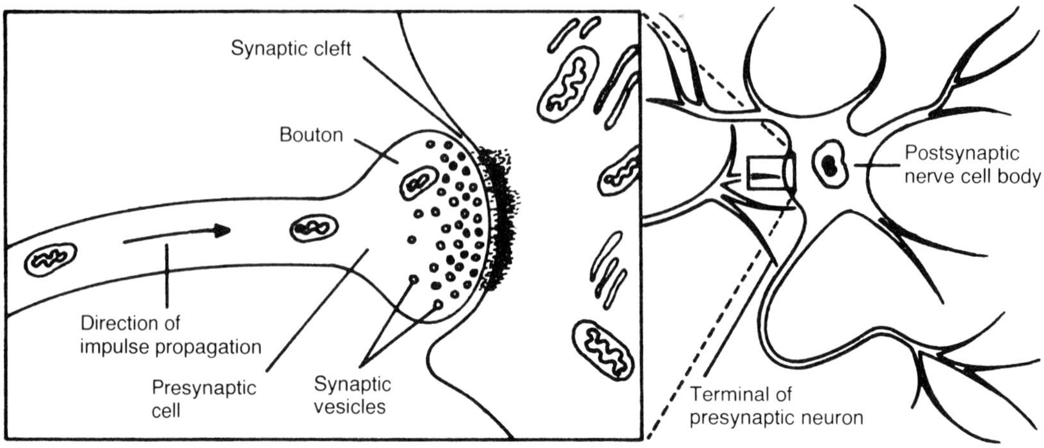

FIG. 13-1. A schematic diagram of a synapse indicating the pre- and postsynaptic elements with synaptic specializations.

TABLE 13-1. KNOWN AND PUTATIVE TRANSMITTER SUBSTANCES IN THE MAMMALIAN NERVOUS SYSTEM

SUBSTANCE	PRESUMED ACTION	LOCATIONS OF MAXIMUM CONCENTRATIONS	MODE OF ACTION	BLOCKING AGENTS
Acetylcholine	Excitation	Interpeduncular, dorsal raphe and caudate nuclei, nucleus accumbens, and ventral horn of spinal cord	Ionotropic metabotropic, cGMP†	Curare, atropine
Glycine	Inhibition	Spinal cord, medulla, pons	Ionotropic	Strychnine
γ-Aminobutyric acid	Inhibition	Cerebellum, cerebral cortex, spinal cord, retina	Ionotropic	Bicuculline
Norepinephrine	Excitation, inhibition	Pons, medulla	Metabotropic, cAMP†	Propanolol, phentolamine
Dopamine	Excitation, inhibition	Putamen, caudate, locus ceruleus, hypothalamus	Metabotropic, cAMP†	Phenoxybenza-mine
Serotonin	Excitation, inhibition	Amygdala, hypothalamus, septum, striatum	?	LSD†
L-Glutamate	Excitation	Temporal cortex, basal ganglia, cerebellum, amygdala	Ionotropic	?
L-Aspartate	Excitation	Substantia nigra, occipital cortex, thalamus, cerebellum, hypothalamus	Ionotropic	?
Epinephrine	?	Thalamus, hypothalamus	Metabotropic, cAMP†	Propanolol, phentolamine
Substance P*	Excitation	Substantia nigra, trigeminal nucleus, dorsal horn of spinal cord, limbic system	Metabotropic, (?)	?
Enkephalins*	Inhibition	Globus pallidus, caudate, nucleus accumbens, hypothalamus	?	Naloxone
Endorphins*	Inhibition	Pituitary, striatum, spinal cord	?	Naloxone
Histamine	Inhibition	Hypothalamus, thalamus	Metabotropic, cAMP†	Ethanolamine, butamide

Others: Taurine, neurotensin, carnosine, angiotensin II, hypothalamic releasing factors, serine, proline, N-acetyl-L-aspartate, adenosine, P-tyramine, tryptamine.

* Peptides
† cAMP = cyclic adenosine monophosphate
cGMP = cyclic guanidine monophosphate
LSD = lysergic acid diethylamide

TABLE 13-2. STATUS OF PUTATIVE TRANSMITTER SUBSTANCES

Criterion	Acetylcholine	Norepinephrine	γ-Aminobutyric acid	Glycine	Glutamate	Aspartate	Dopamine	Serotonin	Substance P	Enkephalins + Endorphins	Histamine
1. Present in presynaptic terminals—precursors and enzymes present	√	√	√	*	√	*	√	√	√	√	√
2. Released from terminals by nerve impulses	√	√	√	x	√	√	√	√	?	?	√
3. Rapid inactivation mechanism	√	√	√	?	?	?	?	√	√	?	?
4. Known action—local application mimics natural transmitter	√	√	√	√	?	?	?	?	?	?	?
5. Pharmacologically similar to natural transmitter	√	√	√	√	?	?	√	?	?	?	?

Key: √ = Property demonstrated
* = Labeled substance is taken up by synapses *in vitro* or *in vivo*, but it is not known that synapses normally contain it.
x = Exogenous, labeled substance is released, but release of endogenous substance has not been shown.
? = Property not examined experimentally or results hard to interpret.

No one of these criteria is sufficient by itself to define a transmitter substance. For example, a compound, present in nerve terminals, could not be a transmitter substance unless it was released and unless it influenced the postsynaptic cell. It is also possible that a compound serves as a transmitter substance in one neuron, but serves a different purpose in another one. Table 13-1 contains a list of some of the substances that have been suggested as chemical transmitter substances, their presumed actions, locations of highest concentration within the central nervous system, modes of action (we will have more to say about this later), and agents that block their actions.

It is difficult to establish the validity of all five criteria at synapses within the central nervous system because the cells involved can rarely be seen; because only small quantities of transmitter substance are released and even these are rapidly degraded if they are not protected from enzyme action; and because it is impossible to know if the putative transmitter substance is being applied near the postsynaptic membrane. Thus, acetylcholine (ACh) and norepinephrine (NE) have been identified as transmitter substances at synapses in the peripheral nervous system, ACh at the neuromuscular junction, at all autonomic ganglia, and at some sympathetic and all parasympathetic postganglionic synapses, and NE at most sympathetic postganglionic synapses. Table 13-2 shows the validity of all five criteria for both of these substances and for gamma aminobutyric acid (GABA), an inhibitory transmitter substance in the central nervous system. The remaining compounds in Table 13-2 meet one or more of the five criteria. These compounds must still be considered as putative transmitter substances though some people ignore the deficiencies and incorrectly call them transmitter substances.

Several new types of connections between cells have been discovered. These junctions, thought to be substrates for chemical transmissions, occur between two dendrites **(dendrodendritic synapses),** a dendrite and an axon **(dendroaxonic**

synapses), a dendrite and a soma **(dendrosomatic synapses)**, and any part of a neuron and a node of Ranvier **(nodal synapses)**. In some cases, synapses have been described in which a single element is both pre- and postsynaptic to a second element. This arrangement, a reciprocal synaptic arrangement, is illustrated in Figure 13-2. Its function is unknown. The physiology of these new synaptic arrangements has not been studied in detail yet, but it can be presumed for now that they behave like any other chemical synapse. Their presence certainly broadens the possibilities for interactions between neurons in the central nervous system.

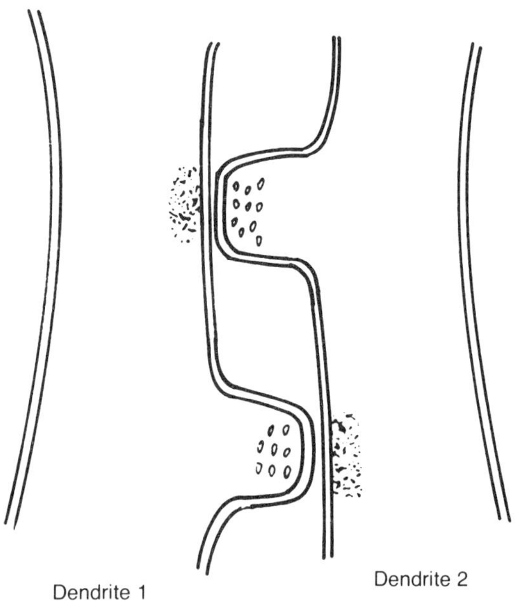

FIG. 13-2. A reciprocal synaptic relationship between two dendrites. Note the accumulations of synaptic vesicles on what is presumed to be the presynaptic side of the synapses.

Another type of synaptic arrangement that has received a great deal of attention lately is the **electrotonic synapse** or **electrical synapse**, the substrate for which is thought to be the tight junction. An example of a tight junction is shown in Figure 13-3A. The membranes of the two cells involved come extremely close or may actually fuse together; some investigators even claim that there are small channels between the two neurons by which their cytoplasms could communicate (Fig. 13-3B). Tight junctions are most frequently seen in dendrodendritic, dendrosomatic, and somatosomatic synaptic arrangements, but they do occur in other types of synapses.

The vast majority of the synapses in the vertebrate central nervous system are of the axosomatic and axodendritic types and of the chemically transmitting type. It is therefore a small wonder that chemical transmission is the most thoroughly understood. There are now many reports of tight junctions and presumed electrotonic coupling between neurons in vertebrates, especially in mammals. Yet, two important mor-

FIG. 13-3. Two conceptions of the structure of an electrical synapse. **A.** The membranes of the cells are simply shown as fused together. **B.** Actual cytoplasmic connections are shown.

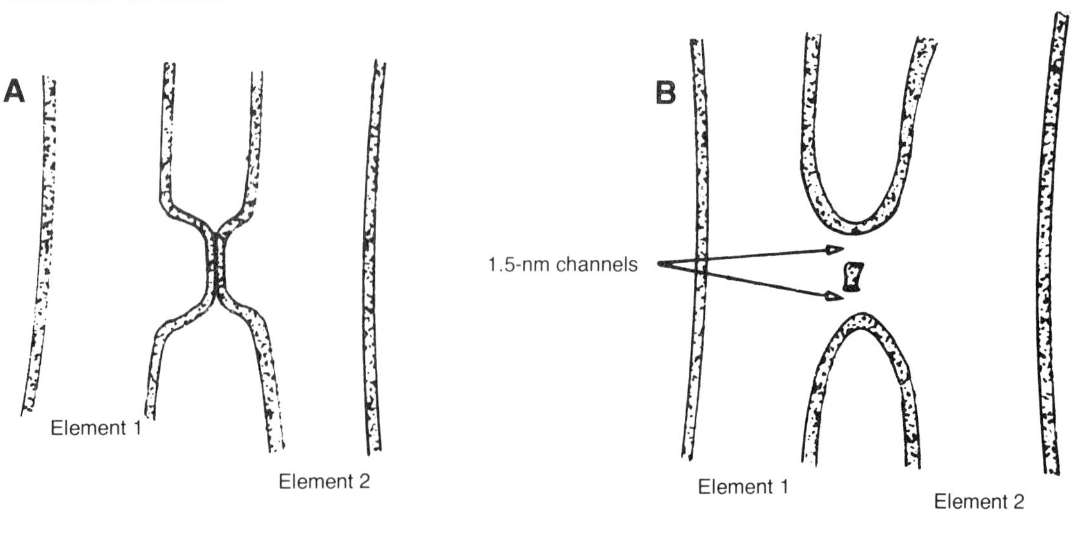

phologic questions still remain unanswered: (1) Is every structure that looks like a chemical synapse really a chemical and not an electrical synapse, or for that matter a synapse at all? (2) Is every tight junction an electrical synapse and not a chemical synapse, or for that matter a synapse at all? These questions are made important by the observations that vesicles (possibly synaptic vesicles) are found in conjunction with both chemical synapses and tight junctions and that tight junctions are characteristic of epithelia, in general, and not limited to the nervous system, which is epithelial in origin. It is not clear that answers to these questions are even possible.

PHYSIOLOGY OF A CHEMICAL SYNAPSE

An action potential, initiated in an afferent axon, arrives at a bouton and depolarizes it. Boutons depolarize in the same way as axons. At this point the action potential itself can go no farther, but the depolarization of the bouton somehow causes some of the synaptic vesicles in the region to fuse with the presynaptic membrane whereupon the fused membrane breaks and spills the contents of the vesicles into the synaptic cleft. The release of transmitter depends upon several factors, including the magnitude of the depolarization, the number of available vesicles, and, importantly, the concentration of calcium in the extracellular fluid. Reduced calcium blocks synaptic transmission. Likewise, increased manganese, a calcium inhibitor, leads to depression or block of transmission. Calcium is necessary for depolarization–release coupling. It is thought that depolarization leads to opening of voltage-gated Ca^{2+} channels and entry of Ca^{2+} into the terminal. Once inside, Ca^{2+} promotes fusion of the vesicles with the terminal membrane and release of the transmitter substance. The released transmitter substance diffuses across the cleft in a fraction of a millisecond and interacts with the postsynaptic membrane, changing its permeability and, ultimately, the membrane potential at that point on the membrane. The action of the transmitter substance is terminated by its removal from receptors on the postsynaptic membrane. Some transmitters are then degraded, for example, acetylcholine, whereas others are taken up by the presynaptic terminal, for example, norepinephrine. This entire process, from presynaptic spike to the termination of the postsynaptic response, usually requires only 10 to 20 msec.

Chemical transmitter substances all act by producing changes in the transmembrane potential of the postsynaptic cell. Some produce their effects noticeably more slowly than others. For example, the interval between the arrival of the presynaptic spike at the synapse and the change in membrane potential, the **synaptic delay,** is shorter at the neuromuscular junction, where acetylcholine is the transmitter substance, than at sympathetic postganglionic synapses, where norepinephrine is the transmitter substance. Surprisingly, acetylcholine acts faster at the neuromuscular junction than at the parasympathetic junctions at the heart. At ganglionic synapses of the sympathetic nervous system acetylcholine has both a fast action (4- to 7-msec latency and a 200-msec duration) and a slow action (200- to 300-msec latency and a 5-sec or longer duration). Both effects occur on the same postsynaptic cell! The rapid-onset, briefer effects of acetylcholine at skeletal muscle are apparently the consequence of changed ionic conductances, resulting from conformational changes in the membrane. These conformational changes result from the interaction of the transmitter substance with receptors (a term used here in the sense of a molecule or molecules that bind specifically to the transmitter substance) in the postsynaptic membrane. This is called **ionotropic transmission,** and it is illustrated schematically in Figure 13-4A. The longer latency and duration of norepinephrine effects on sympathetic postsynaptic structures have been explained by invoking a **second messenger,** in this case, cyclic adenosine monophosphate (cAMP). The model proposed for this kind of transmission, called **metabotropic transmission,** is shown schematically in Figure 13-4B. According to the model, the transmitter substance interacts with the receptor on the postsynaptic membrane, activating adenylate cyclase and producing cAMP. The cAMP activates a protein kinase, phosphorylating a protein. It is the phosphorylation of the protein that produces the change in membrane potential, either through a change in membrane

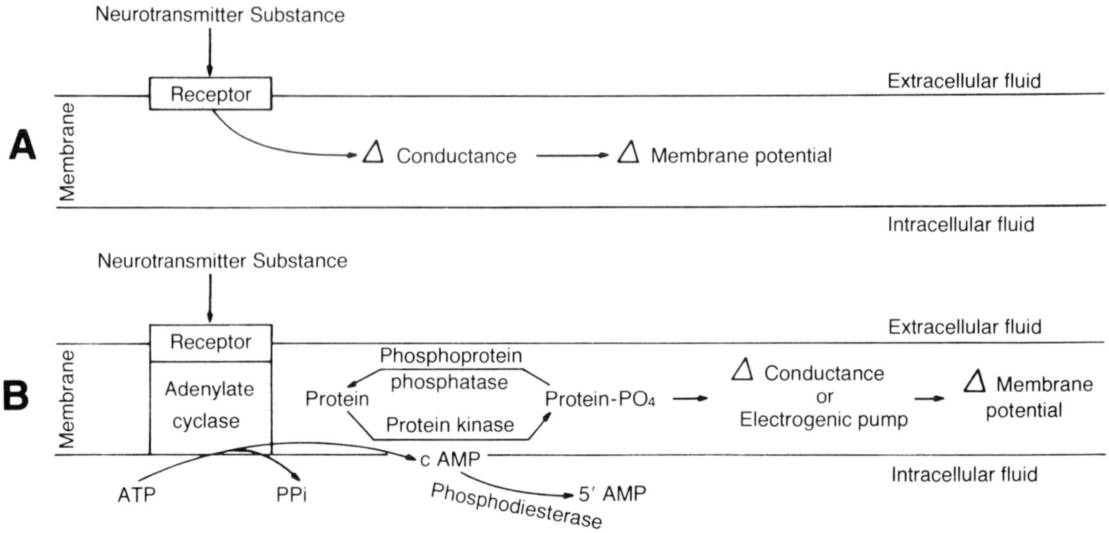

FIG. 13-4. Models of ionotropic **(A)** and metabotropic **(B)** synaptic transmission. Here the second messenger is shown as cAMP, but cGMP or another substance could serve as well. (McGeer PL, Eccles JC, McGeer EG: Molecular Neurobiology of the Mammalian Brain. New York, Plenum Press, 1978)

ionic conductance or through stimulation of an electrogenic pump. The process is reversed by dephosphorylating the protein and hydrolyzing cAMP. Associated with metabotropic transmission is an *increase* in membrane resistance, not a decrease as in ionotropic transmission.

Table 13-1 shows that glycine, GABA, L-glutamate, and L-aspartate are probably ionotropic transmitter substances. Norepinephrine, dopamine, serotonin, epinephrine, histamine, and probably substance P are metabotropic. Acetylcholine is sometimes ionotropic (at nicotinic cholinergic synapses; see Chapter 17 for a discussion of nicotinic and muscarinic synapses), and sometimes metabotropic (at muscarinic cholinergic synapses). The second messenger at metabotropic (muscarinic) cholinergic synapses is thought to be cyclic guanidine monophosphate (cGMP).

THE EXCITATORY POSTSYNAPTIC POTENTIAL

The postsynaptic cell can either hyperpolarize or depolarize in response to the transmitter substance. It is possible to study the postsynaptic events by puncturing the soma of a cell with a microelectrode (historically this has been done most often with α motoneurons because of their large size) to pick up the changes in membrane potential that result from activity in a presynaptic axon. The arrangement for doing this is shown in Figure 13-5 along with some sample records. If we stimulate a peripheral nerve at weak intensity while recording from a motoneuron, we see in the record a depolarization with a latency of 1 to 2 msec, followed shortly by a repolarization of the cell. This response is the **excitatory postsynaptic potential,** or **EPSP,** shown in Figure 13-5B. It has a time constant of about 4 msec and, like the generator potential, is a local or nonpropagated event. The EPSP is in fact a generator potential; it is sufficiently important to warrant special consideration and a name of its own. The amplitude of the EPSP varies with the strength of the stimulus (that is, with the number of fibers stimulated) as shown in Figure 13-5C–E, and if it depolarizes the membrane to or beyond its critical firing level, the motoneuron will discharge an action potential (Fig. 13-5E).

THE NEUROMUSCULAR JUNCTION: AN EXAMPLE OF EXCITATORY TRANSMISSION

We can use transmission at the neuromuscular junction as an example of excitatory transmission because it displays many of the important features of such transmission.

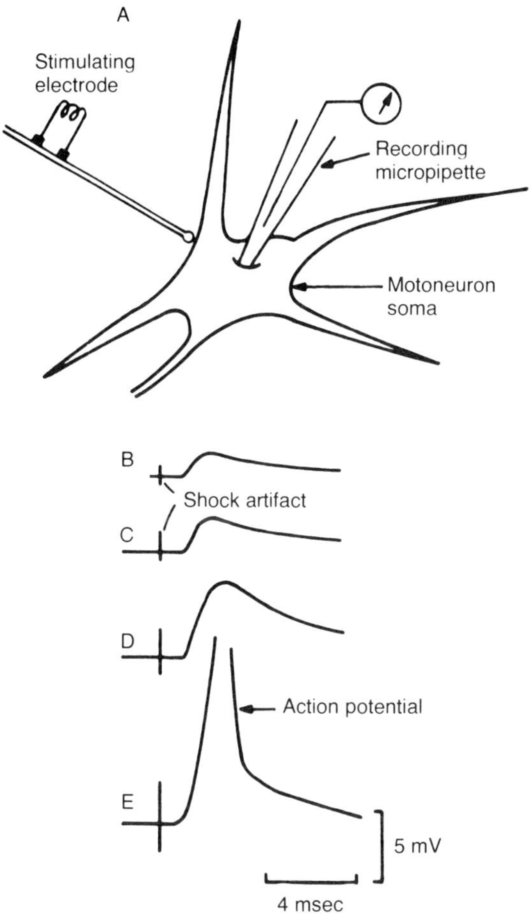

FIG. 13-5. A. The method of recording the postsynaptic potential with a micropipette. **B–E.** EPSPs elicited in a motoneuron by stimuli to a peripheral nerve at increasing strengths. Note that the critical firing level is achieved and that the action potential is initiated in **E.** (Eccles JC, Eccles RM, Lundberg A: J Physiol (Lond) 136:527–546, 1957)

It is also of historic interest because it was in the neuromuscular junction that most of the early studies of synaptic transmission were done. It is easily accessible, and the postsynaptic cell is large and easily penetrated by recording electrodes. The **neuromuscular junction** or **motor end-plate** is morphologically much like any other synapse except that it is larger. The axon of the motoneuron loses its myelin sheath near its termination and expands greatly, forming a bouton that is 10 μm or so in diameter. It contains synaptic vesicles, known to contain the transmitter substance, acetylcholine, in its terminal. The postsynaptic element in this synapse is a skeletal muscle cell whose membrane is specialized at the end-plate by numerous deep infoldings. Only the peaks of these folds are near the motoneuron terminal, but the depths of the folds are in contact with the fluid of the synaptic cleft. The structure of the neuromuscular junction is shown in Figure 13-6.

It is possible to remove the muscle and its nerve from an organism and put it into a bath of Ringer's solution (a balanced ionic solution, the ionic constituency of which is similar to that of blood). The nature of such a preparation is shown in Figure 13-7. When a microelectrode is used to penetrate the muscle, a resting membrane potential (V_r) of about −70mV is recorded as described in Chapter 3.

When the axon of the motoneuron is stimulated, it can be excited to discharge a spike that conducts down to the terminal. Depolarization of the terminal by the action potential opens the voltage-gated Ca^{2+} channels, Ca^{2+} enters the terminal, the synaptic vesicles fuse with the terminal membrane, and acetylcholine is released into the synaptic cleft. The acetylcholine diffuses across the synaptic cleft in less than 100 μsec and interacts with the acetylcholine receptors on the folded postsynaptic muscle membrane. This opens chemically gated channels, permeable to small ions—Ca^{2+}, Na^+, K^+, and Cl^-. As a result, ionic currents begin to flow, comprised mainly of Na^+ current because of its large electrochemical gradient at the resting membrane potential. Inward Na^+ current depolarizes the membrane and, when the membrane potential crosses the critical firing level, an action potential is initiated in the muscle membrane. In Figure 13-8, the instant when the stimulus is applied to the nerve is signaled by the stimulus artifact (a nearly instantaneous spread of stimulus current from stimulating to recording electrodes) and then, after a suitable time for conduction along the axon and for synaptic delay, the membrane depolarizes, leading to the action potential.

If the preparation has been bathed in a solution containing the drug curare, a substance used experimentally as a muscle relaxant and used by South American Indians as a poison that is applied to arrowheads, the stimulus to the nerve leads to a change in potential, called the **end-plate potential.** The end-plate potential looks and behaves

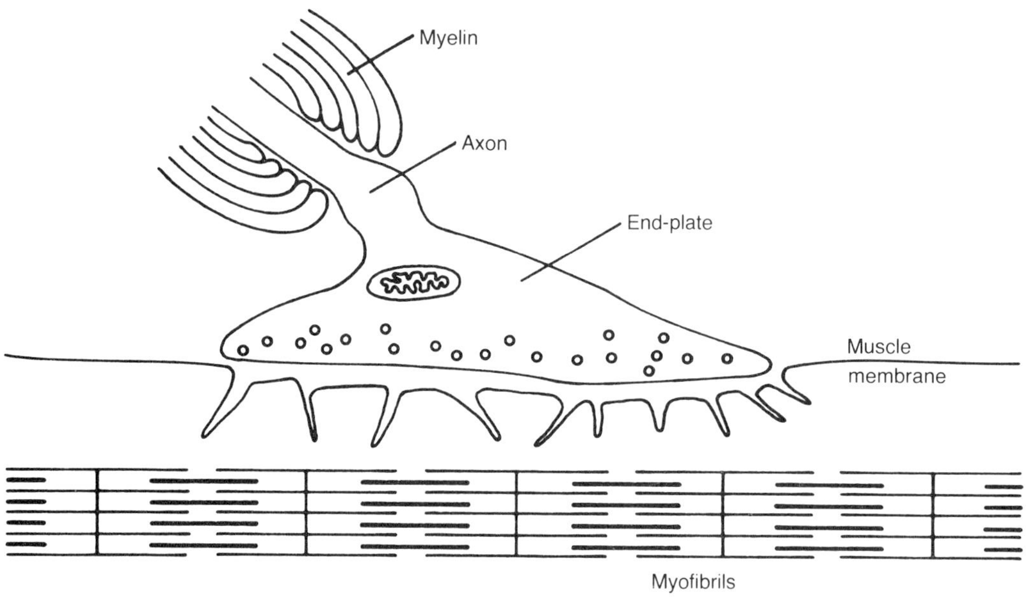

FIG. 13-6. Structure of the neuromuscular junction. The terminal of the motoneuron is expanded over the synaptic cleft. Muscle membrane is deeply infolded under the terminal.

FIG. 13-7. Recording setup for the end-plate potential. Muscle is bathed in Ringer's solution containing curare, and motor axon is placed on stimulating electrodes. A recording micropipette penetrates the muscle membrane at 1-mm intervals away from the end-plate. Sample records show the nature of the recording at each site.

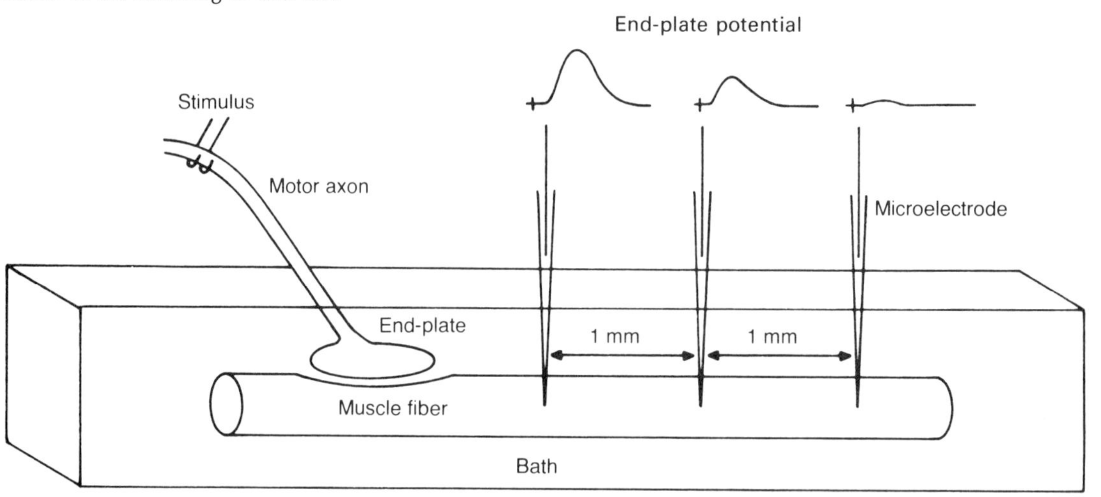

much like EPSPs in nerve cells; an example is shown at the right of Figure 13-8. Like the EPSP, the end-plate potential is graded and nonpropagated, as shown in Figure 13-7. As the electrode is moved farther and farther along the muscle membrane away from the end-plate, the potential drops in amplitude because it conducts electrotonically. As in other synapses, the receptor region of the postsynaptic membrane contains no voltage-gated channels and therefore does not discharge spikes, but the end-plate potential has only to bring the adjacent membrane to critical firing level to initiate an action potential there. Normally, in the absence of curare, the end-plate potential is more than large enough to bring the membrane to the critical firing level; an action potential is initiated in the muscle fiber for each spike in the motoneuron connected to it.

Acetylcholine acts to open the ionic channels in the postsynaptic membrane for only 1 to 2 msec; the remainder of the end-plate potential is simply due to the passive properties of the muscle membrane. After 1 to 2 msec, the acetylcholine is removed from the receptor and hydrolyzed by the enzyme **acetylcholinesterase,** which is found on the postsynaptic membrane mainly in the region of the synaptic cleft. Most of the transmitter substance is hydrolyzed and the products are taken up again by the motoneuron terminal, but some of the acetylcholine escapes from the cleft and is carried away by the blood. There is no danger that this escaped transmitter can reexcite the muscle because it is only effective in changing the membrane potential when applied to the membrane within the cleft, that is, there are no active receptors on the muscle membrane except in the cleft.

Within the motoneuron terminals, acetylcholine is stored in the synaptic vesicles, each vesicle containing about 10,000 molecules of acetylcholine. Because the transmitter substance is stored in this fashion and because the entire content of a vesicle is released or none of it is released, it is reasonable to assume that the end-plate potentials must be made up of some multiple of the potential change caused by a single vesicle's contents. Actually, when recordings are made from a nerve–muscle preparation (Fig. 13-7) at rest, small, spontaneous depolarizations are seen in the membrane potential. These have a time course and configuration reminiscent of the end-plate potential, and they are termed **miniature end-plate potentials** or **MEPPs.** Pharmacologically and physiologically, it has been demonstrated that MEPPs have the same properties as the end-plate potential and that they are caused by spontaneous release of small quantities of acetylcholine. MEPPs tend to have the same amplitude or multiples of their smallest amplitude, so it is surmised that they are caused by release of nearly equal-sized packets of acetylcholine, called **quanta.** It seems reasonable to assume that a quantum is the amount of transmitter substance in a single vesicle. It also seems reasonable that the end-plate potential is always composed of integral multiples of a MEPP.

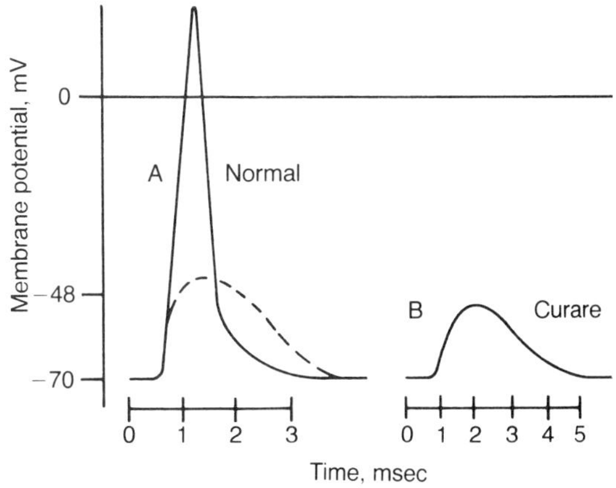

FIG. 13-8. The spike and the end-plate potential. **A.** The spike recorded by a transmembrane micropipette from the muscle. **B.** The end-plate potential recorded after the spike has been blocked with curare.

MEPPs occur spontaneously at irregular intervals with a low rate of occurrence at the resting end-plate. The motoneuron spike increases the rate of occurrence of MEPPs for a short time, 1 to 2 msec, during which 200 to 2000 quanta, depending upon the particular nerve–muscle preparation, are released. Each quantum opens up to 2000 channels and each channel can admit as many as 20,000 Na^+ ions. The potential for change in the membrane potential of the muscle is therefore always more than enough to cause a spike in normal, healthy muscle.

Because the process of transmission at the neuromuscular junction contains so many different steps, the possibilities for interference with the process are numerous. Curare has already been mentioned as a blocker; curare competes with acetylcholine for the receptor sites, but is incapable of activating them. Other competitive blockers, such as decamethonium or succinylcholine, not only compete, but activate the receptor. Their paralyzing effect is due to the tenacity with which they bind the receptor and the difficulty with which they are removed from the receptor and hydrolyzed.

The toxin of botulinus bacteria, found in some spoiled food, is an extremely powerful neuromuscular blocker that works by preventing the release of the transmitter substance from the motoneuron terminals. Low

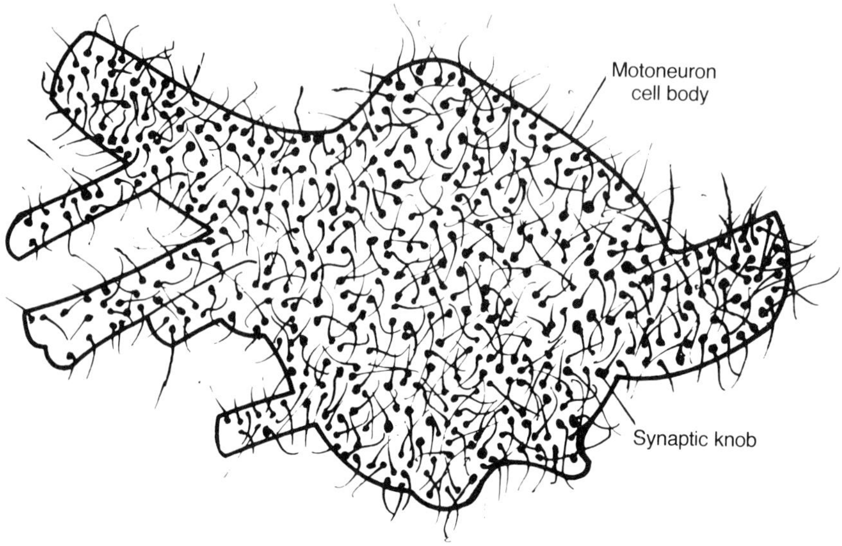

FIG. 13-9. The surface of a motoneuron soma studded with boutons terminaux. (Schadé JP, Ford DH: Basic Neurology. Amsterdam, Elsevier, 1965)

FIG. 13-10. Spatial and temporal summation of EPSPs. **A.** EPSPs elicited by stimulation of two fibers afferent to a motoneuron both separately and simultaneously. Notice the algebraic summation. **B.** EPSPs elicited by a single stimulus to a fiber afferent to a motoneuron and two stimuli applied in rapid succession (2 msec apart).

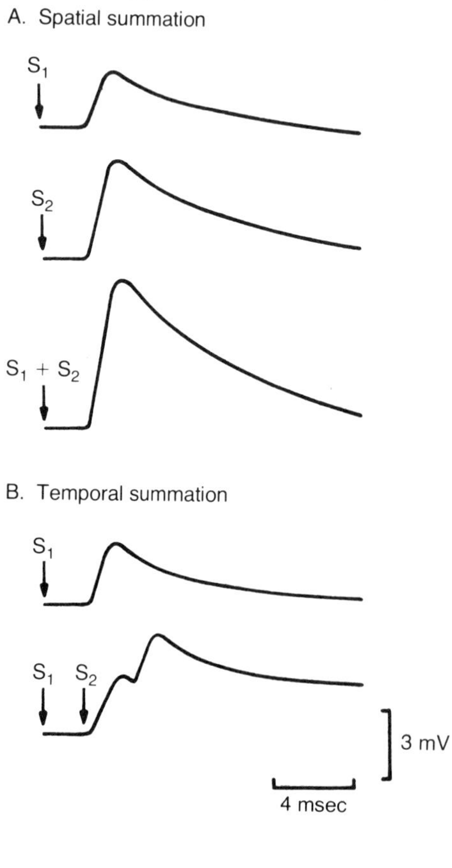

Ca^{2+} concentrations in the extracellular fluid also prevent transmitter substance release. Elevated Mg^{2+} or Mn^{2+} levels also block release, but they work by competition with Ca^{2+}.

Neuromuscular blocks can also be created by interfering with the action of the ACh-degrading enzyme acetylcholinesterase. Cholinesterase inhibitors, such as neostigmine, block the removal and hydrolyzation of acetylcholine; thus, the muscle membrane stays depolarized for too long a period and the muscle cannot relax. This is the principle of action of many insecticides and nerve gases. Prolonged depolarizations lead to convulsions, then to paralysis and death, usually caused by paralysis of the diaphragm.

The disease myasthenia gravis is characterized by muscle weakness after repeated activation of the neuromuscular junction, but not for a single activation. Patients typically are strong in the morning, but become progressively weaker as the day goes on. The problem with the myasthenic patient appears to be a decreased ability to resynthesize acetylcholine from the acetate and choline taken up into the terminals. With repeated activation of the synapse, the vesicular stores of acetylcholine are depleted, not replenished as they normally would be, and after a while the junction fails to transmit.

SYNAPTIC TRANSMISSION BETWEEN NEURONS

Synaptic transmission between neurons is basically the same as at the neuromuscular junctions. Transmitter substance release is triggered by terminal depolarization and is dependent upon Ca^{2+}. The release process is quantal in nature, and transmitter release occurs spontaneously. Synaptic transmission is terminated by removal of the transmitter substance from the synaptic cleft through reuptake or hydrolysis. One fundamental difference is that in synaptic transmission between neurons, and EPSP in the postsynaptic neuron, caused by a single spike at a single synapse, seldom is large enough to trigger a spike. In general, the EPSPs caused by a single presynaptic action potential are small, only 1 to 2 mV of depolarization, and cannot bring the postsynaptic cell to critical firing level. For the postsynaptic cell to be excited to discharge requires spatial and temporal summation, the same two phenomena discussed previously. Figure 13-9 shows a sketch of the soma of a motoneuron, literally encrusted with boutons from afferent fibers of various sources, to show how extensive neural interconnections are. Estimates of the density of synapses on motoneurons have indicated that boutons cover 40% to 50% of the somatic and 50% to 80% of the dendritic surfaces. If we stimulate more than one of these afferent fibers with a single stimulus, then each active fiber will release its transmitter substance onto the membrane of the motoneuron and cause its own EPSP, and we see the algebraic sum of them. In Figure 13-10A are illustrated the EPSPs elicited in a motoneuron by two action potentials in two different afferent fibers, when stimulated separately and when stimulated together. The response to simultaneous stimulation is clearly seen to be the algebraic sum of the two single responses. This is an example of spatial summation.

Like all generator potentials, EPSPs can show temporal summation. If the same afferent axon is stimulated twice in rapid succession, the response to the first stimulus is not yet over before the response to the second begins. The potential changes again summate, but because they do not start at exactly the same time, the sum is a bit irregular in shape (Fig. 13-10B). This is an example of temporal summation. The membrane potential can be brought to firing level by summation, either spatial or temporal, or both. Any number of EPSPs, from a variety of types of presynaptic neurons, can be summed by a single postsynaptic cell.

Synapses that require a lot of summation to reach firing level are called **integrative synapses,** and they make up the bulk of the synapses in the nervous system. A few synapses require only one presynaptic action potential to bring the postsynaptic membrane to critical firing level, and these are called **obligatory synapses.** An example of an obligatory synapse is the neuromuscular junction. A single action potential in a single α motoneuron causes a postsynaptic action potential in every extrafusal muscle fiber in the **motor unit** (a motoneuron plus all the muscle fibers it innervates is a motor unit) of that neuron. Generation of the action potentials in the α motoneurons themselves requires considerable summation, and therefore synapses on motoneuron somata or dendrites are integrative. Not all neurons behave exactly like motoneurons, but most use this same basic mechanism for transmission at junctions with other cells.

THE INHIBITORY POSTSYNAPTIC POTENTIAL

Another difference between neuronal and neuromuscular synapses is the possibility of inhibition at neuronal synapses. Inhibition is not seen in mammalian neuromuscular junctions. With an appropriate stimulus, the response of the motoneuron can be a hyperpolarization, beginning 3 to 4 msec after the stimulus, followed by a return to the resting potential, again with a time constant of about 4 msec. This response is called the **inhibitory postsynaptic potential,** or **IPSP,** because it drives the membrane 1 to 4 mV away from the critical firing level and therefore reduces the frequency or, alternatively, the probability of firing of the postsynaptic cell. Figure 13-11 shows that as the stimulus strength increases, so does the amplitude of the IPSP. Like the EPSP, the IPSP is a nonpropagated event. IPSPs can sum either spatially or temporally to hyperpolarize the cell to an even greater extent than a single IPSP. IPSPs are never seen in mammalian muscles.

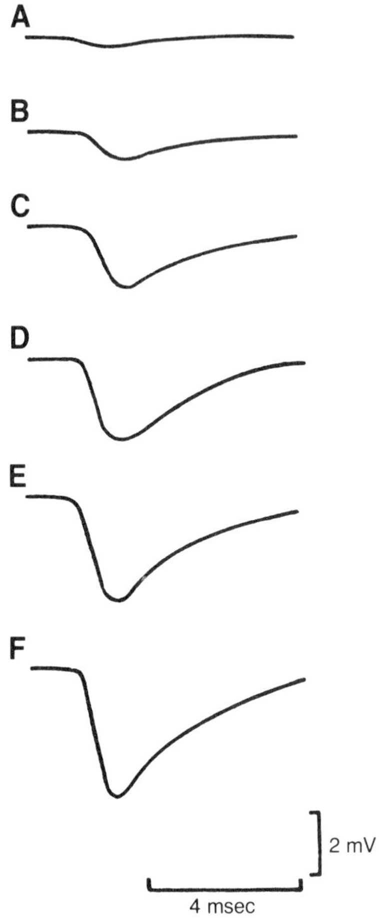

FIG. 13-11. An IPSP elicited by a single stimulus applied to a peripheral nerve at increasing strengths from top to bottom.

IONIC MECHANISMS OF POSTSYNAPTIC POTENTIALS

It appears that the excitatory transmitter substances responsible for the EPSP act at the postsynaptic membrane by increasing the permeability of the membrane to all small ions, including sodium, potassium, calcium, and chloride ions; there is an increase in net flux of ions with all ions moving down their electrochemical gradients. The major contributor to the change in potential is sodium current because of the large driving force (membrane potential minus equilibrium potential) on sodium ions and the large change in sodium conductance. It is also apparent that the change in the membrane's permeability to sodium is much larger than the change for potassium, because the potential that the membrane is seeking during the EPSP, the equilibrium potential of the EPSP, is 0 to +30 mV, the exact value depending upon what synapse is being studied. It should be recalled that the resting membrane's permeability to sodium is only $^1/_{30}$ of that to potassium, making the resting potential near the potassium equilibrium potential. If the membrane is suddenly made 30 times more permeable to sodium ions, the membrane potential will shift to a level halfway between the sodium and potassium equilibrium potentials, about −15 mV. In fact, during the EPSP, the membrane potential shifts farther, to 0 to +30 mV, so the relative change in sodium permeability must make the permeability ratio much greater than 1 : 30, in fact, greater than 1 : 1. Apparently, chloride plays no major role in this process, but any chloride current would tend to hold the membrane near ϵ_{Cl^-}, that is, near V_r.

The IPSP, on the other hand, is produced by increased permeability of the membrane to chloride or potassium or both. In either case, an increase in permeability would allow the ion to flow down its concentration gradient and result in hyperpolarization. Chloride and potassium are nearly in electrochemical equilibrium, and therefore their driving forces are small, but then the amplitude of the IPSP is also small.

It is important that the inhibitory effect of the IPSP is not due simply to the hyperpolarization, driving the membrane away from the critical firing level, but includes another process. If the effect were simply due to the hyperpolarization, then summation between EPSPs and IPSPs would still be linear, IPSPs summing with a negative sign. The maximum change in voltage of the EPSP is 8 to 10 mV, whereas that for the IPSP is 2 to 4 mV; yet an IPSP can reduce the amplitude of an EPSP by more than its own amplitude, that is, they do *not* sum algebraically. This is shown in Figure 13-12. When the appropriate pathways to a cell are stimulated, an EPSP and IPSP are initiated in the cell, as shown in A and B. If the EPSP and the IPSP are initiated at the same time, the resulting change in potential is a small hyperpolarization as shown in C, not the small depolarization that would be expected if there were algebraic summation. An EPSP (D) much larger than the IPSP (in terms of amplitude) must be added to the response to depolarize the cell to the same level as the original EPSP, as shown in E. This happens because the IPSP results from an increased membrane conductance for K^+ and Cl^-. This means that the membrane resistance ($R = 1/g$) is decreased. The inward Na^+ current of the EPSP therefore produces a smaller voltage drop across the smaller membrane resistance ($V = iR$) and a smaller EPSP. The IPSP inhibits both by virtue of the decreased membrane resistance and the hyperpolarization. The hyperpolarization forces a greater amount of depolarization to achieve critical firing level and the decreased membrane resistance reduces the size of the EPSP. For this reason, inhibition always makes itself felt. Equal excitatory and inhibitory presynaptic inputs to a cell always result in inhibition of its discharge.

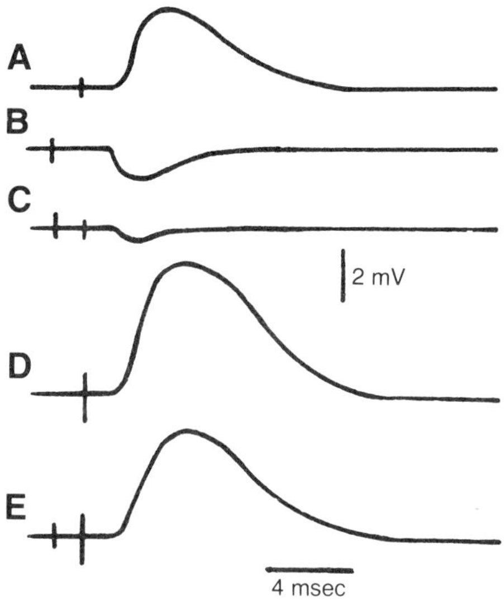

FIG. 13-12. The effectiveness of an IPSP in reducing EPSPs. **A.** The EPSP by itself. **B.** The IPSP by itself. **C.** The EPSP and IPSP initiated at the same time. **D.** A much larger EPSP by itself. **E.** The EPSP in **D** with the IPSP in **B.**

The postsynaptic membranes at all synapses are electrically inexcitable; the action potential is initiated somewhere else on the membrane. Most people think that the spike in most neurons is initiated in the region where the axon is connected to the soma, the **axon hillock.** The axon hillock is thought to have an electrical threshold about half that of the soma and dendrites, so that the spike is initiated there first. Figure 13-13 shows a drawing of the neuron showing the axon hillock and synaptic junctions on the soma and dendrites. EPSPs and

FIG. 13-13. Current flow at synapses. Excitatory and inhibitory synapses are indicated on the soma and proximal dendrites and currents initiated at each, flowing through the postsynaptic membrane and the region of the axon hillock, where the spike is thought to be initiated.

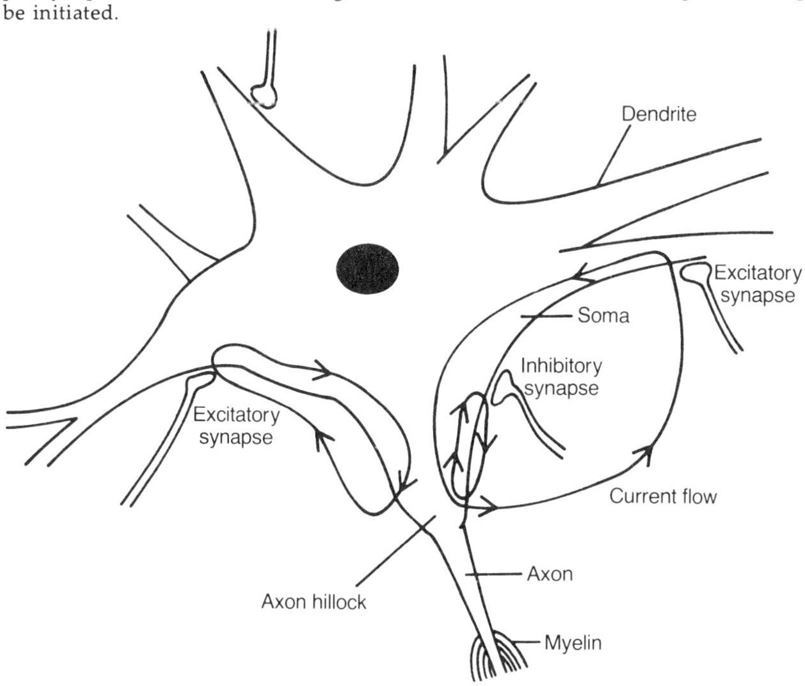

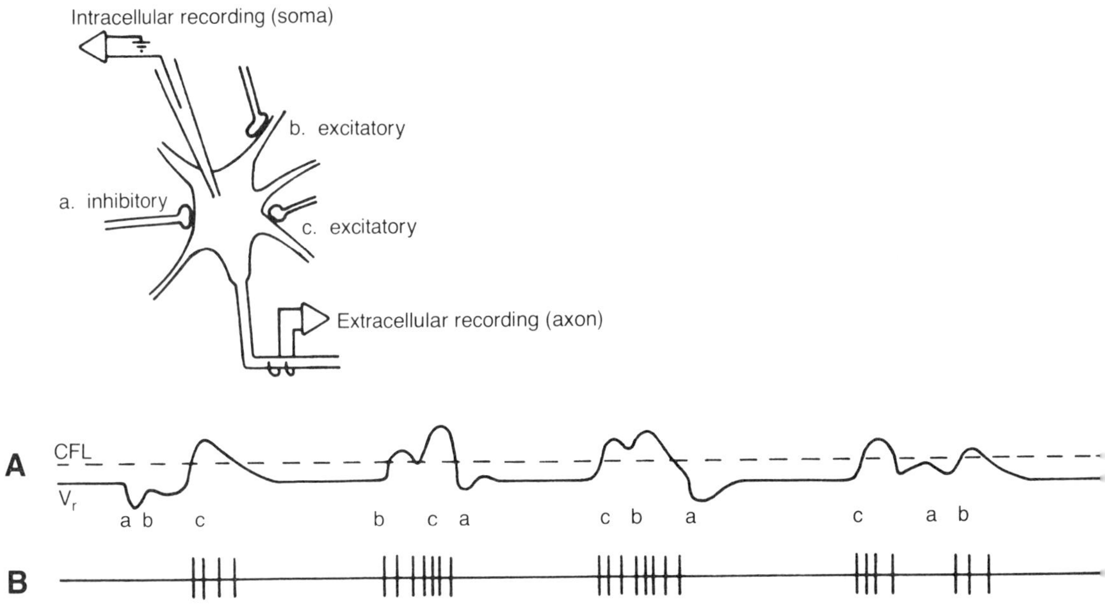

FIG. 13-14. The combination of EPSPs and IPSPs to generate different patterns of spike discharge. **Inset** shows a neuron with three synaptic junctions—two on the soma and one on a proximal dendrite. Two of the synapses are excitatory; one is inhibitory. **A.** Transmembrane potential recorded with the micropipette, with different temporal arrangements of a single postsynaptic potential at each synapse (indicated by letters under trace). For the purpose of illustration, EPSPs and IPSPs are shown larger than normal; they can cause the membrane potential to cross the critical firing level **(CFL)**. **B.** The spike trains that would be recorded from the axon of the cell as generated by the synaptic potential patterns in **(A)**.

IPSPs are not propagated, but spread electrotonically into the region of the hillock. This means that, for synapses producing equal changes in membrane potential at the synapse, the one closer to the hillock has the greatest influence on the firing of the cell. However, synapses on dendrites tend to generate particularly large EPSPs, somewhat offsetting their greater distance. Inhibitory synapses, synapses that produce IPSPs, also tend to be located closer than excitatory synapses to the axon hillock (the spike-generating region). This arrangement may also add to the great influence of IPSPs on the neuron membrane.

The firing pattern of the neuron is completely determined by the sum of its synaptic bombardment, both excitatory and inhibitory. This is especially important in cells with integrative synapses. It was pointed out in the earlier discussion of generator potentials that there is a linear relationship between generator potential amplitude and the frequency of discharge in the receptor or its nerve. The EPSP is a generator potential, and it also is related to discharge frequency in a linear way. The depolarization at the axon hillock is increased by summation of EPSPs from different synapses and decreased by summation of IPSPs. As a result, the firing frequency increases or decreases. Figure 13-14 shows some different configurations of synaptic potentials at the axon hillock (A) and the resulting patterns of discharge in the axon hillock (B). The same synapses are involved in generating each pattern; only the order and timing are changed. Even small changes result in noticeably different patterns of spike discharges, with great consequences for behavior.

If the precise timing required to produce spatial and temporal summation is altered, the precise firing patterns of interneurons and motoneurons required to produce even the simplest of movements are no longer possible. In fact, the real impact of certain demyelinating diseases such as **multiple sclerosis** is not due to destruction of neurons or even blockage of conduction; they still conduct (at least initially), although at reduced velocities after the myelin is removed. The slowed conduction in a demyelinating disease means that some impulses do not arrive on time at synapses on motoneurons. Considering the time constant of an EPSP, a slowing of conduction that produces even a 0.5-msec delay in the arrival of an impulse at the synapse can have devastating effects on movement.

RECTIFICATION*

In the initial discussion of the initiation of an action potential in axons, it was noted that, with electrical stimulation, once the critical firing level is reached, the action potential propagates in both directions away from the point of stimulation. The direction normally taken by action potentials is the **orthodromic** direction; the reverse is the **antidromic** direction. If the action potentials can travel down an axon both ways, why is there a "normal" direction? The answer lies in the synapse. When the action potential reaches a synapse it can go no further, but it can cause a release of transmitter substance from a presynaptic element. There is no transmitter mechanism in the postsynaptic element; therefore, synapses act as rectifiers, allowing transmission in only one direction.

PHYSIOLOGY OF AN ELECTROTONIC SYNAPSE

In known examples of electrotonic synapses in invertebrates, the anatomic substrate of transmission is a tight junction in which the joined membrane is of lower resistance than surrounding membrane, that is, the cell-to-cell resistance is less than the cell-to-extracellular fluid resistance, and it is electrically inexcitable, that is, it does not generate action potentials. An impulse propagates into the region of the junction, and the resulting current flows across the junctional membrane, out of the presynaptic cell and into the postsynaptic cell. That current must again flow out of the postsynaptic cell (according to Kirchhoff's current law), this time through electrically excitable membrane, causing a depolarization, which, if large enough, can cause the postsynaptic cell to discharge. Usually, though, the resulting depolarization is small, on the order of 1 to 2 mV.

Figure 13-15 shows recordings made intracellularly from two spinal motoneurons that drive the electric organ of the electric fish, *Gnathonemus.* The electric organ emits electrical impulses of 0.3-msec duration at frequencies of up to 100/sec and presumably is used by the fish for guidance or perhaps communication. The recording arrangement is shown in A. Histologically, these motoneurons have been shown to be interconnected by thick dendritic or somatic processes, as shown. A hyperpolarizing current was applied to neuron 1, and responses were recorded from both in Figure 13-15B. Both cells were hyperpolarized. A similar result occurred when a hyperpolarizing current was applied to neuron 2 (Fig. 13-15C). A depolarizing current, applied to either cell, depolarized both or, in some cases, caused both to discharge action potentials (Fig. 13-15D–G). Notice that the latency of the discharge was longer in the cell that did not receive the current injection directly. This is due to the slower rate of rise of the electrotonic potential farther from the current source, causing a delay in reaching the critical firing level (Fig. 13-15F,G). The sort of reciprocal relationship shown in Figure 13-15 is just what one would expect for such an electrotonic synapse. Current flows as easily from neuron 1 to neuron 2 as from neuron 2 to neuron 1, that is, the junction is not rectifying. There are a few examples in invertebrates of electrotonic synapses that do rectify. This can be the result of the two cells having greatly different membrane resistances, membrane areas, or voltage thresholds, the latter being the voltage at which the synapse begins to transmit.

CHEMICAL AND ELECTROTONIC SYNAPSES COMPARED AND CONTRASTED

INHIBITION

It should be clear that chemical synapses can produce either depolarizations (excitation) or hyperpolarizations (inhibition) in

* Here the term rectification is used in the engineering sense of a lower resistance to transmission in one direction than in the opposite direction.

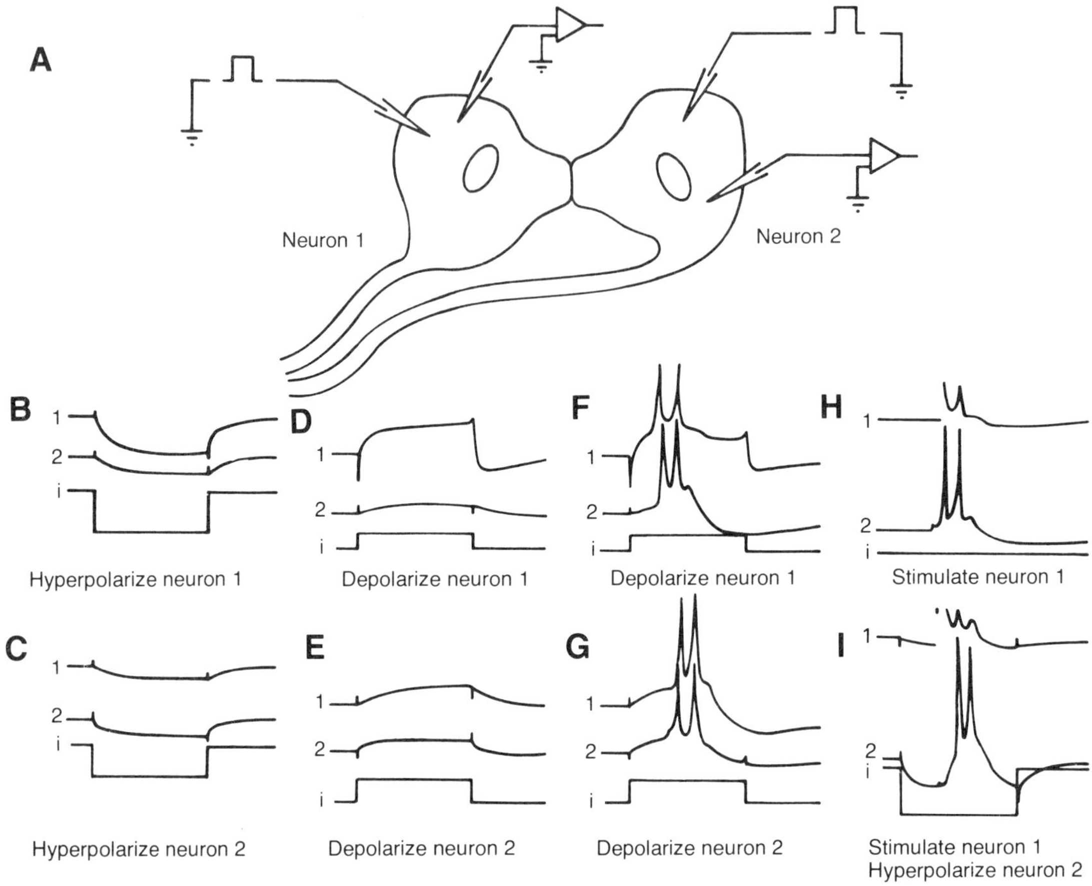

FIG. 13-15. Electrotonic spread between spinal neurons in an electric fish. **A.** Recordings are made simultaneously of the membrane potentials of two neurons while either one is depolarized or hyperpolarized through an intracellular electrode. **B–G.** The responses of both cells are shown to hyperpolarization of neuron 1 (**B**) or neuron 2 (**C**), depolarization of neuron 1 below (**D**) and exceeding its critical firing level (**F**), and depolarization of neuron 2 below (**E**) and exceeding its critical firing level (**G**). **H.** An impulse is initiated by a brief stimulus to neuron 1 and it spreads to neuron 2. **I.** The same as in **H** except that neuron 2 is strongly hyperpolarized; this fails to block spread of the spike from neuron 1 to neuron 2. (Bennett MVL, Pappas GD, Aljure E et al: J Neurophysiol 30:180–208, 1967)

the postsynaptic cell. As far as we know, axons do not carry propagated hyperpolarizations in any nervous system, and therefore simple hyperpolarizing postsynaptic potentials will not occur at electrical synapses. There is the possibility of transmission of hyperpolarizing after-potentials at electrical synapses, especially if transmission at the junction were rectified in the proper direction. If the polarity of rectification is such that depolarizations pass more easily from pre- to postsynaptic and hyperpolarizations from post- to presynaptic, a large hyperpolarizing after-potential in the postsynaptic cell would then produce a feedback inhibition to the presynaptic cell with little feedback excitation (Table 13-3). Such a possibility has been suggested for synapses in *Aplysia*.

The advantages of chemically mediated inhibition are that it can be larger in size, that is, a greater hyperpolarization, longer in duration, and not limited in its site of application. Electrically mediated inhibition occurs more rapidly because of the lack of synaptic delay, but this need not be a big advantage. The CNS could easily produce small time compensations.

TABLE 13-3. PROPERTIES OF SINGLE CHEMICAL AND ELECTRICAL SYNAPSES

	CHEMICAL	ELECTRICAL
1. Rectification	Always	Sometimes, usually not
2. Amplification	Yes	No
3. Delay	Yes	No
4. Inhibition	Yes	Yes
5. Summation	Yes	Yes
6. Influenced by membrane potential	Yes	No

SYNAPTIC DELAY

Transmission at a chemical synapse requires mobilization of synaptic vesicles, exocytosis, diffusion of transmitter substance, reaction of transmitter substance with postsynaptic receptor sites, and production of changes in membrane permeability, either directly or through a second messenger. All of these steps take time. This time is called the **synaptic delay**, and it is measured as the time between arrival of the impulse at the presynaptic terminal and the start of the postsynaptic response. In mammals, the ionotropic synaptic delay is of the order of 0.1 to 0.3 msec. At the neuromuscular junction, most of the delay consists of the time required for release of the chemical transmitter substance. Diffusion time and onset of permeability changes apparently contribute little to it.

The process of electrical transmission occurs with minimal delay, usually less than 0.05 msec. It is this short delay that gives electrical synapses their usefulness as neural synchronizers. The electrical interconnection of neurons causes them to tend to fire synchronously. This is presumably of advantage when rapid movements or high-frequency events, such as electric organ discharges, are being controlled. What other advantages it may confer on a system are not known.

RECTIFICATION

Because of the locations of synaptic vesicles and receptors for transmitter substance at chemical synapses, the latter are, of necessity, rectifying junctions, that is, they allow transmission in only one direction, as we have already discussed. In cases of reciprocal synapses, there is a mechanism for removing rectification, but it is not known how pervasive this mechanism may be. It is known to exist in the retina and the olfactory bulb. As we have already mentioned, most electrical synapses appear to be nonrectifying; however, the study of rectification requires intracellular recording and stimulation of both the pre- and postsynaptic elements of the synapse, which is seldom possible in vertebrates.

SUMMATION

The processes of spatial and temporal summation in chemical synapses are general integrative properties of neurons and fundamental to operation of the nervous system. They are also properties of electrical synapses. The major difference between summation by chemical and by electrical mechanisms is the longer time course of chemical summation. The postsynaptic potentials at chemical synapses typically last 10 msec or longer, whereas those at electrical synapses seldom outlast the duration of the presynaptic spike, that is, about 1 msec. Therefore, summation can occur over a period 10 times (or more) longer at chemical synapses.

AMPLIFICATION

At chemical synapses, there can be an effective **amplification** of the transmitted signal such that the electrical energy of the postsynaptic response is greater than that of the presynaptic response. This can occur if the resistance of the postsynaptic membrane is higher than that of the presynaptic membrane or if the change in membrane permeability, brought about by a single presynaptic spike, is extremely large. This may manifest itself as an increase in the number of action potentials discharged by the postsynaptic cell. Amplification has been observed for neurons in the dorsal horn of the spinal cord that are connected to cutaneous primary afferent neurons (Tapper, Mann, 1968). It probably also occurs at the synaptic junctions between receptors and other cells that do not generate action potentials themselves and neurons that do generate action potentials, for example, bipolar and gan-

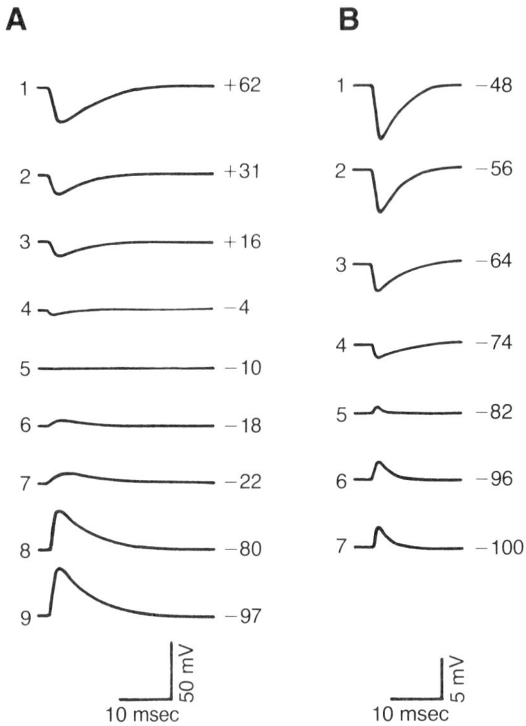

FIG. 13-16. Demonstration of the equilibrium potentials of the EPSP and IPSP. **A.** The influence of changes in membrane potential (indicated at the end of each trace), induced by passing current through an intracellular electrode, on the EPSP recorded from a frog sympathetic ganglion cell is shown. The resting potential for this cell was −80 mV, and the equilibrium potential for the EPSP (*A5*) was −10 mV. (Nishi S, Koketsu K: J Cell Comp Physiol 55:15–30, 1960) **B.** The influence of membrane potential on the IPSP recorded from a motoneuron in the cat. The resting membrane potential for this cell was −74 mV, and the equilibrium potential for the IPSP was −81 mV. (Coombs JS, Eccles JC, Fatt P: J Physiol (Lond) 130:326–373, 1955)

glion cells in the retina. No such amplification has ever been seen in an electrical synapse.

INFLUENCE OF MEMBRANE POTENTIAL

Because the postsynaptic potentials at chemical synapses result from changes in permeability of the postsynaptic membrane to sodium, potassium, chloride, or other ions, their amplitude and polarity are greatly affected by the polarity and magnitude of the membrane potential. An example of the influence of membrane potential upon both EPSPs and IPSPs is shown in Figure 13-16. In Figure 13-16, A8 and B4 show the normal configurations of the EPSP and IPSP, when initiated with the cell at resting membrane potential. If the cell is depolarized, the IPSP gets larger (Fig. 13-16, B4-1) because the driving forces get larger as the membrane potential gets further removed from the equilibrium potentials of the ions whose permeability is changed, that is, chloride and potassium. The EPSP, on the other hand, gets smaller as the membrane is depolarized (Fig. 13-16, A8–6), until it disappears (Fig. 13-16, A5) and is replaced by a negative-going potential (Fig. 13-16, A4). The value of the membrane potential at which the EPSP disappears is called the **equilibrium potential for the EPSP,** ϵ_{EPSP}, and it is determined by the equilibrium potentials for the ions whose conductances change during the EPSP, that is, Na^+ and K^+, with a weighting factor related to the amount of conductance change, as indicated in equation 10 of Chapter 3. If the permeabilities for both Na^+ and K^+ change, then the equilibrium potential for the EPSP is somewhere between the sodium equilibrium potential, ϵ_{Na^+}, and the potassium equilibrium potential ϵ_{K^+}. The squid giant synapse, has a reversal potential of +20 mV, the cat motoneuron, 0 mV, and the neuromuscular junction, −15 mV, indicating that different relative permeability changes for Na^+ and K^+ ions occur at different synapses. The relative change in potassium conductance is larger for the neuromuscular junction than for either the cat motoneuron or squid giant synapse. With further depolarization, a new driving force develops, but this time in the opposite direction, moving the membrane back toward ϵ_{EPSP} (Fig. 13-16, A4–1).

One can see that the IPSP decreases in amplitude and reverses to a depolarizing potential as the membrane is hyperpolarized (Fig. 13-16, B4–7), whereas the EPSP gets larger (Fig. 13-16, A5–7). The IPSP gets smaller either because i_{Cl^-} and i_{K^+} exactly balance each other (if both ions are involved) or because $i_x = V_m - \epsilon_x = 0$ (if only one ion, **x**, is involved). At the equilibrium potential for the IPSP, the amplitude of the IPSP is zero because there is no net membrane current. As the equilibrium potential is exceeded (Fig. 13-16, B5–7), a net current (two ions) or new driving force (one ion) develops, but it is in the opposite direction, so the polarity of the

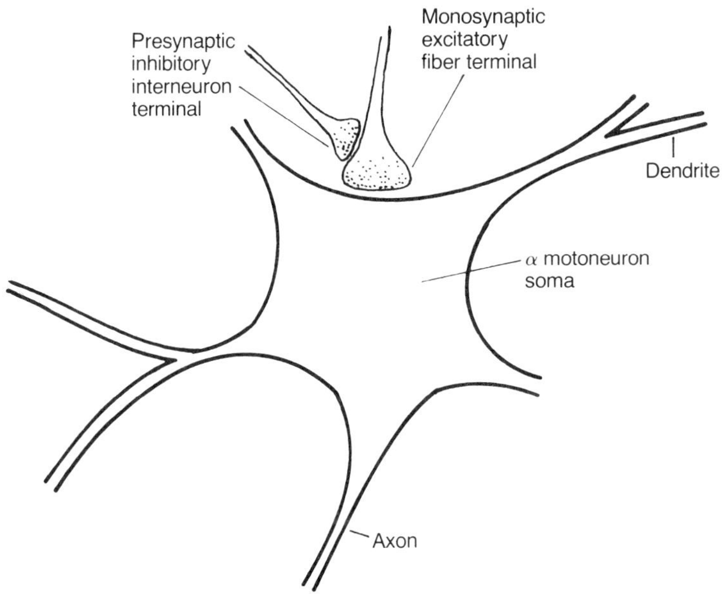

FIG. 13-17. The anatomic arrangement of an axoaxonic synapse showing the pre- and postsynaptic axons. Also shown is the axosomatic synapse of the group Ia afferent fiber on the motoneuron. (Eccles JC: The Understanding of the Brain. New York, McGraw-Hill, 1973)

IPSP reverses. The EPSP gets larger with membrane hyperpolarization, primarily because the driving force on Na^+ increases as the membrane potential moves further from the equilibrium potential of the EPSP.

The postsynaptic potential at an electrical synapse is due to a flow of current through the membrane resistance with no concomitant change in membrane permeability, although an EPSP may lead to a permeability change in adjacent, electrically excitable membrane. Because the EPSP is a simple ohmic voltage change (*iR* drop), it is not influenced by membrane potential, and therefore it has nearly the same size at any membrane potential. This is shown in Figure 13-15, H and I. (Of course, if the cell is near critical firing level, the EPSP may have a disproportionate effect, that is, the cell may discharge.)

PRESYNAPTIC INHIBITION

The sort of inhibition of impulse discharge through a pathway, which is mediated by IPSPs, is called **postsynaptic inhibition,** because the effect is exerted directly on the postsynaptic cell. Postsynaptic inhibition reduces the cell's excitability to all synaptic inputs. In the last 20 years a new mechanism for inhibition has come to light, mainly through the work of two groups led by Sir John Eccles and Karl Frank. This form of inhibition is called **presynaptic inhibition** because in this case the effect is exerted on a presynaptic axon terminal.

To illustrate this inhibition, let us examine the primary afferent fibers of group Ia. These enter the spinal cord and go, among other places, to the ventral (anterior) horn, where they make synaptic contacts on α motoneurons that innervate the muscle from which the afferent fibers originated. (This, as we shall see in Chapter 15, is the anatomic basis of the monosynaptic, stretch reflex.) There are synapses on the boutons of the Ia afferent fibers, the presynaptic terminal of which comes from interneurons that are driven by group Ia afferent fibers from another muscle. This arrangement is shown in Figure 13-17. The synapse between the two axons, the axoaxonic synapse, is excitatory in that the presynaptic (interneuronal, in this case) action potential produces an EPSP in the terminal of the group Ia afferent fiber.

If the group Ia afferent fiber terminal membrane is maintained in a slightly depolarized condition and then stimulated to

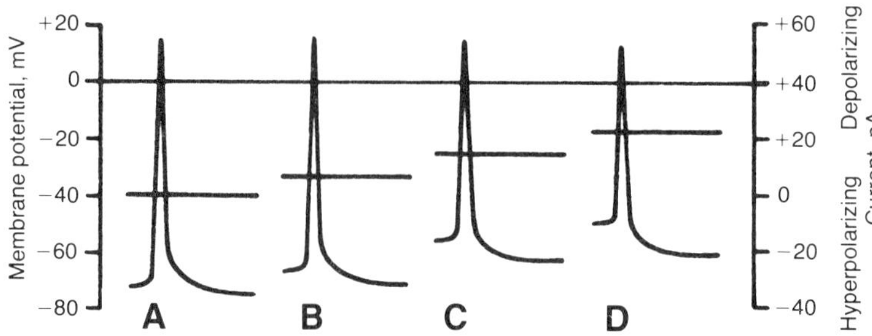

FIG. 13-18. Effect of membrane polarization level on the action potential. **B.** Action potential initiated with membrane at resting potential. **A.** Spike configuration when cell was previously hyperpolarized by 10 mV. When spike is initiated in a depolarized membrane, the spike is reduced in amplitude. Examples are shown for 10 mV **(C)** and 20 mV **(D)** depolarization. Horizontal line through each record indicates the current passed through membrane to change membrane potential before spike was initiated; values on right ordinate. Membrane potential on left ordinate. (Eccles JC: The Physiology of Nerve Cells. Baltimore, Johns Hopkins Press, 1968)

initiate an action potential, the action potential will be smaller than one that is initiated when the membrane is at its resting potential, V_r. This result is illustrated in Figure 13-18. Trace B shows the action potential initiated at $V_r = -65$ mV. The smaller spikes in C and D were obtained when the membrane started at depolarized values, $V_m = -55$ mV and -50 mV. The trace in A shows a larger than normal spike initiated when $V_m = -70$ mV, that is, the membrane was hyperpolarized. (Actually, these records were made in a motoneuron, but the same thing would presumably happen in the axon terminal.) The spike in C and D is reduced partly because it arises from a more positive level of membrane potential and partly because the depolarization (previous to the spike) increased the K^+ conductance and partially inactivated the Na^+ conductance (accommodation) in the membrane. The increased K^+ conductance and Na^+ conductance inactivation reduced the ratio of conductances and therefore the positive overshoot potential as predictable from equation 10 of Chapter 3. The spike is, therefore, smaller both because it starts closer to zero and because it does not overshoot as far. This phenomenon is the basis for the presynaptic inhibitory action. Activity at the axoaxonic synapse partially depolarizes the terminal so that, when an action potential comes down the Ia afferent fiber, its amplitude is reduced in the bouton. Because the amount of transmitter substance released by a bouton is proportional to the amplitude of the action potential in it, less transmitter substance is released, resulting in a smaller EPSP and less excitation of the postsynaptic cell, in this case the motoneuron. Some measurements indicate that a 15-mV reduction in the amplitude of the presynaptic spike will reduce the transmitter substance released to 1/10 of its original value.

It is usually said that presynaptic inhibition has no direct effect on the postsynaptic cell, but this is not entirely true. The EPSP initiated in the Ia bouton causes the release of a small amount of transmitter substance that raises the level of excitability of the motoneuron slightly. It is possible that this slight increase in excitability may offset a small amount of the decrease in transmitter output caused by the spike in the group Ia afferent fiber. In any case, the increased excitability of the motoneuron will add to the excitatory synaptic activity from other uninhibited boutons on the same cell. This could give the nervous system a rather subtle way of modulating excitability in certain pathways, a possible function of this "presynaptic inhibitory circuit" that has received little attention.

Pre- and postsynaptic inhibition not only differ in their mechanisms but also in their consequences for the system. With postsynaptic inhibition, the postsynaptic cell is silenced or at least reduced in its excitability to all inputs no matter what their source. The consequence for the muscle is that it relaxes because there is no alternate pathway to it. With presynaptic inhibition, the excitation of the postsynaptic cell (in this case, the α motoneuron) through one synapse is reduced, but all other synapses

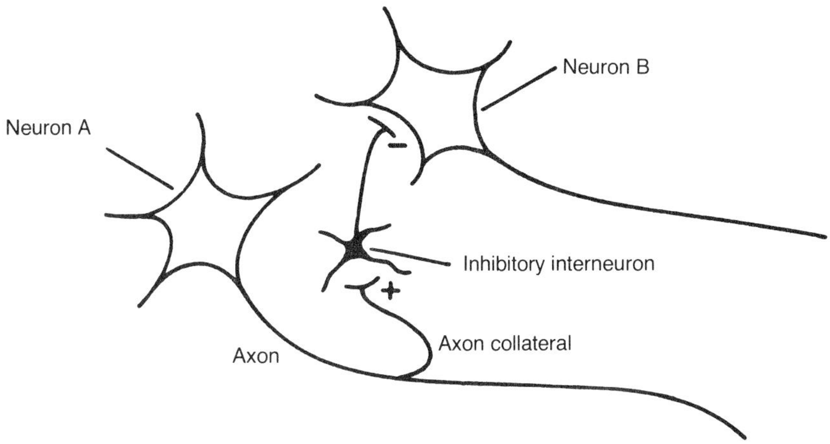

FIG. 13-19. A collateral inhibitory circuit. Spike initiated in neuron A invades the collateral to excite the inhibitory interneuron that produces IPSPs in neuron B.

FIG. 13-20. Circuit for Renshaw inhibition. Spike **(A)** generated in the axon at the top of the figure invades the axon collateral, exciting the Renshaw cell. The Renshaw cell discharges a train of spikes **(B)** in response to a single presynaptic spike (an example of synaptic amplification). The train of spikes in the Renshaw cell produces summed IPSPs in the motoneuron **(C).** (Eccles JC: The Physiology of Nerve Cells. Baltimore, Johns Hopkins Press, 1968)

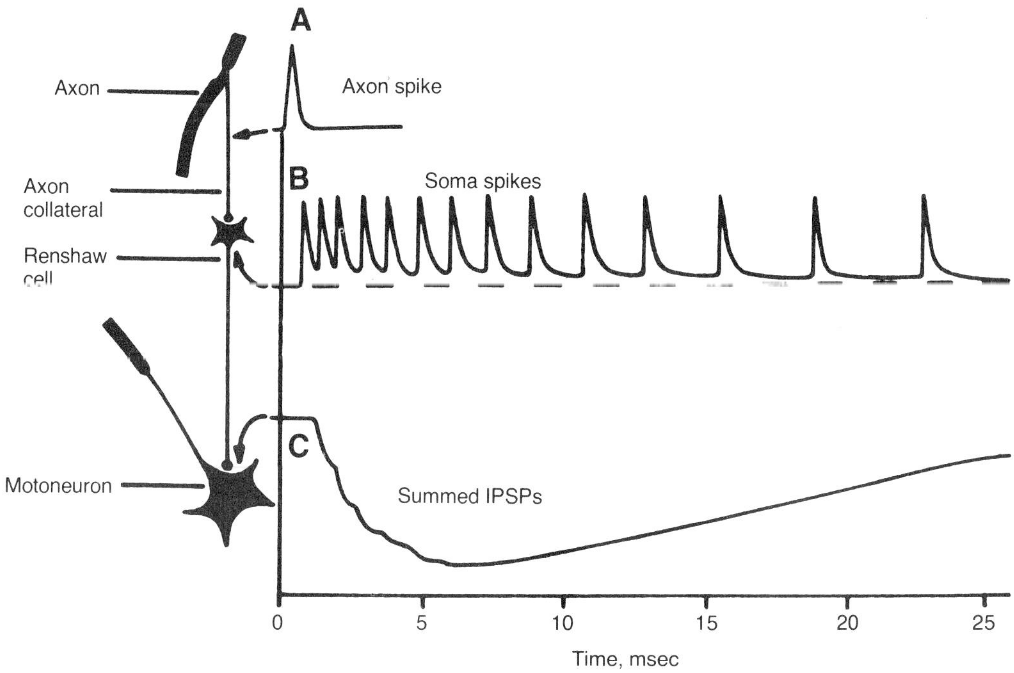

perform normally or perhaps even supranormally (see previous paragraph). For the motoneuron, this means that transmission through group Ia afferent fibers is reduced, but transmission through polysynaptic and supraspinal pathways is still possible.

With a few exceptions, presynaptic inhibition has been found only on the terminals of primary afferent neurons, and all types of primary afferent fibers seem to receive presynaptic inhibition from one source or another. The terminals of pyramidal tract fibers in the brain stem have been shown to be depolarized in the same manner. The significance of this effect is unknown. Presynaptic inhibition may be found to be more widespread as information accumulates in the future. Postsynaptic inhibition has been found in every structure of the central nervous system, and our ideas of its importance and ubiquity seem to be increasing. The function of presynaptic inhibition on primary afferent neurons may be to modulate sensory inputs to the spinal cord at the earliest possible point, before they can influence spinal cord activity. In this way, the central nervous system can eliminate unwanted sensory information. By reducing some sensory inputs, presynaptic inhibition may be useful in certain kinds of contrast enhancement.

RECURRENT INHIBITION

A special case of postsynaptic inhibition is **recurrent inhibition,** the circuit for which is shown in Figure 13-19. The output of a neuron, neuron A, conducts along its axon and out one axon collateral to excite an interneuron that inhibits another neuron of the same type as neuron A, in this case neuron B. Many people draw this circuit showing that the inhibitory interneuron inhibits neuron A, making neuron A inhibit itself. Although this is possible, there is no evidence that it occurs. The evidence does suggest that neurons inhibit other neurons of the same type. Thus, neuron A inhibits neuron B and, similarly, neuron B inhibits neuron A. Thus, the inhibition may more appropriately be termed **collateral inhibition.** This is a type of **feedback inhibition,** in which the output of a neuron is used to inhibit at an earlier point in the pathway.

Recurrent inhibition has been found in nearly every major nucleus in the central nervous system, notably in the cuneate and gracile nuclei, thalamic nuclei, cerebellar nuclei, cerebellar cortex, and cerebral cortex. One theory suggests that recurrent inhibition in the thalamus may play a role in synchronizing thalamic activity to produce the cortical alpha rhythm (see Chap. 20). It is not known whether this theory can stand empirical tests nor what this kind of inhibition might be doing elsewhere.

A special case of recurrent inhibition is **Renshaw inhibition.** This form of inhibition involves the same circuit as in Figure 13-19, in which neurons A and B are α motoneurons, whose axons innervate skeletal muscles. The Renshaw circuit is shown in Figure 13-20. The axon collateral that activates the inhibitory interneuron is short, remaining within the ventral horn of the spinal cord and releasing acetylcholine at its terminal. (Acetylcholine is also released at the muscle.) The inhibitory interneuron, called a **Renshaw cell** in honor of its discoverer Birdsey Renshaw, discharges a burst of spikes (B) in response to a single motoneuron spike (A), releasing a transmitter substance, perhaps glycine, at terminals on other α motoneurons. This leads to a large, summed IPSP in these motoneurons (C). Again, there is no evidence that an α motoneuron inhibits itself through Renshaw inhibition. It has been speculated that Renshaw inhibition may serve to limit motoneuron firing rates. It is unlikely that this is an important control mechanism for normal motor activity; motoneurons do not discharge at high rates anyway and, at least during walking, this kind of inhibition is suppressed. It is possible, however, that this kind of inhibition may play an important role in preventing or limiting certain kinds of pathologic or seizure discharges. What else it might be doing for an organism is not known.

SUGGESTED READING

Bennett MVL: Similarities between chemically and electrically mediated transmission. In Carlson FD [ed]: Physiological and Biochemical Aspects of Nervous Integration. Englewood Cliffs NJ, Prentice-Hall, 1968

Curtis DR, Johnston GAR: Amino acid transmitters in the mammalian central nervous system. Ergebn Physiol 69:97–188, 1974

Horcholle-Bossavit G: Transmission électrotonique dans le système nerveux central des mammifères. J Physiol (Paris) 74:349–363, 1978

Krnjević K: Chemical nature of synaptic transmission in vertebrates. Physiol Rev 54:418–540, 1974

McGeer RL, Eccles JC, McGeer EG: Molecular Neurobiology of the Mammalian Brain. New York, Plenum Press, 1978

Pappas GD, Waxman SG: Synaptic fine structure-morphological correlates of chemical and electrical transmission. In Pappas GD, Purpura DP [eds]: Structure and Function of Synapses. New York, Raven Press, 1972

Schmidt RF: Presynaptic inhibition in the vertebrate central nervous system. Ergebn Physiol 63:19–101, 1971

Tapper DN, Mann MD: Single presynaptic impulse evokes postsynaptic discharge. Brain Res 11:688–690, 1968

14

Muscle Contraction

It is impossible to overemphasize the importance of muscle in vertebrates. The very life style of every one demands movement, impossible without muscle. In fact, in man about 40% of the body mass is striated muscle, making it the most abundant tissue. **Striated muscle** is so named because of its characteristic cross-striped appearance. Most striated muscle is skeletal muscle, involved in rotation of bones around joints and therefore responsible for most of the movements of which we are aware. Other striated muscles move the eyes and serve as valves to check the flow of blood or other fluids, for example, the bulbospongiosus aids erection of the penis or clitoris by compressing the deep dorsal vein. **Cardiac muscle** is also striated in appearance, but it differs significantly from other striated muscle in both its structure and its behavior. Still other muscles, called **smooth muscles,** lack the characteristic cross-striations but contain the same contractile proteins. The smooth muscles are important as linings of the gastrointestinal tract that churn and propel food through the tract, as linings of blood vessels that control their diameters and thus flow through them, as valves that control the passage of gases and fluids in the body, and as controllers at many other places in the body.

Of the three types of muscle, skeletal and cardiac muscle have been studied most thoroughly. It is presumed that the mechanism of contraction is the same for both types and that only the details of initiating and controlling the contraction differ. Not all striated muscle, however, behaves in the same way. For example, skeletal muscles of vertebrates all appear to initiate contractions with sodium spikes, whereas striated muscles of some invertebrates initiate contractions with calcium spikes. We will confine our discussion primarily to vertebrate skeletal muscle, pointing out the distinctive features of structure and function of cardiac and smooth muscle.

MUSCLE STRUCTURE

Skeletal muscles are composed of masses of fibers, each an individual cell. There are several types of muscles, differing in terms of the arrangement of their fibers, but these can be divided into two major classes: those with fibers arranged in parallel and those with a pennate arrangement. Figure 14-1 shows these two classes. In the parallel arrangement, each muscle fiber, or a small group of fibers, is attached to its own tendon, the tendons converging on a common point (A). The muscle fibers are side by side, that is, in parallel, but the name of the class comes from the fact that the muscle fibers shorten in a direction (double-headed arrow, f) parallel to the direction of shortening of the muscle (single-headed arrow, F).

The pennate muscle fibers attach to a common tendon (B), so that the direction of shortening of the individual fibers (double-headed arrow, f) is different from the direction of shortening of the whole muscle (single-headed arrow, F). As a result, the pennate muscle cannot shorten as much as the parallel muscle. Pennate muscles are located in positions requiring small but powerful movements; parallel muscles

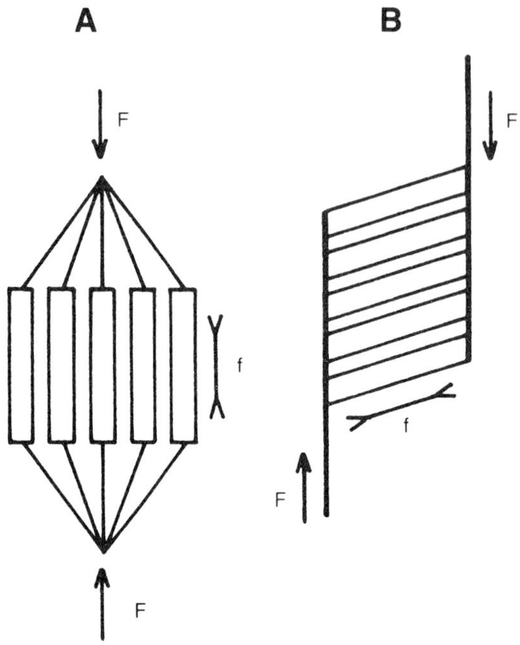

FIG. 14-1. Two arrangements of muscle fibers within a muscle. A. Parallel arrangement: Tendons are lines radiating from rectangles (muscle fibers) at each end. B. Pennate arrangement: Tendons are vertical lines extending from the two sides of the parallelogram. Double-headed arrows (f) indicate direction of force exerted by individual muscle fibers; single-headed arrows (F) indicate direction of force exerted by whole muscle. (Zierler KL: Mechanism of muscle contraction and its energetics. In: Mountcastle VB [ed]: Medical Physiology, 13th ed, Vol. 1. St. Louis, C.V. Mosby, 1974)

are located in positions requiring longer movements with less power or faster movements.

MUSCLE FINE-STRUCTURE

Our understanding of the mechanism of contraction of muscle depends upon an understanding of the fine-structure of muscle cells, because it is the internal parts of the cells that do the work. Muscle cells contain the usual complement of nucleus, mitochondria, and so forth, but, in addition, they contain bundles of **myofibrils.** The myofibrils have a characteristic striated appearance, and, because the myofibrils are more or less in register (the same stripes are lined up), they give the whole muscle a striated appearance. Figure 14-2 shows, on the left, the whole muscle, a bundle of muscle fibers, and their subunits, the myofibrils. Note the striated appearance of all three. Each muscle fiber contains about 1000 myofibrils that are 1 μm in diameter and run the length of the fiber. Myofibrils have no membrane, being simply surrounded with cytoplasm.

The cross-striations of the myofibrils are serially repeating units called **sarcomeres.** A sarcomere (Fig. 14-3A) can be from 1.5 to 3.5 μm in length, depending upon the contractile state of the muscle, and it is bounded on each end by a disc, called the **Z disc** or **Z line.** Each sarcomere contains an anisotropic (doubly refractive, therefore dark in phase microscopy) band bounded by two isotropic (singly refractive, therefore light) bands. The anisotropic band is called the **A band;** the isotropic band is called the **I band.** Actually, each sarcomere contains two half I bands because a single I band straddles the Z line and therefore is part of two adjacent sarcomeres. In the center of the A band, there is a lighter region known as the **H zone** or **H band.** During contraction it is observed that the A band does not change length,* though the sarcomere shortens, the distance between Z lines lessens, and the I and H bands narrow. Any theory of muscle contraction must account for these observations.

The myofibrils, as shown in Figure 14-2, are composed of **myofilaments** that are proteinaceous. One filament is thick, about 11 nm in diameter and 1.5 μm long, whereas the other is thin, 5 nm in diameter and 1 μm long. These filaments are referred to as the **thick filaments** and **thin filaments,** respectively. Thick filaments are made up of several hundred **myosin** molecules, proteins of a molecular weight of about 500,000. The myosin molecule has a tail region that is rodlike, and a head region, with two globular subunits projecting out at approximately a right angle with the tail. Drawings of a myosin molecule and its position within the thick filament are shown in Figure 14-2. The myosin molecules of thick filaments are arranged in a sheaf with heads oriented toward each end and tails toward the center. Each subsequent myosin molecule attaches 14 nm further toward the end of the filament and is rotated 60° around the filament from its predecessor. Thus, the thick filament is studded with projections except at its center, which contains only myosin tails.

* Actually, it is generally accepted that in *Limulus*, the horseshoe crab, the A bands do change length when contractions occur at lengths less than the resting length. They apparently do not in mammalian muscle.

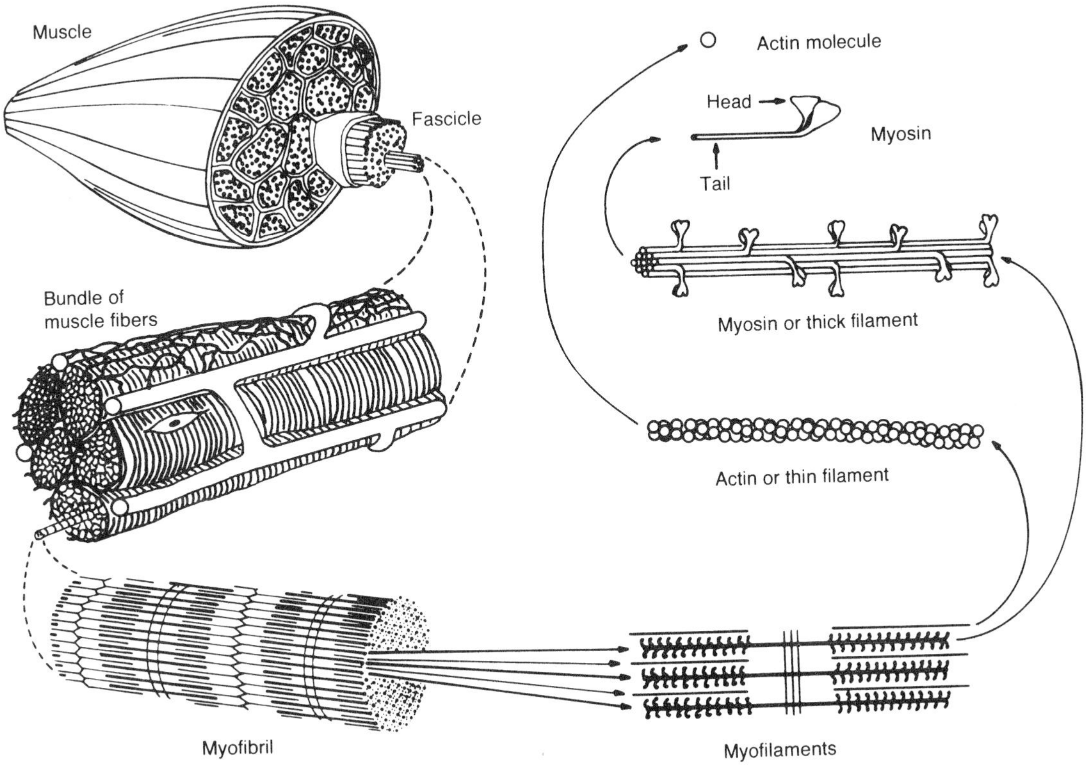

FIG. 14-2. Levels of organization within a skeletal muscle, including (counterclockwise from top left) whole muscle and fascicles, bundles of muscle fibers, myofibrils, myofilaments, thin and thick filaments, and myosin and actin molecules. (Warwick R, Williams PL [ed]: Gray's Anatomy. 35th British ed, Edinburgh, Churchill Livingstone, 1973; modified from a drawing by Professor D Fawcett)

The thick filaments are coincident with the A band of the sarcomere.

The thin filaments contain three protein molecules: **actin, troponin,** and **tropomyosin.** A single thin filament is composed of 300 to 400 actin molecules and 40 to 60 troponin and tropomyosin molecules. Actin is a small, nearly spherical molecule that is arranged in the filament into two helical strands, as shown in Figure 14-2, with about 13 actin molecules per complete turn of the helix. Tropomyosin is a filamentous protein that is thought to form two strands that lie in the grooves formed between the actin strands. Troponin, a globular protein, binds to tropomyosin at only one site and therefore is thought to sit astride the tropomyosin molecule strand at regular intervals approximating 40 nm. Figure 14-4 shows the relationships between the three proteins as they are currently thought to exist. The thin filaments attach to the Z disc, a flat protein structure.

The relatively high anisotropocity of the

FIG. 14-3. Organization of the sarcomeres. **A.** Pattern of cross-striation in skeletal muscle with bands labeled. **B.** Arrangement of thick and thin filaments that accounts for the pattern of cross-striations. **C.** Hexagonal arrays of thick and thin filaments in cross sections through the sarcomere in the A band, H band, and I band.

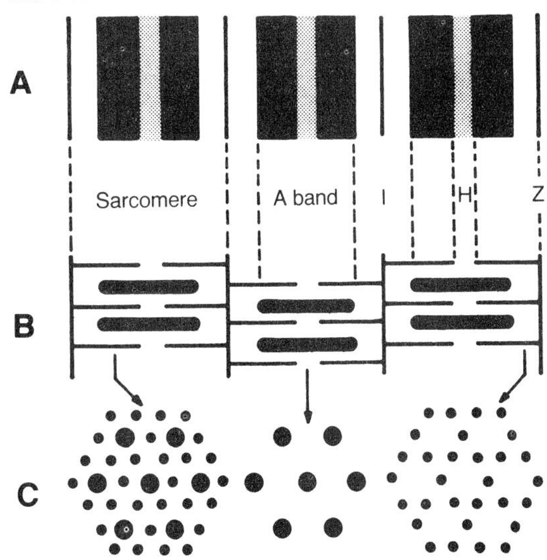

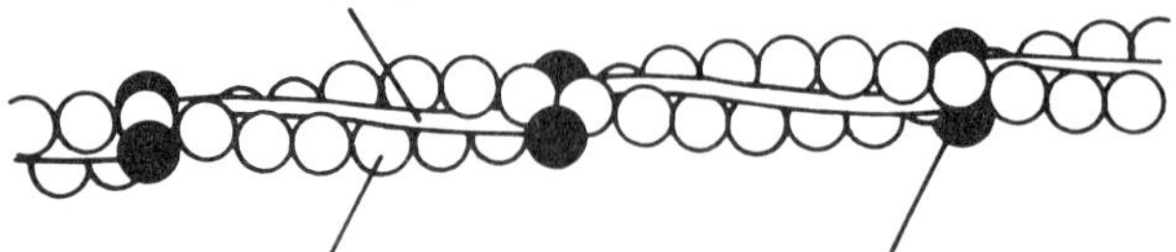

FIG. 14-4. Thin filament structure. Proposed structure of thin filament with relative positions of actin, troponin, and tropomyosin indicated. (Ebashi S, Endo M, Ohtsuki I: Quart Rev Biophys 2:351–384, 1969)

FIG. 14-5. Three-dimensional reconstruction of skeletal muscle illustrating organization of myofibrils, endoplasmic reticulum, and T tubules. (Warwick R, Williams PL [ed]: Gray's Anatomy, 35th British ed, Philadelphia, W.B. Saunders, 1973)

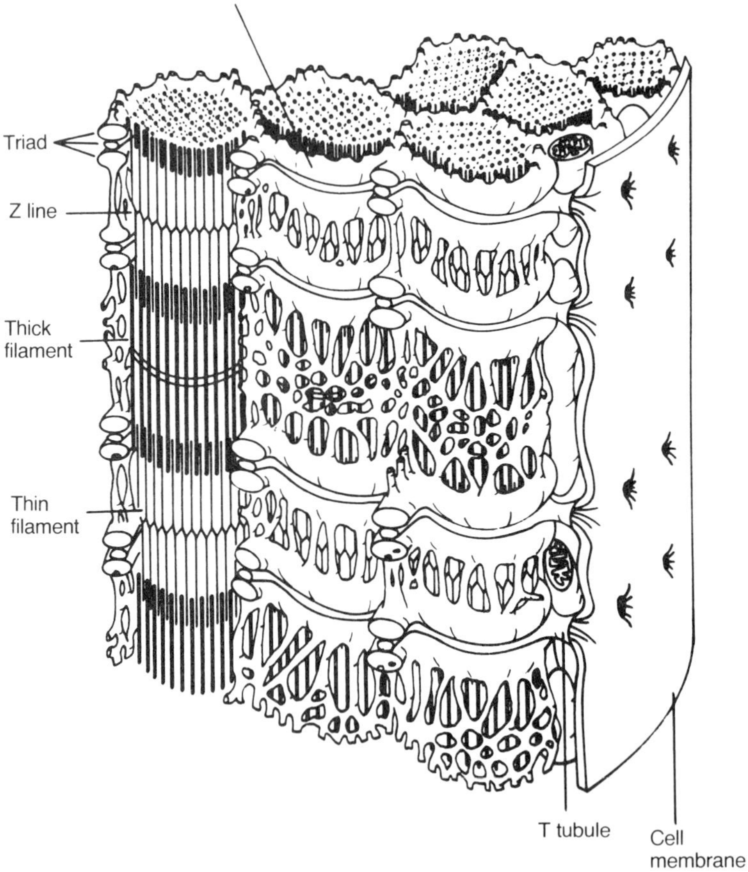

A band results from the presence of both thin and thick filaments (Fig. 14-3B). The I band is only slightly anisotropic because it contains only thin filaments. The H band is not optically as dense as the rest of the A band because it does not contain any thin filaments when the muscle is at rest. As can be seen in cross section in Figure 14-3C, the thin filaments are organized into regular hexagonal arrays within the myofibrils, with a thick filament at the center of each array in the A band. Three thick filaments are equidistant from each thin filament, whereas six thin filaments are equidistant

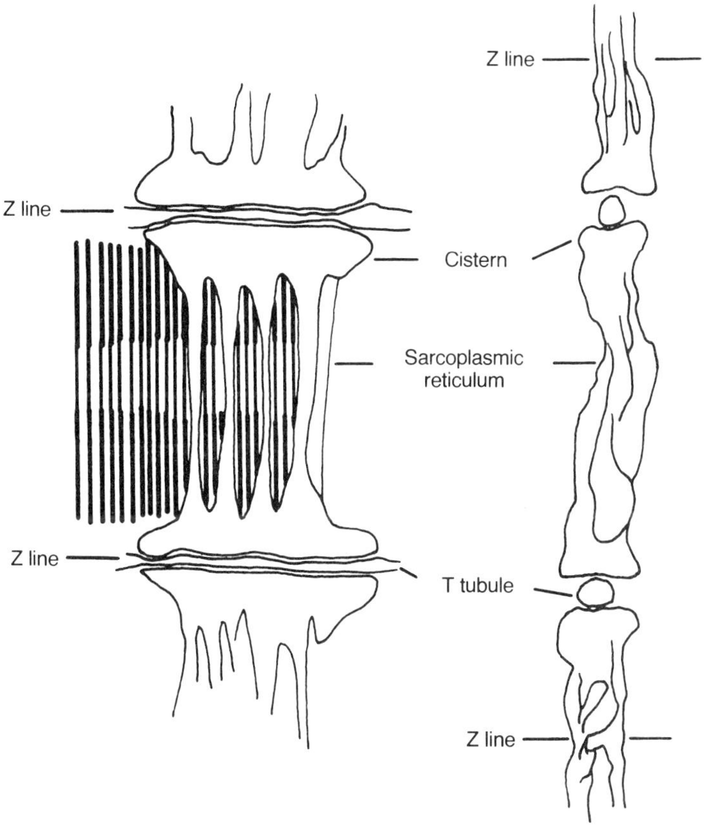

FIG. 14-6. Fortuitous sections through triads, one at right angles to the other. Relative positions of T tubules and sarcoplasmic reticula at the triad are shown clearly.

from each thick filament as shown in the left panel. A cross section through the I band shows only the thin filament array (right panel); a section through the H band shows only the thick filament array (center panel).

The myosin heads project out from the thick filaments toward the thin filaments at intervals of about 43 nm. Because they are staggered around the thin filament at 60° intervals, each projects in the direction of a thin filament and each thin filament has projections toward it from three thick filaments. These projections have been termed either **cross-bridges** or **cross-projections,** depending upon whether the heads are thought to contact and bind thin filaments or not. As we shall see, there are two schools of thought, in fact, two different mechanisms proposed to account for the generation of the mechanical force of contraction.

Muscle cells have a unique membrane structure, called the transverse tubule or simply the T tubule. The T tubule is an invagination of the muscle membrane, much like the invagination produced in a balloon by pushing a finger into its side without puncturing it, but the T tubules are long and tortuous. The T-tubule system forms a ring around every myofibril either at the Z line, in which case there is one per sarcomere, or at the A–I-band junction, in which case there are two per sarcomere. These perifibrillar rings are interconnected, forming a kind of honeycomb arrangement, as shown in Figure 14-5. The position of the T tubule with respect to the sarcomere is somewhat species specific; frog skeletal muscle has only one tubule per sarcomere, whereas human skeletal muscle has two. It should be noted that in human cardiac muscle there is only one tubule per sarcomere as shown in Figure 14-17. The inside of the T tubule is continuous with the extracellular space and presumably contains a fluid like extracellular fluid, but, because the tubular space is small and not well stirred, it is likely that ionic movements across the tubule membrane produce sig-

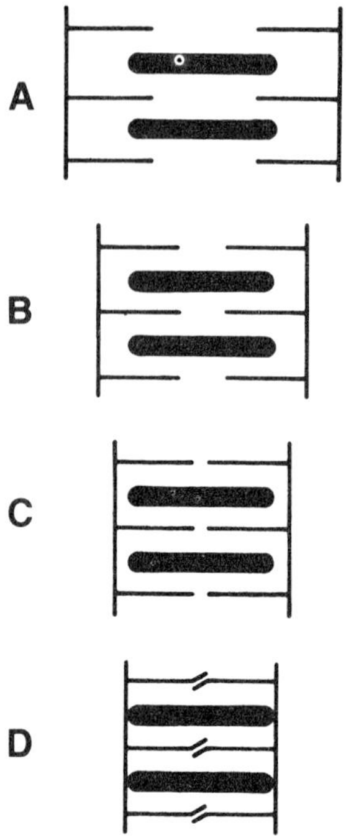

FIG. 14-7. Sliding filament model of muscle contraction. A single sarcomere is shown stretched, with little overlap between thick and thin filaments (A), with greater overlap (B), with complete overlap (C), and extremely shortened with thin filaments shown buckled (D). Another possibility, not shown, is that at extreme shortening, the buckling occurs at the Z line.

nificant changes in ion concentration, at least on a short-term basis.

Another intracellular structure of special significance to contraction is the sarcoplasmic reticulum, the muscle cell version of the endoplasmic reticulum. The sarcoplasmic reticulum is made up of tubules that run parallel to the sarcomeres and run from T tubule to T tubule (see Fig. 14-5 and 14-17); thus, there are two sets of sarcoplasmic reticulum tubules per sarcomere in muscles with two sets of T tubules per sarcomere. The sarcoplasmic reticulum is a sack with its ends expanded (the cisternae) adjacent to the T tubules and with narrow, longitudinal channels connecting these expansions. In fortuitous sections, one can find a section of T tubule bounded on two sides by sort of dumbbell-shaped sarcoplasmic reticula as illustrated in Figure 14-6. The T tubule with its two adjacent regions of sarcoplasmic reticulum is often called a triad. Because the T tubules and the cisternae of the sarcoplasmic reticulum run together for such a long way, a large proportion of the sarcoplasmic reticulum is in contact with the sarcolemma, but the region of contact is not a tight junction as has been suggested. Rather, there is a space of about 12 nm between the membranes.

The sarcoplasmic reticulum serves as a repository for Ca^{2+}. In rested muscle, Ca^{2+} is found in high concentration in the cisternae at the triad. On the other hand, in recently active muscle, the calcium is found in the narrowed, longitudinal portion from which it moves to the triad as time passes. During contraction, Ca^{2+} is found in high concentration among the myofilaments.

SLIDING FILAMENT MODEL

Observations that during muscle contraction, the sarcomere, the I and the H bands become narrower but the A band does not, coupled with the observation that thick and thin filaments do not shorten (although at very short lengths the thin filaments may either push through the Z line or fold up like an accordian), suggested the *sliding filament model of contraction*. According to the model, the thick and thin filaments simply slide past each other. Figure 14-7 shows several positions in the shortening of the muscle, illustrating the sliding of the filaments. At the maximum length there is little or no overlap of the filaments (A), but as the muscle shortens there is more and more overlap until the fibers completely overlap (D). There is general agreement that the sliding filament model is an accurate description of what happens during muscle contraction.

EVENTS LEADING TO CONTRACTION

Although muscle contraction can be initiated by direct electrical stimulation of the muscle, it usually results from activity in the motoneurons innervating the muscle. An action potential initiated in an α motoneuron propagates into the motoneuron terminals and releases acetylcholine into the synaptic cleft. The acetylcholine induces an end-plate potential in the muscle that, in normal muscle, always leads to an action potential in the muscle. The muscle spike is very much like the nerve spike but slightly longer in duration and with a de-

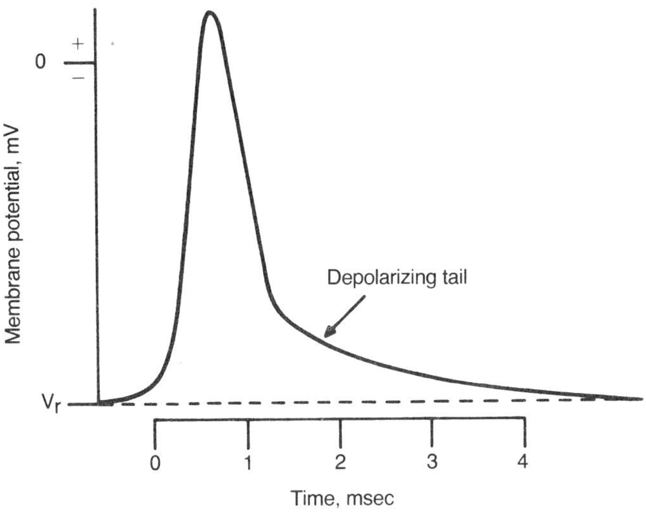

FIG. 14-8. The skeletal muscle action potential. The spike is followed by a depolarizing tail that lasts 4 to 5 msec.

polarizing tail on the falling phase that prolongs the spike by 3 to 4 msec. An example of a muscle spike is shown in Figure 14-8. The mechanism of generation of the spike in mammalian striated muscle is the same as that described for nerve in Chapter 3. The long depolarizing tail of the muscle action potential is probably the electrotonic reflection of the action potential as it conducts into the T tubules. At least, the tail disappears from the spike when the muscle is treated with glycerol and then returned to Ringer's solution, a treatment that more or less specifically ruptures T tubules, leaving the surface membrane intact, with a resting potential. The muscle still generates a spike but does not contract. Conduction of the spike into the T tubules is probably an active process as elsewhere on the membrane, and it is the depolarization of the T tubule that leads to contraction.

It is reasonable to ask why there exists such an elaborate system of tubules. The answer may lie in the synchronization of contraction of sarcomeres along the length of the muscle and in its depths. The myofibrils are located throughout the muscle fiber, but in mammalian muscle there is usually only one neuromuscular junction per fiber. If there were no way for the depolarization of the spike to get into the center of the fiber, the myofibrils on the surface would contract before those in the center. With the T-tubule system, the spike is conducted rapidly to all parts of the cell, reaching all of the myofibrils at nearly the same time.

No one knows whether the spike is propagated into the sarcoplasmic reticulum from the T tubule, but somehow the spike leads to a release of calcium from the cisternae into the region of the myofilaments. This is an essential step in the contraction mechanism; muscles depleted of calcium do not contract. The calcium diffuses to the thin filaments and binds to troponin. Each head of the myosin molecule (a molecule has two) is an ATPase, capable of hydrolyzing ATP to ADP and inorganic phosphate, releasing energy; however, according to current thought, tropomyosin inhibits the ATPase. The combination of troponin with Ca^{2+} removes the tropomyosin inhibition, perhaps by inducing a conformational change in the thin filament.

CROSS-BRIDGE THEORY

To this point, most theories of contraction agree. There are, however, two plausible theories of how the force of contraction develops. The first, the cross-bridge theory, suggests that an actual physical binding of the myosin head to the thin filament occurs, that the hydrolysis of ATP causes a rotation of the head toward the tail, pulling on the compliant arm of the cross-bridge. This pull results in a relative movement of thin and thick filaments and tension and shortening of the sarcomere. In detail, ATP binds to myosin and then, in the presence of Ca^{2+},

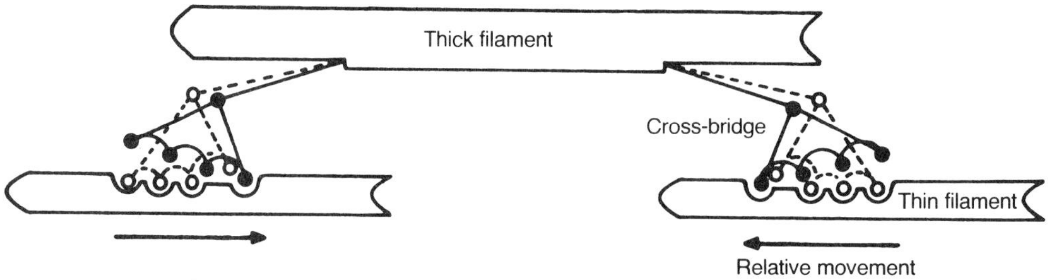

FIG. 14-9. Production of force according to the cross-bridge theory. Cross-bridges, projecting from the thick filament, are shown attached to the thin filament and swiveled **(dashed outline).** Directions of force and translation are indicated by **arrows.** (Noble MIM, Pollack GH: Circ Res 40:333–342, 1977)

troponin, and tropomyosin, there is a physical link formed between actin and myosin. The ATPase activity of the myosin is then exerted, cleaving a phosphate bond of the ATP, releasing energy, and causing the myosin head to swivel. Figure 14-9 shows the way in which the myosin head is thought to rotate and the relative movement of the filaments that results. Because the heads of the myosin molecules are oriented in opposite directions at opposite ends of the thick filament, each pulls its adjacent thin filament toward the center of the sarcomere and the sarcomere shortens.

When the depolarizing stimulus of the spike in the T tubules is over, calcium ceases to be released by the cisternae of the sarcoplasmic reticulum and is somehow taken up by the longitudinal portion of the reticulum. Some investigators believe there is a calcium pump that transports the ion back into the tubules; all that is known is that it gets back inside and eventually makes its way back to the cisternae. When calcium is removed from the myofibrils, ATP replaces ADP on the myosin complex and the myosin–actin bond is broken. Because the muscle has some elasticity, it will be restored to its resting length in the absence of a further stimulus to release calcium.

A single cycle of attachment, swivel, and detachment of the myosin head will produce a linear translation of the myofilaments of about 10 nm. If all cross-bridges in a myofibril cycle once synchronously, a relative movement equal to about 10% of the muscle length will occur, but obviously muscles shorten by more than 10%. The total shortening of a sarcomere during contraction may exceed 1000 nm; therefore the relative movement of a thin and thick filament would be half this amount or 500 nm. To achieve this magnitude of change in total length when each cross-bridge cycle produces a 10-nm shortening, a minimum of 50 cycles must occur. The flexor muscles of the human upper arm can contract at the rate of 8 m/sec (Wilkie, 1949), during which they can shorten by as much as 10 cm. This contraction rate gives a contraction rate for the sarcomere of 160 nm/msec. If a stroke of the cross-bridge is taken to be 10 nm, then at this rate there will be a minimum of 16 strokes/msec. Thus, we can see that swivel time for the cross-bridge must be of the order of 60 μsec. Calculations for the frog's sartorius muscle, which can shorten at up to 4 cm/sec, indicate a swivel time of about 1 msec, but this contraction occurs at a lower temperature. In any case, it is clear that the swiveling of the cross-bridge must be a fast mechanical process.

The cross-bridge theory assumes that the force generated by the muscle is proportional to the number of cross-bridge linkages formed at that time and that the probability of formation of a cross-bridge is proportional to the speed of shortening, that is, the probability is great when attachment sites move slowly past one another, small when they move rapidly. If tension is a function only of the number of cross-bridges, then there should be a linear relationship between length and tension such that tension increases with decreasing length because of the greater overlap of thick and thin filaments at shorter lengths. The force required to stretch the muscle at any time is therefore also proportional to the number of cross-bridges—it is the force required to break the actin–myosin bonds.

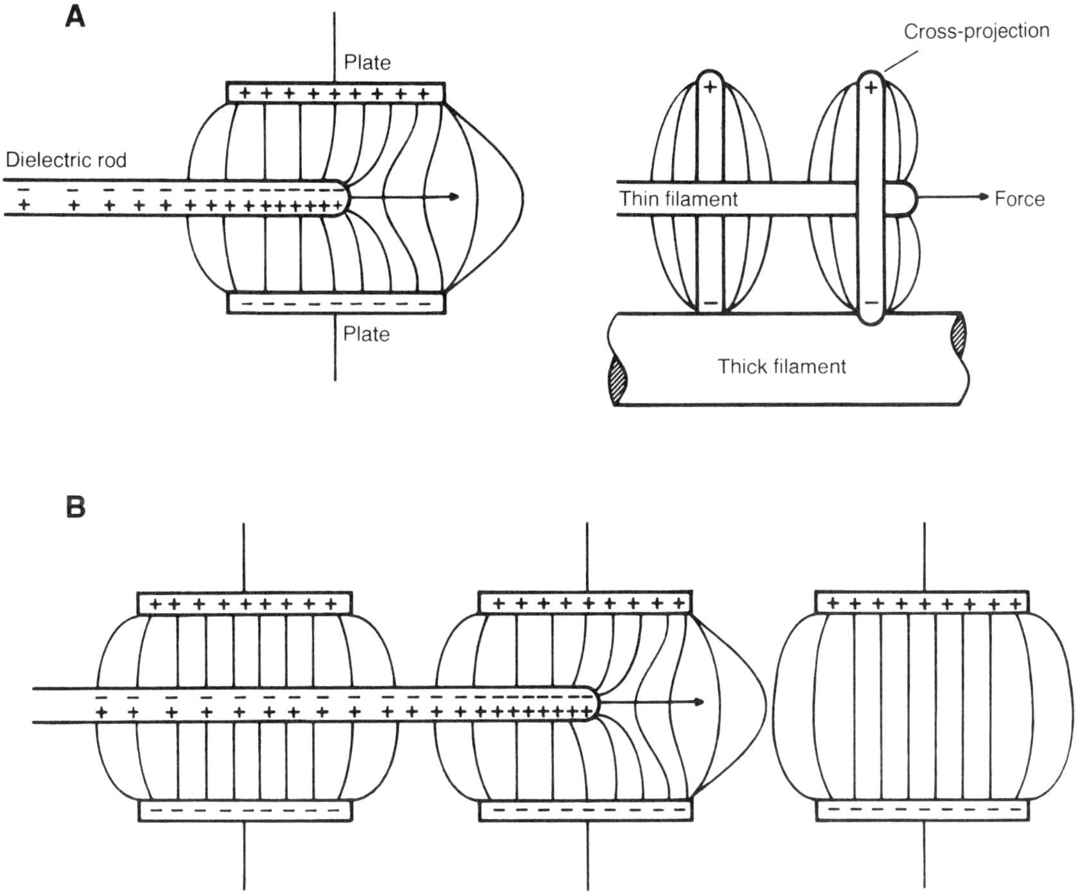

FIG. 14-10. Force generation according to the electrostatic theory. A. A dielectric rod within the electric field between the plates of a charged capacitor experiences a force indicated by the **arrow.** Lines of force of the electric field are shown between the plates of the capacitor. The equivalent diagram for the muscle filaments is shown at the right. The cross-projection is the capacitor and the thin filament is the dielectric rod. B. Capacitors along the rod induce a symmetric charge distribution and thus no force (left capacitor), except that capacitor near the tip of the filament (center capacitor). (Noble MIM, Pollack GH: Circ Res 40:333–342, 1977)

ELECTROSTATIC THEORY

There is considerable support for the cross-bridge theory; however, there is no compelling evidence that thick and thin filaments ever bind to each other in living muscle. X-ray diffraction studies of muscles in rigor mortis suggest that such cross-bridges are formed, but the diffraction picture of muscle in rigor is not like that of living muscle. Another plausible scheme of force generation in muscle involves the properties of a dielectric rod in an electric field between the plates of a capacitor. According to this theory, the thin filament is a dielectric rod, that is, a rod that does not conduct electricity. The positive and negative charges in a dielectric material are not free to move very far, but they can be displaced slightly under the influence of an external electric field. This causes the charge to be distributed asymmetrically, and the dielectric material becomes polarized.

According to the theory, the cross-projection is a capacitor, charged negatively near the thick filament, positively away from the filament. By this separation of charge, an electric field is generated on each projection and the field is maintained by hydrolysis of ATP. Because the charge on the dielectric rod is asymmetric, there is always an attractive force tending to pull the rod into the field. Figure 14-10A shows the nature of the charge separation in the capacitor and the polarization of the dielectric rod as well as the direction of the force on the rod. The right drawing shows the assumed equivalent arrangement for the thin and thick filaments. In an electric field, force is only exerted upon the tip of the rod because the charge induced by other capacitors (cross-projections) in the overlap zone is symmetric as shown in Figure 14-10B. Thus, for the electrostatic theory, force depends upon the interaction of the tip of the thin filament with the field of the local cross-projection.

According to the electrostatic theory, the force of contraction can be varied in four ways:

1. *Variation in calcium concentration in the vicinity of the tip of the thin filament.* Calcium released by the muscle spike increases the activity of the myosin-ATPase. The higher the ATPase activity, the greater is the strength of the electric field and, therefore, the greater is the force it exerts on the tip of the thin filament. During relaxation, calcium is withdrawn from the myofilaments and charge leaks off the capacitor, to be restored in the next calcium activation of the ATPase.

2. *An inductance effect of the dielectric rod as it moves through the capacitor changing capacitor voltage and thus field strength.* Just as a magnetic field induces a voltage in a moving coil of wire, so the dielectric rod induces a voltage in the capacitor as it moves between the plates. This voltage changes the electric field strength of the capacitor and the force it exerts on the dielectric rod.

3. *Variation in calcium concentration along the sarcomere.* The electrostatic theory assumes that calcium concentration within the sarcomere is lowest at the center of the thick filaments and that it rises to a maximum at the end of the thick filament (at the A–I-band boundary), an assumption not inconsistent with what is known about muscle. As a result of this distribution, when the muscle is stretched, the tip of the thin filament is pulled into a region of higher calcium concentration and, when stimulated, the muscle contracts more forcefully. Conversely, when the muscle is shortened, the tip of the thin filament moves into a region of lower calcium concentration and the force of contraction is reduced.

4. *Variation in position of the tip of the thin filament with respect to the nearest cross-projection.* The electric field strength is greatest in the immediate vicinity of the cross-projection, and it decreases with distance away from the projection. Thus, the force is greatest when the tip of the thin filament is exactly aligned with the cross-projection and it is zero when the tip is halfway between two cross-projections. However, there is always a force generated upon the thin filament because, due to the helical arrangement of the myosin heads on the thick filament, some thin filament tips are always within the field of a cross-projection while others are passing through regions of zero field.

COMPARISON OF ELECTROSTATIC AND CROSS-BRIDGE THEORIES

As pointed out earlier, the proponents of both the cross-bridge and electrostatic theories agree upon the molecular mechanisms of contraction except with regard to the actual mechanism for generating the force. Table 14-1 summarizes the mechanisms, including points of agreement and disagreement. The two theories differ in three fundamental ways:

1. Tension is developed by physical bonds between thick and thin filaments in the cross-bridge theory and by electrostatic fields in the electrostatic theory.
2. Tension depends upon the degree of overlap between thick and thin filaments in the cross-bridge theory and is unrelated to overlap, but depends upon Ca^{2+} concentration in the region of the tip of the thin filament in the electrostatic theory.
3. The cross-bridge originates at the thick filament and terminates at the thin filament, whereas the cross-projection spans most of the gap between thick filaments.

With such striking differences between the two theories, it would seem that they could be easily tested empirically, but this has not proved to be the case. For example, electron micrographs of muscle cannot resolve the cross-projections clearly enough; sometimes they appear as cross-bridges, some-

TABLE 14-1. SUMMARY OF EVENTS IN MUSCLE CONTRACTION AND RELAXATION

CROSS-BRIDGE THEORY ⟷ AGREEMENT ⟷ ELECTROSTATIC THEORY

Arrival of motoneuron action potential
↓
Synaptic transmission at neuromuscular junction
↓
Action potential propagates along sarcolemma
↓
Depolarization of T tubules
↓
Ca^{2+} released into sarcoplasm from sarcoplasmic reticulum
↓
Ca^{2+} bound by troponin
↓
Cooperative configurational change in troponin and tropomyosin
↓
Release of inhibition of myosin-ATPase
↙ ↘

Cross-bridge theory	Electrostatic theory
Link between thick and thin filaments, swivel of myosin head	Electric field develops on cross-projection, dielectric thin filament is pulled into field

↘ ↙
Tension exerted
↓
Shortening by sliding filament
↓
Ca^{2+} removed from sarcoplasm
Mg^{2+}-ATP bound by actinomyosin
↙ ↘

Cross-bridge theory	Electrostatic theory
Cross-bridges disconnected	Charge leaks off cross-projection, field reduced

↘ ↙
Actinomyosin-ATPase inhibited
↓
Active tension disappears
↓
Series elastic elements restore resting length

times as cross-projections. Both theories are able to account for most of the behavior of living muscle as we shall see, although the cross-bridge theory often requires additional assumptions. Nevertheless, the cross-bridge theory is still most widely accepted, perhaps because of its seniority. The only real comparison of the two theories that has been published led the reviewers to the conclusion that existing evidence does not favor one theory over the other (Noble and Pollack, 1977).

PROPERTIES OF CONTRACTING MUSCLE

When a muscle is stimulated either directly or synaptically, it develops tension and, if allowed to, it contracts, that is, it shortens. In this section we will discuss the ways in which a muscle contracts.

ISOMETRIC VS. ISOTONIC CONTRACTION

When a muscle is stimulated after its ends or tendons have been fixed, it contracts but cannot shorten. This is called an **isometric** (iso = same, metric = measurement or length) contraction. The muscle develops tension, but because it does not shorten, it does no external work (recall: work = force × distance moved). Careful observation reveals that during an isometric contraction some sarcomeres of the muscle shorten, stretching other sarcomeres and, in addition, some sarcomeres shorten, stretching elastic elements of the muscle. Figure 14-11A is a schematic diagram of the mus-

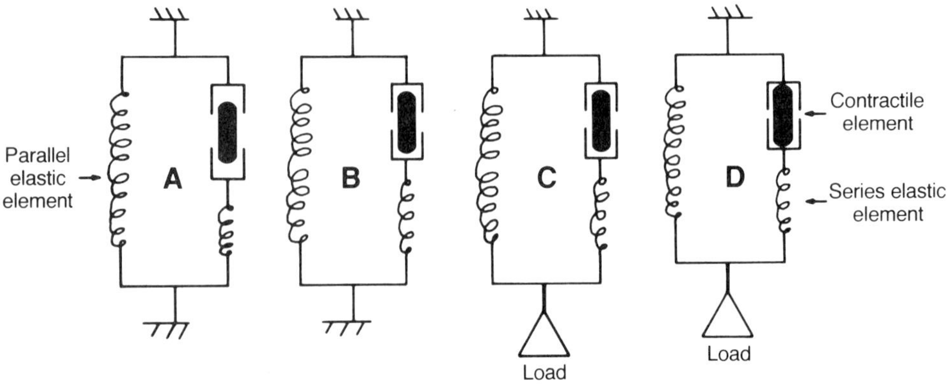

FIG. 14-11. Series and parallel elastic elements in muscle. **A.** Resting muscle contains elastic elements in series with the contractile elements (sarcomeres) and in parallel with them. **B.** During an isometric contraction, the muscle does not change length, but sarcomeres shorten, stretching the series elastic elements. **C.** During isotonic contraction, the contractile elements shorten, stretching the series elastic elements, before they develop tension to lift the load. **D.** Muscle begins to shorten when contractile elements shorten further.

cle, showing elastic elements both in series and in parallel with the contractile elements (the myofibrils) of the muscle. When a whole resting muscle or a single resting muscle fiber is stretched, it opposes the stretch with a force that increases with increased stretch. This elasticity is due to the parallel elastic elements that lie, for the most part, outside the contractile elements in elastic tissues, including tendons and the sarcolemma. When the muscle contracts, the shortening of the muscle lags behind the shortening of the sarcomeres because of the series elastic elements. Therefore, in the isometric contraction, the sarcomeres shorten and stretch the series elastic component even though the muscle as a whole does not shorten, as shown in Figure 14-11B. Even though there is no external work being done by the muscle, there is internal work being done.

If only one end of the muscle is fixed, the muscle shortens and, if it shortens with a constant load, the contraction is **isotonic** (iso = same, tonic = tension). When the contractile elements shorten they must first stretch the series elastic elements and develop a tension equal to the load before the next increment in tension causes the load to be lifted. All of the contraction that occurs before the load is lifted is isometric. Even if the muscle carries no external load, it still must develop a tension equal to its own weight before it can shorten. When contractile forces exceed the load, shortening begins; tension remains slightly larger than the load throughout shortening. Shortening stops when active tension drops to the point where it equals the load. At this point, contraction again becomes isometric. The muscle lengthens (is stretched) when the tension falls below the load. Figure 14-11C and D shows the changes in both series and parallel elastic elements and in the contractile elements during an isotonic contraction. In C, the contractile elements have shortened, stretching the series elastic elements, but the muscle has not shortened. This is the isometric phase of the isotonic contraction. In D, the further shortening of the contractile element leads to shortening of the muscle because the series elastic elements are already stretched.

TWITCH AND TETANIC CONTRACTIONS

If a brief stimulus is applied to the muscle or a single stimulus is applied to the nerve, a single action potential will be elicited in the muscle and the muscle will contract. The time course of this contraction, called a **twitch contraction**, is shown in Figure 14-12A. The tension in the muscle rises rapidly to a maximum, about 50 to 80 msec after the stimulus and then returns to resting tension over the next 100 to 200 msec or so, depending upon the particular muscle. In B, the muscle action potential is reproduced for comparison with the twitch, which lasts about 100 times longer. The muscle whose contraction is shown in the figure, the adductor pollicis muscle of the thumb, is a **fast muscle.** As we shall see, mammals also have **slow muscles** that require 200 msec or more to attain their maximum twitch tension.

A second stimulus, applied before the muscle has completely relaxed, induces another contraction that adds to the first, the sum of the tensions being greater than that of a single twitch. This event, as you probably have guessed, is called **summation.** An example is shown in Figure 14-13. A single stimulus evokes the twitch at the left in A. Repeated stimulation at a rate of 10/sec evokes the summed tensions in B. When the stimulus frequency is increased to 50/sec, the tension rises to a more-or-less steady value, much greater than the twitch tension. This summation, as in C, is called **tetanus** or **tetanic contraction.** Because individual twitch contributions to the tetanus can still be seen as bumps in the record, this tetanus is called **unfused** or **incomplete.** At even higher rates of stimulation, the maximum tension the muscle can sustain is obtained, and there is no sign of individual twitches in the record. This is called **fused** or **complete tetanus,** and it is shown in Figure 14-13D for a 100/sec stimulation rate. Fast and slow muscles, as defined by their twitch times, also differ in the least stimulus frequency at which their contractions produce fused tetanus. Fast muscles may not fuse until stimulus rates equal or exceed 60/sec, whereas slow muscles may fuse at rates of only 16/sec.

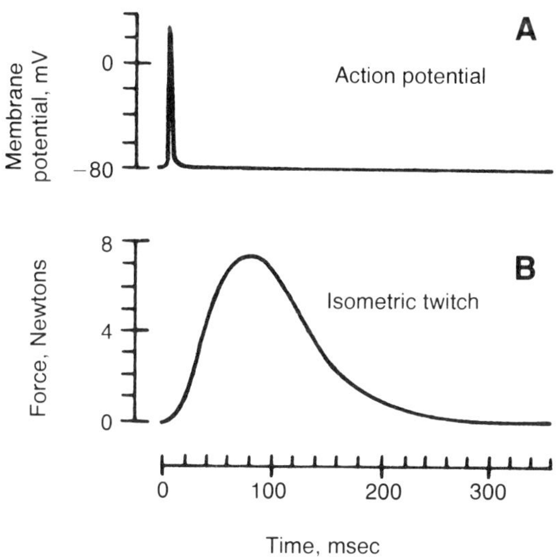

FIG. 14-12. Relation between muscle action potential and twitch contraction. The time course of the action potential is indicated in **A** and the longer development of tension (ordinate) of the twitch contraction is shown in **B**. (Dudel J: Muscles. In Schmidt RF [ed]: Fundamentals of Neurophysiology, 2nd ed. New York, Springer-Verlag, 1978)

LENGTH–TENSION RELATION

When a resting muscle is stretched from its resting length, that is, its length at rest in the body, the parallel elastic elements are stretched and tension increases along the dotted curve in Figure 14-14. In this figure, length is plotted on the abscissa against tension on the ordinate. If the muscle is stretched to about 180% of its resting length (this is about the maximum stretch without damage), and the length is held constant at this value while a contraction is induced, the maximum isometric tension of the muscle is obtained. This tension is the sum of the parallel elastic tension and the contractile tension. At any length less than 180% of

FIG. 14-13. Isometric contractions during repeated stimulation. **A.** Tension development during a single twitch contraction in a fast skeletal muscle. **B.** Summation of twitch contractions when stimulation is repeated at 10 per sec; note greater tension. **C.** Unfused tetanus evoked by stimulation at 50 per sec. **D.** Fused tetanus evoked by stimulation at 100 per sec; note maximum tension developed. (Vander AJ, Sherman JH, Luciano DS: Human Physiology: The Mechanisms of Body Function. New York, McGraw-Hill, 1970)

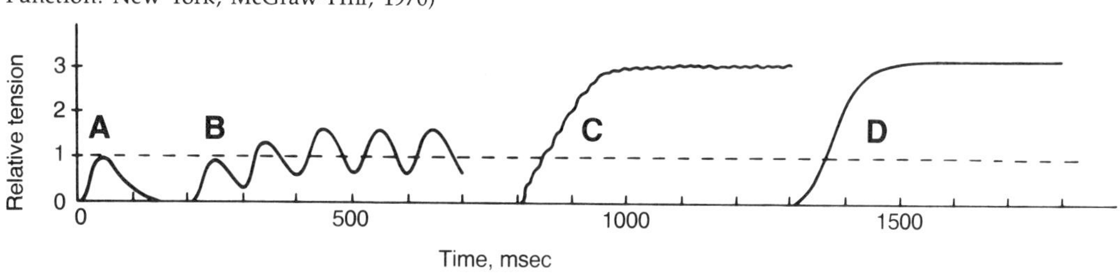

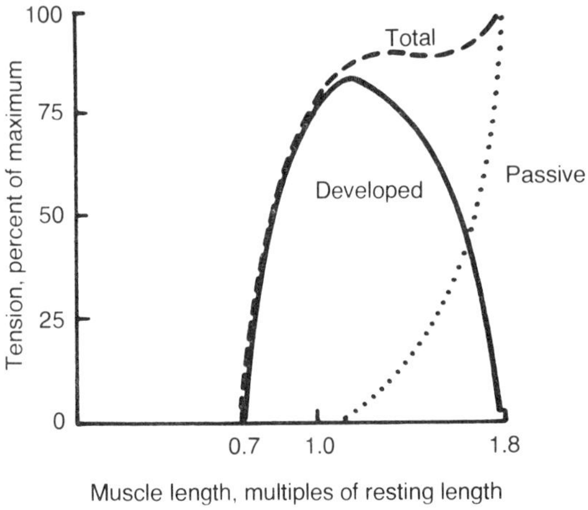

FIG. 14-14. Length–tension curve. Isometric tension (ordinate) is plotted against muscle length (abscissa) expressed as a fraction of resting muscle length, 1.0. The muscle's elasticity resists stretch, developing tension that follows the dotted curve; this is passive tension. When the muscle's length is fixed at a value on the abscissa and then it is stimulated to contract, it develops tension that lies on the dashed curve. This is the total tension or the sum of passive tension and developed tension. The difference (solid curve) between the dashed and dotted curves is the tension developed by the muscle when it contracts. This is maximum at the resting length. (Dudel J: Muscles. In Schmidt RF [ed]: Fundamentals of Neurophysiology, 2nd ed. New York, Springer-Verlag, 1978)

the resting length, the total tension developed by the muscle during an isometric contraction will be less and will follow the dashed curve in Figure 14-14. To compute the contractile tension, the tension developed by the contractile elements, we simply subtract the dotted curve from the dashed curve. The result is the solid curve, sometimes referred to as an isometric length–tension curve.

Obviously, the maximum isometric contractile tension occurs when the muscle is at its resting length. At shorter or longer lengths, the isometric tension produced by the contractile elements is less. The exact shape of the curve for lengths longer than the resting length depends upon when and how the tension is measured (for a discussion see Noble and Pollack, 1977). At lengths less than about 70% of resting length, the muscle develops no tension at all when stimulated. It follows that, during an isotonic contraction, a muscle can only shorten to about 70% of its resting length, and it can only develop tension at lengths between 70% and 180% of resting length. The isotonic length–tension curve approximately superimposes upon the isometric curve; hence during an isotonic contraction the muscle shortens to a length appropriate for the tension developed.

The length–tension curve can be explained by both the cross-bridge and electrostatic theories. Instead of the length of the whole muscle, we could just as accurately have plotted sarcomere length on the abscissa of Figure 14-14, with resting length equal to about 2 μm. At resting length, the thin and thick filaments are in relative positions as shown in Figure 14-7C, with nearly the whole thick filament overlapped by thin filaments. In this position, all of the myosin heads are overlapped by the thin filament, and therefore all are available to form cross-bridges. Recall that in the cross-bridge theory the force of contraction is proportional to the number of cross-bridges formed. At longer lengths, such as those in A and B of Figure 14-7, some of the myosin heads are not overlapped by actin and therefore are not available to form cross-bridges. As a consequence, the tension developed will be less. At shorter lengths, such as D, the actin filaments from opposite ends of the sarcomere begin to interfere with each other and at shortest lengths the Z disc may block movement of the thick filament.

According to the electrostatic theory, the length–tension curve is a simple result of the variation in calcium concentration and, therefore, in electrostatic field strength along the sarcomere. As the muscle is shortened from its resting length, the tip of the thin filament moves from the region of the end of the thick filament, where the Ca^{2+} concentration is assumed to be high, toward its center, where the Ca^{2+} concentration is assumed to be low. Because the field strength is proportional to the Ca^{2+} concentration, the field strength and tension drop. As the muscle is lengthened so that the tip of the thin filament is beyond the last cross-projection of the thick filament, that is, outside the A band, the tension will fall as a function of distance away from that cross-projection, just as the field strength of the capacitor falls with distance.

FORCE–VELOCITY RELATION

Even though the conditions are right for an isotonic contraction, that is, the muscle is fixed at only one end and a weight is attached to the other, the velocity of shortening will be zero (or negative, *i.e.*, the muscle will lengthen) when the weight applied to the muscle is more than the muscle can lift. On the other hand, when there is no weight on the muscle, it will shorten at its maximum velocity. These are the boundary conditions of the force–velocity relation. Between these two extremes, the velocity of shortening decreases as the load increases. Earlier measurements of the velocity of shortening during isotonic contractions indicated that the velocity was an hyperbolic function of the load being lifted, as shown in Figure 14-15. Newer measurements indicate that this is not usually the case (Hill, 1970). In both skeletal and cardiac muscle, the relationship, measured at the sarcomere level, is clearly not hyperbolic. The exact shape of the curve is, however, less important for this discussion than the fact that velocity decreases with increased load. Notice that the solid curve does not intersect the ordinate. This is because it is difficult experimentally to make the load zero in a practical way. We can extrapolate the curve back to the ordinate to find out what the velocity at zero load would be (dashed line, extending curve in Figure 14-15). This is the maximum velocity or V_{max}.

Actually, because the force exerted by the muscle is also related to its length, there will be a family of curves like that in Figure 14-15. The curve shown was obtained when the muscle started to contract at its resting length. The force generated at greater or lesser initial lengths will be less than that at the resting length. Therefore, all of the curves for lengths other than the resting length will be roughly parallel to, but below that shown in Figure 14-15. They will be roughly parallel except near zero load, where all the curves will converge onto the same value of V_{max}.

The cross-bridge theory is able to account for the force–velocity curve by assuming that the rate constants for the processes of attachment and detachment of the cross-bridges are dependent upon the instantaneous position of the cross-bridge relative to the attachment site on the thin filament. The rate of attachment is zero after the cross-bridge passes the attachment site, but the rate of detachment is high. When approaching the attachment site, the cross-bridge cannot attach unless it is within a certain distance; beyond that distance, the rate of attachment is zero, but the rate of detachment is not. Detachment requires a certain minimum time. At low velocities, there is sufficient time for detachment, but at higher velocities, there may not be. Thus, the cross-bridge may remain attached longer than it should and actually oppose the movement of the thin filament in the direction it has just propelled it. This will cause a force opposite in direction to that caused by sarcomere shortening and, therefore, reduce the effective contractile force. The greater the velocity, the greater the effect of the detachment failure.

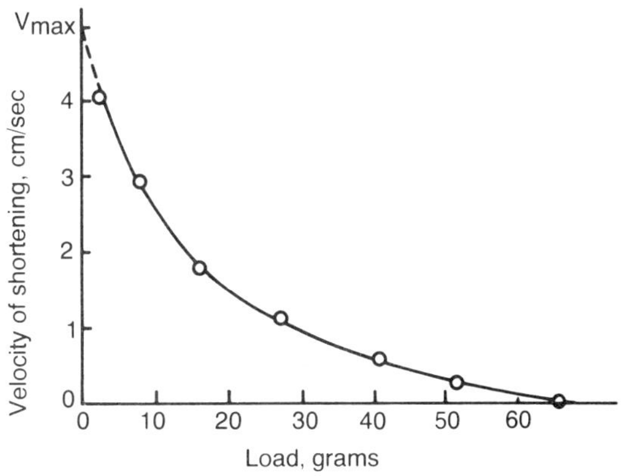

FIG. 14-15. Force–velocity curve. Velocity of shortening (ordinate) is plotted against the load (force) applied to the muscle (abscissa). As the load increases, the velocity of shortening decreases. The curve is extrapolated back to zero load, yielding the maximum velocity the muscle can achieve, V_{max}. (Aidley DJ: The Physiology of Excitable Cells. Cambridge, Cambridge Univ Press, 1971)

In the field theory, there are two factors that reduce force at higher velocities. First, whenever a dielectric rod enters between the plates of a capacitor, it increases its capacitance, thus reducing its voltage (recall from Chapter 3 that $C = Q/V$) and the electric field strength. This effect reduces the force exerted on the tip of the thin filament. At slow shortening rates, the tip of the thin filament stays within the capacitor longer, and there is sufficient time for the capacitor voltage to recover from the transient decrease in field strength. At higher rates, the tip of the filament spends less time in each capacitor and there is less time for recovery; therefore, the force produced is less than for an isometric contraction.

The second factor to influence force–velocity relations is the longitudinal positions of the thin filament tips relative to the cross-projections. When velocity is zero, that is, during an isometric contraction, the tips and cross-projections are aligned. In this position, the field strength and force are greatest. When the velocity is not zero, some of the thin filament tips will not be aligned with cross-projections; hence, they will experience less force. The greater the velocity, the greater will be the proportion of unaligned elements and the smaller the force.

MECHANISMS FOR GRADING FORCE OF CONTRACTION

We have already discussed one mechanism for grading muscle force, that is, by grading the frequency of discharge in the motoneurons and thus the temporal summation of twitch contractions. The end points of this continuum are, of course, a single twitch in the weakest element and a fused tetanic contraction in the strongest. Each muscle fiber is contacted by only one motoneuron, but a motoneuron can contact many muscle fibers. When a motoneuron discharges, it activates all of the muscle fibers with which it makes synaptic contact. A motoneuron and the muscle fibers it contacts are called a **motor unit.** A motor unit for muscles of the lower leg may contain as many as 1700 muscle fibers, whereas a motor unit for the extrinsic muscles of the eye may contain only 7 fibers. The fibers that make up a motor unit are not grouped together in a single bundle, but are scattered in small bundles of a few fibers. Thus, forces produced by contraction of a single motor unit are distributed throughout the muscle. Because all of the muscle fibers of a motor unit contract simultaneously, it is more difficult to achieve fine gradations in the force of contraction when motor units are large. Suppose a motor unit contains 20 fibers and another only 5 and each fiber can produce 1 gram of force. The minimum forces producible by the motor units would be 20 grams and 5 grams in a twitch, and temporal summation would produce forces graded in 20- and 5-gram increments. When fine gradations are necessary, as they are in eye movements, the motor units are usually small.

The force of muscle contraction can also be varied by varying the number of motor units that are active, that is, by spatial summation. Because the muscle fibers are connected in parallel and exert force on the same tendon, the forces produced in all the fibers will be summed at the tendon. Therefore, the greater the number of motor units active, the greater is the force on the tendon. With strong stimulation at rates higher than 5/sec, the force of contraction will increase over that of the twitches evoked by weak, lower-frequency stimulation. This is the result of both spatial and temporal summation. The maximum tension a muscle can develop obviously occurs when all motor units produce fused tetanic contractions. This occurs at stimulation frequencies over about 50/sec, well within the discharge rate capabilities of motoneurons. This brings the limits of control of muscle tension to a minimum of the tension produced by a single twitch in the smallest motor unit and a maximum of the tension of a fused tetanic contraction in all motor units. Nearly any force in between can be produced by some combination of contraction of different motor units and different motoneuron discharge rates.

Tension develops smoothly during normal muscle contractions, not at all like the subtetanic contractions that we have seen. Yet, motoneurons have stable firing rates over a wide range of developed tensions, and they often fire at rates below those necessary to produce tetanic fusion. At these low frequencies, the motor units must behave in a twitchlike fashion. This means that the smoothness of development of tension is due to the asynchrony in contraction of different motor units.

FAST AND SLOW MUSCLES

There are two different types of skeletal muscle fibers in vertebrates, the **red** and **white muscle fibers.** Red muscle fibers are red because they contain the protein myoglobin that, like hemoglobin, contains the iron-rich heme group. It is the heme group that gives both hemoglobin and myoglobin a red color and the ability to bind oxygen. White muscles are white because they contain little myoglobin. Red muscles are the more slowly contracting twitch muscles, the slow muscles, whereas white muscles are the more rapidly contracting fast muscles.

TABLE 14-2. PROPERTIES OF WHITE AND RED MUSCLE FIBERS*

PROPERTY	WHITE FIBERS	RED FIBERS
Twitch contraction time, msec	Fast, 50–80	Slow, 100–200
Minimum tetanic frequency	60/sec	16/sec
Myoglobin content	Low	High
Primary source of ATP	Glycolysis	Oxidative phosphorylation
Glycogen	High	Low
Myosin-ATPase activity	High	Low
Capillary blood flow	Low	High
Fatiguability	Easy	Difficult
Nerve fiber size	Large	Small
Nerve fiber activity	Intermittent, high frequency	Continuous, low frequency

* Vander AJ, Sherman JH, Luciano DS: Human Physiology: The Mechanisms of Body Function. New York, McGraw-Hill, 1970

As already noted, slow muscles also require a lower minimum rate of stimulation for tetanic fusion.

The concentration of myosin is about the same in both red and white muscle, but the concentration of myosin-ATPase is much higher in white muscle fibers. Red muscle contains many mitochondria and gets most of its ATP from oxidative phosphorylation. This source supplies ATP rapidly, and thus the red muscles are able to sustain contractions longer without fatiguing. In addition, red muscle is highly vascularized, receiving and using more oxygen than white muscle. This may also be a function of the high concentration of myoglobin. White muscle, on the other hand, contains few mitochondria and gets most of its ATP from glycolysis, the breakdown of glycogen (which occurs in high concentration in white muscle) into lactic acid. This source of ATP is not as efficient as oxidative phosphorylation, and therefore white muscles fatigue more rapidly than red muscles. White muscle is also more poorly vascularized. These deficiencies may not be a big problem because white muscles tend to be active for only short periods in normal behavior. In addition, although a motor unit consists of only one kind of muscle fiber, most muscles are mixtures of both red and white muscle fibers. The soleus muscle contains almost exclusively red fibers, whereas the gastrocnemius has about 50% red and 50% white fibers. Muscles seldom contain more than 50% white fibers.

The red and white muscle fibers also receive different innervation. Red muscle fibers are innervated by motoneurons of small diameter, thus lower conduction velocity, that discharge nearly continuously at low frequency. White muscle fibers receive innervation from larger motoneurons that have longer periods of silence between discharges, but discharge at high frequencies.

The properties of both red and white muscle fibers are summarized in Table 14-2. The properties of slow muscle fibers make them most suited to extended periods of contraction where a minimum force is required, for example, in maintenance of posture. Fast muscle fibers are better suited to short periods of rapid contraction at higher forces, for example, in sprint running. In fact, during exercise training there may be a differential effect on the two types of muscles. Strength training leads to hypertrophy of mainly white muscle fibers. The number of fibers does not increase, but the size of fibers and the number of myofibrils do increase. This increases both the strength and velocity of contraction. Endurance training apparently affects mainly red muscle fibers, causing an increase in concentration of the enzymes of oxidative phosphorylation and in the vascularization of the muscle, but no change in muscle size.

ELECTROMYOGRAPHY

When muscles contract, they generate action potentials. The action potentials result from transmembrane currents in muscle fibers that can be recorded extracellularly. This may be done in unanesthetized humans using small metal electrodes on the skin over the muscle or using hypodermic

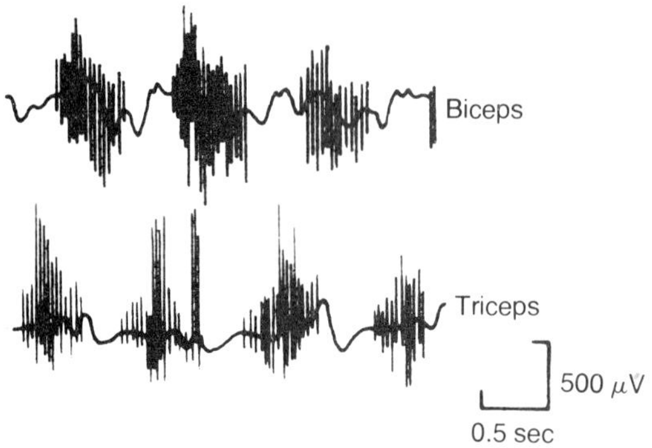

FIG. 14-16. Electromyographic records of activity in the human arm during alternate flexion and extension of the elbow. The **upper trace** shows the EMG from the biceps, and the **lower trace,** the EMG from the triceps muscle. (Ganong WF: Review of Medical Physiology, 7th ed. Los Altos, CA, Lange, 1975)

needle-electrodes inserted into the muscle. The record of the muscle contraction obtained in this way is the **electromyogram,** abbreviated **EMG.** When needle electrodes are used, it is often possible to detect the discharges in single muscle fibers near the electrode. Discharges in different fibers can sometimes be distinguished on the basis of the amplitudes of their spikes. Figure 14-16 shows the EMGs from human biceps and triceps muscles during alternate flexion and extension of the elbow. Note the spikes of different amplitudes and the general increase in spike density with each contraction.

CARDIAC MUSCLE

Structurally, cardiac muscle is similar to skeletal muscle in that it is striated, having both thick and thin filaments. It has a well-

FIG. 14-17. Three-dimensional reconstruction of cardiac muscle, showing organization of myofibrils, T tubules, and sarcoplasmic reticula. Compare with Figure 14-5. (Warwick R, Williams PL [ed]: Gray's Anatomy. 35th British ed, Philadelphia, WB Saunders, 1973)

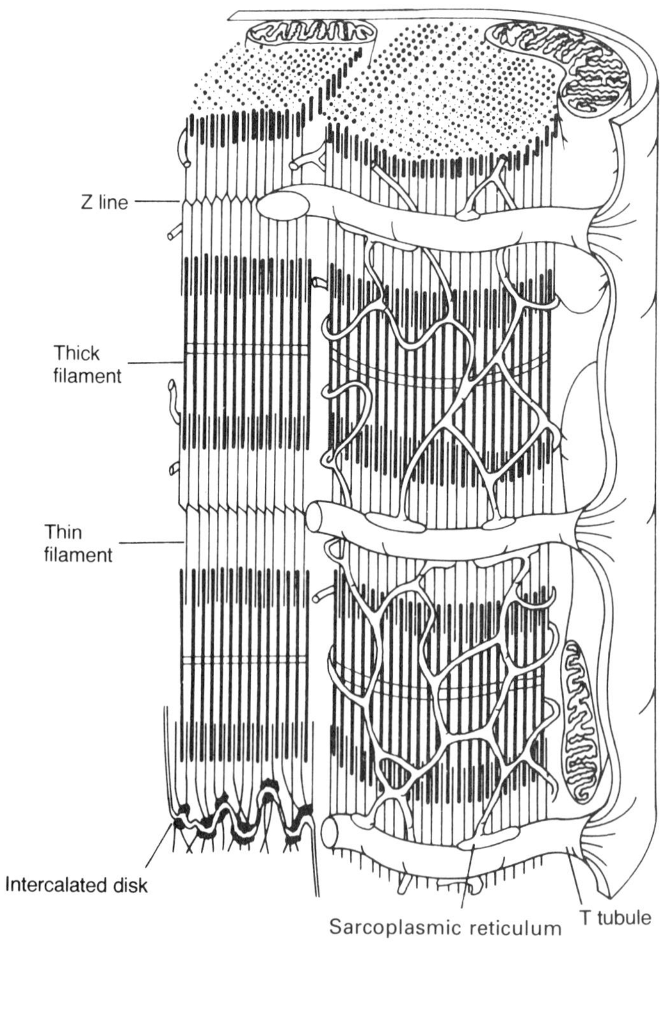

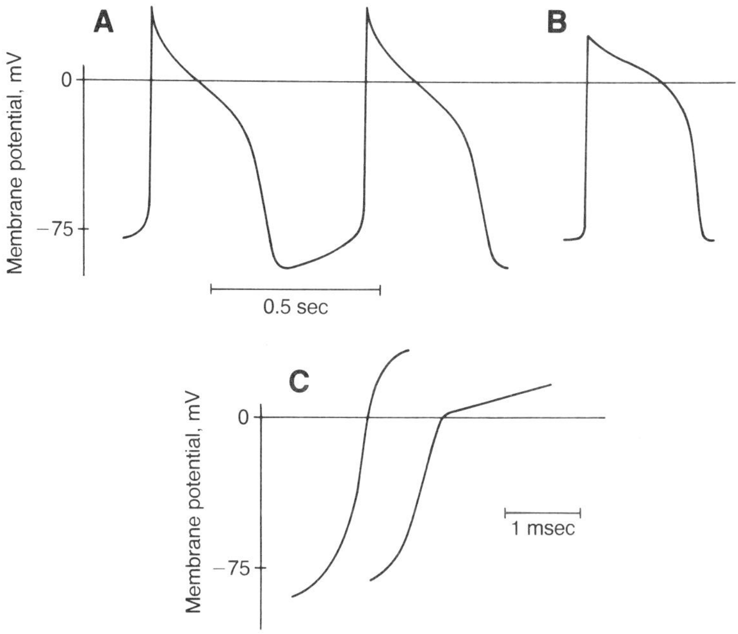

FIG. 14-18. Cardiac muscle action potentials. **A.** Two consecutive action potentials from a pacemaking Purkinje fiber. **B.** Action potential from a contractile fiber. **C.** The upstrokes of Purkinje fiber and contractile fiber action potentials shown in expanded sweeps.

developed T-tubule system, although the sarcoplasmic reticulum is not as large or as extensive as in skeletal muscle. Figure 14-17 shows the basic structure of cardiac muscle. Unlike those in skeletal muscle, the triads of cardiac muscle of humans are located at the Z line, giving only one per sarcomere. The mechanism of excitation–contraction coupling is the same as for skeletal muscle: The membrane action potential leads to a release of Ca^{2+} from the sarcoplasmic reticulum that activates myosin-ATPase and leads to sliding of the thin and thick filaments.

There are a large number of different kinds of cells in cardiac muscle. These include cells of the sinoatrial node, the atrioventricular node, the atrium, the bundle of His, and the ventricle, each with a differently shaped action potential. The details of these differences are beyond the scope of this treatment. For our purposes, it is convenient to distinguish two kinds of cardiac muscle cells: pacemaker cells, like the Purkinje fibers,* and contractile cells. Examples of a Purkinje fiber action potential (A) and a contractile cell action potential (B) are shown in Figure 14-18. Both action potentials are much longer than spikes in nerve cells and skeletal muscle cells, 0.5 sec compared to 0.5 to 5.0 msec. The depolarizing phase of the Purkinje fiber's action potential is not different from that in skeletal muscle, and it appears to have the same ionic mechanism, that is, a dramatic increase in sodium conductance. The rising phase of the contractile cell's action potential is shown in an expanded sweep in Figure 14-18C along with that of the Purkinje fiber for comparison. The contractile cell's action potential has two rising phases, a rapidly rising phase, like that in the Purkinje fiber, and a more slowly rising phase. The fast phase has the same mechanism as the rising phase of Purkinje fiber action potentials, but the slower phase is the result of a slow inward current, carried mostly by Ca^{2+}. Calcium current activation occurs at a more depolarized level of the membrane potential than does sodium activation, and the inactivation of the calcium current is less rapid by about two orders of magnitude.

The long plateau of the action potential in cardiac muscle serves two functions: It provides a more prolonged contraction without resorting to tetanus and it provides a longer refractory period to prevent the heart from

* Do not confuse the Purkinje fibers (muscle) of the heart with Purkinje cells (nerve) of the cerebellum.

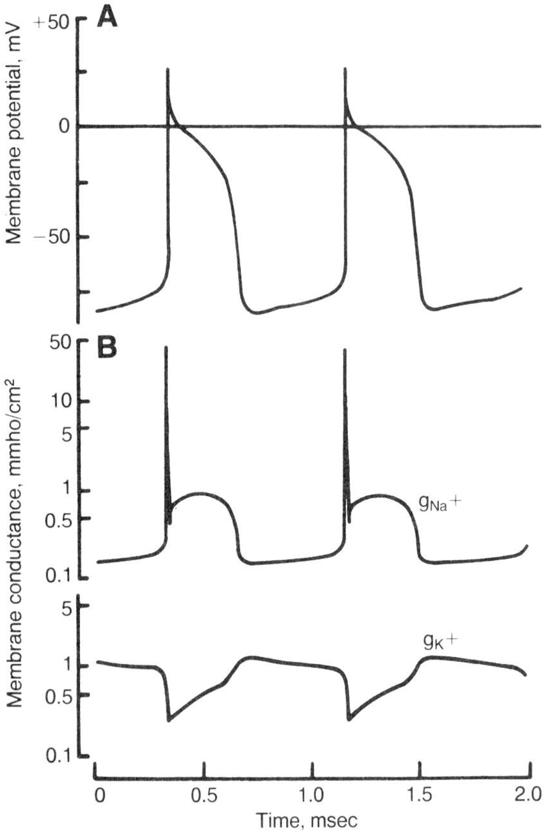

FIG. 14–19. A scheme that explains the form of the Purkinje fiber action potential and the pacemaking activity. Two consecutive Purkinje fiber action potentials are shown in **A.** Changes in sodium and potassium conductances during the action potential are shown in **B.** The ordinates are membrane potential **(A)** and membrane conductance **(B)**; abscissa is time. (Noble D: J Physiol (Lond) 160:317–352, 1962)

contracting prematurely. This plateau is produced by a number of factors, the most important of which is a *decrease* in potassium conductance with depolarization, followed by a slowly developing increase that brings the potassium conductance to a final value just slightly greater than resting levels in Purkinje fibers and to resting levels in contractile cells in about 300 msec. Changes in sodium and potassium conductances are shown in Figure 14-19B on the same time scale as the Purkinje fiber action potential in A. A change in membrane conductance with changes in membrane potential is called rectification by biophysicists. This change in potassium conductance is called **anomalous rectification.** During the plateau of the action potential, membrane resistance is high. Thus, after the peak of the action potential, g_{Na^+} begins to decrease, albeit more slowly than in skeletal muscle and nerve, and in contractile cells the slow inward current persists. In addition, there may be a small inward current due to chloride ions. These currents would be effectively canceled by a big outward K^+ current if the potassium conductance remained normal, but, because g_{K^+} is depressed, the outward i_{K^+} is just slightly larger than $i_{Na^+} + i_{Ca^{2+}} + i_{Cl^-}$ and the membrane repolarizes only very slowly. However, as g_{K^+} increases during the spike, i_{K^+} increases while g_{Na^+} and $g_{Ca^{2+}}$ are decreasing, and the membrane begins to repolarize faster and faster until the resting membrane potential, V_r, is reached.

In Purkinje fibers, the membrane really has no V_r because the membrane potential is constantly changing. This is a property of **pacemaker cells.** As soon as one action potential is completed, the membrane immediately begins to generate another, even in the absence of any neural connections. This kind of behavior is never found in skeletal muscle; the muscle does not contract in the absence of innervation. When the Purkinje fiber membrane repolarizes, it returns to the maximum negative diastolic membrane potential, V_d, where membrane current is zero, $i_m = 0$, but it stays there only for an instant before the membrane begins to depolarize again. The reason why the membrane begins to depolarize is that the potassium conductance, after its initial decrease and slow rise to a level just higher than resting level, begins to decrease toward resting level. As it does so, the potassium current decreases and a point is reached where i_{K^+} no longer balances the inward currents and the net inward current depolarizes the membrane. When the critical firing level is reached, the action potential is initiated. The pacemaker rhythm that develops is **myogenic** (of muscle origin) rather than **neurogenic** (of neural origin) but it can be influenced by neurotransmitters; these decrease or increase the rate of formation of action potentials by decreasing or increasing the rate of depolarization after the action potential. With increased rate, the succeeding action potential begins sooner; with decreased rate, it begins later.

Not all muscle cells are pacemaker cells, but the whole heart must behave as a unit for it to be an effective pump. Contractions are probably synchronized by electrotonic spread of action potentials from one cell to another. Heart muscle is a network of branching muscle fibers connected to each other by tight junctions that are strung together in a structure called the intercalated disk. An intercalated disk is shown in Figure 14-17. The tight junction is thought to be a low impedance pathway, much like an electrotonic synapse. It seems likely that transmission of the action potential from cell to cell in cardiac muscle is the same as transmission from cell to cell at an electrotonic synapse.

Cardiac muscle behaves much like skeletal muscle, but it exerts a passive tension when stretched at much shorter lengths. In fact, when the muscle is stretched from a length even shorter than resting length, there is a resistance to the stretch. In other words, cardiac muscle experiences elastic tension even at resting length (skeletal muscle does not). The result is that the length–tension curve does not have the dip at longer lengths as shown for skeletal muscle in Figure 14-14. In addition, the maximum tension in cardiac muscle occurs, not at the resting length, but when it is stretched beyond resting length. The result is that when more blood returns to the heart from the veins, the blood will automatically be pumped out more forcefully than when the heart is just normally full.

The force–velocity curve for cardiac muscle has the same shape as that for skeletal muscle, and similar parallel curves are generated for different initial lengths, with a constant V_{max}. Increasing the amount of blood in the heart therefore does not increase the contractile ability or contractility of the muscle. On the other hand, actions of certain agents like norepinephrine include increasing V_{max} or contractility of cardiac muscle.

SMOOTH MUSCLE

There is considerable diversity among smooth muscles but all share a lack of the cross-striations characteristic of cardiac and skeletal muscle and an innervation by fibers of the autonomic nervous system like cardiac muscle. This is unlike skeletal muscle that is innervated by fibers of the somatic system. Smooth muscle fibers are smaller than skeletal muscle fibers and are filled with filaments oriented approximately along the long axis of the fiber. There are both thick, myosin-containing filaments and thin, actin-containing filaments, but they are not interdigitated like those in striated muscle. The thin filaments appear to be attached to the plasma membrane or to some structure in the cytoplasm. In general, there is twice as much actin but only one-third as much myosin in smooth muscle as in striated muscle.

Smooth muscles develop tension that varies with muscle length in a manner similar to that in skeletal muscle, but over a much wider range of muscle lengths, nearly twice that of skeletal muscles. This property is appropriate for their functions as linings of hollow organs; even when the organ is greatly distended, smooth muscles can still exert considerable tension. Many people assume that the presence of a length–tension curve implies that contraction occurs by a sliding filament mechanism, but how this occurs is not known. It has been shown that substantial tension can be developed in myofibrils to which myosin heads have been added in the presence of Ca^{2+} and ATP, but in which thick filaments are absent (Oplatka, Gadasi, Borejdo, 1974). This could be related to the contraction mechanism in smooth muscle.

Stretching a denervated smooth muscle causes it to contract, a phenomenon never seen in skeletal muscle. Presumably, stretching, like the occurrence of an action potential, causes an increase in intracellular Ca^{2+} that comes either from the sarcoplasmic reticulum or directly across the cell membrane. Smooth muscle contraction is much slower than that of skeletal muscle. This may be due to slow diffusion of Ca^{2+} from outside the cell or to the slow rate of ATP hydrolysis or both.

Smooth muscle, like cardiac muscle, undergoes spontaneous, rhythmic contraction, driven by activity in certain pacemaker cells that behave like pacemaker cells in cardiac muscle. This pacemaker activity is conducted through tight junctions to neighboring smooth muscle fibers that do not generate pacemaker activity. This is typical of a type of smooth muscle called **single-unit smooth muscle.** Contractile activity of single-unit smooth muscle can be altered by nerve activity or hormones. This kind of smooth muscle also contracts in response to rapid stretching. Single-unit smooth muscles are found in intestinal tract, uterus, and blood vessels.

Multi-unit smooth muscles are found in the lungs, arteries, and erectile tissues of hair follicles. These smooth muscles contain few tight junctions, and therefore contractions do not spread from cell to cell as in single-unit smooth muscle. Multi-unit smooth muscle is richly innervated, with each cell receiving innervation from more than one nerve fiber and each fiber innervating several cells. The response of the whole muscle depends upon the number of motor units active and the frequency of discharge in the fibers. Multi-unit smooth muscle activity can be initiated by hormones but not by rapidly stretching the muscle.

SUGGESTED READING

Bendall JR: Muscles, Molecules and Movement. New York, American Elsevier, 1970

Carlson FD, Wilkie DR: Muscle Physiology. Englewood Cliffs, NJ, Prentice-Hall, 1974

Ebashi S, Endo M, Ohtsuki I: Control of muscle contraction. Q Rev Biophys 2:351–384, 1969

Gordon AM, Huxley AF, Julian FJ: Tension development in highly stretched vertebrate muscle fibres. J Physiol (Lond) 184:143–169, 1966

Gordon AM, Huxley AF, Julian FJ: The variation in isometric tension with sarcomere length in vertebrate muscle fibres. J Physiol (Lond) 184:170–192, 1966

Hill AV: First and Last Experiments in Muscle Mechanics. London, Cambridge Univ. Press, 1970

Huxley AF, Simmons RM: Proposed mechanism of force generation in striated muscle. Nature 233:533–538, 1971

Huxley AF: Muscular contraction. J Physiol (Lond) 243:1–43, 1974

Julian FJ, Moss RL, Solens MR: The mechanism for vertebrate striated muscle contraction. Circ Res 42:2–14, 1978

Noble MIM, Pollack GH: Molecular mechanisms of contraction. Circ Res 40:333–342, 1977

Oplatka A, Gadasi H, Borejdo J: The contraction of "ghost" myofibrils and glycerinated muscle fibers irrigated with heavy meromyosin subfragment–1. Biochem Biophys Res Comm 58:905–912, 1974

Wilkie DR: The relation between force and velocity in human muscle, J Physiol (Lond) 110:249–280, 1949

Zierler KL: Mechanism of muscle contraction and its energetics. In: Mountcastle VB [ed]: Medical Physiology, 13th ed. Vol. 1. St. Louis, Mosby, 1974

15

Reflexes

If you look at every textbook of neurophysiology and neurology in the library, you will not find many that give a definition of the term **reflex.** It is difficult to define the term in a way that includes everything we call a reflex, yet says anything that allows one to decide if any particular event is a reflex. We will follow suit in a sense and define a reflex as "a relatively stereotyped movement or response elicited by a stimulus applied to the periphery, transmitted to the central nervous system and then transmitted back out to the periphery." Most reflexes involve activities that are nearly the same each time they are repeated, but no activity of an organism is fixed and independent of either the state or the history of the organism. Most reflexes involve the simplest of neural circuits, some only two or a few neurons; but many, like the scratch-reflex in a dog, are so complicated that their organization remains a mystery. Most reflexes are "involuntary" in the sense that they occur without the person willing them to do so, but *all* of them can be brought under "voluntary" control.

There are a number of ways of classifying reflexes. One is in terms of the systems that receive the stimulus and give the response. There are **viscerovisceral reflexes,** for example the decrease in heart rate that follows distension of the carotid sinus; **viscerosomatic reflexes,** like the abdominal cramping that accompanies rupture of the appendix; **somatovisceral reflexes,** such as the vasoconstriction that results from cooling the skin; and **somatosomatic reflexes,** like the knee jerk that follows tapping of the patellar tendon. Another way to classify reflexes is in terms of the number of neurons or synapses between the primary afferent neuron and the motor neuron. We distinguish two types, the **monosynaptic reflex** and the much more common **polysynaptic reflex.**

THE TENDON JERK REFLEX

The simplest reflex is the monosynaptic reflex or the two-neuron reflex, an example of which is the **tendon jerk reflex,** sometimes called the **stretch reflex** or **myotatic reflex.** This is the reflex that is elicited by tapping the tendon just below the patella. The tap, applied to the tendons of the quadriceps muscles, stretches the muscles and their muscle spindles. A brisk tap excites the group Ia afferent fibers, because of their velocity sensitivity, ultimately causing the muscle to contract. The neural circuit for this reflex is shown in Figure 15-1. The group Ia afferent neuron enters the spinal cord through the dorsal root, penetrates into the ventral horn, and then synapses on an α motoneuron. (This is the only synapse in the pathway within the spinal cord, thus the reflex is monosynaptic.) The α motoneuron then exits the spinal cord through the ventral root and innervates the extrafusal fibers of the muscle from which the group Ia afferent fiber originated, that is, the **homonymous muscle.** Note that the drawing shows only one neuron of each type, afferent and efferent, but that one represents many. For example, the cat soleus muscle contains about 50 group Ia afferent fibers and each soleus α motoneuron appears to have a synaptic connection with each one of those 50 group Ia afferent fibers.

Tapping the tendon of the rectus femoris muscle of the quadriceps group produces a brief stretch of that muscle that acts as a powerful stimulus for the group Ia afferent fibers of the muscle, causing them to give a brief, synchronous discharge. Each dis-

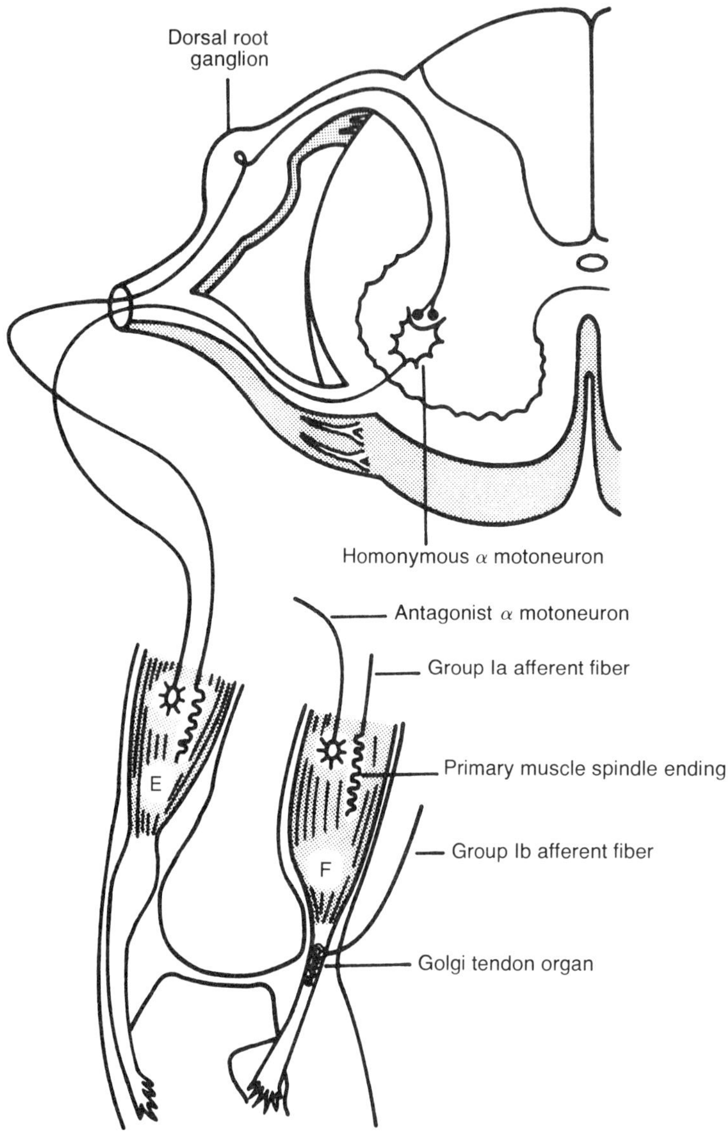

FIG. 15-1. The tendon jerk reflex. A circuit diagram of the elements of the tendon jerk reflex: the muscle spindle, group Ia afferent fiber, α motoneuron, and extrafusal muscle fiber. Note that this is a monosynaptic reflex. **F** and **E** indicate flexor and extensor muscles. (Schadé JP, Ford DH: Basic Neurology. Amsterdam, Elsevier, 1965)

charge, after propagating down the axon to its termination, produces an EPSP in the rectus α motoneurons. Because there are many EPSPs from many group Ia afferent fibers occurring nearly simultaneously in some α motoneurons, the membrane potentials reach critical firing level (by spatial summation) with depolarization to spare, and the motoneurons discharge an action potential. The action potentials travel out by way of the ventral root to the muscle and, because the neuromuscular juction is an obligatory synapse, the muscle contracts. The contraction in turn causes the spindle to be unloaded or shortened passively, its equatorial region to relax, the group Ia afferent fiber to turn off, and the muscle to relax. This is the tendon jerk reflex.

Many of the homonymous α motoneurons are not discharged by the group Ia afferent fiber input, but have EPSPs evoked in them that do not achieve the critical firing level. The excitability of the motoneuron is therefore increased. This group of excited neurons is called the **subliminal fringe.** The presence of the subliminal fringe accounts for enhancement of the reflex response under certain circumstances, for example with the Jendrassik maneuver. If one hand pulls against the other while the tendon tap reflex is evoked, the reflex will be stronger than in the absence of the maneuver. (Interestingly, mental arithmetic and a number of other activities will do the same thing!) The increased muscle contraction is due to activation of more motoneurons primarily because of activity descending to the spinal cord from above. This activity by itself does not cause the muscle to contract, but when added to the subcritical-firing-level-excitation of the subliminal fringe, it causes the neurons that were in the subliminal fringe to discharge. There may also be some influence of increased γ-motoneuron activity, increasing the sensitivity of the primary spindle endings, but this influence should be small because the stimulus for the reflex is very brief.

The value of the stretch reflex mechanism may not be clear at first, but some reflection may clarify its role in motor control. It is unlikely that muscles undergo such rapid stretches very often, with the possible exception of when a person jumps off a wall or jumps up and down on a pogo stick. However, in these instances, the rapid stretch that results when landing causes a reflex contraction that helps prevent the gluteus from being overly bruised. Usually, the postural muscles experience relatively slow, sustained stretches and the antigravity muscles, of which the quadriceps is an example, are pulled upon by gravitational forces. This steady force sets up a sustained discharge in each group Ia afferent fiber, but the discharges in different fibers are not synchronized as they are when the tendon is tapped. This asynchronous discharge sums in the α motoneuron with other activity from within the CNS to produce a contraction that just balances the gravitational force. If an additional force is applied, stretching the muscle, additional tension is developed by the stretch reflex to counteract that force. In this way, the stretch reflex serves as a mechanism for maintaining an upright body orientation under a variety of load conditions; the mechanism is automatic ("unconscious") and fast (19–24 msec for the quadriceps in man).

In addition to the monosynaptic connections of the group Ia afferent fibers with the homonymous α motoneurons (*e.g.*, rectus femoris Ia with rectus α motoneuron), there are also monosynaptic connections with synergistic α motoneurons, those innervating muscles that act in the same way at the same joint, but the effects are not as strong in the **synergists** as they are in the homonymous α motoneurons. Thus, the rectus group Ia afferent fibers also excite the vastus α motoneurons, though not as strongly as they do the rectus α motoneurons. Fewer of the synergistic α motoneurons actually discharge, and the subliminal fringe is larger than for homonymous α motoneurons.

Most skeletal muscles exhibit a tendon tap reflex, but the reflex is strongest in the **antigravity** or **physiologic extensor muscles.** This makes some sense in light of the discussion of the last paragraph. Note that physiologic extensors are not necessarily anatomic extensors. The biceps brachii are a case in point; they are anatomic flexors of the elbow but they are physiologic extensors, moving the forearm against gravity.

RECIPROCAL INNERVATION

When the extensor muscle contracts during such a reflex, there is usually a relaxation of its **antagonists,** the flexor muscles crossing the same joint. If this did not occur, the reflex movement would be resisted and diminished by the force of the antagonist muscle. The neural mechanism underlying this relaxation of the antagonist muscles is shown in Figure 15-2. The group Ia afferent fiber, after entering the spinal cord, gives off a collateral branch that synapses on an interneuron. This interneuron, in turn, synapses on the antagonist α motoneuron, in the case of our previous example, the hamstring motoneurons. Its effect on the hamstring α motoneuron is inhibitory, that is, it causes an IPSP in the α motoneuron that is ultimately manifested as a relaxation of the muscle. This is **reciprocal inhibition.** Notice that this is a polysynaptic reflex pathway. It is a general principle that anything that has an excitatory (or inhibitory)

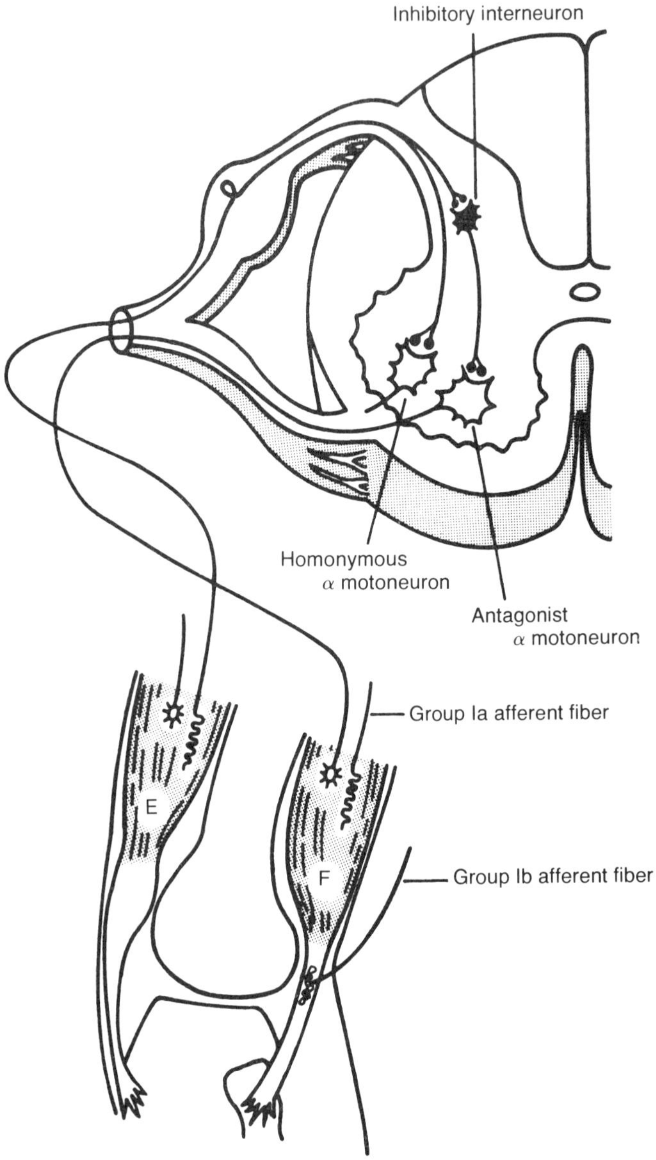

FIG. 15-2. Reciprocal innervation. A circuit diagram showing the collateral of the group Ia afferent fiber synapsing on an inhibitory interneuron that synapses on the α motoneuron of the antagonist muscle. **E** and **F** indicate extensor and flexor muscles. (Schadé JP, Ford DH: Basic Neurology. Amsterdam, Elsevier, 1965)

influence on an α motoneuron also inhibits (or excites) its antagonist α motoneurons. This is the principle of **reciprocal innervation.** Thus, for example, excitation of the hamstring α motoneurons by group Ia afferent fibers is accompanied by inhibition of quadriceps α motoneurons. Reciprocal inhibition is a specific example of the more general principle of reciprocal innervation.

DALE'S PRINCIPLE

At this point, it is appropriate to bring up the reason for interneurons in pathways such as that in Figure 15-2. **Dale's principle** (formulated by Sir Henry Dale) states that a single neuron synthesizes only one transmitter substance. Therefore, if a neuron secretes acetylcholine at one of its terminals, it

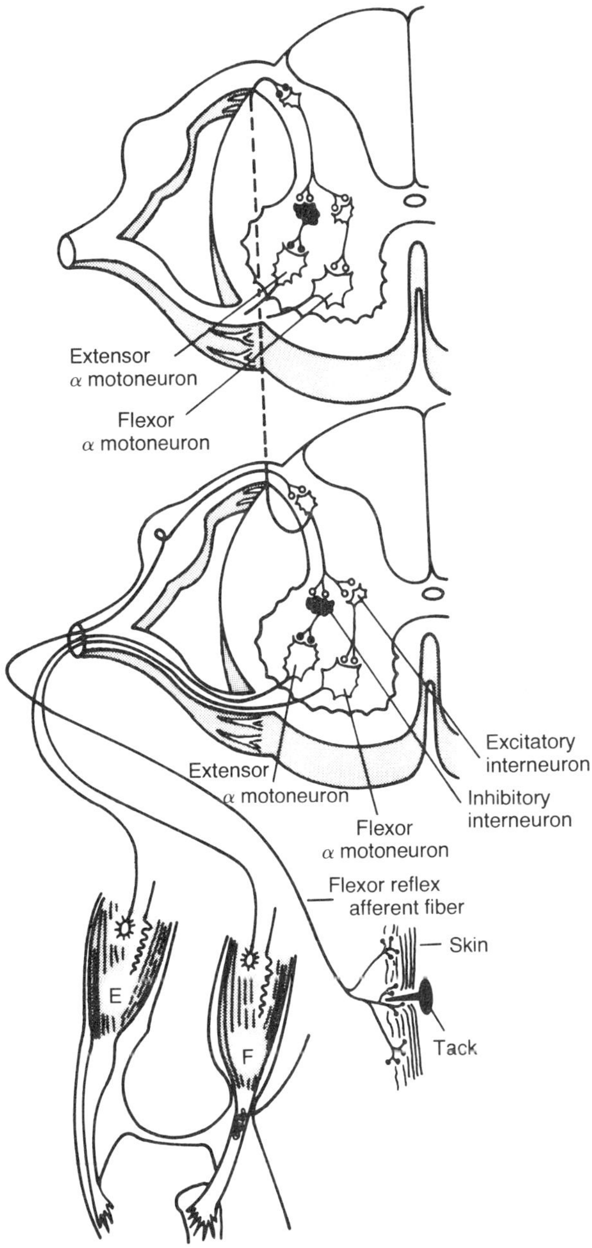

FIG. 15-3. Flexion reflex. A circuit diagram of the flexion reflex showing afferent fibers from skin, interneurons, and flexor α motoneurons in two spinal cord segments. Note that some interneurons are intersegmental. **E** and **F** indicate extensor and flexor muscles. (Schadé JP, Ford DH: Basic Neurology. Amsterdam, Elsevier, 1965)

secretes acetylcholine at all of its terminals. Eccles has extended this notion to say that the effect of the transmitter released by a single fiber is the same at all its terminals. This would imply that the net result of activity in all group Ia afferent fibers is excitation and only excitation. Thus, if it is necessary to have inhibition in a pathway involving group Ia afferent fibers, then an inhibitory interneuron must be interposed.

There is some evidence that a neuron makes, or at least contains, more than one of the putative transmitter substances discussed in Chapter 13. However, it is not known whether all of the substances made by a neuron are actually used as transmitter substances by that neuron. Therefore, it is not clear that this is a violation of Dale's principle. On the other hand, the idea that the effect of a transmitter is everywhere the same is not tenable. It is now known that certain neurons in *Aplysia californica*, the sea slug, secrete acetylcholine at synapses with two different postsynaptic cells, and, in one cell, the transmitter substance evokes an EPSP and, in the other, an IPSP. Thus, the action of the transmitter substance on a neuron depends upon that neuron. Whether this behavior is also a characteristic of mammalian neurons is not yet certain. However, the usual approach in neurophysiology has been to interpose an interneuron whenever the sign of the effect changes, whether there is direct evidence of an interneuron or not.

THE FLEXION REFLEX

If you have ever touched a hot object or stepped on a sharp object and withdrawn your hand or foot, you have experienced a **flexion reflex,** a **nocifensive reflex,** or a **withdrawal reflex,** all terms describing the same event. The protective result of this reflex is obvious; it quickly removes the part of the body from the vicinity of the offending object by contracting the appropriate muscles, usually flexors, and relaxing extensor muscles (again, reciprocal innervation). The vigor of the reflex depends upon the strength of the stimulus. A weak pinch produces flexion of the foot; a slightly stronger one, flexion of both the foot and the lower leg; and a very strong one, flexion of foot, leg, and even hip. This spread of the reflex with stronger stimulation is called **irradiation.**

The pathways for the flexion reflex are illustrated in Figure 15-3. The afferent limb (the part going to the spinal cord) of this reflex consists of nociceptors with Aδ or C fibers and fibers of groups II, III, and IV of muscle. These are sometimes referred to collectively as the **flexor reflex afferent fibers.** They enter the spinal cord and synapse on interneurons, whose axons distribute to other interneurons that affect α motoneurons within the same and in different segments of the spinal cord. Notice that this is a polysynaptic reflex. Activity in the nociceptive afferent fibers in the common peroneal nerve serving the first and second toe leads to discharge of the peroneus α motoneurons, which, in turn, leads to dorsiflexion of the foot. If the nociceptive activity is strong enough, it is able to activate other peroneus α motoneurons, further increasing the flexion of the foot, and also to bring in α motoneurons of synergistic muscles of the foot, as well as other related muscle groups, for example the hamstrings, to lift the leg. This may involve transmission to spinal segments other than the segment of entry.

THE CROSSED-EXTENSION REFLEX

If protection of the limb requires it to be elevated, then the rest of the body is imperiled by removal of the support it normally provides, unless some compensation is made. The reflex contraction of flexor muscles on one side of the body is always accompanied by contraction of the extensor muscles of the contralateral limb. This gives increased antigravity support on the contralateral side to hold the body upright and is called the **crossed-extension reflex.** The circuit for this reflex is illustrated in Figure 15-4. The flexor reflex afferent fibers also synapse on interneurons that decussate (cross the midline) and terminate on contralateral extensor α motoneurons. This pathway is polysynaptic and purely excitatory. In addition, there is the usual reciprocal inhibitory effect on the contralateral flexor α motoneurons.

AUTOGENIC INHIBITION

Activity in the group Ib afferent fibers, associated with Golgi tendon organs, inhibits the homonymous α motoneurons. The inhibition is disynaptic involving one interneuron and two synapses between the afferent fiber and the motoneuron. The effect is called **autogenic inhibition** (sometimes written autogenetic inhibition). Like the group Ia excitation, group Ib inhibition is exerted not only on the homonymous α

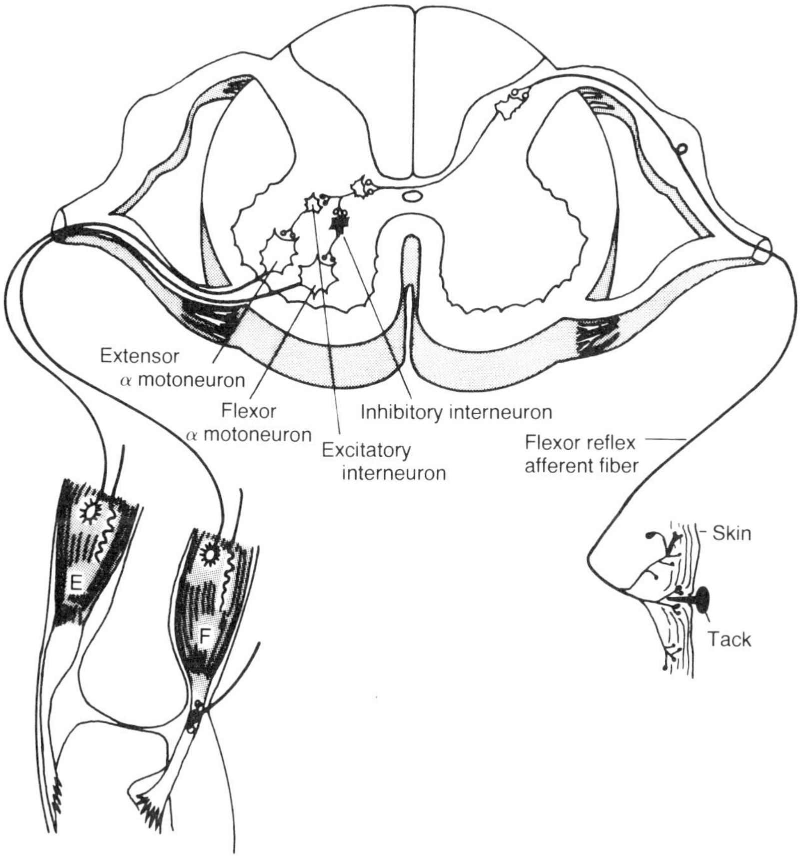

FIG. 15-4. Crossed-extension reflex. Circuit diagram showing branching of the flexor reflex afferent fibers and their termination on an interneuron that decussates and terminates on contralateral extensor α motoneurons. The circuit for the contralateral reciprocal inhibition of flexor α motoneurons is also shown. **E** and **F** indicate extensor and flexor muscles. (Schadé JP, Ford DH: Basic Neurology. Amsterdam, Elsevier, 1965)

motoneurons, but also on the α motoneurons of synergistic muscles. Reciprocal innervation is also present here, with group Ib activity exciting the α motoneurons of the antagonist muscles.

It was originally thought that this inhibition served only to protect the muscle from being injured by contracting against too heavy a load. This concept came from two sources: (1) the supposed high threshold of group Ib fibers to tension (not true for developed tension) and (2) the existence of a clasp-knife reflex. This reflex exists only in certain pathologic conditions, for example, "upper motoneuron" disease. Under these conditions, there is an extensor spasticity that resists any attempt to flex the limbs, especially the arms. If the arm is gradually, forceably flexed by someone other than the patient, a point will be reached when the resistance to flexion suddenly melts away, and the limb collapses easily into full flexion. This is the **clasp-knife reflex** or the **lengthening reaction.** It is probably mediated by autogenic inhibition and was thought formerly to occur near the threshold for group Ib activation by tension. Now it is thought that it occurs at the point where autogenic inhibition is great enough to overcome the stretch reflex excitation, that is, when the membrane potential of the extensor motoneuron falls below the critical firing level and the muscle relaxes. Actually, Golgi tendon organ activity cannot entirely account for the clasp-knife reflex. As the spastic muscle is lengthened, the group Ia discharge continually increases and, because the tension is increasing, the group Ib discharge also increases. The result, at the α motoneuron, is excitation from the group

Ia fiber input and inhibition from the group Ib fiber input, the inhibition finally taking dominance and silencing the α motoneuron. The muscle relaxes. This accounts for the relaxation of the spastic muscle, but it does not account for the failure of its immediate return. When the muscle relaxes, the tension falls and with it the group Ib fiber discharge. This should decrease the autogenic inhibition and allow group Ia fiber input to reestablish the spasticity, but the muscle stays relaxed until the joint is extended again, whereupon the spasticity reappears. Evidence suggests that group Ia fibers from muscle spindles also contribute to autogenic inhibition (Fetz, Jankowska, Johannisson, et al, 1979). Because the muscle does not shorten, but lengthens when the spasticity disappears, the group Ia fibers will discharge even more briskly, increasing both excitation and autogenic inhibition of the α motoneurons. Apparently, the inhibition predominates.

In the normal person, it is certain that the Golgi tendon organ contributes to control of muscle activity over the whole range of movement, not just at its extremes. There is no reflex movement associated with stimulation of Golgi tendon organs in isolation, so that nothing can be said with certainty about their reflex function. Perhaps they do serve a protective function, but they may also be supplying tension information for complicated tension-maintaining reflexes or supplying inhibition at the appropriate moment to swtich from flexion to extension movements in walking or running.

OTHER REFLEXES

There are a number of other reflexes that are commonly tested in the clinic, whose mechanism we do not understand thoroughly. The **extensor thrust reflex** involves extension of the lower limb when a tactile stimulus is applied to the plantar surface of the foot. This may play some role in walking or standing by maintaining contact with the surface. The **Babinski sign** is a reflex that is pathologic in adults but normal in infants. Scraping the sole of the foot of a normal adult with a tongue depressor results in plantar flexion of the toes. In the infant and the spinal adult (with a spinal cord transection), the same stimulus leads to dorsiflexion of the toes. This pathologic change is called Babinski's sign, and, as we shall see, it is a sign of pyramidal tract damage.

There are a great many other reflexes that could be mentioned here. We have already discussed reflex control of pupil diameter and lens shape in the eye and auditory sensitivity by the middle ear muscles and olivocochlear bundle. In addition, there are stretch receptors in the lungs, probably in the bronchi and bronchioles, that are activated by lung inflation. The activity of these receptors enters the medulla by way of the vagus nerve (Xth cranial nerve) to produce inhibition of inspiratory neurons. This effect, called the **Hering-Breuer reflex,** has the effect of terminating inspiration when a certain level of inflation has been attained. It is mediated through the nucleus solitarius and the reticular formation.

There are other respiratory reflexes as well. For example, the stretch reflex and autogenic inhibition play a major role in control of the intercostal muscles during inspiration. The gamma motoneuron loop appears to provide an important facilitation of discharges in α motoneurons to the external intercostals in particular. A most important reflex pathway regulates the concentrations of oxygen and carbon dioxide in arterial blood by adjusting respiratory parameters. Chemoreceptors in the carotid and aortic bodies increase their discharge rates in response to a decrease in arterial oxygen concentration or an increase in arterial carbon dioxide concentration (or, alternatively, a decrease in *p*H). Sensory fibers from these receptors enter the brain stem through the glossopharyngeal nerve (IXth cranial nerve), where they make connections with cells whose activity results in an increase in respiratory volume and rate, with certain changes in peripheral vasculature, to elevate blood oxygen or decrease blood carbon dioxide levels. In addition, there are chemoreceptors in the CNS that are excited by elevation of the carbon dioxide level of the cerebrospinal fluid or a decrease in its *p*H. Their activity results in the same changes in respiration, apparently without much change in the cardiovascular system.

There are also reflexes involving the heart. Baroreceptors in the carotid sinus, in the aortic arch, and perhaps elsewhere, increase their discharge rates in response to elevated blood pressure. This increase in activity leads reflexly to a decrease in sympathetic discharge, resulting in peripheral vasodilatation and in an increase in parasympathetic discharge primarily through the vagus nerve, resulting in decreased heart rate. The net result is a decrease in blood pressure. Stimulation of high threshold (small diameter) primary afferent fibers in cutaneous and muscle nerves also leads to a reflex increase in blood pressure.

Vomiting is the result of a reflex arc involving receptors in the region of the pharynx, supplied by the IXth and Xth cranial nerves and also involving receptors in the medulla. The medullary receptors, located in a region with high permeability of the blood–brain barrier, are sensitive to chemical agents in the blood. The efferent limb of the reflex involves somatic innervation of the abdominal muscles and autonomic innervation of the stomach (smooth) muscles and the cardiac sphincter. During vomiting, the cardiac sphincter relaxes while the abdominal and stomach muscles contract, expelling the stomach contents through the esophagus.

Swallowing is also a reflex activity. The reflex is triggered by tactile stimulation of the mucosa of the palate, pharynx, and epiglottis. Receptors in these regions, perhaps free nerve endings, send their activity through the IXth cranial nerve, the superior laryngeal branch of the Xth cranial nerve, and perhaps also the Vth cranial nerve. The reflex pathway involves synapses in the nucleus solitarius and efferent fibers to the tongue in the hypoglossal nerve (XIIth cranial nerve) and to the palate, pharyngeal, and esophageal musculature through the IXth, Xth, and XIth cranial nerves from the nucleus ambiguous.

Temperature regulation (see also Chap. 17) is a complicated reflex activity, involving both peripheral thermoreceptors and central thermoreceptors located in the anterior hypothalamus and perhaps elsewhere. The reflex pathways are not well understood, but they involve hypothalamic activation of the autonomic system, resulting in peripheral vasoconstriction, piloerection, and shivering, if heat needs to be generated or conserved, and in sweating, increased respiration, and peripheral vasodilatation, if heat needs to be lost in maintaining body core temperature at around 37°C.

Micturition is a reflex activity that depends upon stretch receptors located in series with smooth muscle cells of the bladder wall. This mode of attachment allows the receptors to discharge both when the muscles are stretched and when they contract. Fibers from these receptors are carried in the pelvic nerves to the S2–S4 spinal cord segments. Somatic afferent fibers to these same segments play a role in the reflex as well. Bladder emptying is produced by contraction of the detrusor muscle of the bladder and also muscles of the abdominal wall, with relaxation of the internal (smooth muscle) and external (striated muscle) sphincters. Reflex emptying can be accomplished with an isolated sacral spinal cord, provided that the sacral roots, especially ventral root S3, are intact, but usually the reflex is under strong descending control.

The reflex emptying of the colon, that is, defecation, is accomplished in a way similar to micturition. Here, the receptors are located in series with smooth muscle of the rectal wall. Tactile receptors in the skin and anus also facilitate defecation, as does the simultaneous occurrence of a micturition reflex. Emptying is under parasympathetic control from the S2–S4 spinal cord segments, producing contraction of the smooth muscle lining the rectum and relaxation of the sphincters. Evacuation is also assisted by contraction of the diaphragm and abdominal muscles with the glottis closed (Valsalva's maneuver), increasing the pressure in the abdominal cavity.

There are also sexual reflexes whose organization is partially understood. The afferent fibers for erection and ejaculation reflexes arise from the genitalia and course through branches of the pudendal nerve, again, to spinal cord segments S2–S4, although many other stimuli can elicit sexual responses under appropriate circumstances. Many of these other stimuli must act through higher centers. Both somatic and autonomic efferent fibers are involved in producing erection, with parasympathetic fibers producing vascular engorgement and somatic motoneurons to the bulbocavernous and ischiocavernous muscles producing contraction that compresses the venous outflow from erectile tissues. Sympathetic fibers also play a poorly understood role; bilateral sympathectomy reduces or eliminates both erections and ejaculations. Sympathetic, parasympathetic, and somatic motor activity are all involved in producing ejaculation.

These are a few of the many reflexes mediated by the nervous system. Some are mediated by the spinal cord and can occur when the spinal cord is isolated, but some require intact connections with the brain stem or diencephalon for their operation. All, however, are under the influence of cortical and subcortical structures in their normal operation.

THE FUNCTION AND UTILITY OF REFLEXES

For the most part, the reflexes are artifacts of the way we stimulate the body (although some, like the eye blink reflex, are essential to protect body parts from injury). However, they tell us two useful things: (1) how the nerve circuits of the spinal cord or brain stem are put together and (2) the condition of various parts of these circuits. The first piece of information is useful to the neurophysiologist, who ultimately wants to know how the nervous system works. However, we will see in the next chapter that many reflexes are suppressed or modified during phases of the stepping cycle in order to prevent muscles from contracting at the wrong times. The state of a reflex circuit may be highly variable depending upon the condition of a person, for example, awake, asleep, comatose; upon what he is doing, such as walking, running, thinking; upon his position in space or posture; and upon other factors. Therefore, the reflex pattern at any one time may not be a good indicator of the neural circuits available in the nervous system or of how they behave under a variety of conditions.

The second piece of information is useful to the clinician, who wants to know what is wrong with a patient. An example may help to show how the reflexes are used clinically. A patient complains of **paresis** or weakness of the right leg. There are three possible causes for this paresis: (1) He is suffering from disease of descending tracts having to do with leg function; (2) he is suffering from disease of the α motoneurons themselves; or (3) something is wrong with the muscle. A normal tendon tap reflex rules out the last two alternatives, because the α motoneurons and muscle must be functional to give a normal reflex.

REFLEX PATHWAYS AS CONTROL SYSTEMS

One way to think of the function of reflexes is as **control systems,** systems that regulate the various parameters of muscle contraction. The essential feature of this type of system is the more-or-less continuous flow of information from the element controlled back to the device that controls it. This is called **feedback.** An everyday example of feedback is the continuous information your eyes give you about the course your automobile is taking. Without visual information, you are likely to run off the road before you can detect errors in your steering. With visual feedback, small corrections can be made in your steering before you leave the road.

A convenient way of illustrating a control system is to use a block diagram such as that shown in Figure 15-5. In a block diagram, boxes indicate the components of the system, and arrows indicate the direction of flow of signals in the system. The controlled system has an input that can be varied by a controller. This input interacts with influences from outside the system, called disturbances, in producing the output of the system, which is the parameter to be controlled. In the automobile example, the input is the position of the steering wheel, the output is the position of the car on the road, and a disturbance might be a sudden gust of wind that forces the car off its intended course. The sensor is a device that measures the output of the system and its measurement is the feedback signal to the error detector. The feedback signal is compared with the control signal (the signal that specifies the intended output) by the error detector, which, when it finds a difference between the two signals, sends an error signal to the controller to increase its output and reduce the amount of error. The actual output is brought closer to the intended output, the new output is again sensed by the sensor, and a new correction is made, bringing the system even closer to the intended output, and so on. In our car example, the error detector, sensor, and controller

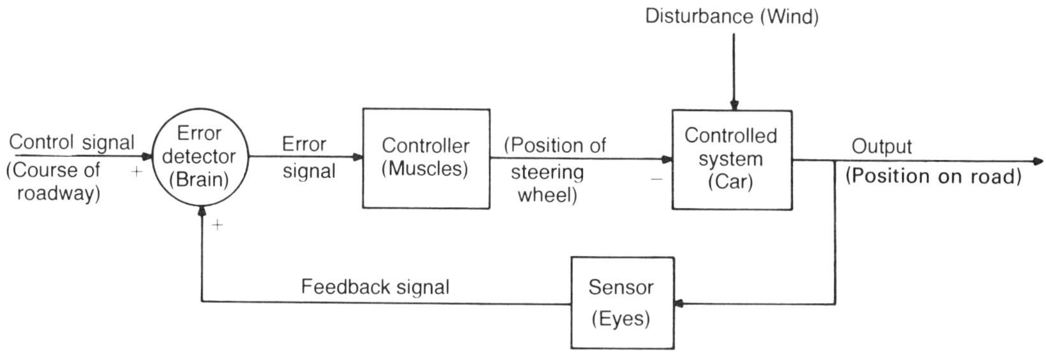

FIG. 15-5. Block diagram of a generalized feedback control system. The operation performed by each component is indicated by its name. **Arrows** indicate the unidirectional flow of information. Any feedback control system can be drawn in this form. Terms indicated in parentheses refer to the car analogy used in the text. (Houk J, Henneman E: Feedback control of muscle: introductory concepts. In Mountcastle VB [ed.]: Medical Physiology, 13th ed., Vol. 1. St. Louis, Mosby, 1974)

FIG. 15-6. Block diagram of the control system involving the stretch reflex. This system controls muscle length. (Houk J, Henneman E: Feedback control of muscle: introductory concepts. In Mountcastle VB [ed.]: Medical Physiology, 13th ed., Vol. 1. St. Louis, Mosby, 1974)

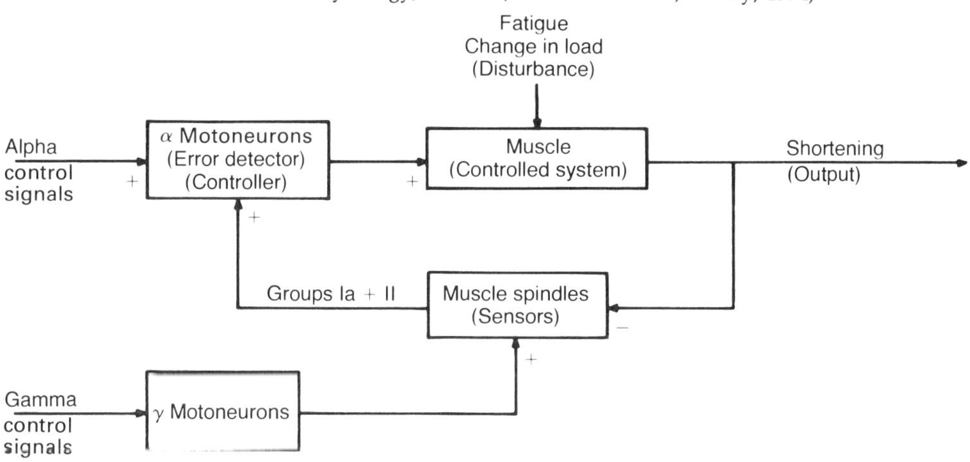

are all within the human operator. He senses the position of the car with his eyes (sensor), compares that with the course of the road (control signal), and, if they are not the same (an error exists), uses his muscles (controller) to turn the steering wheel to bring the car (controlled system) back to the appropriate position on the road (output). When the wind gusts, the car deviates from the course that would ordinarily be determined by the position of the wheel; the driver senses this and corrects for the disturbance.

It is possible to view the control of the driver's muscles in the same way. The muscle spindle receptors and their reflex connections form a feedback system to control muscle length, as shown in the block diagram of Figure 15-6. In this case, the control signal is a command from some supraspinal center to maintain the biceps muscle at some fixed length in order to hold a chair at a fixed distance off the floor. This signal is fed to spinal neurons, which are the error detectors, with the α motoneurons as the controller that signals the muscle (controlled system) to contract, producing enough force to decrease its length (output) and lift the chair off the floor. The muscle spindle endings (length and velocity sensors) sense the length of the muscle and transmit its length (feedback signal) back to the α motoneuron, where it is compared with the control signal. If the length of the muscle (or the height of the chair) is not as intended, a new error signal is generated, commanding more force and so on, around the system loop until the actual and intended muscle lengths are the same. Small deviations from the length specified by the control signal, for example due to fatigue, are sensed and quickly corrected in the same way.

Suddenly, someone drops a heavy book onto the chair and a disturbance of the system is produced by the sudden downward movement of the chair and the lengthening of the muscle. The spindle receptors sense the increased length and signal this increase to the α motoneurons, which detect the error and command more force to be generated by the muscle and the load to be lifted back to the intended height. In this manner, the system helps to maintain the length of the muscle in the face of changes in the load being lifted. Other disturbances are, of course, possible. The lifter's other hand could touch a hot object, evoking a flexion reflex and a crossed-extension reflex, or the ground could suddenly tilt due to an earthquake, yet the length of the muscle will be maintained constant until a new control signal comes to the α motoneuron. Suppose a new control signal orders the chair to be held higher. This new control signal will produce a large error signal, because it is quite different from the feedback signal. As a consequence, the controller will increase its output, resulting in more force that tends to decrease the error. There will be a continuous cycling around the loop until the error is reduced to zero and the new intended length is achieved.

Notice that the γ motoneurons affect the sensitivity of the sensors, so that any input that excites the γ motoneurons will result in an increase in the feedback signal because of the increase in spindle activity. The γ motoneurons also receive their own control signals, perhaps independent of those to α motoneurons, especially from cutaneous receptors and many supraspinal pathways, including the corticospinal, reticulospinal, and rubrospinal tracts. However, in general, pathways that influence α motoneurons also influence γ motoneurons **(alpha-gamma coactivation),** with the striking exception that group Ia afferent fibers do not influence γ motoneurons.

It has been suggested that some movements are initiated, not by control signals to α motoneurons, but by control signals to γ motoneurons. An increase in γ-motoneuron activity would result in a shortening of the intrafusal muscle fibers and an increase in the discharge of group Ia afferent fibers. This, in turn, would lead to an increase in α-motoneuron activity causing contraction of the extrafusal muscle fibers and shortening of the whole muscle. This mechanism is called the **follow-up length servo mechanism** of contraction, because the length of the spindle controls the length of the muscle and the changes in the length of the muscle *follow* the changes in the length of the spindle. It is not likely that this is the only mechanism by which contractions are initiated because of the alpha–gamma coactivation from most sources. Contractions are probably initiated mainly by direct action on the α motoneurons, but perhaps in some situations they are initiated by the follow-up length servo mechanism.

When a movement is initiated by α–γ coactivation, the coactivation can act as a servo-assistor. If the estimated load, as determined by the command signal, is correct, that is, if the actual load equals the estimated load, the spindle discharge will remain constant and no further reflex α-motoneuron excitation will occur. If the actual load exceeds the estimated load, there will be a misalignment of the intra- and extrafusal fibers, a large spindle discharge, and an increased α-motoneuron discharge with increased tension. On the other hand, if the actual load is less than the estimated load, there will be a different misalignment of the intra- and extrafusal fibers and a reduced spindle discharge leading to reduced α-motoneuron activation. In any case, α–γ coactivation ensures that the spindles will continue to act as length detectors even when the muscle shortens.

SUGGESTED READING

Fetz EE, Jankowska E, Johannisson T et al: Autogenetic inhibition of motoneurones by impulses in group Ia muscle spindle afferents. J Physiol (Lond) 293:173–195, 1979

Granit R: The Basis of Motor Control. New York, Academic Press, 1970

Henneman E: Spinal reflexes and the control of

movement. In Mountcastle VB [ed]: Medical Physiology. 13th ed., Vol. 1. St. Louis, Mosby, 1974

Homma S [ed]: Understanding the Stretch Reflex, Vol. 44. Progress in Brain Research. Amsterdam, Elsevier, 1976

Houk J, Henneman E: Feedback control of muscle: introductory concepts. In Mountcastle VB [ed]: Medical Physiology, 13th ed., Vol. 1. St. Louis, Mosby, 1974

Hunt CC, Perl ER: Spinal reflex mechanisms concerned with skeletal muscle. Physiol Rev 40:538–579, 1960

Matthews PBC: Mammalian Muscle Receptors and their Central Actions. Baltimore, Williams and Wilkins, 1972

16

Initiation and Control of Movement

Control over movement is exerted by *all* parts of the nervous system, not just those identified as "motor" in textbooks. The participation of α motoneurons in motor control is obvious; without them there can be no movement! Considering our knowledge of reflex pathways, the roles of the primary afferent neurons, certain interneurons, and the γ motoneurons seem fairly evident. Most of the nerve fibers that innervate a muscle are there to sense and control the length and tension of the muscle, not to make it contract. This is clearly seen in Table 16-1. In the cat soleus muscle, there are about 50 group Ia fibers, 50 group II fibers, 40 group Ib fibers, and 100 γ motoneurons compared with only 150 α motoneurons. This means the muscle has 240 nerve fibers for control and only 150 for contraction. Clearly the bias is in favor of control.

At the spinal cord segmental level, a considerable amount of organization of movement is already apparent as indicated by reflex patterns in spinal animals. Reciprocal innervation is the sort of mechanism of coordination one might expect to find in the spinal cord to "allow" movement to occur, but other reflex patterns, such as the compensation contributed by the crossed-extension pathway, may not be entirely expected. In addition, in the spinal cord, there are even higher levels of coordination. The scratch reflex in animals, for example, is mediated entirely at the spinal cord level, and patterns of movement reminiscent of walking, that is, a series of alternating flexions and extensions of the limbs, can be seen in the spinal human or animal. It has been shown that the stepping cycle in experimental animals depends upon rhythmic activity that is generated in the spinal cord itself and not by primary afferent fibers or descending influences. This is not to say that walking is entirely a spinal cord event, but many of the neural circuits for the behavior are there. There is more to walking, however, than just the generation of the stepping cycle. It is also necessary to coordinate the movements of upper and lower limbs during walking or running and, to a certain extent, this also appears to be mediated at the spinal cord level. The stepping must be performed in relationship to the environment so that the foot is put on level ground and not in a hole, so that walking is in relationship to the intended course, and so that moving obstacles can be avoided. These adjustments and corrections are the province of supraspinal structures. We will have more to say about this subject later.

SPINAL CORD TRANSECTION

A view of the net effect of supraspinal pathways (pathways descending from structures above the spinal cord) upon the spinal cord circuits can be seen in experimental cord transections or in cases of accidental cord transection in humans. With modern car traffic, this is not a terribly rare event in humans, and if it occurs below the level of the spinal roots containing fibers of the phrenic nerve (C3–C5), the chances of survival without life-support systems are good because the diaphragm still functions. Immediately after transection of the spinal cord, all movement as well as all sensation and all reflexes is lost in the parts of the body innervated by the segments below the cut. This temporary condition is called **spinal shock.** The duration of spinal shock is variable, though usually of the order of several weeks in humans, less long in other species. Spinal shock is understandable in terms of the excitability of central neurons, among them the α motoneurons, which is determined by the sum total of the excitatory and inhibitory synaptic inputs to them. Apparently, the net effect of removing all supraspinal influences on motoneurons is the elimination of a significant excitation. Under these conditions, even the normally powerful group Ia afferent fibers are without their usual effect as indicated by the **areflexia,** that is, the absence of reflexes. This points out again the importance of summation in setting the excitability levels and firing patterns of neurons.

An indicator of the onset of the period of recovery from spinal shock is the appearance of flexion reflexes, which are mediated by polysynaptic pathways. One of the earliest to appear is the Babinski sign, which is a symptom associated with pyramidal tract disorder. Over time, the flexion reflexes become stronger and usually become hyperactive to the point that a small stimulus sets off a generalized flexion reflex. During this increase in flexor reflex activity, the stretch reflexes make their appearance and grow in excitability until they are exaggerated. With the **hyper-reflexia** (greater than normal reflex activity) in extensors, a **spasticity** develops. Spasticity is a strong and persisting contraction of either flexors or extensors but not both and should not be confused with **rigidity,** which is a resistance to movement due to hyperactivity of both flexors and extensors at the same joint. With the spasticity comes the clasp-knife reflex, **clonus** (rhythmic, alternating contraction and relaxation of a rapidly and briefly stretched muscle), and brisk tendon jerk reflexes.

During spinal shock, the bladder wall is atonic, with increased sphincter tone, resulting in extensive dilatation of the bladder. During recovery, there is a gradual increase in wall tone, and emptying may occur with exaggerated flexion reflexes. Vasomotor control (control of blood vessel diameter) is also lost below the transection during spinal shock, and postural hypotension (reduced blood pressure when standing) becomes a problem for the "spinal" patient. During recovery, the automatic control of vessel diameter returns and the problem disappears.

TABLE 16-1. INNERVATION OF THE CAT'S SOLEUS MUSCLE

Afferent	
50 group Ia fibers	50 spindle primary endings
40 group Ib fibers	45 Golgi tendon organs
50 group II fibers	50 spindle secondary endings
Efferent	
100 γ motoneurons	300 intrafusal muscle fibers in 50 spindles
150 α motoneurons	25,000 extrafusal muscle fibers

When the transection occurs at higher spinal cord levels, the control of body temperature is lost. The more of the spinal cord left connected to the brain by a transection, the more temperature regulation returns after spinal shock, presumably because more of the exit pathways from the spinal cord are available. Endocrine function will be impaired to the extent that it is mediated by the autonomic nervous system or requires sensory information carried by the nervous system for its regulation. The more spinal cord there is connected to the brain stem, the more of the thoracicolumbar and craniosacral efferent fibers are available for use in regulating both temperature and endocrine function.

DISRUPTIONS OF THE HIGHER NEURAXIS

A strikingly different pattern of effects is produced by lesions at higher levels of the central nervous system. Table 16-2 gives a summary of the experimental lesions and their effects. The levels of the lesions are shown in Figure 16-1. The decerebrate and decorticate conditions are seen in humans, though the decorticate is uncommon. Sectioning the brain stem and certain vascular lesions at the anterior border of the

TABLE 16-2. BRAIN-STEM CONTROL OF MOVEMENT

LESION OR PREPARATION	FLACCIDITY	EXTENSOR SPASTICITY	STANDS	RIGHTS	WALKS	TEMP. H_2O ENDO CONTROL	SHAM RAGE
1. Spinal	Early in spinal shock	Later after recovery	No	Depends on level	No	Depends on level	No
2. Low decerebrate* (bulbospinal)	No	Yes	Not by itself	No	No	No	No
3. Sherringtonian* (midcollicular)	No	Yes, extreme	Not by itself	Reflexes present, but not the full behavior	No	No	No
4. High decerebrate (mesencephalic)	No	Yes, but less than above and not during movement	Yes	Yes	Yes	No	Yes, but less violent than below
5. Hypothalamic	No	Yes, but less	Yes	Yes	Yes	Yes	Yes
6. Decorticate	Only if decortication is limited to cortical area 4	Yes, but least	Yes	Yes	Yes	Yes	Yes

* Usually comatose in human

FIG. 16-1. The locations of lesions of the neuraxis whose consequences are listed in Table 16-2. Numbers correspond to the numbered lesions in the table. The lesions are drawn on the brain of a cat.

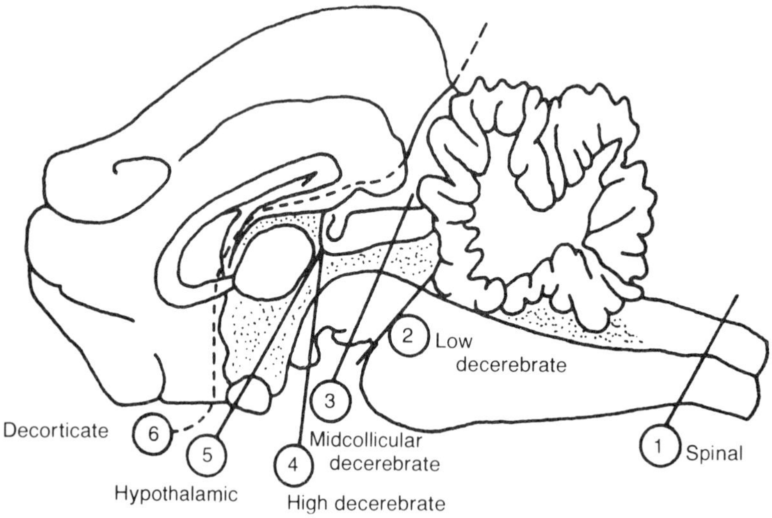

trapezoid body produces what is known as a "low decerebration." The low decerebrate human is usually comatose and shows extensor spasticity as in the later stages of spinal transection, but of more severity. The low decerebrate animal cannot stand by itself in spite of the heightened extensor tone, partly because it lacks vestibular control to maintain upright posture. It cannot right itself if turned upside down; it cannot walk; and it cannot regulate its temperature or endocrine function.

A slightly higher lesion, at midcollicular levels, produces a "Sherringtonian" decerebration. The lesion in the human is often caused by impact on the vertex as a result of a fall or, commonly, as a result of flying over the handle bars of a motorcycle that has made a sudden stop! Extensor spasticity is extreme in the Sherringtonian patient, causing it to be termed **decerebrate "rigidity,"** but in truth the condition is a spasticity. Extensor muscles are in extreme contraction, giving off large amounts of heat, driving the body temperature up, and throwing the person into a posture with the head thrown back and back arched **(opisthotonos)** and the arms, legs, and digits extended. The Sherringtonian decerebrate animal resembles the low decerebrate animal except for the severity of the spasticity and the presence of certain postural reflexes. Rotation of the head increases extensor contraction on the side toward which it is turned and decreases it on the other side, but the animal still cannot stand or right itself.

Decerebrate rigidity requires intact dorsal roots. Cutting the roots eliminates the spasticity, producing a flaccid paralysis, but this is not a reasonable treatment, because the spasticity either goes away by itself or the patient never regains consciousness; in either case cut roots would be of no advantage. The low decerebrate condition depends upon activity descending mainly through the lateral vestibulospinal tract from Deiters' nucleus, whereas the Sherringtonian condition also depends upon activity in the pontine reticulospinal tract. Presumably, the lesions that produce the spasticity remove an ongoing net inhibitory influence, exerted upon these tracts by structures above them, allowing them to excite the extensor motoneurons continuously. With the return of function of the higher structures in recovery, the vestibulo- and reticulospinal tracts are again brought under control. Elimination of the spasticity by dorsal root section implies that descending influences are exerted upon γ motoneurons, not α motoneurons; thus it is called **gamma spasticity.** Removal of the cerebellum during gamma spasticity increases the spasticity, but the spasticity is no longer abolished by dorsal root transection, implying that the effect is due to strong activation of α motoneurons, that is, that it is an **alpha spasticity.**

Transections above mesencephalic and hypothalamic levels rarely occur in humans, but they can be produced in animals. Extensor spasticity is present following lesions at both levels, but it is less severe when more tissue is left intact. Animals with experimentally induced lesions at either level can stand unaided, right themselves when inverted, and walk. The high decerebrate or mesencephalic spasticity disappears when the animal moves by itself. The hypothalamic animal regulates its temperature and endocrine function to some extent, because important autonomic centers in the hypothalamus are spared. Both mesencephalic and hypothalamic lesions lead to a phenomenon known as **sham rage,** which is characterized by biting and hissing when the tail is pinched, but this behavior is not directed toward the offending object (it is thus *sham* rage).

If the cerebral cortex is destroyed or separated from the rest of the system by a lesion of the internal capsule, a constellation of symptoms similar to that in the animal with a hypothalamic lesion is seen. With large-scale removal of cortex, extensor spasticity develops, but it is less severe than in any of the other conditions. If, on the other hand, the lesion is limited to cortical area 4, the "motor" cortex, **flaccidity** develops instead of spasticity. Possibly, the reduced severity of the spasticity with lesions at higher levels indicates that the activity of the vestibulospinal and reticulospinal tracts is more inhibited when more tissue is left in connection with them, but there are other tracts that originate at higher levels, for example, the rubrospinal tract, which could be exerting inhibitory effects directly upon extensor α motoneurons or indirectly upon extensor γ motoneurons through excitation of flexor α motoneurons or flexor γ motoneurons and reciprocal innervation.

SUPRASPINAL MOTOR CENTERS

Many structures above the spinal cord have been referred to as motor structures, and it is to them that we turn our attention. In this section, anatomic and physiologic circuits within each structure are discussed, along with current concepts of their role in movement. In addition, clinical manifestations of diseases involving these structures are presented. A later section of this chapter presents a synthesis of the control of movement, involving all these structures.

THE BRAIN STEM

Brain-stem pathways usually recognized as motor include those arising from the vestibular nuclei (vestibulospinal), the interstitial nucleus of Cajal (interstitiospinal), the pontine and medullary reticular formation (reticulospinal), and the red nucleus (rubrospinal). In addition to these well-known motor centers, the brain-stem motor systems involve areas of the hypothalamus and the limbic system (see Chap. 17 for further discussion of the hypothalamus and Chap. 21 for the limbic system).

Lesions that selectively interrupt the vestibulo-, interstitio-, and reticulospinal tracts in humans are rare if they ever occur at all, but they can be produced in animals. Such interruptions in monkeys lead to a flexion bias of the trunk and limbs that is manifested in forward slumping in sitting postures, retraction of the shoulders, and slight flexion of the elbow joint. (This picture contrasts sharply with the extensor bias resulting from transection of the neuraxis as discussed previously.) The monkeys stand with a crouched posture, walk with an unsteady gait, and have some impairment of righting ability, at least early after the surgery. They often miss their targets in jumping and show ataxia (a lack of fluidity of movement) involving mainly axial and proximal muscles, those of the trunk and proximal parts of the extremities. On the other hand, these animals show no impairment of ability to use their hands and fingers.

The effects of rubrospinal tract (and, as we shall see later, also pyramidal tract) interruption are quite different. Following rubrospinal lesions there is no unsteadiness of gait and no proximal ataxia or flexion bias. Rather, the impairments are found in independent finger and hand movements and ability to flex the extended limb. By contrast, animals with rubrospinal tract interruption reach for objects using mainly the proximal arm and trunk muscles, whereas those with vestibulo-, interstitio-, and reticulospinal interruption reach using the distal muscles of the limb more than the proximal muscles.

These observations have led to the suggestion that the ventromedial brain-stem pathways—vestibulo-, interstitio-, and reticulospinal—are especially concerned with maintenance of erect posture and integrated movements of body and limbs, and with directing the course of movement. The lateral brain-stem pathway—rubrospinal—is suggested to be responsible for the capacity for independent use of the extremity, particularly the hand. The corticospinal pathway would then provide a capacity similar to that provided by the rubrospinal tract, but, in addition, would provide for further independence of movement, especially by individual fingers. As we shall see when discussing the pyramidal tract in detail, the picture of movement control is not quite this simple. The ventromedial brain-stem pathways also exert some influence on distal musculature, and the lateral brain-stem pathway and corticospinal tract also influence proximal musculature. In addition, the foregoing suggestion does not easily explain the small size of the red nucleus and rubrospinal tract in man or the very well developed pyramidal tracts in some animals, notably seals, that do not have independent finger movements, but it serves at least to summarize the main deficiencies that occur when these pathways are interrupted.

Movements can be evoked by electrical stimulation of many sites within the central nervous system. Electrical stimulation of the cerebral neocortex leads to movements of parts of the body or, if suitably small stimuli are used, contractions of individual muscles, but complex behaviors (patterns of movements) are usually not evoked by neocortical stimulation. In contrast, stimulation of certain areas of the brain stem leads to complex motor patterns, involving sequential performance of a variety of movements. This suggests that the brain stem contains "hard-wired circuits," specific, permanent neural connections, for such complex motor patterns. Some examples may help to illustrate the types of motor patterns evoked by brain-stem stimulation. Stimulation within the lateral hypothalamus leads to eating, possibly because it induces sensations of hunger. Electrical stimulation of other points within the lateral hypothalamus leads to nest building, paper gathering, and gnawing (not eating, just chewing, for example on wooden blocks) behavior in rats. Sexual activity in rats can be induced by stimulation of certain sites in the posterior and anterior dorsolateral hypothalamus. Attack and escape

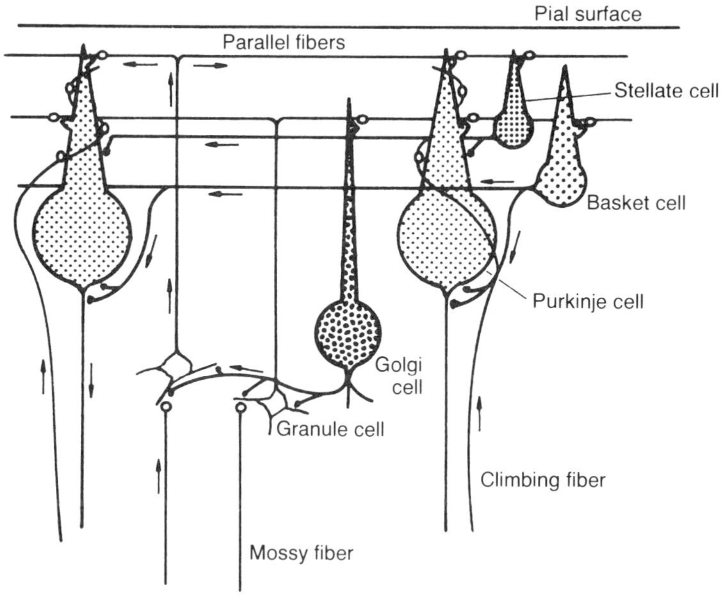

FIG. 16-2. Circuit diagram of the cerebellar cortex. Two sources of afferent impulses, mossy and climbing fibers; one efferent cell, Purkinje cell (two are shown); one excitatory interneuron, granule cell; and three inhibitory interneurons, Golgi, basket, and stellate cells, are shown. (Allen GI, Tsukahara N: Physiol Rev 54:957–1006, 1974)

behaviors can similarly be elicited by stimulation of regions of the amygdala (the amygdala is cortical tissue, but not neocortical), hypothalamus, and mesencephalon.

It seems likely that these sorts of stereotyped behaviors are permanently "wired" into the nervous system and simply triggered or both triggered and modulated by activity from the peripheral receptors and from the cerebral cortex or elsewhere within the central nervous system. Exactly where the neural circuits for these behaviors may be localized, if in fact they are, is not known.

THE CEREBELLUM

The cerebellum lies over the brain stem and is connected to the medulla by three thick connectives, the inferior, middle, and superior cerebellar peduncles. The outer surface, called the cortex, is highly convoluted and covers a region of white matter, containing inputs and outputs from the cortex, and a region of nuclei: the fastigial, dentate, globose, and emboliform nuclei. (The last two are indistinct in animals other than apes and man and together are termed the nucleus interpositus.) The cortex is divided into three zones: the vermis, the hemisphere, and the flocculonodular lobe. The flocculonodular lobe is completely buried in man; it is phylogenetically the oldest part of the cerebellum, and comparative anatomists say it has changed little throughout its evolution. The vermis constitutes the majority of the cerebellum in most animals, but in apes and man it is quite overshadowed by the hemispheres. Anatomists divide the vermis into many parts; for our purposes it suffices to treat it as a single unit lying along the midline of the cerebellum. The hemispheres, on the other hand, can be usefully divided into an intermediate zone (also called pars intermedia or paravermis), flanking the vermis, and a lateral zone (or pars lateralis).

The cellular structure of the cerebellar cortex is practically identical throughout, and therefore it is possible to draw a circuit diagram for the cerebellum as shown in Figure 16-2. The cortex has two kinds of afferent fibers: the climbing fibers, so named because they ascend into the cortex and climb along the Purkinje cells' dendrites, and the mossy fibers, named for their microscopic appearance. Most (some say all) of the

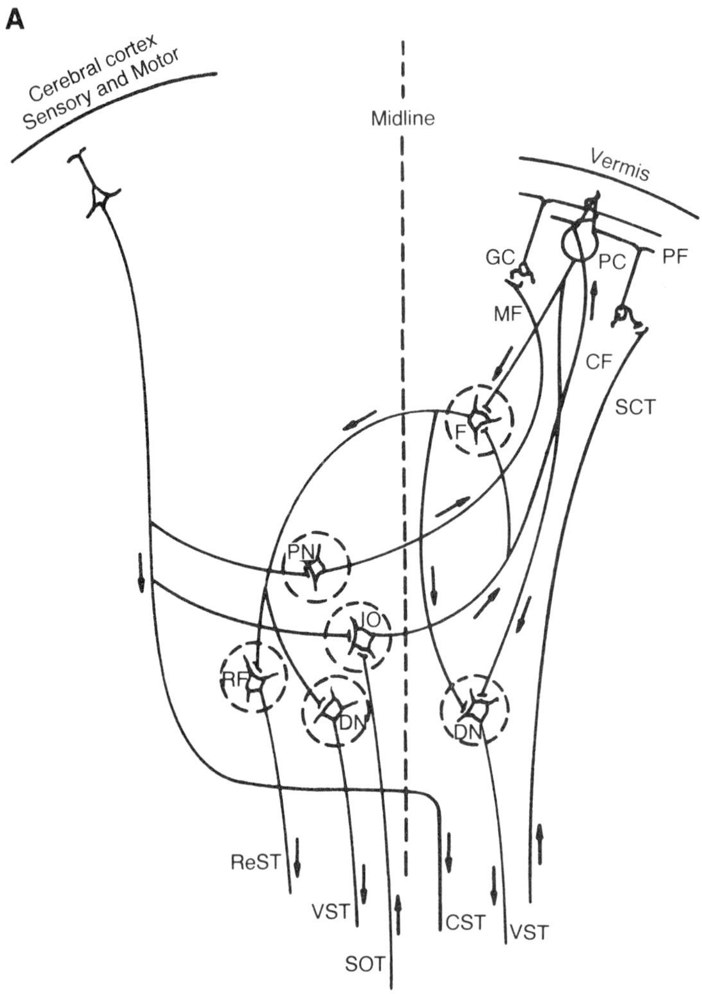

FIG. 16-3. Cellular connections of the cerebellar cortex. Synaptic connections of cerebellar vermis **(A)**, hemisphere, pars intermedia **(B)**, and hemisphere, pars lateralis **(C)** are shown with the cerebral cortex and descending tracts. Abbreviations are as follows: CF = climbing fiber; CST = corticospinal tract, D = dentate nucleus; DN = Deiters' nucleus; F = fastigial nucleus; GC = granule cell; IO = inferior olive; IP = interpositus nucleus; LRN = lateral reticular nucleus; MF = mossy fiber; PC = Purkinje cell; PF = parallel fiber; PN = pontine nucleus; ReST = reticulospinal tract; RF = reticular formation; RN = red nucleus; RST = rubrospinal tract; SCT = spinocerebellar tracts; SOT = spino-olivary tracts; VL = nucleus ventralis lateralis of thalamus; VST = vestibulospinal tract. (Allen GI, Tsukahara N: Physiol Rev 54:957–1006, 1974)

climbing fibers come from the inferior olive, whereas the mossy fibers come from the pontine nuclei, the lateral reticular nucleus, the spinocerebellar tracts, and perhaps elsewhere. There are two "straight-through" pathways in the cerebellar cortex: one involving direct excitation of the output neurons, the Purkinje cells, by the incoming climbing fiber activity, the other involving indirect excitation of Purkinje cells by incoming mossy fiber activity by way of the granule cells and their axons, the parallel fibers. The interneurons of the cerebellar cortex, other than granule cells, are all thought to be inhibitory to Purkinje cells or to the mossy fiber–granule cell relay. These interneurons, called basket cells, Golgi cells, and stellate cells, are excited by mossy fiber activity through the granule cells and perhaps also by climbing fiber activity. As a result of the circuit shown in Figure 16-2, the mossy fiber input excites the Purkinje cells and then inhibits them by a **feedforward inhibition** (inhibition at a subsequent site in the pathway) mediated by stellate and basket cells and inhibits their subse-

B

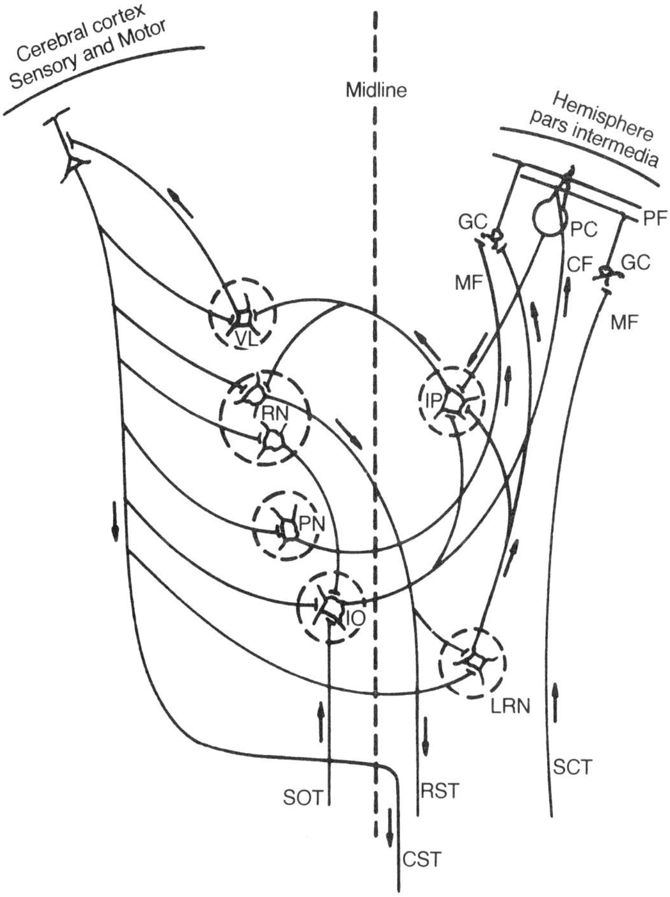
Cerebral cortex
Sensory and Motor
Midline
Hemisphere
pars intermedia
GC
PC
PF
CF
GC
MF
MF
VL
RN
IP
PN
IO
LRN
SOT
RST
SCT
CST

C

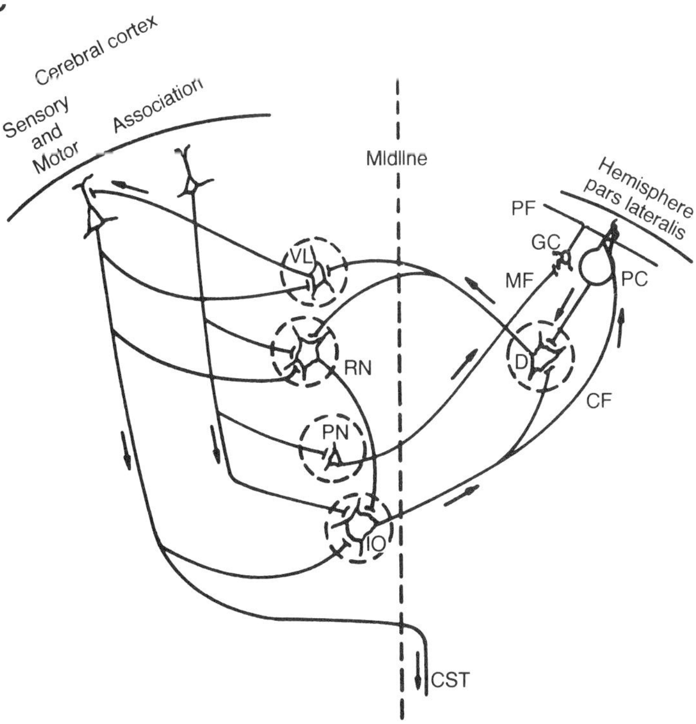
Cerebral cortex
Sensory
and
Motor
Association
Midline
Hemisphere
pars lateralis
PF
GC
MF
PC
VL
RN
D
CF
PN
IO
CST

quent inputs through mossy fibers by a **feedback inhibition** (inhibition at a previous site in the pathway) mediated by Golgi cells. The only output of the cerebellar cortex is by way of Purkinje cell axons that inhibit their target neurons in the cerebellar nuclei and elsewhere.

The major differences between the various portions of the cerebellar cortex are the origin of the mossy fibers that enter them and the destinations of the Purkinje cells leaving them. This is shown schematically in Figure 16-3. Mossy fibers to the vermis originate in the spinocerebellar tracts and the lateral reticular nucleus. The vermal Purkinje cells send their axons to the fastigial nucleus and to Deiters' vestibular nucleus. For comparison, the mossy fibers to the pars intermedia of the hemisphere come from the lateral reticular nucleus, the pontine nuclei, and the spinocerebellar tracts; the pars lateralis receives mossy fibers only from the pontine nuclei. The Purkinje axons of the intermediate lobe project to the globose and emboliform (interpositus) nuclei, whereas those from the lateral lobe project to the dentate nucleus.

The pontine nuclei receive inputs from the cerebral cortex both through collaterals of pyramidal tract axons and through corticopontine fibers. The lateral reticular nucleus receives its inputs from the cerebral cortex, from spinoreticular pathways, from the red nucleus, and the fastigial nucleus. The inferior olive, the source of most climbing fibers, receives its input from the cerebral cortex, the spino-olivary tract, the red nucleus, and perhaps the caudate nucleus.

Because the neuronal circuit is the same throughout the cerebellar cortex, its mode of operation can be indicated using the lateral hemisphere as an example. The same sort of analysis will presumably apply to any of the other components. The pontine fibers, on their way to the lateral cortex, give off a collateral to the dentate nucleus. This is an excitatory connection. In the cortex, the pontine mossy fibers excite granule cells that, in turn, excite (through their axons, the parallel fibers) Purkinje cells and inhibitory interneurons. Thus, the Purkinje cells are first excited and then inhibited. The Purkinje cell output thus inhibits the dentate nucleus for a short time. The result, for the cerebellar nuclei, is first excitation (through direct mossy fiber inputs) and then inhibition (through the cortical circuits). The same pattern also holds for climbing fibers: the climbing fiber first excites the nuclear cells and then they are inhibited by climbing fiber activation of the inhibitory Purkinje cells.

This detailed discussion of cerebellar anatomy and physiology was presented to illustrate the detail in which anatomic connections of parts of the CNS are known and to illustrate how knowledge of the anatomic and physiologic relationships can be used to suggest the role of the cerebellum in movement. Table 16-3 presents a summary of the inputs to and outputs from the various parts of the cerebellum. The vermis and the associated fastigial nucleus get their major inputs from the peripheral sensory receptors and send their outputs back to the spinal cord by way of the reticulospinal and vestibulospinal tracts. We have already seen how powerful these outputs can be in decerebrate rigidity. It has been argued that this close connection with the spinal cord motor nuclei makes the vermis well suited for making follow-up corrections, corrections necessary to bring the actual movement into line with the intended movement. The hemisphere pars intermedia, on the other hand, gets both cerebral cortical and peripheral sensory inputs and sends outputs back to the cerebral cortex and to the peripheral motor apparatus by way of the rubrospinal and pyramidal tracts. The suggestion has been made that the intermediate lobe of the cerebellum participates in movement correction or modification *before* the movement is completed. The output through rapidly conducting rubrospinal and corticospinal fibers is consistent with this idea, but fibers in the reticulospinal and vestibulospinal tracts also conduct rapidly.

The pars lateralis of the hemisphere apparently does not receive a significant input from peripheral sensory receptors, instead receiving its inputs from the sensory, motor, and association cortices. It sends its output, through the dentate nucleus, back to the sensory and motor cortices. The suggestion has been made that the lateral hemispheres work with the association cortex in planning movements rather than in executing and correcting them. There is, however, little or no compelling evidence that either the association cortex or the cerebellar hemi-

TABLE 16-3. SUMMARY OF CEREBELLAR CONNECTIONS

	VERMIS	HEMISPHERE: PARS INTERMEDIA	HEMISPHERE: PARS LATERALIS	FLOCCULONODULAR LOBE
Source of afferent fibers	Peripheral receptors: via spinocerebellar tracts; via lateral reticular nucleus; via inferior olive Sensory and motor cortex: via pontine nuclei	Peripheral receptors: via spinocerebellar tracts Sensory and motor cortex: via pontine nuclei; via lateral reticular nucleus; via red nucleus and inferior olive	Sensory and motor cortex: via pontine nuclei; via inferior olive	Same as vermis
Destination of nuclear fibers	Fastigial to reticular nucleus and reticulospinal tract Fastigial to Deiters' nucleus and vestibulospinal tract Direct Purkinje cell influence on Deiters' nucleus	Interpositus to thalamus, nucleus VL, sensory and motor cortex and pyramidal tract Interpositus to red nucleus and rubrospinal tract*	Dentate to thalamus, nucleus VL, sensory and motor cortex and pyramidal tract Dentate to red nucleus and rubrospinal tract*	Direct Purkinje cell influence on all vestibular nuclei

* This pathway may not be of great significance because of the reduction in size of the red nucleus in man.

spheres actually participate in movement planning. Cooling the dentate nucleus makes monkeys move more slowly, require more sensory cues to guide performance, and make more errors. Similar deficits are seen in some patients with parkinsonism, a disease of the basal ganglia.

Clinical manifestations of cerebellar disease are consistent with a role in coordination of muscle contraction and in prediction and correction of motor events in order to achieve proper force, direction, and rate of movement. Decerebellation is apparently without effect on sensation and intelligence, but the resulting motor deficits are profound. Patients with lesions in the cerebellar peduncles or with cerebellar degeneration, the most common cause of which is excessive chronic alcohol intake **(alcoholic cerebellar degeneration),** may show any or all of these symptoms: (1) cerebellar ataxia, (2) hypotonia, (3) asthenia, (4) decomposition of movement, (5) dyssynergia, (6) dysmetria, (7) dysdiadochokinesia, (8) scanning speech, and (9) intention tremor. The patient with cerebellar disease may show **ataxia,** a lack of fluidity in movement that is manifested in walking as a wide-based gait with staggering and reeling, a characteristic seen also in the acute drunken state. The patient with cerebellar disease has **hypotonia,** a decrease in muscle tone that shows up as excessive pendular, back-and-forth oscillations of the lower limb when the patellar tendon is tapped, and **asthenia,** a muscle weakness that is usually moderate. He has impaired cooperation of all muscle groups so that movements normally made up of many parts in a fluid, continuous whole, are broken up into a series of unitary movements. For example, in stepping over an object, the patient may first raise his leg to the correct height, then move it forward past the object, and only then start to put it down. This is **decomposition of movement.**

A similar abnormality is **dyssynergia,** a term that refers to lack of cooperation between closely related muscle groups. The usual test for dyssynergia is to have the supine patient touch one knee with the opposite heel and then slide the heel down the leg to the ankle, a movement requiring cooperation of a number of muscles. The cerebellar patient shows a great deal of difficulty doing this. **Dysmetria** is an abnormality in the range of movement. The patient is unable to start and stop the movement at appropriate times so that he undershoots or overshoots intended targets. The common clinical task for the patient is to touch alternately the examiner's finger and his own nose. It is an easy task for a normal person. Rapid, alternating movements are also impaired with cerebellar disease. Alternate pronation and supination of the hand, for example, done slowly and with difficulty is a common sign, termed **dysdiadochokinesia.**

Patients with cerebellar disease often have difficulties speaking, using irregular volume or speech rhythms, due to inability to control accurately the rate of flow of air past the vocal cords. This is termed **scanning speech.** In addition, the patient may demonstrate a tremor, but it is subdued, perhaps even unnoticeable, except when the person is actively engaged in some movement. This is **intention tremor,** which should be distinguished from the tremor at rest of the patient with basal ganglion disease.

Damage to the cerebellum caused by wounds instead of disease, presents a slightly different picture. Surgeons have occasion to remove a part of the lateral aspect of the cerebellum in surgery for tumors of the VIIIth cranial nerve, and they normally find only minor and transient deficiencies. On the other hand, even minimal damage to the dentate nucleus can produce the symptoms described above. Cerebellar symptoms can also be produced by a medulloblastoma, a tumor that arises from the fourth ventricle in children and involves mainly flocculonodular tissue producing dysequilibrium, nystagmus (rapid lateral eye movements), and obstruction of cerebrospinal fluid flow. It is difficult, however, in this case to rule out involvement of the deep cerebellar nuclei, which appears to be more detrimental than involvement of the cerebellar cortex alone. It should also be stressed that removal of a section of tissue is quite different from having the tissue present but functioning abnormally. Malfunctioning tissue can be expected to have more severe consequences than the absence of tissue. Perhaps a good analogy is an electronic computer. If you go around behind it and remove a small part, it will probably have a smaller, more predictable, and more easily compensated effect on the functioning of the computer than if you were to stand there and intermittently short-out a part of the circuit. Apparently, other parts of the nervous system can "fill in" for the cerebellum, because an occasional child is born without one (at least, without the vermis) and without cerebellar symptoms (Dandy-Walker syndrome). Whatever the function of the cerebellum is, that function can apparently be assumed by other parts of the nervous system if the cerebellum fails to develop or is damaged in a young child.

THE BASAL GANGLIA

The term basal ganglia has been applied to a number of structures but is now reserved for six specific structures: the caudate nucleus, putamen, globus pallidus, claustrum, subthalamic nucleus, and substantia nigra. The basal ganglia appear to be part of a neural loop involving cerebral cortex, basal ganglia, thalamus, and cerebral cortex again. The major anatomic connections through the basal ganglia appear to be from the cerebral cortex to the caudate nucleus and putamen, then to the globus pallidus, to the thalamus, and back to the motor and premotor cortex. It is particularly the motor cortex that gets the output from the basal ganglia, but a number of cortical areas provide inputs to the basal ganglia. The globus pallidus is interconnected with both the subthalamic nucleus and the substantia nigra. A dopamine-containing pathway from the substantia nigra to the caudate nucleus and putamen has received attention for its role in production of parkinsonism. The basal ganglia do not influence α motoneurons directly; their influences on movement are exerted only indirectly through the cerebral cortex. Information from the basal ganglia and the cerebellum could possibly be integrated in the thalamic nucleus ventralis lateralis, which relays activity from both sources to the motor cortex. We have no idea what the basal ganglia do, but, because of their connections and the nature of the syndromes associated with them, we say they have some motor function.

The **choreas** (dancelike movements) are a group of basal ganglion disorders characterized by rapid involuntary movements **(dyskinesia),** largely restricted to muscles of the distal extremity and face, though others may be involved. These are usually accompanied by a decrease in muscle tone. Huntington's chorea is a devastating disease with progressive dyskinesia and **dementia** (loss of intellectual function). The disease is inherited (autosomal dominant pattern) and of late onset, usually after the child-bearing years. Histologically, the brains of patients with Huntington's chorea show profound loss of neurons and gliosis in the basal ganglia and the cerebral cortex, but this is particularly notable in the caudate nucleus. Evidence has been presented that Huntington's disease is accompanied by a decrease in glutamic acid decarboxylase, the enzyme responsible for converting L-glutamic acid to γ-aminobutyric acid, a putative inhibitory transmitter substance. Whether this reflects a specific enzyme defect or just a reduced amount due to to the reduced cellular population is unknown.

Ballisms are involuntary movement disorders that are normally unilateral and characterized by violent flailing and swinging of the extremities due to activity in proximal muscles. They are frequently of sudden onset, which may suggest a vascular origin, a suggestion supported by pathologic findings of small infarctions in or near the contralateral subthalamic nucleus in patients with ballism.

Unlike the choreiform or ballistic movements, those characterizing **athetosis** are slow and twisting movements of the extremities including the hands and feet. Pathologic examination usually reveals atrophy of the putamen, and there is usually a history of perinatal hypoxia. The hypoxia can sometimes be the result of hemolysis due to Rh or other incompatibility between the blood of the mother and the fetus.

The most common and, therefore, most well-known of the basal ganglia disorders is **parkinsonism.** The patient with Parkinson's disease has true rigidity, in contrast to the spasticities of brain-stem disorders. Both flexors and extensors contract together, and resistance to stretch is present throughout the entire range of passive movement and at any speed. When the rigid muscle is extended passively, it lengthens in steps as if it were a stick being dragged over a series of notches in a piece of wood. This is called **cogwheel rigidity.** Tremor in parkinsonism usually involves the extremities, but may also involve the face. The tremor is a **tremor at rest;** the amplitude of the tremor is often reduced during active movements, but usually does not disappear. In the hand, the tremor takes the form of the extension of the interphalangeal joints and flexion of the metacarpalphalangeal joints so the fingers beat against the thumb about five times per second.

Patients with parkinsonism usually either do not move much **(akinesia)** or they move only slowly **(bradykinesia).** However, their startle responses are normally quite rapid. They lack facial expressions, being described as having **masklike faces,** but they can generate a happy or sad face if they are requested to do so. They show **postural fixations,** in which they assume abnormal postures in spite of their ability to assume normal ones. For example, the posture of a parkinsonian patient normally involves flexion of head and neck, in contrast to the straight head and neck of an unaffected person. The gait of these patients is usually a shuffling one with small steps and a wide stance, without swinging of the arms. Because they cannot make rapid postural reflex movements, most of the patients easily lose their balance, so the wide stance and small steps are understandable.

It is rare that a specific pathologic condition can be associated with parkinsonism. Sometimes the disease develops after (up to 10 years after) cases of encephalitis and is part of the syndromes of both manganese and carbon monoxide poisoning. A reversible form of the disease is induced in some patients by the phenothiazine tranquilizers used in treatment of some psychiatric disorders. A consistent finding is a depigmentation of the substantia nigra that may be correlated somehow with a reduction in dopamine concentration. However, the dopamine concentration is highest in the caudate nucleus and putamen and shows largest reductions in these nuclei during parkinsonism. Eighty percent of the dopamine in brain is found in the basal ganglia. It has been suggested that dopamine is an inhibitory transmitter substance released by neurons of the substantia nigra onto caudate neurons. The symptoms of the disease, according to this hypothesis, are the result of the unchecked activity of neurons in the caudate nucleus. However, there are some people who are beginning to doubt

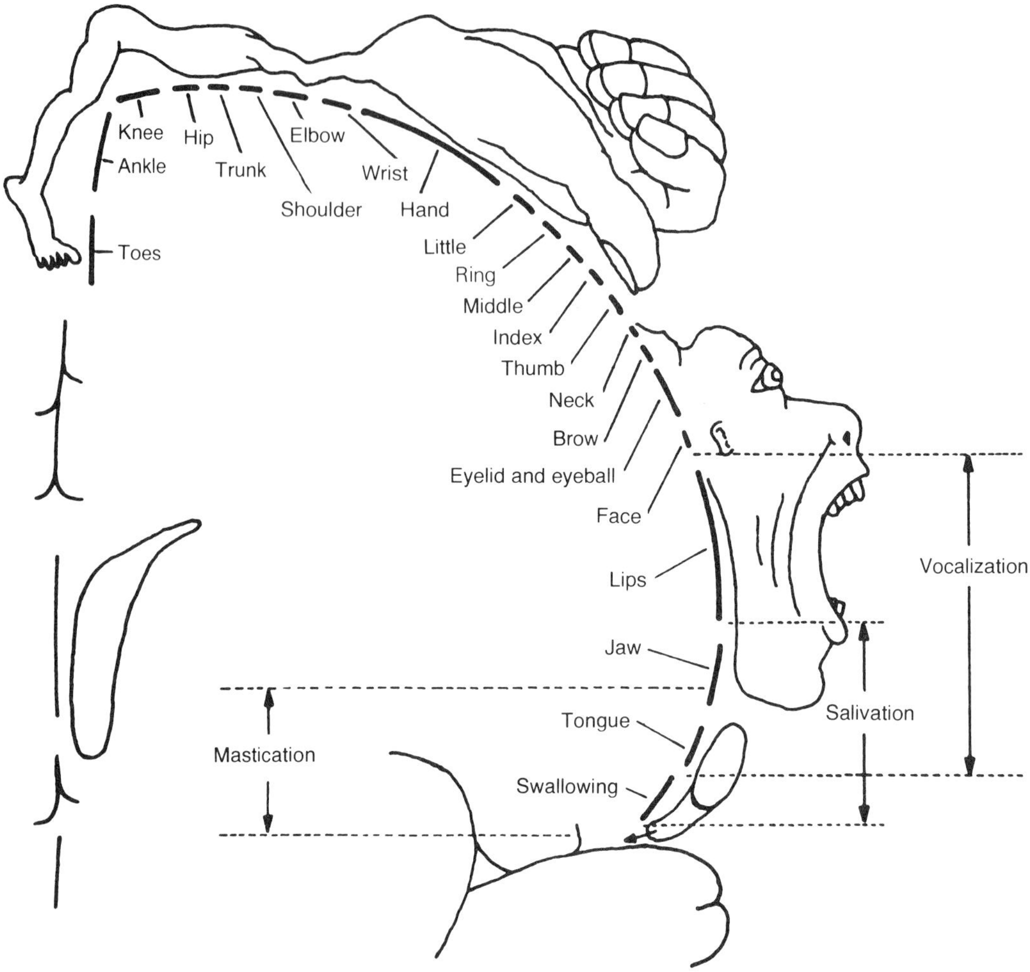

FIG. 16-4. The somatotopic representation in the electrically excitable motor cortex. Note the positions and relative sizes of the representations of different parts of the body on a cross section through the brain at the precentral gyrus. (Penfield W, Rasmussen T: The Cerebral Cortex of Man. New York, Macmillan, 1950)

that dopamine is an inhibitory transmitter substance in the caudate nucleus.

In spite of this doubt, a frequently used therapeutic measure for parkinsonism has been to administer to the patient extraordinary doses (about 4 *grams* per day) of L-dopa, the immediate precursor of dopamine. Dopamine is one of those substances that will not cross the blood-brain barrier, but L-dopa will and, once across, it is converted to dopamine. The dosage can be reduced slightly if L-dopa is given with decarboxylase inhibitors. Some patients who were previously unable to take care of themselves have improved significantly following L-dopa treatment. Others have not been helped, and still others have suffered side-effects. Observations over a period of 5 to 6 years suggest that L-dopa treatment does not halt the progression of the disease, but merely treats the symptoms. For many patients this is enough. It is noteworthy that injection of catecholamines produces immediate remission of symptoms in most patients, but it is short-lived.

CORTICAL CONTROL OF MOVEMENT

Movements can be initiated by stimulation of the surface of the cerebral cortex in awake humans during surgery for epilepsy. This fact is of importance because it defines the

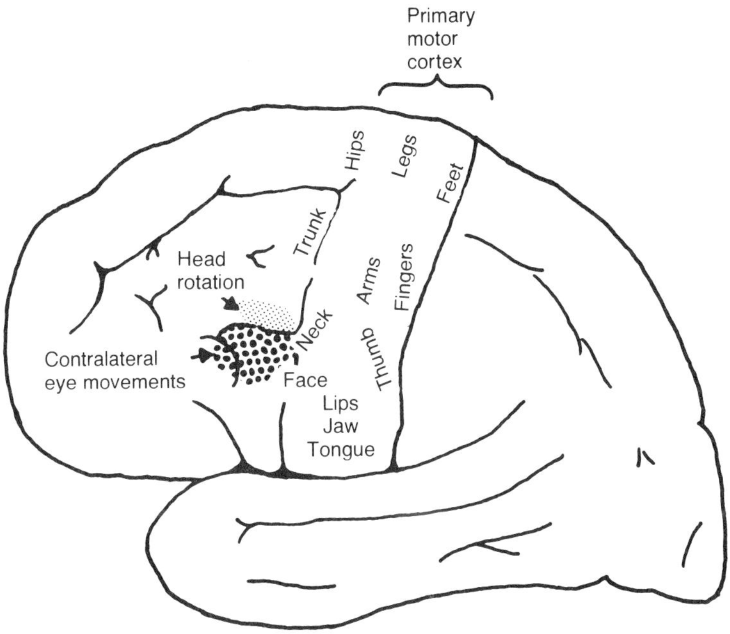

FIG. 16-5. A lateral view of the cerebral hemisphere showing the positions of the primary motor area, the frontal eye fields, and the head movement area. (Guyton A: Textbook of Medical Physiology. Philadelphia, WB Saunders, 1975)

electrically excitable motor cortex, or more commonly, just **motor cortex.** When the cortex is exposed through a small opening in the skull, it all looks pretty much the same, so the position of the motor cortex in the precentral gyrus, identifiable with electrical stimulation, serves as an important landmark for the surgeon.

When the surface of the motor cortex is stimulated electrically, different parts of the body move depending upon the site of stimulation. There is a somatotopic motor representation that resembles the sensory representation on the other side of the central sulcus in somatosensory cortex. Figure 16-4 shows the representation. Movements of the face are elicited by stimulation near the Sylvian fissure. Slightly more medially (toward the midline), stimuli evoke movements of upper extremities, then the trunk, and finally, on the medial surface of the hemisphere, the leg. Notice that the motor representation of the hand and fingers is much larger than for the trunk, much as in the postcentral sensory representation. This perhaps reflects the greater use and dexterity of the hand.

In addition to the precentral or primary motor area, there are other cortical points from which movements can be evoked by electrical stimulation. Figure 16-5 shows the approximate location of some of these. Just anterior to the precentral face representation, on the posterior aspect of the middle frontal gyrus (area 8), lies a part of the cortex from which eye movements can be evoked, the **frontal eye fields.** The frontal eye fields in humans may extend back at least as far as the lip of the central sulcus. Stimulation in the frontal eye fields typically causes conjugate movements of the eyes toward the opposite side, and ablation produces a fixation of gaze on an object such that a person reports he cannot move his eyes toward a different object without first closing them. Why this strange effect occurs is not known, but apparently this area has something to do with "voluntary" eye movements, in contrast to the more automatic visual tracking. Slightly more medially on the cortex is an area, the stimulation of which evokes rotation of the head, again toward the contralateral side. The proximity of this area to the frontal eye fields suggests that they may work together.

Not shown in the figure is an area on the

medial aspect of the hemisphere just anterior to the lower leg and foot representation of the primary motor cortex. This area of the superior frontal gyrus (area 6) is called the supplementary motor area. Stimulation here produces bilateral movements that are one of three types: (1) postural movements, (2) complex patterned movements, and (3) rapid incoordinate movements. Unilateral ablation of this area produces no permanent deficits in either posture or movement; bilateral ablations in animals produce flexor **hypertonia,** myotatic hyper-reflexia, and clonus with some postural deficits. The function of this area remains a mystery.

PYRAMIDAL VS. EXTRAPYRAMIDAL CONTROL

Cortical motor systems have traditionally been divided into pyramidal and extrapyramidal systems, but this distinction is overemphasized. To the pyramidal system is normally assigned the function of initiation and control of "voluntary" movements, whereas the extrapyramidal system is said to control the "involuntary" movements, a distinction that is gradually disappearing from major textbooks. First, let us examine the concepts of "voluntary" and "involuntary" movements. Try to think of an involuntary movement! Let us take a hard one: contraction of the diaphragm, producing inspiration. It goes on night and day without any participation of volition, but it is possible to control the diaphragm and change the breathing rhythm whenever you want to do so. Thus, what was an "involuntary" movement becomes a "voluntary" movement. There is no reason to believe that the neural pathway for ongoing control is different from that in this special circumstance, and certainly the movement itself is no different. Therefore, from this point of view, it makes no sense to distinguish voluntary and involuntary movements. If it makes no sense to distinguish them, it makes no sense to assign different structures to control them. This is an important idea for our understanding of the organization of the nervous system.

There is a distinction that does make some sense in this context. All movements involving the limbs are complex movements. Adduction of the arm not only involves contraction of the arm and shoulder muscles, but also subtle reactions in the axial muscles to compensate for the changes in weight distribution that result from the movement. These postural changes are important components of every movement that are usually overlooked or disregarded. There is considerable evidence that the extrapyramidal tracts (with the exception of the rubrospinal tract) exert their influences most strongly on the proximal or axial musculature, whereas the pyramidal tract exerts its strongest influence on distal musculature. This is perhaps the distinction that should be emphasized.

THE PYRAMIDAL SYSTEM

The pyramidal system receives its name from its only constituent, the pyramidal tract, a bundle of fibers on the ventral surface of the medulla, whose cell bodies are located in the pre- and postcentral gyri in areas 1,2,3,4, and perhaps also 6. The pyramidal tract fibers, defined by having an axon in the medullary pyramids, pass through the internal capsule and the basis pedunculi on their way to the medullary level. The tract is composed mostly of small fibers, less than one micrometer in diameter, about 1 to 1.5 million in number in man. It has been said that man is what he is because of his pyramidal tract. If this is so, then the human is distinguished by his small pyramids; the human has fewer pyramidal tract fibers per unit of brain than one would expect for a mammal of his body size (Towe, 1973b).

Some people equate the pyramidal tract with the corticospinal tract, an entirely inappropriate custom because only a fraction of pyramidal tract fibers ever reach the spinal cord. The nature of the terminations of the pyramidal tract is indicated in Figure 16-6. Some of the same cells that project into the medullary pyramids also send collaterals into the nucleus ventralis lateralis of the thalamus and the red nucleus before even reaching the pons. Other pyramidal tract fibers terminate in the pontine nuclei, the midbrain tegmentum, inferior olive, lateral and medial reticular formations, dorsal column nuclei, and the main and spinal nucleus of the fifth nerve. In man, though not in the cat, some fibers even end in the motor nuclei of the cranial nerves. If the number of fibers entering the pons is taken

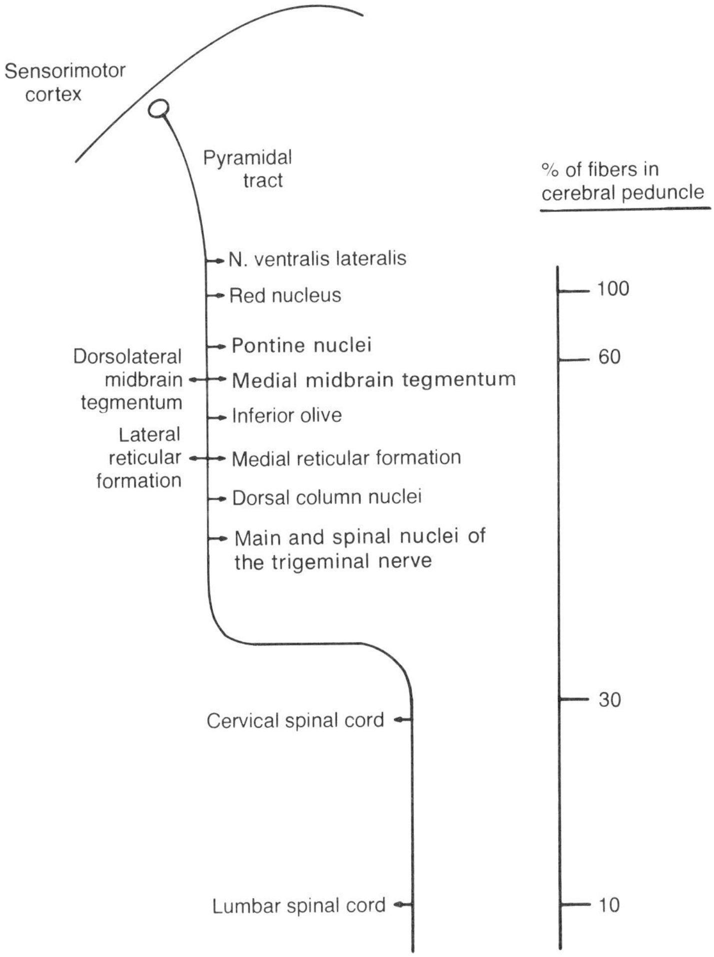

FIG. 16-6. The known termination sites of pyramidal tract axons. It is not meant to be implied that a single fiber ends in all of these nuclei; quite the contrary is true. Also indicated is the approximate percentage of fibers in the basis pedunculi that is still present in the tract at various levels. Notice the rapid decline at the pons and also in the brain stem. Not shown are possible terminations in the cranial nerve nuclei in man that do not occur in animals.

as 100%, then only 30% make it as far as the cervical spinal cord and only 10% make it to the lumbar spinal cord. Most of the pyramidal tract fibers end, in fact, in the brain stem, a strange behavior for a tract that is supposed to be *the* tract mediating "voluntary" movements. (See Towe, 1973a for a thorough discussion of pyramidal tract terminations.)

Look carefully at the distribution of pyramidal tract terminals in Table 16-4. Termination sites are found in as many "sensory" as "motor" nuclei. It is not known why the pyramidal tract has these terminations in sensory nuclei. At the spi-

TABLE 16-4. TERMINATIONS OF PYRAMIDAL TRACT FIBERS

MOTOR	SENSORY
Red nucleus	Dorsal column nuclei
Medial reticular formation	Medial reticular formation
Nucleus ventralis lateralis	Trigeminal nuclei
Ventral horn, spinal cord	Dorsal horn, spinal cord
Medial midbrain tegmentum	Cranial nerve nuclei

CEREBELLUM
Pontine nuclei
Red nucleus
Lateral reticular formation

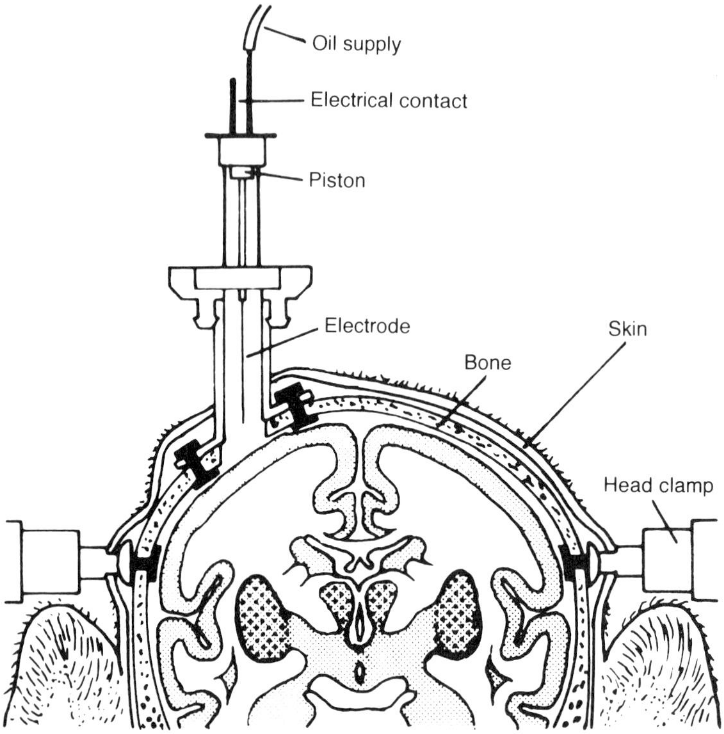

FIG. 16-7. The physical setup for recording from awake, moving monkeys. A chamber is attached to the skull in which a small hole has been made. The electrode and its drive mechanism are attached to the chamber, and the electrode, usually a sharpened tungsten or platinum-alloy wire, is driven through the meninges to the vicinity of a single cell. Note that the head is fixed during recording. (Evarts EV: Sci Am 229:96–103, 1973)

nal cord level, some pyramidal tract axons end directly on α motoneurons and, thus, exert a direct effect on motor output, but the majority end on interneurons in the dorsal horn. The tract could still play a major role in initiating and controlling movement if it had a powerful excitatory effect on α-motoneuron circuits.

It is true that stimulation of the precentral cortex elicits movements (by definition of electrically excitable motor cortex), but it requires several (4–5) stimuli, applied at high frequency (500/sec), to obtain the movement through the pyramidal tract. The question is, Do pyramidal tract fibers fire at these high frequencies during movements? They must if they are going to initiate movements by themselves. It is possible to record from single pyramidal tract neurons in an awake monkey, who is free to move, at least in a limited way. Figure 16-7 shows how a chamber is fixed over the recording site and how the electrode is driven into the cortex. The monkey is seated in a chair and able to move a lever in a certain way in order to get a fruit juice reward (Fig. 16-8). The neuron's activity is recorded at the same time as the monkey is moving the lever. Figure 16-9 shows the records obtained in this experiment. Notice that the neuron begins to discharge before the movement occurs and even before the muscle begins to contract, but does not generate a train of spikes at 500/sec or more. In fact, if you generate a train of stimuli that matches the timing of the discharges in the figure and apply it to the cortex, no movement will be evoked.

The pyramidal tract does have special properties. Figure 16-10 shows a recording, from inside an α motoneuron, of the EPSP evoked by a single pyramidal tract stimulus. If two such stimuli are applied at an interval of 10 msec or less, the resulting EPSP is larger than would be predicted from simple temporal summation (Fig. 16-10).

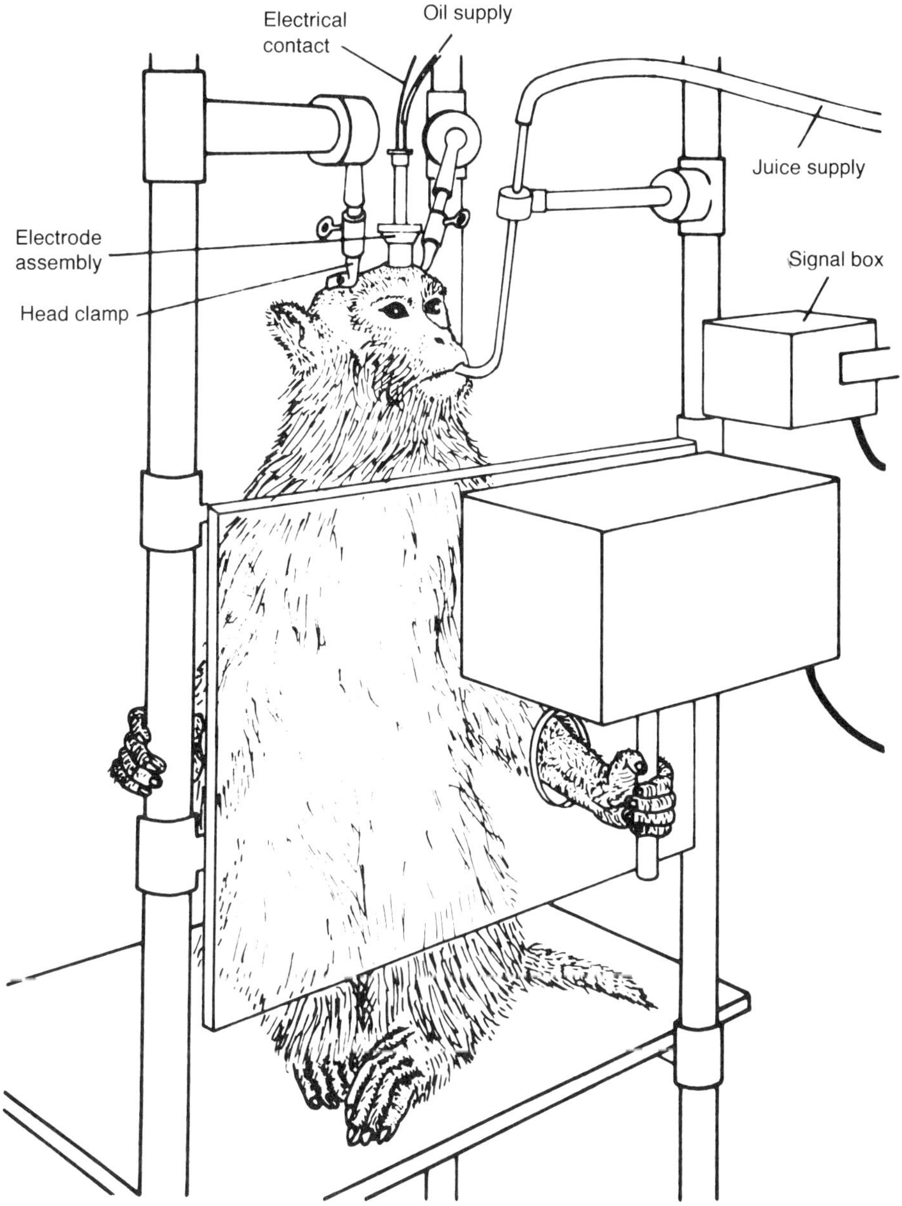

FIG. 16-8. A typical primate chair in which the monkey sits unrestrained except at the head. The hand can reach through a hole to grasp a lever. When the monkey moves the lever in a particular way a reward of a small amount of fruit juice is delivered through the tube near his mouth. (Evarts EV: Sci Am 229:96–103, 1973)

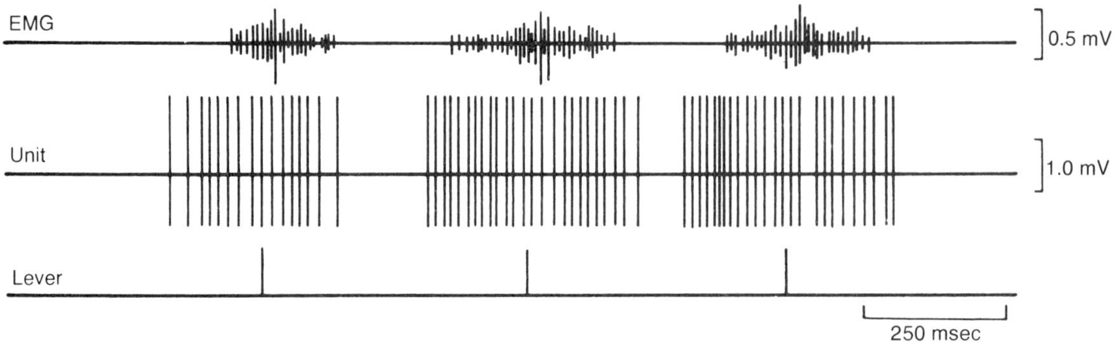

FIG. 16-9. Records from a pyramidal tract neuron in an awake monkey. The **upper trace** shows the EMG recorded from one of the muscles the monkey uses to move the lever. Notice that the amplitude of the EMG record increases just before and while the lever is moved in three separate trials as indicated in the **bottom trace.** The cell begins discharging **(middle trace)** long before the EMG record shows any change. Notice that the interval between action potentials within any one of the three trials first decreases to some minimum value and then increases again, but never reaches 2 msec (equivalent to a frequency of 500/sec). (Porter R, Lewis M McD, Horne M: Brain Res 34:99–113, 1971)

This phenomenon is called **facilitation** and appears to be a special property of pyramidal tract synapses on α motoneurons. For simple temporal summation, R_2 would be less than or equal to R_1; for facilitation, R_2 is greater than R_1. The EPSPs evoked by group Ia afferent fibers from muscle spindles do not show facilitation in α motoneurons. This is shown in Figure 16-11A for stimuli at 5-msec intervals; there is no increment in successive EPSPs. Compare this pattern with the facilitation of corticomotoneuronal EPSPs shown in Figure 16-11B. Clearly, each successive EPSP in the series of six is larger. What good is facilitation?

It appears that no one group of fibers is capable of bringing a motoneuron to the critical firing level by itself in normal functioning of the system. We have just seen that the pyramidal tract cannot do it, and we saw before that in spinal shock even group Ia afferent fibers cannot do it. The critical firing level is achieved by summing all the inputs over different pathways. Figure 16-12 illustrates the positions of the important descending tracts in the spinal cord and the way in which the dendrites of α motoneurons "reach out" toward them. Distal muscles are influenced most strongly by pyramidal and rubrospinal fibers, whereas proximal muscles are influenced most strongly by vestibulo- and reticulospinal fibers, though both groups of muscles are influenced from all four tracts. There is even evidence that different inputs to a single cell may come in on their own dedicated dendrites.

What then is the pyramidal tract doing? Again, no one knows for certain, but consider this hypothesis: The pyramidal tract tells the muscles the precise time when they should begin to contract. Figure 16-13 provides a closer look at the discharge of a pyramidal tract cell during a movement. Notice that there is one interspike interval (the time between two spikes) in the train that is less than 10 msec in duration, the maximum time over which facilitation occurs. In every such train of spikes from a pyramidal tract cell, there is always one interval in this range of durations, so there will always be facilitation at some motoneurons. If all the other inputs to the α motoneuron have brought it near the critical firing level, then the addition of this more powerful (by facilitation) input could drive it over the critical firing level. It turns out that there is a rather high correlation between the time of occurrence of this short interspike interval and the time of onset of the movement. This would seem to support the hypothesis. The time when the pyramidal tract fiber discharges at this short interval may signal the muscle to start the contraction. This is undoubtedly not the only function of the pyramidal tract, but it may be one of them.

If the pyramids of monkeys are sectioned at the medullary level, the results are paresis *not* paralysis, flaccidity *not* spasticity, **hyporeflexia,** and interestingly, the Babinski sign. Impairments of movement observed following pyramidotomy have been described variously, descriptive terms

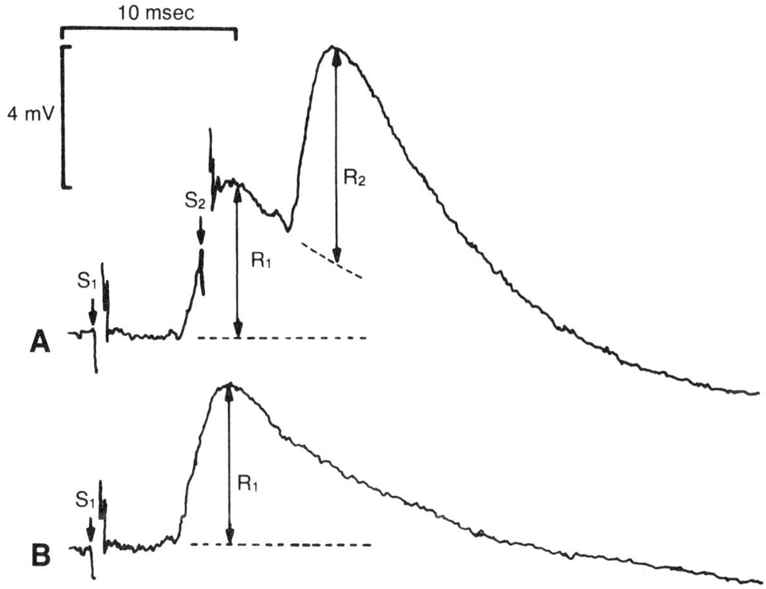

FIG. 16-10. Intracellular recordings of facilitation of a corticomotoneuronal EPSP in an α motoneuron. Two identical stimuli, S_1 and S_2, were delivered to the cortex about 6 msec apart; the resulting EPSP is shown in **A**. When only S_1 was delivered, the EPSP was as shown in **B**. Notice the facilitation ($R_2 > R_1$), not summation ($R_2 \neq R_1$). (Porter R: J Physiol (Lond) 207:733–745, 1970)

FIG. 16-11. Intracellular recordings from a motoneuron of the median nerve. **A.** Simultaneous records of dorsal root volleys evoked by stimulation of muscle afferent fibers at 200/sec **(upper trace)** and monosynaptic EPSPs in the motoneuron. **B.** Simultaneous records of corticospinal volleys at 200/sec **(upper trace)** and monosynaptic EPSPs on the motoneuron. Cortical stimulus strength was adjusted to give an EPSP the same size as the group I EPSP in A. (Phillips CG: Proc Roy Soc B 173:141–174, 1969)

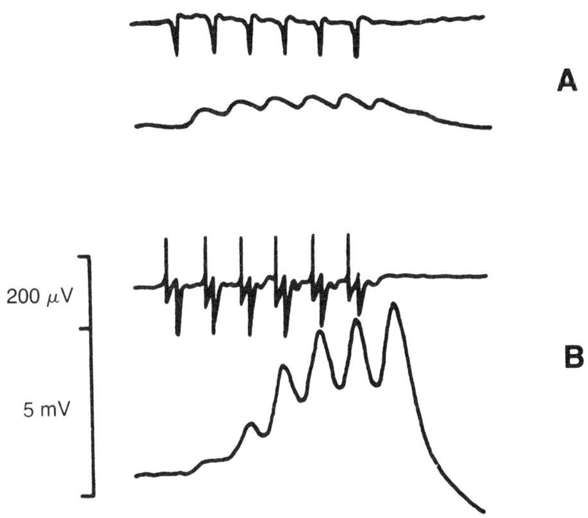

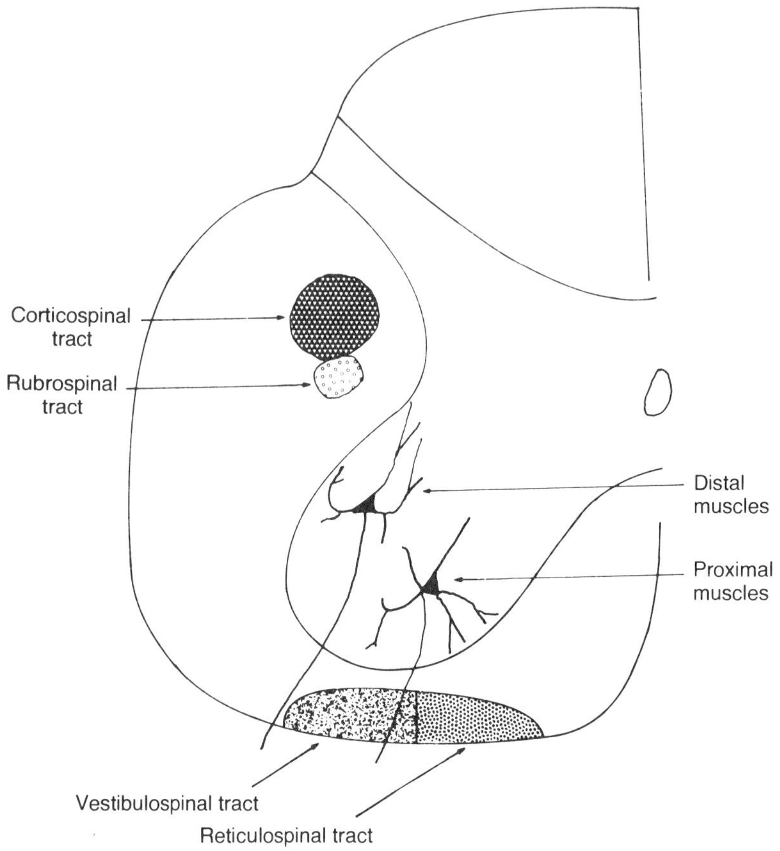

FIG. 16-12. A cross section through the lumbar spinal cord indicating the approximate positions of the cortico-, rubro-, vestibulo-, and reticulospinal tracts and the approximate positions of the motor cell columns for proximal and distal muscles.

FIG. 16-13. An enlarged record of the discharge of a pyramidal tract cell during a movement of the lever by the monkey as shown in Figure 16-9. (Porter R, Lewis M McD, Horne M: Brain Res 34:99–113, 1971)

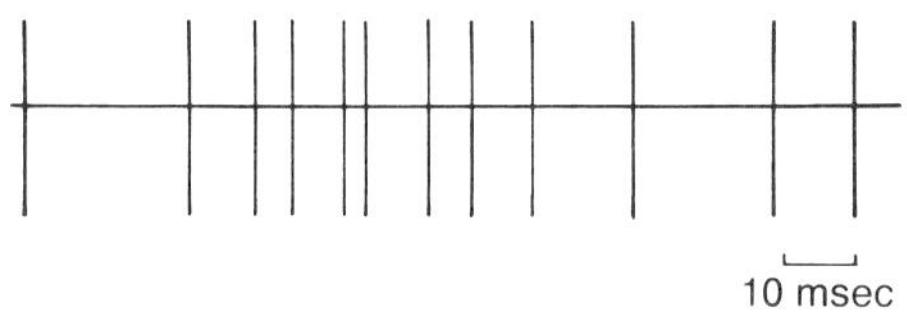

ranging from "grave impairment" to "no obvious deficit." The reasons for this variation in results may be partly differences in surgical skill, in completeness of transection, in the range of movements tested, in time allowed for recovery, and, in some cases, in species. It is usually said that the pyramidal tract exerts its influence mainly upon the distal musculature because the greatest deficits are seen in digital movement. Deficits in thumb–index finger apposition and in grasping are clearly seen following pyramidotomy, but there are, at the same time, deficits involving proximal musculature. These are less often seen because they are more difficult to test. Grasping objects, without at the same time flexing the arm (proximal contraction), is difficult. Deficits are also seen in hip and shoulder movements.

With a pyramidal tract lesion or, alternatively, an appropriately placed area 4 cortical lesion, a flaccid **paralysis** of the upper limb results in monkeys. A similar effect also occurs following limited stroke in man. Under these circumstances, the limb usually dangles at the side and is not used for purposive movements; however, if the other, unaffected, limb is immobilized or if a threat can only be warded off with the affected limb, or in certain training situations that the animal has been exposed to before the lesion, then the affected limb can make required responses. The movements are by no means normal—they lack precision, they are clumsy, and they are not guided throughout their entire course. It is interesting that a complete unilateral cervical dorsal rhizotomy has almost the same effect on the use of the ipsilateral upper limb in monkeys. The affected arm is dangled at the side and unused except when forced or in certain training situations and, under those circumstances where it is used, the movements are clumsy, imprecise, and not fully guided. Yet in the former case the loss is usually described as motor, and in the latter case it is usually described as sensory. Perhaps these results best serve to illustrate our lack of adequate understanding of the distinction between sensory and motor activity or perhaps the nervous system makes no such distinction.

Recovery of movements following pyramidotomy has also varied in different experiments, probably for the same reasons as the variation in initial deficit. The terms, descriptive of the recovery, have ranged from "none" to "almost complete." In fact, in cases of verified, complete pyramidotomy, recovery may be almost complete, with the only lingering signs, a slight paresis and a loss of fluidity and ease of movement, and even the paresis may disappear with time. In general, the permanent losses appear to be in fine-tuning of movements, particularly those involving the distal musculature.

THE EXTRAPYRAMIDAL SYSTEM

The pyramidal system is defined in terms of the pyramids, whereas the extrapyramidal system is defined by default in that anything that is not pyramidal is extrapyramidal. Usually, the red nucleus and rubrospinal tract, the pontine and medullary reticular formations and the reticulospinal tracts, the lateral and medial vestibular nuclei and the vestibulospinal tracts, and the tectum and tectospinal tract are included as part of the extrapyramidal system along with fibers originating in the cerebral cortex but not part of the pyramidal tract. Often the basal ganglia are included, but this is not appropriate, because they have no real outlet to the spinal cord except by way of one of these other pathways or the corticospinal tract. Most of the cortical elements that synaptically activate these extrapyramidal centers have no direct connection with α motoneurons.

The distinction between pyramidal and extrapyramidal systems is purely artificial. Table 16-4 shows that pyramidal tract fibers have terminations in many extrapyramidal structures, and it is known that they have profound effects there. The pyramidal tract also indirectly influences all of those extrapyramidal structures that it does not influence through direct connections. The systems are clearly inseparable at the level of the cortex, the internal capsule, the basis pedunculi, and certainly at the pons. It is only in the pyramids themselves where a clear separation occurs.

UPPER AND LOWER MOTONEURON DISEASE

The only ways to study extrapyramidal effects are to attempt to make lesions in the individual nuclei of the system or to compare the effects of damage to the cerebral cortex with those of pyramidal tract section. The resulting deficits from lesions in some extrapyramidal nuclei were discussed previously.

Clinicians like to refer to **upper motoneuron symptoms** and **lower motoneuron symptoms** in motor deficits. The lower motoneurons are, of course, the α motoneurons. The upper motoneurons, in this context, are all the neurons of descending tracts whose activity impinges upon α motoneurons. We may take this as both pyramidal and extrapyramidal influences together. The characteristic symptoms of both upper and lower motoneuron disease are listed in Table 16-5 along with the symptoms of experimental pyramidal tract section. Note that most of the symptoms of upper motoneuron disease are not symptoms seen in controlled pyramidal tract section and are thus assignable to extrapyramidal tracts alone or to some interaction between pyramidal and extrapyramidal tracts. These effects are more impairing and more permanent than those resulting from pyramidal tract section alone.

It is possible to have both upper and lower motoneuron symptoms at the same time. For example, a lesion in the region of the cervical enlargement of the spinal cord that damages the cervical motoneurons and

TABLE 16-5. COMPARISON OF UPPER AND LOWER MOTONEURON AND PYRAMIDAL TRACT SYMPTOMS

UPPER MOTONEURON DISEASE	LOWER MOTONEURON DISEASE	PYRAMIDAL TRACT SECTION
Paralysis or paresis	Paralysis	Paresis
Spasticity	Flaccidity	Flaccidity
Hyper-reflexia	Areflexia for that muscle	Hyporeflexia
Babinski sign	None	Babinski sign
Clonus	None	None
Absence of abdominal reflexes	Depends on motoneurons affected	Absence of abdominal reflexes
None	Fasciculations	None
None	Atrophy	None

the descending fibers of the vestibulo- and reticulospinal tracts in the ventral white matter, will produce lower motoneuron symptoms, including **fasciculations** and atrophy, in the upper limbs and upper motoneuron symptoms, including Babinski's sign, in the lower limbs. Of course, the cervical motoneurons are also separated from supraspinal influences, but the lower motoneuron symptoms are the only ones seen. Functional disconnection of the muscle from the nervous system is much more devastating.

It is important to note that Table 16-5 lists symptoms of upper motoneuron disease. The results of ablation of the cortex may be quite different. Recall that ablation limited to area 4 produces flaccidity, not spasticity. An even more striking effect occurs in those rare cases in which an entire hemisphere was removed right down to the thalamus. This procedure produces no obvious motor deficits in the clinical sense, but one patient with superior athletic skills preoperatively, did not have such skills postoperatively. This apparent confusion may be resolvable by conjuring up the computer analogy again. The more "abnormal" tissue there is present, the more the abnormality in movement. Complete removal is far less devastating than partial removal. It may be useful in the clinical setting to have committed Table 16-6 to memory. It gives some useful tools for distinguishing between possible levels of lesions involving motor deficits.

CORRELATES OF MOVEMENT

Experiments have begun to show what various parts of the central motor systems are doing when animals are actually moving. A cat can walk almost normally on a flat, horizontal surface after removal of the forebrain and rostral thalamus. As we have already noted, there is no spontaneous walking in a cat when the brain stem is sectioned, but, if the section is made rostral to the superior colliculus and the animal is stimulated in the region of the nucleus cuneaformis, the animal walks, maintaining its equilibrium. The stimulus used is a continuous train of shocks, but the movement is an alternation in the limbs at 1 to 2 Hz. The head and spinal column of the animal can be rigidly fixed because the brain-stem section deprives the animal of nociception. Thus, recordings can be made of the activity of any remaining neurons while the animal is walking.

Walking in the mesencephalic cat, a cat with its brain stem sectioned rostral to the superior colliculus, is very close to normal in terms of joint movements and muscle activity, and, like in normal walking, the movement of any limb can be divided into a stance phase and a swing phase. The stance phase begins when the foot touches the ground and ends when it is removed from the ground. During the stance phase, the limb exerts a force on the substrate, the horizontal component of which propels the animal forward. The swing phase begins when the animal removes its foot from the substrate and ends when it replaces it. During the interim between these two activities, the limb is lifted and swung forward to be in position to contact the ground for the next stance phase. This sequence is reminiscent of walking in humans as described in Chapter 2, except that the knee and ankle of the cat move in phase, the knee and ankle of man do not. As in humans, the movements of the hindlimbs of the cat alternate, but because the cat is quadripedal the forelimbs also participate in locomotion.

Movement of the joints in the mesencephalic cat is shown schematically in Figure 16-14A. In this figure, the joints are flexing when the trace deflects upward, extending when it deflects downward. The upper trace shows movements of the hip joint and the lower trace, movements of the ankle and

TABLE 16-6. SUMMARY OF CLINICAL SIGNS OF DAMAGE AT DIFFERENT SITES ALONG THE NEURAXIS

			CLINICAL SIGNS			
LESION SITE	Reflexes	Muscle Tone	Spasticity	Rigidity	Flaccidity	Additional Clues
Spinal—Shock	Areflexia	Atonic			√	Postural hypotension, atonic bladder
Recovery	Hyper-reflexia	Hypertonic	√			Clonus
Trapezoid body—Low decerebrate	Hyper-reflexia	Hypertonic	√			May lack doll's eyes, comatose
Midcollicular—Sherringtonian	Hyper-reflexia	Hypertonic	√			May lack doll's eyes, postural reflexes present, comatose
Mesencephalic—High decerebrate	Hyper-reflexia	Hypertonic	√			Conscious, may lack light reflex
Hypothalamic	Hyper-reflexia	Hypertonic	√			Conscious, may lack light reflex, controls temperature
Decorticate	Hyper-reflexia	Hypertonic	√			Clonus, Babinski
Motor cortex—Area 4 only	Hyporeflexia	Hypotonic			√	Babinski
Pyramidal tract	Hyporeflexia	Hypotonic			√	Babinski
Cerebellar	Hyporeflexia	Hypotonic				Ataxia, intention tremor, dyssynergia
Basal ganglion	Hyper-reflexia	Hypertonic		√		Bradykinesia, tremor at rest (hyperkinesia with ballism)

knee. The latter two joints are plotted together because they move in phase in the cat. The hip joint is extending throughout the stance phase and the hip and leg are moving backwards relative to the trunk. The knee and ankle are flexing during the first half of the stance phase as they yield to body weight. At the end of the stance phase, all three joints are extending because of active extensor muscle contractions and forward movement of the animal.

The swing phase begins when the limb reaches the most caudal position, with activity in both flexors and two-joint muscles, resulting in flexion of all three joints. Flexion terminates earlier in the knee and ankle and they begin to extend before the hip. The sequence of muscle activity can be seen in relationship to the stepping cycle in Figure 16-14B. In this figure, the muscle is identified at the left and its action is indicated at the right. The horizontal lines indicate the times when the EMG activity for the muscle increases above its resting level. Many limb extensor muscles are strongly activated *before* the limb touches the ground. The fact that extensor activity occurs before the footfall implies that it is *not* a reflex elicited by foot contact. The shortest latency from receptor activation to onset of an autogenetic reflex change in tension in ankle extensor muscles is about 30 msec. Considerably longer might be required to balance tension among motor units, exceeding the durations of the various phases of the step cycle at least at fast rates of locomotion. Therefore, it is unlikely that reflexes play an important role.

Stepping, in the mesencephalic cat, continues as long as the stimulation continues (a train of pulses is used to drive stepping). Increasing the strength of stimulation results in increased stepping frequency due to increased force developed by the limb (apparently through recruitment of additional motoneurons rather than through increasing motoneuron firing rate), but does not change the phase relationships of the joint movements or the muscle contractions. Changing the frequency of pulses within the train has little effect. Walking or trotting in the cat is characterized by alternating movements in both fore- and hindlimbs with each forelimb moving in phase with the contralateral hindlimb. As the strength of stimulation increases, the animal changes from a walk to a trot and, with even higher strengths, the animal gallops, with both hindlimbs moving in phase and alternating with both forelimbs. This same sequence

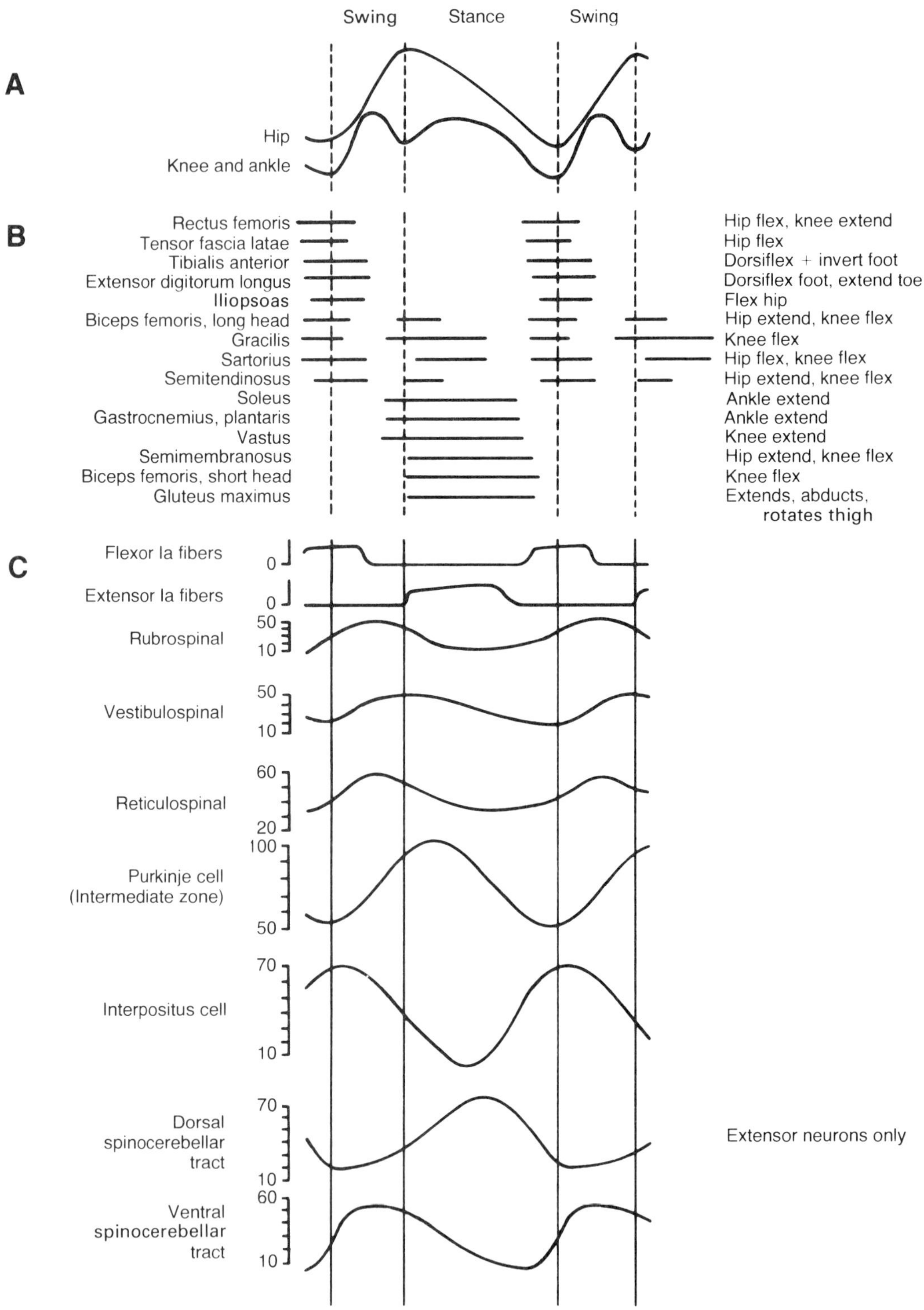

FIG. 16-14. The stepping cycle in the mesencephalic cat. **A.** Movements of the hip, knee, and ankle during the swing and stance phases of stepping. Flexion is indicated by an upward deflection of the curve; extension, by a downward deflection. **B.** Contractions of various muscles during the stepping cycle. Time of contraction is indicated by the position of the horizontal bar; the action of each muscle is indicated at the right. **C.** Activity of neurons in various parts of the motor system during the stepping cycle. Frequency of discharge is indicated on the ordinates. (Orlovsky GN, Shik ML: Control of locomotion: A neurophysiological analysis of the cat locomotor system. In Porter R [ed]: International Review of Physiology. Vol. 10, Neurophysiology II. Baltimore, University Press, 1976)

can be observed in an intact cat, moving spontaneously.

It should be emphasized that this region of the brain stem, the region whose stimulation leads to stepping, is not required for stepping to occur; animals with spinal cord transections are also capable of walking under certain circumstances. This implies that the stepping cycle itself is generated within the spinal cord. The alternation of limb movements does not depend upon crossed reflexes because one limb will continue to step if the contralateral ventral roots are cut, and alternating activity can still be recorded from the ventral roots when ventral roots on both sides are cut distal to the recording site. Dorsal roots are likewise not required for stepping, but after dorsal rhizotomy limb movements are not adapted to the real speed of locomotion (when the animal is on a moving treadmill), and the limbs do not change the force they develop when the load is changed. Thus, although stepping can occur without sensory feedback, the feedback does play a role in normal walking. There are, however, movements in which feedback is not only not required but is not desirable. Ballistic or rapid, pendular movements (such as removing the hand rapidly from a telegraph key) are performed more rapidly without sensory feedback. Sensations from the moving part of the body are greatly reduced just before and during such a movement (Luschei ES: Personal communication). In fact, there would not be time for the information to be used during the movement anyway.

Many of the spinal cord reflexes discussed in Chapter 15 are either modified or eliminated during stepping. For example, Renshaw inhibition, feedback inhibition from collaterals of α motoneurons resulting in decreased frequency of discharge in neighboring α motoneurons, disappears when stepping begins. Likewise, reciprocal inhibition can only be observed at certain appropriate times during the stepping cycle. Thus, stimulation of group Ia fibers of the antagonist muscle will only inhibit the agonist motoneurons when they would normally be silent (their muscle relaxed) during the cycle (in Fig. 16-14B, when there is *no* horizontal bar).

The behavior of muscle spindle afferent fibers during stepping is also a bit surprising. These muscle receptors are frequently silent as their muscle is being lengthened, but they discharge vigorously as the muscle is actively shortening. This can be seen in the upper two traces of Figure 16-14C. The activity of flexor Ia fibers increases at the beginning of the swing phase when most flexors are actively contracting; the extensor Ia discharge increases early in the stance phase when extensor muscles are contracting. This behavior is surprising because we are accustomed to thinking of muscle spindle afferent fibers as length detectors; however, in this case they increase their discharge when the muscle shortens. The observed behavior of the receptors could occur as a result of α–γ coactivation and, in fact, γ motoneurons are active at the same time during the stepping cycle as the homonymous α motoneurons. The increased sensitivity of the spindle receptors during muscle contraction allows their activity to influence the α motoneuron when it is active, whereas the withdrawal of γ-motoneuron activity during the relaxation phase for the muscle prevents the α motoneuron from being activated by the group Ia afferent input during the wrong phase, that is when the muscle is being passively stretched. The Golgi tendon organs are more active during the isometric or lengthening contractions of the stance phase than in the passive stretches of other phases. Therefore, they discharge together with group Ia fibers from extensor muscles.

Similarly, supraspinal descending influences on α motoneurons are variable during the stepping cycle. At rest, that is, when the animal is not walking, the vestibulospinal tract exerts an excitatory action on extensor muscles and an inhibitory action on flexor muscles; the reticulospinal tract excites flexor and inhibits extensor muscles; and the rubrospinal and corticospinal tracts excite flexors. (These are not the only actions of these tracts, but they are statistical statements of the most frequently observed effects.) During the stepping cycle, stimulation of Deiters' nucleus leads to an increase in EMG activity of extensor muscles, but only during the phases of the cycle when they would normally be active, that is, in the stance phase. Stimulation of the pontine reticulospinal tract leads to increased flexor EMGs and decreased extensor EMGs, whereas stimulation of rubrospinal and corticospinal tracts leads mainly to increased flexor EMGs. These influences are also only exerted during the appropriate time during the stepping cycle.

The neurons in many parts of the central nervous system show rhythmic changes in their discharge frequencies in phase with stepping. Some of these changes are illustrated in Figure 16-14C. Many rubrospinal tract neurons increase their firing rates during the swing phase and decrease their rates during the stance phase. Similar changes are also seen in reticulospinal neurons. Vestibulospinal neurons begin increasing their discharge rates at the beginning of the swing phase, but peak rates occur at the transition from swing to stance and early in the stance phase. These changes in activity of tract neurons are consistent with influences discussed in the last paragraph; the neurons increase their discharge when the target motoneurons are active during the step cycle. It is interesting that this rhythmic variation in discharge rate disappears if the cerebellum is removed, even though stepping continues. Apparently, the modulation in discharge rate reflects rhythmic input from the cerebellum.

In the cerebellar intermediate lobe, Purkinje cells show similar rhythmic changes in discharge rate, and these changes are reflected in discharge of cerebellar nuclear neurons. Both changes are shown in Figure 16-14C. Notice that the changes in the cortex and nuclei are out of phase, as expected from the inhibitory influences of Purkinje cells on nuclear neurons. We have seen that rhythmic changes in descending pathways are due to rhythmic changes in the discharges of cerebellar neurons. The latter changes reflect similar rhythmic changes in spinocerebellar tracts. Such changes are indicated in the lower two traces of Figure 16-14C. The dorsal spinocerebellar tract receives inputs from muscle spindle receptors among others, and rhythmic activity in the tract neurons simply reflects rhythmic changes in receptor activity (compare the dorsal spinocerebellar tract rhythm with that for extensor Ia fibers). The ventral spinocerebellar tract rhythm probably reflects rhythmic inputs from the spinal cord stepping generator mechanism because the rhythms are not disturbed by deafferentation of the limb.

In summary, there appears to be an automatic system for control of locomotion, located within the spinal cord, that can be set into motion by descending impulses and under certain circumstances by impulses from sensory receptors. Presumably, this system is also used in locomotion of the intact animal and perhaps, with appropriate modification for the different gait pattern, in man. This automatic system works by modification of basic reflex mechanisms and alteration of at least some sensory mechanisms. Descending influences in mesencephalic animals operate to strengthen contractions of certain muscles in certain phases of stepping, but do not change the basic locomotor pattern. Presumably, in the intact system, descending influences also modify the pattern to compensate for changes in elevation or contour of the substrate and for changes in the goal of the movement, for example, deviation of the target.

THE INITIATION OF MOVEMENT

One can criticize the preceding experiments on grounds that the locomotion was artificially driven by the experimenter, not generated by the animal. It is true that the experiments tell us nothing about how the animal initiates movements or where in the central nervous system they might begin. A very old idea suggests that movements are conceived in the association cortex, which relays the command for the movement to the motor cortex. The motor cortex relays the command to the muscles and at the same time to the cerebellum and basal ganglia. These structures generate corrections or commands for subsequent movements, based in part upon sensory information from receptors, and feed these back to the motor cortex. In addition, sensory information is conducted to sensory cortex and relayed to association cortex for use in generating future movements. A newer idea, discussed previously, suggests that movements are planned or programmed by the association cortex with the cooperation of the lateral cerebellar hemisphere and the basal ganglia. The plan is then fed to the motor cortex, which issues the command for the movement. The nucleus interpositus updates the movement based upon its continuous monitoring of current limb position and velocity. The interpositus update lags slightly behind the corticospinal command in reaching the motoneurons and modifies

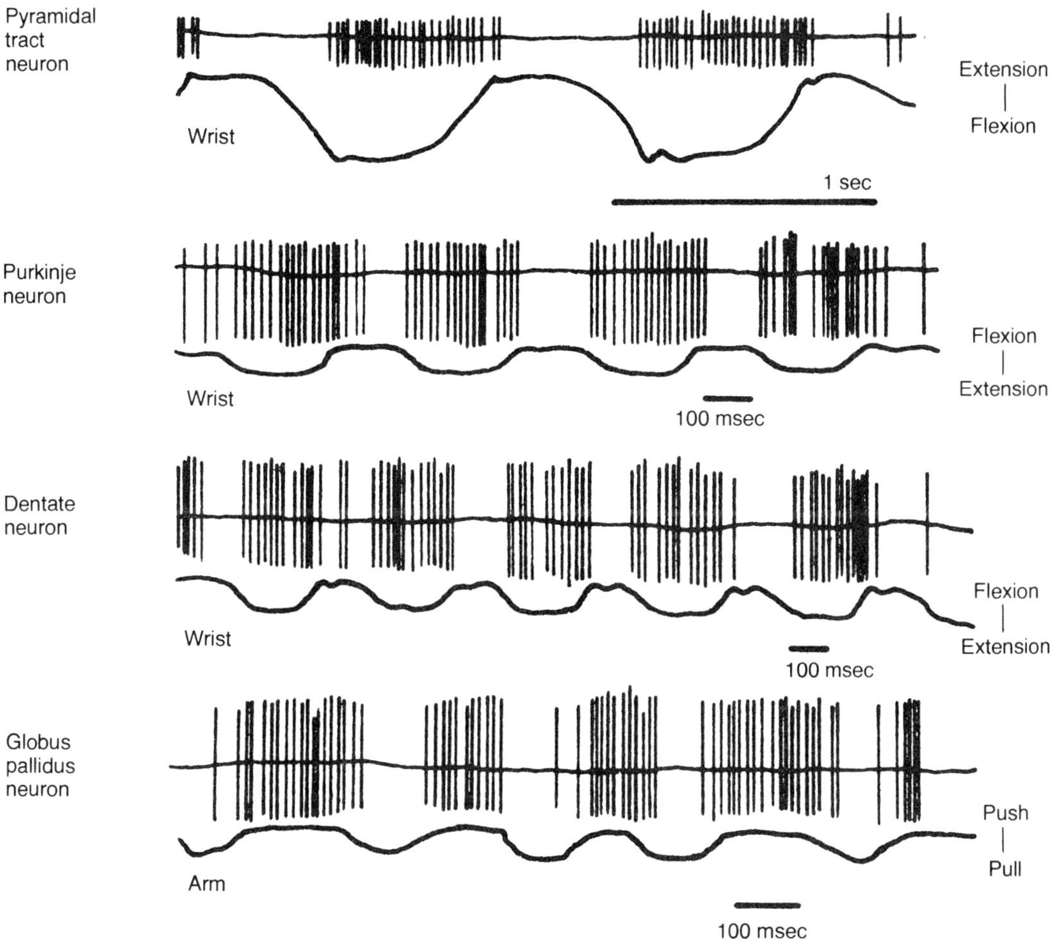

FIG. 16-15. Discharges of neurons in motor centers during wrist or arm movements in monkeys. Spikes were recorded in chronic preparations from a pyramidal tract cell, a Purkinje cell, a dentate nucleus cell, and a globus pallidus cell, the first three during wrist flexion and extension and the fourth during push and pull with the arm. The **upper trace** in each pair is the spike record; the **lower trace** is a monitor of the movement. (Data from Evarts EV: J Neurophysiol 31:14–27, 1968; Thach W: The behavior of Purkinje and cerebellar nuclear cells during two types of voluntary arm movements in the monkey. In Fields WS, Willis WD [eds]: Cerebellum in Health and Disease. St. Louis, Warren Green, 1970; DeLong MR: Brain Res 40:127–135, 1972)

the cortically designated motor discharge. As a result of the movement that occurs, sensory signals are generated in receptors and conducted to the cortex, cerebellum, and elsewhere to be used in generating subsequent movements or corrections.

Using the chronic recording setup shown in Figure 16-7 and 16-8, recordings have been made in various motor regions in an attempt to find out how the neurons discharge in relation to movements. Unfortunately, studies of the responses of neurons in association cortex have not emphasized the timing of the discharges with respect to the start of the movements. Some neurons in parietal areas 5 and 7 of monkeys do fire before movements of the hand, some up to 400 msec before. Some of these neurons do not appear to respond to sensory stimuli, but discharge at high rates when the animal attempts to reach for an object. Apparently, the same movements performed without a goal (an object) are not accompanied by firing in these neurons. Just what the relationship between these neurons and the movements might be is still to be worked out.

At other places in the central motor system the time relationships of neuron discharges and some movements are better known. Figure 16-15 shows recordings from a pyramidal tract neuron in a monkey's

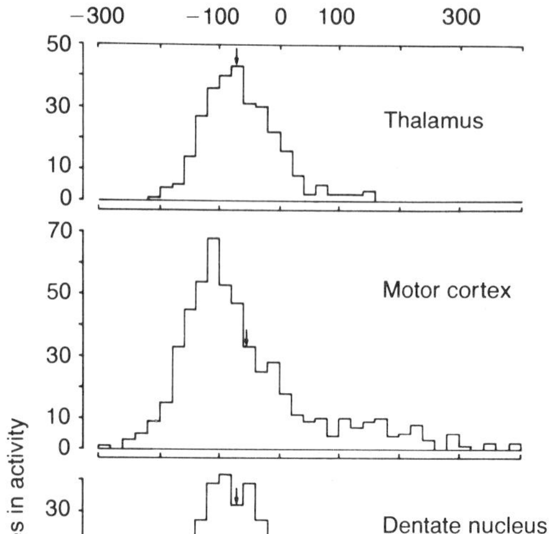

FIG. 16-16. Discharges of neurons in motor centers near the time of a movement. The time of the first change (either increase or decrease) in the discharge frequency of the neurons is plotted relative to the start of a movement. On the ordinate is the number of times a neuron was observed to change its discharge at each time before (time in negative numbers) and after (time in positive numbers) the movement. Movement began at time zero. The **arrow** above each histogram shows the median time of the first change in discharge for neurons in that center. The lower record shows the same kind of plot indicating when forearm muscles begin to discharge. (Data from Evarts EV: J Neurophysiol 31:14–27, 1968; Thach W: The behavior of Purkinje and cerebellar nuclear cells during two types of voluntary arm movements in the monkey. In Fields WS, Willis WD [eds]; Cerebellum in Health and Disease. St. Louis, Warren Green, 1970; DeLong MR: Brain Res 40:127–135, 1972)

motor cortex, a Purkinje cell in the cerebellar hemisphere, a neuron in the dentate nucleus, and a neuron in the globus pallidus of the basal ganglia. Note that each of these neurons fires in relation to a particular phase of a repeated movement of a handle by the monkey. The pyramidal tract neuron begins firing before the animal starts a movement of the handle requiring wrist extension; other pyramidal tract neurons might fire before flexion. Many neurons in the motor cortex, the cerebellar cortex and nuclei, the thalamus, and the red nucleus begin to discharge, increase their discharge rates, or decrease their discharge rates before movements. The discharges in the basal ganglia are usually not related to movement, but a few cells do discharge in relation to movements. The movement-related discharges in motor cortex and the dentate nucleus appear to be related to (1) the pattern of muscular activity required to hold the limb in a certain position, (2) the angle of a particular joint, or (3) the direction of the intended next movement. Neurons in the nucleus interpositus of the cerebellum appear to discharge in relationship only to the pattern of muscular activity [number (1) above].

Figure 16-16 shows the timing of the discharges in neurons of the thalamic nucleus ventralis lateralis, the motor cortex, dentate nucleus, nucleus interpositus, and cerebellar cortex related to the time of onset of muscle activity and the time of movement of the wrist. On the abscissa is plotted time before (negative numbers) and after (positive numbers) a movement beginning at time zero. The values on the ordinate are the number of changes in firing rate (either increases or decreases) that occurred in relation to that movement. Thus, the first changes in thalamic neuron discharges were seen slightly more than 200 msec before the movement. Clearly, neurons at each recording site change their discharges before the movement begins, but the earliest changes are seen in the motor cortex and dentate nucleus. The arrow in each histogram plots the median time of the first change in activity. This indicator of central tendency puts the first discharge in the thalamus, then later in the dentate nucleus, motor cortex, interpositus nucleus, and Purkinje cells. Neurons in the red nucleus (not shown) begin discharging between interpositus and Purkinje neurons. These data do not really allow one to say where a movement begins; neurons everywhere dis-

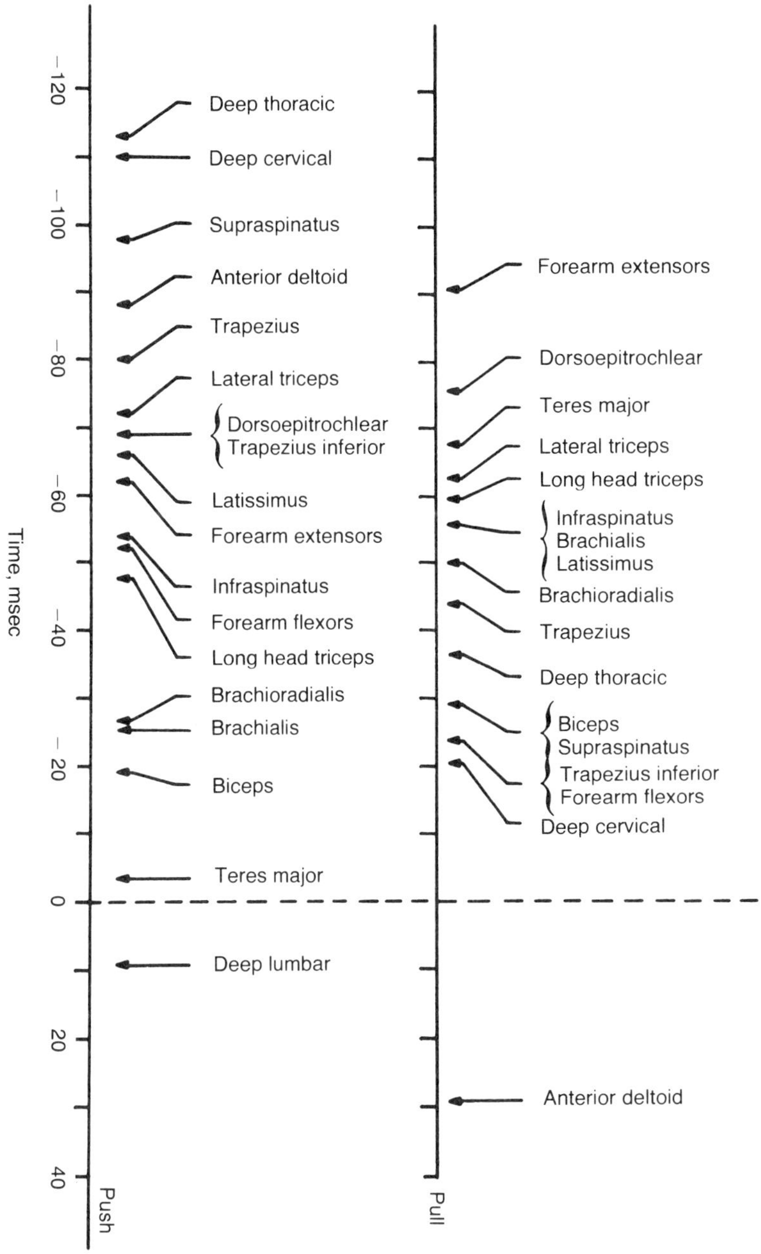

FIG. 16-17. Time of contraction in various muscles during a push–pull movement by a monkey. The movement (push, **left;** pull **right**) began at time zero; negative time is before movement; positive is after. (DeLong MR, Strick PL: Brain Res 71:327–335, 1974)

charge before, during, and after the movement.

One should always keep in mind that a movement of any part of the body involves contractions in muscles other than those intrinsic to that part. Thus, movement of the wrist involves more than just flexors and extensors of the wrist. Figure 16-17 shows some of the muscles that contract when a monkey pushes a lever away from himself or pulls it toward himself. With a rapid pull, the arm extensors contract first about 90 msec before the lever moves. This is followed by contractions in the dorso-

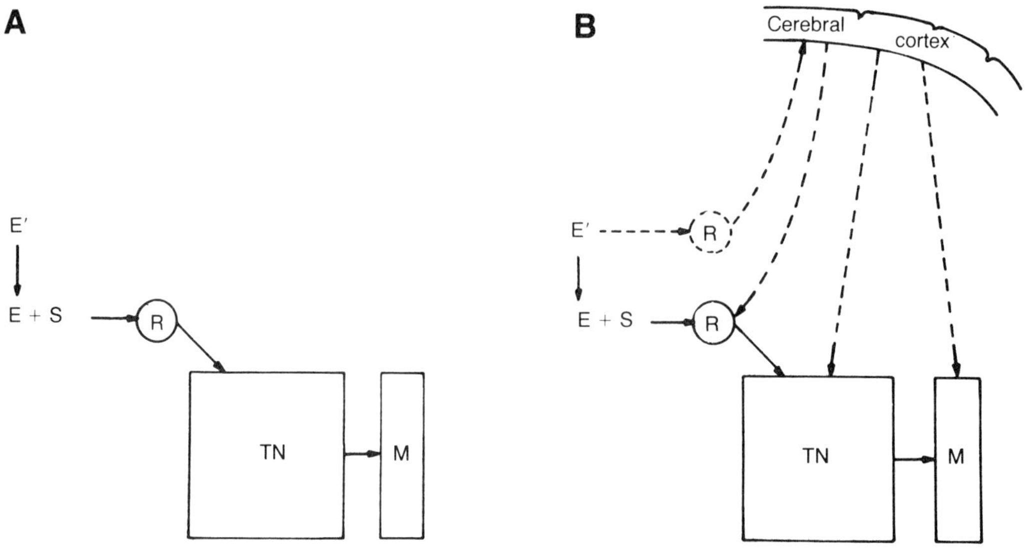

FIG. 16-18. A. Basic fly-detecting and catching circuitry of a frog. B. Basic fly-catching circuitry of a "smarter" frog and perhaps the schema for motor organization in mammals. R = exteroceptors and related sensory circuits; E and E′ = environments; S = the trigger stimulus, in this case the fly; TN = the automatic triggered network whose activity results in the behavior; and M = the motor apparatus that produces the behavior (Towe AL: Neurosci Res Prog Bull 9:42–48, 1971)

epitrochlear muscle at 75 msec and so on. Muscles that actually adduct the arm, the latissimus and biceps, do not begin contracting until 75 and 30 msec before the movement. With a rapid push, the sequence begins earlier, at about 170 msec before the movement, with contractions of the deep thoracic muscles and other muscles that do not move the arm. In fact, the muscles that extend the forearm, pushing the lever away, do not begin to contract until 90 msec (deltoid) and 70 msec (triceps muscles) before the movement. It cannot be ascertained to which muscle contractions in the sequence a given neuronal discharge may be related. Perhaps part of the variability in histograms of Figure 16-16 may be due to this involvement of many muscles in even the simplest movements.

THE FUNCTION OF SUPRASPINAL CONTROL OF MOVEMENT

If much of motor control and muscular coordination takes place at the spinal cord level, why have all this other machinery involved in movement? The frog, after all, moves perfectly well (for a frog) without a lot of brain. The answer lies in the smoothness, range, complexity, and plasticity of movements that are possible with these added controls. It is clear that a frog catches flies without a pyramidal tract and he escapes predators pretty well without large basal ganglia or large cerebellar hemispheres, but with these his repertoire of behaviors is nearly exhausted. The basic neural circuitry of the frog fly-catching apparatus is schematized in Figure 16-18A. The frog sits in some environment, E, that contains a flying insect, S; the insect is detected by an exteroceptor, R, activating an automatic, triggered network, TN, resulting in activation of the motor apparatus, M, for fly-catching behavior. The whole event is played out rapidly, but without any elements of prediction. If the nervous system of the frog were "smart," it would soon discover that there are places where flies are likely to be and places where they are not likely to be. Actually, frogs are able to do this, at least to a limited extent. If frogs could make extensive use of this information, the chances of successful fly-catching and therefore survival would increase; they would, in short, become better fly traps.

Figure 16-18B is schematic of how such a mechanism might work. Let us say E′ is an environment in which flies are likely to be. The frog's exteroceptors sense the presence of E′ even though S is not present. This information is transmitted to his cerebral cortex (this is a very unusual frog), which increases the excitability of the exteroceptor network (arrow from cerebral cortex to R), the excitability of the triggered-network (arrow from cerebral cortex to TN), and/or the motoneurons producing the movements (arrow from cerebral cortex to M). Now everything is ready: S appears in E, and the fly-catching behavior can occur even more rapidly, increasing the chances of success. Not only that, but the information about the whole event, including the quality of the environment E′, can be saved for future reference. This ability to predict the need for action and to change sensory function as well as motor function in prewired, stereotyped networks is probably what the cerebral cortical influences give the organism that has them. The cortex is incapable of acting on its own, but can call into play other centers to help in modifying the excitability not only of distal muscles, but also proximal, postural muscles. This makes some sense in light of the evolution of the nervous system, as discussed in Chapter 1.

SUGGESTED READING

Allen GI, Tsukahara N: Cerebrocerebellar communication systems. Physiol Rev 54:957–1006, 1974

DeLong MR, Strick PL: Relation of basal ganglia, cerebellum, and motor cortex units to ramp and ballistic limb movements. Brain Res 71:327–336, 1974

Evarts EV: Brain mechanisms of movement. Sci Am 241:164–179, 1979

Glickman SE, Schiff BB: A biological theory of reinforcement. Physiol Rev 74:81–109, 1967

Lawrence DG, Kuypers HGJM: The functional organization of the motor system in the monkey. I. The effects of bilateral pyramidal lesions. Brain 91:1–14, 1968

Lawrence DG, Kuypers HGJM: The functional organization of the motor system in the monkey. II. The effects of lesions of the descending brain-stem pathways. Brain 91:15–36, 1968

Orlovsky GN, Shik ML: Control of locomotion: A neurophysiological analysis of the cat locomotor system. In Porter R [ed]: International Review of Physiology, Vol. 10, Neurophysiology II. Baltimore, University Press, 1976

Porter R: Functions of the mammalian cerebral cortex in movements. In Kerkut GA, Phillis JW [eds]: Progress in Neurobiology. Oxford, Pergamon Press, 1973

Ruch TC: Transection of the spinal cord. In Ruch TC, Patton HD [eds]: Physiology and Biophysics, I. The Brain and Neural Function, 20th ed. Philadelphia, WB Saunders, 1979

Ruch TC: Brain stem control of posture and orientation in space. In Ruch TC, Patton HD [eds]: Physiology and Biophysics, I. The Brain and Neural Function, 20th ed. Philadelphia, WB Saunders, 1979

Towe AL: Untitled quoted contribution in: Central control of movement. Neurosci Res Prog Bull 9:42–48, 1971

Towe AL: Motor cortex and the pyramidal system. In Maser JD [ed]: Efferent Organization and Integration of Behavior. New York, Academic Press, 1973a

Towe AL: Relative numbers of pyramidal tract neurons in mammals of different sizes. Brain Behav Evol 7:1–17, 1973b

17

The Autonomic Nervous System

The **autonomic nervous system** basically is concerned with the regulation of visceral functions. Its peripheral constituents are to cardiac and smooth muscles essentially what α motoneurons are to skeletal muscles. The basic difference is that many of the tissues controlled by the autonomic system have their own intrinsic rhythms of activity, controlled by their own pacemakers. What the autonomic nervous system does in these tissues is speed up or slow down their inherent rhythms. For example, the isolated heart beats by itself, but the intact heart's contraction frequency is altered by autonomic discharge. This is not the only function of the autonomic system, however. It also causes vascular smooth muscle to contract or relax, it causes glands to secrete, it causes changes in certain metabolic functions, and it causes muscles in the eye to contract or relax. The neural mechanisms of these effects are not really different from those we have already considered. The autonomic system is an anatomic curiosity, not a physiologic one. We consider it in some detail here, because understanding its structure and function is essential to the study of moden clinical practices.

ANATOMY OF THE AUTONOMIC SYSTEM

The autonomic nervous system, as it is usually defined, is only an efferent (motor) system; it contains no sensory fibers. There are afferent fibers associated with visceral function that do contact and influence autonomic neurons, but these are usually termed **visceral afferent fibers.** There are some people, however, who prefer to call these autonomic afferent fibers. The visceral afferent fibers, in conjunction with somatic afferent fibers, provide the sensory input for control of the peripheral autonomic system. The autonomic nervous system is usually divided into two subdivisions: the **sympathetic** or **thoracicolumbar** nervous system and the **parasympathetic** or **craniosacral** nervous system. There are a number of differences between the two systems: They originate in different places (as their alternate names suggest); they have their ganglia in different locations with respect to the spinal cord and their target organs; they affect the organs in different, often opposite, ways; and they usually use different transmitter substances in influencing the effector organs. Both systems differ from the somatic motor system in having the cell bodies of their motoneurons in peripheral ganglia, that is, outside the CNS.

THE SYMPATHETIC NERVOUS SYSTEM

The sympathetic system on the periphery consists of a two-cell efferent pathway. The soma of the first cell in the pathway, the **preganglionic cell,** lies in the intermediolateral column of the gray matter of the spinal cord. These somata are distributed over spinal cord segments T1 to L2 (thus the name thoracicolumbar). The axons of these cells are myelinated fibers and usually have conduction velocities in the B-fiber range. The preganglionic axons exit the spinal cord by way of the nearest ventral root, which they soon leave as a bundle.

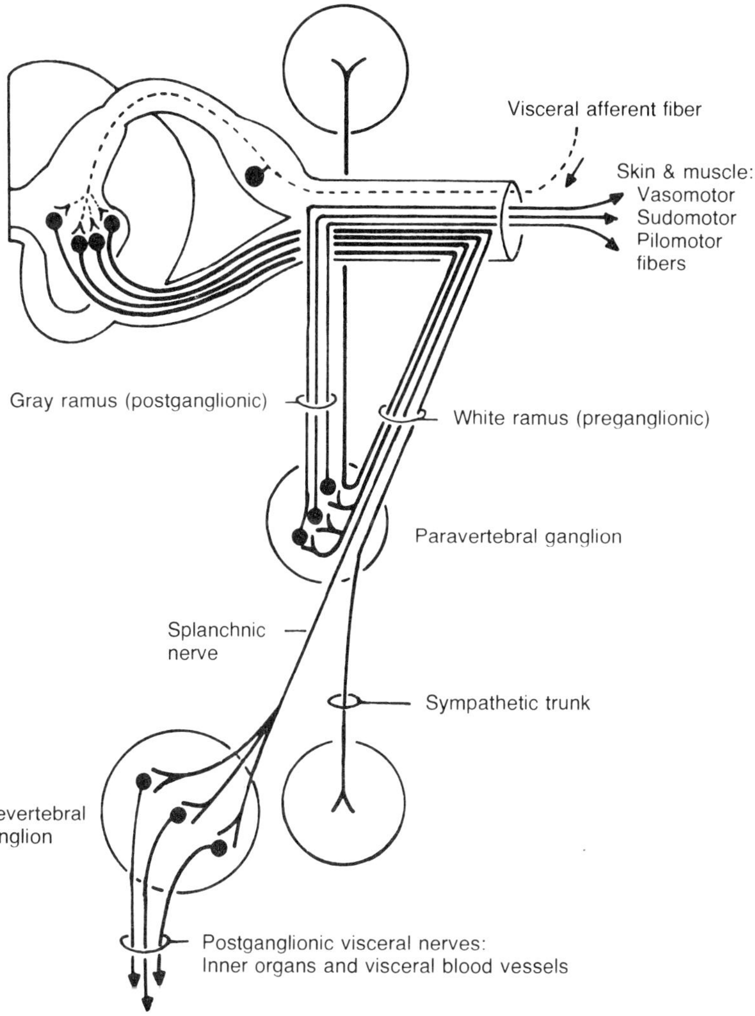

FIG. 17-1. The basic unit of the sympathetic nervous system. Shown are the location of preganglionic somata and the course of their myelinated axons **(heavy lines)** into the ventral roots, white ramus, paravertebral ganglion, sympathetic chain, and splanchnic nerve. Postganglionic cells are shown in paravertebral and prevertebral ganglia with unmyelinated axons **(thin lines)** running into the gray ramus and visceral nerves. Also note the interconnection of adjacent paravertebral ganglia by the sympathetic trunk. (Pick J: The Autonomic Nervous System. Philadelphia, JB Lippincott, 1970)

This bundle, the white (myelin is white) ramus communicans, enters one of the 22 to 23 paravertebral ganglia that happens to be located at the level of that ventral root, as illustrated in Figure 17-1. Within the ganglion an axon may (1) synapse on a soma within that ganglion; or (2) it may turn rostrally or caudally into the sympathetic trunk (which interconnects the ganglia in the paravertebral chain) and synapse on a soma in another ganglion of the chain; or (3) it may pass through the ganglion without forming a synapse, enter a nerve that runs to one of the prevertebral ganglia, and end on a soma there. The cell upon which the terminals of the preganglionic cell form a synapse is called the **postganglionic cell.** The axons of postganglionic cells are, in general, unmyelinated fibers, and they run out to the organ to be influenced. Those that are destined for the blood vessels, glands, and other smooth muscle of the skin and skeletal muscle originate in the paravertebral ganglia and take a course out of the ganglia by way of the gray (unmyelinated fibers are gray) ramus communicans and rejoin

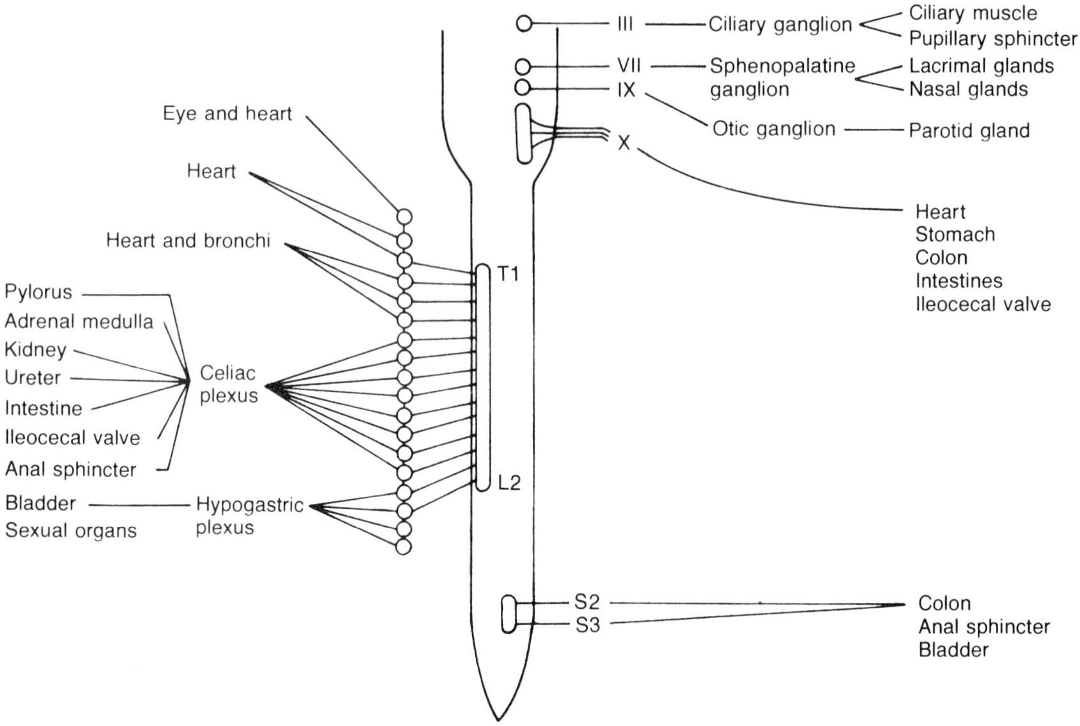

FIG. 17-2. Sites of origin and distribution of autonomic fibers to the various effector organs. On the **left,** the origin of the sympathetic nervous system in the intermediolateral cell column of the T2 to L2 cord segments is shown along with a schematic diagram of the relationship to the sympathetic chain and effector organs. On the **right,** the origin of the parasympathetic nervous system is shown to be in four cranial nerves and in the intermediolateral cell column of the sacral spinal cord. Also shown are the relays and effector organs of the parasympathetic system. Note that the sympathetic and parasympathetic systems both occur bilaterally; thus, what is shown is only half of the systems. (Willis WD Jr, Grossman RG: Medical Neurobiology. St. Louis, CV Mosby, 1977)

the fibers of the ventral root before going to the cutaneous or muscle nerves. This is also shown in Figure 17-1. Those postganglionic axons destined for the visceral organs arise from the prevertebral ganglia and course in the visceral nerves to smooth muscle of the inner organs and visceral blood vessels. An exception to this basic scheme is the sympathetic innervation of the adrenal medulla. Preganglionic fibers, whose activity influences the medulla of the adrenal gland, travel to the celiac prevertebral ganglion, pass through without making any contacts, and contact the adrenal gland directly. Thus, the chromaffin cells (the secretory cells) of the adrenal are postganglionic sympathetic cells.

The arrangement of the paravertebral ganglia is approximately segmental, but some of them have become fused together in development. The end result is that there are usually only two cervical ganglia, the superior and middle cervical ganglia, and the third cervical is fused with the first thoracic, forming the stellate ganglion. Normally, there are 10 to 11 thoracic, 4 lumbar, 4 sacral ganglia, and 1 coccygeal ganglion, with only the thoracic and lumbar ganglia attached to the ventral roots by a white ramus. This is shown diagrammatically in Figure 17-2 (left). The ganglia are joined together to form a chain by the sympathetic trunk. As we have seen, this trunk serves as a pathway for distribution of preganglionic fibers up and down the sympathetic chain, and it is the only source of preganglionic input to the cervical, sacral, and coccygeal ganglia.

The distributions of the postganglionic fibers of the sympathetic system to visceral organs are shown on the left side of Figure 17-2. The superior cervical ganglion sends its fibers to the eye, where they dilate the pupil and innervate the superior tarsal muscle (opens the upper lid), and to the heart. Additional fibers are contributed to the regulation of heart rate and contractility from several others of the rostral ganglia. Preganglionic fibers arising from the T5–T11 ganglia course to the celiac plexus, from which postganglionic fibers contact the stomach, kidney, intestines, and the internal anal sphincter. The hypogastric plexus receives fibers from the most caudal ganglia and sends them to the bladder and sexual organs.

THE PARASYMPATHETIC NERVOUS SYSTEM

Preganglionic fibers of the parasympathetic system arise from the brain stem and exit through four of the cranial nerves (III, VII, IX, and X) and from intermediolateral cell columns of spinal cord segments S1–S4, but mainly S2 and S3 (Fig. 17-2, right). Preganglionic fibers arising in the oculomotor nucleus, specifically the Edinger-Westphal nucleus, form connections with postganglionic cell somata located in the ciliary ganglion. The distribution and functions of these fibers in the eye are discussed in Chapter 7. The facial nerve contains preganglionic fibers that synapse in the sphenopalatine ganglion. Postganglionic fibers from this ganglion innervate glands of the nasal and pharyngeal mucous membranes and the lacrimal glands. The third parasympathetic cranial nerve, the glossopharyngeal (IX), synapses in the otic ganglion and thereby influences the secretions of the parotid salivary glands. Unlike the others, the vagus (X) does not send its preganglionic fibers to a cranial ganglion, but instead sends them directly to ganglion cells in plexuses in the walls of the organs it innervates, specifically, the heart, stomach, colon, intestines, and the ileocecal valve. Like those in the vagus, the preganglionic fibers arising from the sacral spinal cord run directly to organs in the lower abdomen and pelvis, where they form similar connections in the walls of the colon, bladder, and sexual organs.

POSTGANGLIONIC SYNAPSES

The synaptic structures involving postganglionic fibers and their target organs are a bit different from those described in Chapter 13. The axons enter the layers of smooth muscle or cardiac muscle or the parenchyma of glands and simply terminate. They do not seem to enter into any specialized synaptic contacts, but apparently just release their transmitter substances from the terminals as in other synapses. The transmitter substance then diffuses to the receptor sites on the effectors, sometimes over considerable distances. This partially accounts for the rather slow responses of these smooth muscles compared to skeletal muscles.

PHARMACOLOGY OF AUTONOMIC TRANSMISSION

It is important to know something of the pharmacology of autonomic transmission, because drugs that affect autonomic nervous system transmission are widely used clinically. To understand experimental work in these areas, you must know the actions of some of the most common agents. Preganglionic axons, both the short sympathetics and the relatively longer parasympathetics, release acetylcholine at their terminals on postganglionic cells. Synapses that employ **acetylcholine** as their transmitter substance are called **cholinergic synapses.** The synapses formed by the relatively short postganglionic parasympathetic axons are also cholinergic. On the other hand, the majority of the postganglionic sympathetic axons secrete the catecholamine, **norepinephrine,** at their synapses. Synapses that employ this substance are called **adrenergic synapses.** (Adrenergic is a general term used for synapses employing the structurally similar compounds, norepinephrine and epinephrine.) A few sympathetic postganglionic neurons form synapses that are cholinergic. Sympathetic innervation of the sweat glands and blood vessels in skin and skeletal muscle is both adrenergic and cholinergic. In blood vessels, transmission through adrenergic synapses may either constrict (alpha effect) or relax (beta effect) vascular smooth muscle, whereas cholinergic synapses, where they occur, cause vessels to relax. A summary of the basic plans of the two divisions and their transmitter substances is shown in Figure 17-3 for quick reference.

Physiologists have subdivided effects at both cholinergic and adrenergic synapses into two groups each, based upon whether they are elicited by compounds other than acetylcholine and norepinephrine.

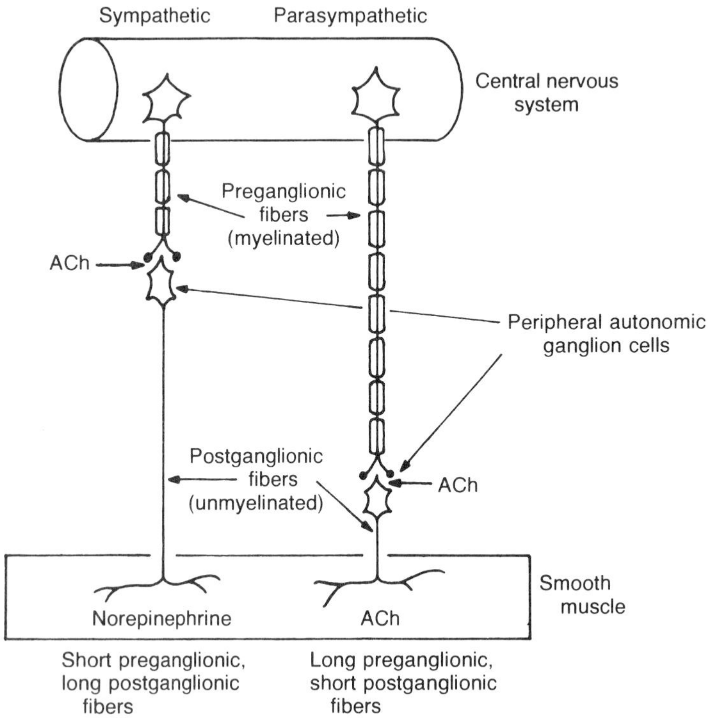

FIG. 17-3. Relative lengths of preganglionic and postganglionic fibers of sympathetic **(left)** and parasympathetic **(right)** systems and transmitters employed at various synapses. Note that preganglionic fibers are myelinated; postganglionic fibers are not. (Willis WD Jr, Grossman RG: Medical Neurobiology. St. Louis, CV Mosby, 1977)

TABLE 17-1. TYPES OF CHOLINERGIC AND ADRENERGIC EFFECTS

CHOLINERGIC SYNAPSES All activated by acetylcholine		ADRENERGIC SYNAPSES All activated by norepinephrine	
↙	↘	↙	↘
Nicotinic Effects All produced by nicotine	**Muscarinic Effects** All produced by muscarine	**Alpha Effects** Greater response to norepinephrine	**Beta Effects** Greater response to isoproterenol
↓	↓	↓	↓
Also produced by: carbamylcholine methacholine	Also produced by: pilocarpine	Also produced by: epinephrine	Also produced by: epinephrine
↓	↓	↓	↓
Blocked by: curare tetraethylammonium ions hexamethonium pentolinium	Blocked by: atropine scopolamine	Blocked by: phenoxybenzamine phentolamine	Blocked by: propranolol
↓	↓	↓	↓
Examples: contraction of skeletal muscle excitation of postganglionic cells	Examples: decreased heart rate salivation penile erection	Examples: cutaneous vasoconstriction sudomotor effects pilomotor effects pupillary dilatation intestinal relaxation	Examples: cutaneous vasodilatation increased heart rate skeletal muscle vasodilatation bronchiolar dilatation muscle glycogenolysis

Table 17-1 summarizes this subdivision. Cholinergic effects are either **nicotinic** or **muscarinic** depending upon whether they are also caused by administration of nicotine, an alkaloid extracted from tobacco, or muscarine, an alkaloid extracted from toadstools. A variety of compounds can produce each type of effect, but muscarine does not produce nicotinic effects and nicotine does not produce muscarinic effects. Examples of both types of cholinergic actions are shown in Table 17-1. The contraction of skeletal muscles by α motoneurons and the excitation of postganglionic autonomic cells by preganglionic fibers are both nicotinic effects. The slowing of the heart by vagal activity and the activation of effectors by parasympathetic postganglionic fibers are both muscarinic effects.

It should be kept in mind that both nicotinic and muscarinic effects are produced by acetylcholine under normal circumstances. Nicotine and muscarine are not naturally occurring substances in animal tissues. The value of the distinction between the two sorts of effects is pharmacologic. Suppose you wanted to slow the heart rate without affecting transmission to skeletal muscles. It would be possible to do this by administration of pilocarpine, which produces only muscarinic effects (see Table 17-1).

The effects of adrenergic activity are divided into alpha and beta effects, depending upon whether they are produced by lower concentrations of norepinephrine as opposed to either isoproterenol or epinephrine. Both types respond to all three agents, but **alpha effects** are produced more readily by norepinephrine than by isoproterenol or epinephrine, and **beta effects** are produced more readily by isoproterenol and epinephrine than by norepinephrine. The magnitude of the responses initiated by epinephrine is usually between the magnitudes of the responses to these other two agents. *Bear in mind: both alpha and beta effects are produced by norepinephrine, epinephrine, and isoproterenol!* It is pharmacologically impossible to produce beta effects without, at the same time, producing alpha effects on some tissue.

As shown in Table 17-1, alpha adrenergic effects are blocked by phenoxybenzamine and phentolamine, whereas beta adrenergic effects are blocked by administration of propranolol. Examples of alpha and beta effects are shown at the bottom of the table. In general, beta adrenergic effects involve relaxation or inhibition of activity except in the heart where the opposite is true. Alpha effects, on the other hand, often involve contraction. Both alpha and beta adrenergic effects are produced by the norepinephrine and epinephrine released from the adrenal medulla when it is stimulated by preganglionic sympathetic activity. This is in addition to the effects produced by catecholamines released at adrenergic synapses. The adrenal medulla, in fact, acts like a postganglionic sympathetic neuron, but it releases it catecholamines directly into the blood.

Many people refer to alpha and beta adrenergic receptors or even alpha and beta adrenergic pathways. This is inappropriate terminology. There is no evidence that there are different receptors for the various catecholamines. These substances differ little in chemical structure, yet they may differ greatly in their sites of action; perhaps one acts inside the cell, the other outside. There is even evidence of a conversion, by temperature changes, of apparent alpha responses to beta responses in the frog heart and also in the mammalian heart, suggesting that there may be in fact only a single receptor type whose conformation and therefore responsiveness to agonists and antagonists is variable (Kunos, Yong, Nickerson, 1973). It is appropriate to refer to alpha and beta adrenergic effects. It is, however, appropriate to speak of nicotinic and muscarinic cholinergic synapses, because here the physical separation has been demonstrated.

EFFECTS OF AUTONOMIC SYSTEM ACTIVITY

The effects of general sympathetic nervous system activity are similar to those seen in an animal that is behaving in an emotional manner that physiologists like to call "fight or flight." The sympathetic system is likely to be very active at times when the organism (human or other) is angry or frightened. Heart rate is increased, blood pressure rises, gastric motility is decreased, pupils dilate, and hair stands on end.

TABLE 17-2. RESPONSES OF EFFECTOR ORGANS TO AUTONOMIC ACTIVITY

ORGAN	TYPE OF EFFECT	SYMPATHETIC EFFECT	PARASYMPATHETIC EFFECT
Eye: Pupil	α	Dilatation	Constriction
Ciliary muscle	β	Slight relaxation	Contraction
Glands: Nasal, salivary lacrimal, gastric and pancreatic		Vasoconstriction, salivary secretion	Secretion, vasodilatation
Sweat glands	α	Sweating (cholinergic and adrenergic)	Secretion
Apocrine glands		Sweating	None
Heart: Muscle	β	Increased frequency of contraction, increased contractility	Decreased frequency of contraction, decreased contractility
Coronary vessels		Dilatation	Dilatation
Lungs: Bronchi	β	Dilatation	Constriction
Blood vessels	α	Mild constriction	None
Gut: Lumen	α, β	Decreased peristalsis and tone	Increased peristalsis and tone
Sphincter	α	Increased tone	Decreased tone
Liver		Glucose release	None
Gall bladder and bile ducts		Relaxation (no secretion)	Contraction (secretion)
Kidney		Decreased output	None
Bladder: Detrusor	β	Relaxation	Contraction
Trigone and sphincter	α	Contraction	Relaxation
Penis		Ejaculation	Erection, ejaculation
Systemic blood vessels: Abdominal	α	Constriction	None
Muscle	β	Dilatation (adrenergic)	None
	α	Constriction (adrenergic) Dilatation (cholinergic)	
Skin	α	Constriction (adrenergic) Dilatation (cholinergic)	Dilatation
Piloerector muscles	α	Contraction	None
Skeletal muscles		Increased glycogenolysis	None

Parasympathetic activity can normally be suspected to be high in an organism that is sated and contented. Heart rate is slowed, pupils constrict, and food is being digested. A catalogue of the effects of sympathetic and parasympathetic stimulation can be seen in Table 17-2. This general scheme can be seen to apply fairly well. The frequent opposition of the two systems can also be seen in the table.

Often people speak about the autonomic nervous system in a manner that suggests that they think that the sympathetic and, to some extent, the parasympathetic systems always act as a unit. Whenever any part of one of them is active, all or most of the system is active. Although this can be the case when an organism is under extreme danger or otherwise highly excited, the majority of the time the two systems do not behave in this way. Examples of activity in isolated portions of the sympathetic system are the initiation of sweating and increased blood flow through the skin without other effects when the body temperature rises and the many reflex activities involving this system, as outlined in Chapter 15. Parasympathetic reflexes normally also act in this isolated fashion, but they, too, can act together as they do, for example, after a large meal when glands secrete, stomach and intestines are active, and micturition and defecation reflexes are active.

SYMPATHETIC AND PARASYMPATHETIC TONE

We have already seen that the α motoneurons have a basal resting discharge rate that results in a continuous resting muscle contraction, called muscle tone.

Likewise, the sympathetic and parasympathetic fibers are continuously active, resulting in what are called **sympathetic** and **parasympathetic tone.** The value of tone in any system lies in the ability of the system either to increase or decrease its activity from the resting levels. Of course, this is not possible if the resting level is zero.

In the peripheral vasculature, sympathetic tone is seen as an ongoing contraction of vascular smooth muscle, such that at rest blood vessels are maintained at about half their maximum diameters. From this rest position, they can decrease their diameters in response to an increase in sympathetic activity or increase them in response to a decrease in sympathetic activity. Sectioning the parasympathetic innervation of the gut by sectioning the vagus can lead to serious gastric and intestinal problems, referred to as atony. This illustrates that the parasympathetic system may also have tone.

SUPRASPINAL CONTROL OF AUTONOMIC FUNCTION

Some autonomic functions are controlled fairly effectively by brain-stem mechanisms whose components lie below the pontine level. Heart function and respiration (a somatic function influenced by the autonomic system) appear, at least superficially, to be normal in the low decerebrate animal. We will see shortly that there are some changes in these functions in the low decerebrate animal, but the heart still beats, blood pressure rises in response to hypoxia, and the animal breathes well enough to regulate its blood gases at normal values. Even these functions are not completely normal, however. It is seldom that autonomic activity occurs in one part of the system in isolation; heart and lungs usually change activity in parallel, and there are cardiovascular and respiratory changes that occur with digestion, temperature changes, exercise, and even sexual behavior. The integration of the autonomic components of these various behaviors appears to be the domain of the hypothalamus.

The hypothalamus consists of the tissues that make up the walls and floor of the third ventricle, including a number of nuclei and fiber tracts. The nuclei are often divided into three groups. Anteriorly are found the supraoptic and paraventricular nuclei, immediately above the optic chiasm. Approximate locations are shown in Figure 17-4 on a parasagittal section of the human brain. The middle group of nuclei consists of the dorsomedial, ventromedial, and lateral nuclei, whereas the posterior group consists of the mammillary nuclei and the posterior nuclei. The hypothalamus receives its afferent input from the olfactory bulbs either directly, as some anatomists claim, or indirectly by way of the amygdala and piriform cortex; from the periaqueductal gray matter of the mesencephalon; from the reticular formation; from the hippocampus by way of the fornix to the mammillary bodies or by way of the septum; from the cingulate cortex through the thalamus; and perhaps also from the retina by disputed direct retinohypothalamic fibers. The hypothalamus is thus supplied with sensory information of olfaction, vision, audition, and somesthesia, from the olfactory bulb and from reticular inputs; with pain and mesenteric sensory information from the periaqueductal gray matter and elsewhere; and perhaps motor and motivation information from the cortex, amygdala, and hippocampus.

The hypothalamus sends its activity to the anterior thalamus by way of the mammillothalamic tract; to the amygdala and septum; to the mesencephalic periaqueductal gray matter, pretectal area, and superior colliculus; and to the brain stem by way of the mammillotegmental tract. In addition to these connections with "neural" autonomic centers, the hypothalamus connects with the "endocrine" autonomic structures by hypothalamohypophyseal fibers to the posterior pituitary and by the hypophyseal portal vasculature to the anterior pituitary. The hypothalamus is thus able to influence autonomic functions directly through its connections with the brain-stem autonomic nuclei and indirectly through the thalamus and periaqueductal gray matter.

Of those functions known to be under hypothalamic control, only temperature regulation, control of cardiovascular function, and control of food and water intake will be discussed here. These three are good examples of how the autonomic nervous system maintains physiologic parameters—blood pressure, body temperature, blood sugar, and water—within normal boundaries.

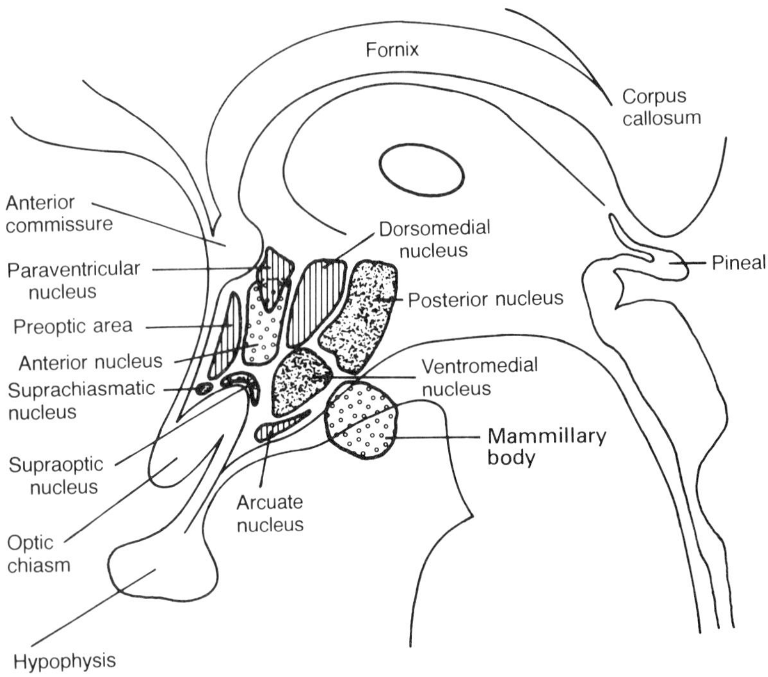

FIG. 17-4. Schematic diagram of the medial hypothalamic nuclei on a parasagittal section of the human brain (anterior is left). The lateral hypothalamic nuclei are not shown but would be located lateral to and approximately dorsoventrally coextensive with the dorsomedial, ventromedial, and posterior nuclei. (Carpenter MB: Human Neuroanatomy, 7th ed. Baltimore, Williams and Wilkins, 1976)

TEMPERATURE REGULATION

The hypothalamus is the major center for the control of body temperature in homeotherms. As we have seen in Chapter 16, animals with transections of the neuraxis below the level of the hypothalamus do not regulate their body temperature and will soon die of exposure if their temperature is not maintained artificially. There are a number of mechanisms used in regulating body temperature. An animal that is hypothermic can create heat by increasing its metabolic rate and by shivering; it can conserve heat by piloerection and peripheral vasoconstriction. A warm animal can lose heat by panting, sweating, and peripheral vasodilatation.

Thermoregulation can be triggered by changes in arterial blood temperature, by changes in skin temperature, by motor activity, by changes in the level of arousal, and by hormonal secretion. Thus, the hypothalamus would be expected to come into play in changes in body temperature that occur with exercise, the sleep–wakefulness cycle, and with ovulation. Its position in the brain and its connections with other structures are well suited to this function.

Bilateral lesions in the anterior hypothalamus produce an animal that does not increase heat loss when brought into a warm room, whereas bilateral lesions of the posterior hypothalamus lateral to the mammillary bodies produce an animal that does not shiver or show vasoconstriction when brought into a cold room. Heating the anterior hypothalamus with a small thermoprobe produces increased heat loss that, in the cat, takes the form of panting. Presumably, in humans, the heat loss would be promoted through sweating and vasodilatation. Thus, the anterior nuclei appear to act mainly in lowering body temperature, whereas the posterior nuclei appear to act mainly in elevating body temperature.

The hypothalamus, including the preoptic area, contains many neurons that are responsive to changes in local brain temperature and to changes in skin temperature. These neurons have been found all over the hypothalamus, but they are more common anteriorly.

It now appears that heat loss responses are induced only upon increases in hypothalamic temperature, whereas heat-producing or -conserving responses are elicted by changes in either peripheral temperature or hypothalamic temperature. The exact pathways by which these effects are produced are not yet known.

CARDIOVASCULAR CONTROL MECHANISMS

The extent of supraspinal control of cardiovascular responses is about as well understood as the supraspinal control of movement, that is, we know what structures (nuclei or larger structures) are involved and we know what happens when we ablate or stimulate them. For example, stimulation of the posterior and lateral aspects of the hypothalamus produces increases in blood pressure and heart rate, whereas stimulation of the anterior aspects produces decreases in blood pressure and peripheral vasodilatation. Many of the areas of the cerebral cortex are involved in autonomic functions, but no area does so exclusively; all have some other function, usually somatic, as well. Stimulation in areas 4 and 6 (the motor and premotor cortices) produces peripheral vasodilatation with constriction of the renal vascular bed. Extirpation of these areas produces vasomotor changes in those limbs that are at the same time made paretic. Stimulation of the fronto-orbital cortex leads to depression of both blood pressure and heart rate which result from decreased sympathetic constrictor tone and increased vagal activity. It is said to be possible to produce sympathetic vasoconstriction in one of the gastrointestinal, renal, muscle, or cutaneous vascular beds without affecting the others, by properly controlling stimulus parameters (*i.e.*, duration, intensity, and frequency).

The posterior hypothalamus contains neurons that respond to changes in blood pressure induced by administration of epinephrine, but do not change activity if the blood pressure is "clamped" or if sinoaortic baroreceptors are denervated. They change their firing rates, either increase or decrease, roughly in proportion to the change in blood pressure. Neurons sensitive to activity in baroreceptors and/or chemoreceptors have also been found in the medial hypothalamus. In addition, neurons in the supraoptic and paraventricular nuclei and in the anterior, lateral, and medial hypothalamic nuclei are responsive to changes in atrial (right or left) volume, presumably through mediation of enteroceptors responsive to atrial stretch. Their role in regulation of cardiovascular parameters is not known, but they may be involved in regulation of blood volume rather than in regulation of blood pressure.

In spite of this responsiveness to changes in the cardiovascular system, there appears to be little involvement of suprabulbar structures in control of heart rate and total peripheral vascular resistance, based on baroreceptor inputs alone; however, many higher centers are capable of modifying baroreceptor reflexes as a part of their role in control of movement or behavior. This conclusion comes from observations made in intact, thalamic, and low decerebrate rabbits (as described in Table 16-2). Resting parameters of respiratory and cardiovascular function in these three preparations are shown in Table 17-3. It can be seen that low decerebrate animals—animals with only pontine and more caudal control centers intact—differ from intact animals in having lower heart rates, higher right atrial blood pressures, lower blood flow in portal vessels, and higher flows in muscle beds. A transection of the neuraxis that leaves the thalamus and hypothalamus intact produces an animal (a thalamic animal) with higher than normal respiration rate, larger respiratory volumes, and greater flows in renal and muscle vascular beds. Otherwise, both low decerebrate and thalamic animals at rest are much like control animals at rest.

The importance of supraspinal control mechanisms is shown when the organism is challenged, as it might be during some behavior. Figure 17-5 shows changes in various cardiovascular parameters during a period of hypoxia induced by forcing the animal to breathe 8% O_2 in N_2. The period of hypoxia is initiated at the downward arrow and terminated at the upward arrow. The responses of a normal animal are shown in the first column, those of a thalamic animal in the second, and those of a low decerebrate animal in the third column. Low decerebrate animals differ in terms of changes in heart rate, skin, and renal vascular resistance, suggesting that structures above the

TABLE 17-3. RESTING VALUES OF CARDIOVASCULAR PARAMETERS IN RABBITS*

	NORMAL	THALAMIC	LOW DECEREBRATE
Arterial Po_2, mm Hg	105 ± 1.9†	109 ± 2.5	109 ± 5.0
Arterial Pco_2, mm Hg	25 ± 0.81	21 ± 0.74	27 ± 1.76
Arterial pH	7.54 ± .022	7.52 ± .042	7.63 ± .039
Respiration rate, per min	65	80	64
Respiratory flow rate ($\dot{V}_E$)‡	1.16	1.68	1.18
Heart rate, per min	302 ± 9.5	295 ± 10.5	246 ± 10.9
Arterial blood pressure, mm Hg	93 ± 2.1	91 ± 4.6	89 ± 3.9
Right atrial blood pressure, mm Hg	−0.8 ± 0.27	−0.9 ± 0.74	+0.1 ± 0.46
Portal blood flow, ml/min	105 ± 15.5	95 ± 13.8	62 ± 7.3
Renal blood flow, ml/min	57 ± 6.8	70 ± 10.4	52 ± 8.8
Muscle blood flow, ml/min/hindlimb	14 ± 3.2	24 ± 6.0	26 ± 8.8
Skin (ear) blood flow, ml/min/100g	16 ± 0.6	14 ± 0.8	14 ± 0.6

* Uther JB, Hunyor SN, Shaw J, Korner PI: Circ Res 26:491–506, 1970.
† Values are means ± standard errors.
‡ Units; liters/min.

FIG. 17-5. Cardiovascular responses to hypoxia induced by breathing 8% O_2 at the **downward arrow** and released at the **upward arrow.** Experiments were done in rabbits sham-operated (control), with cerebral hemispheres removed (thalamic), and with low decerebrations. (Uther JB, Hunyer SN, Shaw J et al: Circ Res 26:491–506, 1970)

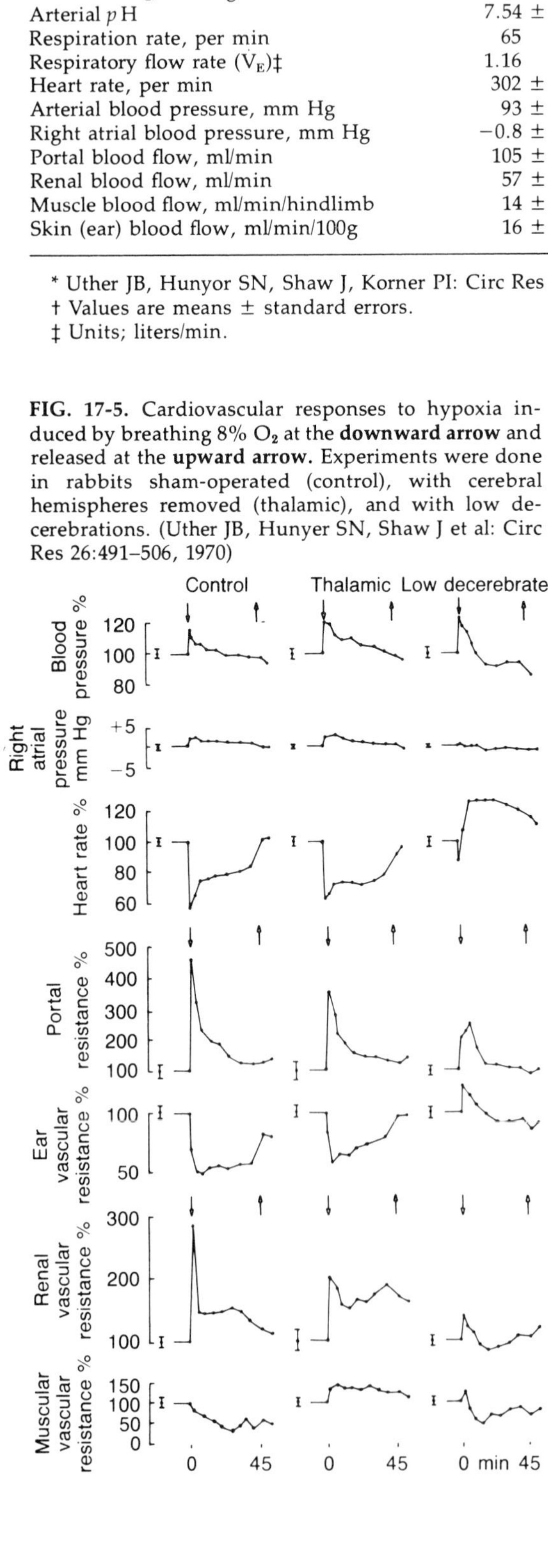

pontine level play a role in these responses. Changes in the various parameters are similar for control and thalamic animals, suggesting that structures above the thalamic level have little role in these responses.

The results of these experiments have been summarized in Figure 17-6, where excitatory effects (effects that tend to increase autonomic activity) are shown as open arrows and inhibitory effects (effects that tend to decrease autonomic activity) are shown as black arrows. Approximate magnitudes of effects are indicated by the size of the arrows. It should be noted that the cerebral cortex exerts a weak excitatory influence only upon the responses to hypoxia of portal and renal vasoconstrictor muscles. The composite effect of all structures above the pons is a strong excitation of vagal cardiac nerves and a strong inhibition of sympathetic actions on the heart, weak excitation of portal vasoconstrictors, strong excitation of renal and muscle vasoconstrictors, and strong inhibition of cutaneous vasoconstrictors in the ear. Presumably, these influences are normally exerted when the supraspinal centers are readying the body for exercise, for strong emotional responses, or for other behaviors mediated by these centers.

CONTROL OF FOOD AND WATER INTAKE

The hypothalamus plays a major role in controlling food and water intake. Obviously, we eat when we are hungry and drink when we are thirsty, but both hunger and thirst

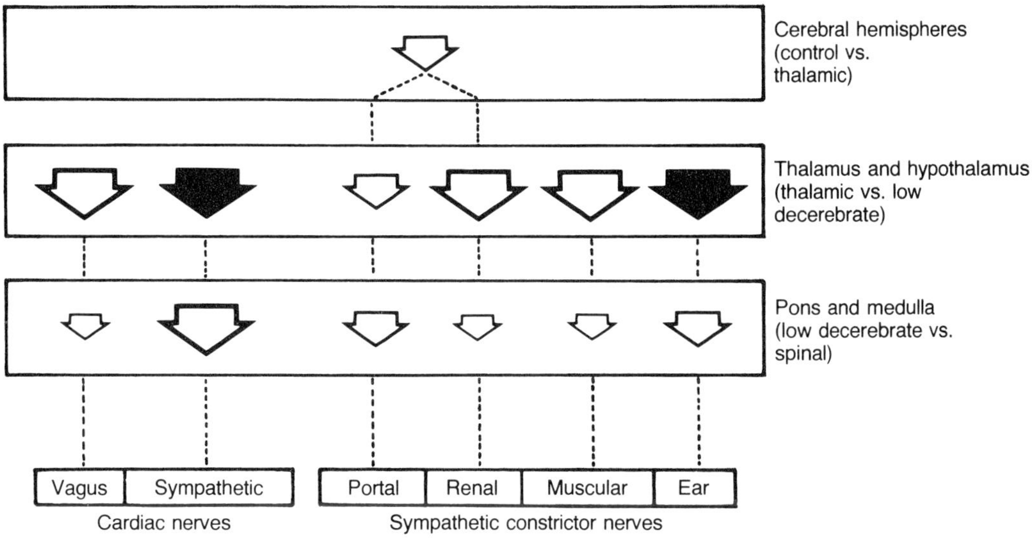

FIG. 17-6. Summary diagram indicating approximate contribution of pons and medulla, thalamus and hypothalamus, and cerebral hemispheres to autonomic responses of rabbit during hypoxia. **Black arrows** indicate inhibition of the autonomic effector to which arrow is pointing; **open arrows** indicate excitation of effectors. Size of arrow is approximately proportional to the magnitude of the effect (Uther JB, Hunyor SN, Shaw J et al: Circ Res 26:491–506, 1970)

are complex sensations that depend upon peripheral and central receptors. Hunger sensations can result from a fall in blood sugar level, but blood sugar level itself does not seem to be the factor that initiates hunger. Some people believe it is the degree of sugar utilization by the tissues that determines hunger. On the other hand, the cessation of hunger depends upon oral and gastric factors involving taste, content, and volume of food but depends little on restoration of blood sugar levels or other nutrient levels. Likewise, thirst involves both central and peripheral receptors. The sensation of thirst is evoked by dryness in the mouth, loss of body fluids, or concentration of body salts. Cessation of drinking can be brought about by elimination of mouth dryness or stomach distention but it occurs before restoration of blood or tissue fluid levels. Animals will drink to restore water levels precisely and stop before any of the water can be absorbed into the blood.

The hypothalamic involvement in food intake is indicated by a number of different types of experiments. Lesions in the ventromedial nucleus lead to **hyperphagia,** in which the animal or human becomes obese. Hypothalamic hyperphagia is not a constant phenomenon, but is an initial transient overeating (2–3 times normal amounts), followed by a reduction in intake to near normal levels while the excess weight gained during overeating is maintained. Lesions in the lateral hypothalamus in animals lead to **aphagia,** in which the animal does not eat and, unless special measures are taken, starves to death. If the animals are fed for some days by tube, they will usually recover to the point of maintaining an adequate intake. They can also be induced to take in enough food by making some reward contingent upon eating. For example, rats love to run in activity wheels. They can be trained to eat in order to run. **Anorexia** occurs rarely in man and is not found in cases of known hypothalamic lesions. Electrical stimulation of the lateral hypothalamus induces eating even in a satiated animal. Similarly, stimulation of the ventromedial nucleus suppresses eating even in an animal near starvation.

Recordings have been made of the activity of single neurons in the hypothalamus that may be involved in initiating or terminating eating. Intravenous infusion of glucose excites some neurons in the ventromedial region, whereas it reduces activity in some neurons of lateral regions. Direct **iontophoresis** of glucose into the recording region produces excitation in about half of the cells recorded from in the ventromedial region, but no effect is seen from iontophoresis of NaCl, suggesting that these neurons may be glucoreceptors—or connected to them—and not osmoreceptors, receptors for sensing fluid osmolality. In the lateral hypothalamus, iontophoresis of glucose produces a decrease in activity in some cells, and NaCl is without effect. In other cells, glucose produces either an increase or decrease in activity and NaCl has the same effect, implying that these cells are associated with osmoreception. Free fatty acids have the reverse effect of glucose on hypothalamic cells. One can, as yet, only speculate upon the exact role of these neurons in control of food intake.

The stimulus for drinking is undoubtedly cellular dehydration. This point is illustrated by the fact that intravenous infusion of a 20% solution of NaCl (hyperosmotic) induces drinking, whereas infusion of an isosmotic solution of urea does not. (The mobility of urea is very high, and thus it equilibrates without any water movement.) Similarly, a 5% solution of glucose injected intraperitoneally will inhibit drinking in a thirsty dog, because it induces cellular hydration. The receptors that detect and signal this dehydration are in the central nervous system. Bilateral carotid infusion of water causes a reduction to predehydration levels in osmolality of blood in the jugular vein (from the brain), but not in the systemic blood, and reduces water intake in dogs that have been water-deprived for 24 hours. This reduction in drinking occurs in spite of the fact that the dog is still hypovolemic and the blood in the peripheral circulation is still hyperosmotic. Infusion of an amount of isosmotic saline sufficient to replace the volume of water lost during the water deprivation, but not sufficient to reduce the elevated osmolality, also reduces the quantity of water consumed; however, the reduction is not as great. Apparently, the drinking control system is sensitive to both changes in blood osmolality and changes in blood volume. The same corrections of osmolality and volume isolated to the systemic circulation do not affect drinking, indicating that the receptors are in the CNS or at least in the regions of the body drained by the jugular vein.

Lesions that produce aphagia in animals, lateral hypothalamic lesions, also produce **adipsia,** absence of drinking. Lesions of the ventromedial nuclear region do not, however, produce **polydipsia** along with hyperphagia. Rather, it is the region of the supraoptic area that seems to be important in stopping drinking. Direct injection of angiotensin, a substance formed by renin (from the kidneys) from a fraction of plasma globulin, into the supraoptic area induces drinking in rats. Conversely, injection of water into the same site reduces drinking induced by systemic injections of hypertonic saline or by water deprivation. There is some disagreement about the exact location of the receptors—some investigators believing that they are supraoptic neurons, others maintaining that they are subfornical organ neurons. At any rate, they appear to be anterior hypothalamic neurons.

CLINICAL ASPECTS OF AUTONOMIC FUNCTION

Autonomic functions are subject to various forms of trauma just as are somatic functions. Lesions involving the lateral funiculus at the L3 level that result from a wound, spinal fracture, tumor, or transverse myelitis, lead to increases in autonomic reflexes, as has already been mentioned in the discussion of spinal shock. Lesions of the pons and medulla may interrupt descending pathways, also inducing spinal shock with early **anhidrosis,** vasodilatation, and, later, **Horner's syndrome.** These symptoms, like the spinal shock, diminish with time. Fracture of the base of the skull can lead to diabetes insipidus, a condition of excessive water loss due to a reduction in antidiuretic hormone released by the pituitary. Though signs of hypothalamic malfunction show up rarely with vascular incidents, they do occur with primary or metastatic tumors, epidemic encephalitis, syphilitic meningoencephalitis, and poliomyelitis. Multiple small hemorrhages are found in the hypothalamus in cases of chronic gastric or duodenal ulcers.

SUGGESTED READING

Anand BK: Nervous regulation of food intake. Physiol Rev 41:677–708, 1961

Fitzsimons JT: Thirst. Physiol Rev 52:468–561, 1972

Koizumi K, Brooks C McC: The autonomic nervous system and its role in controlling visceral activities. In Mountcastle VB [ed]: Medical Physiology, 13th ed., Vol. 1. St. Louis, CV Mosby, 1974

Kunos G, Yong MS, Nickerson M: Transformation of adrenergic receptors in the myocardium. Nature 241:119–120, 1973

Novin D, Wyrwrcka W, Bray GA [eds]: Hunger. Basic Mechanisms and Clinical Implications. New York, Raven Press, 1976

Peters G, Fitzsimons JT, Peters-Haefeli L: Control Mechanisms of Drinking. Berlin, Springer-Verlag, 1975

Pick J: The Autonomic Nervous System. Philadelphia, JB Lippincott, 1970

Teitelbaum P, Epstein A: The lateral hypothalamic syndrome: recovery of feeding and drinking after lateral hypothalamic lesions. Psychol Rev 69:74–90, 1962

18

Neurotrophic Effects and Axoplasmic Transport

Some of the functions that nerve cells have in addition to their ability to send messages in the form of nerve impulses are discussed in this chapter. This subject is just beginning to be explored experimentally, partly because everyone thought they knew the function of nerve cells—to generate and conduct spikes. These newer findings have opened new vistas in neuroscience.

NEUROTROPHIC EFFECTS

Neurotrophic effects are the interactions between neurons and what they connect to, especially other nerve cells, muscles cells, receptors, and glia. Neurotrophic effects are distinguishable from the usual neural control effects by their long-term natures and by the molecular or functional modifications they produce in the other cells.

EFFECTS OF NERVES ON GLIA

We usually do not think of neurons having an influence on glia, but one of the closest interactions between nerve cells and glia appears to be the association between the nerve fibers and the Schwann cells in the periphery and between fibers and oligodendroglia centrally. The nerve fiber has long been known to influence the Schwann cell, because sectioning a nerve leads to disappearance of the myelin covering of its fibers if the nerve does not regenerate. It has been speculated, but not demonstrated, that Schwann cells, in addition to their effects on conduction velocity, provide nutrients to the axon. We now know that the axon is capable of transporting its own nutrients (this will be discussed later), but the glia may also be involved in this function. The formation of the tightly would myelin sheath by the Schwann cells seems to be induced by the axon. Schwann cells will not wrap around glass or metal rods or even unmyelinated nerve cells of approximately the same size, though they will remyelinate the same or similar previously myelinated fibers. The nature of the induction process in myelin formation is not known.

EFFECTS OF NERVES ON RECEPTOR STRUCTURE

It now appears that nerve cells may play a role in the induction of specific receptor structures in several sensory systems. For example, in the gustatory system, the taste buds, whose structure has been discussed previously, disappear from the tongue when the gustatory nerve (*e.g.*, the chorda tympani or lingual nerve) is severed. When the taste nerve grows back and reinnervates the tongue, the taste buds reappear. Only the taste nerve will cause re-formation of new taste buds. The taste buds persist for a longer period of time if their nerve is sectioned farther from the bud (more centrally) than if it is sectioned more distally. If ganglion cell bodies are left connected to the fibers innervating the tongue (by cutting the nerve proximal to the ganglion), there is no degeneration of the receptors at all. Taste buds regenerate if the tongue is reinnervated with either the central or peripheral process of the taste ganglion cells (recall that these are pseudo-unipolar cells), implying that the nerve is not polarized with respect to this function, that is, either the sending or receiving end can induce formation of receptors. Administration of the male sex hormone, testosterone, in male rats induces the formation of taste buds in lingual regions where they normally are not found, but it does this only if the taste nerve is intact and not in tongues reinnervated with nontaste nerves. These observations imply that the nerve regulates the normal, constant differentiation of the germinal taste cells. The nerve cannot, however, do this by itself; the epithelium also plays a role. No taste buds are formed if the taste nerve is allowed to innervate a nongustatory epithelium.

One receptor structure in the skin has received some attention from this point of view. The receptor associated with type I slowly adapting cutaneous afferent fibers is a dome-shaped structure about 150 to 400 μm in diameter (discussed in Chaps. 4 and 5). It is associated with a thickened epithelium, a special blood capillary tuft, and specialized receptor cells, called Merkel cells, that lie at the dermal–epidermal border. The nerve fiber approaches the dome from the dermis and ends in close apposition to the Merkel cell (see Fig. 4-8). If the nerve containing the type I fiber is cut, the dome disappears from the surface and, in histologic preparations, no Merkel cells can be found. When the nerve is allowed to regenerate, new domes appear on the skin, and Merkel cells appear in the domes after the nerve reaches the skin. However, the locations of regenerated domes are not necessarily the same as the original locations of domes before nerve section, implying that the nerve fiber induces the dome formation and the differentiation of some epithelial cells to form Merkel cells.

Even a receptor structure as complex as the muscle spindle is not immune from influence by its nerve fibers. Transection of the sciatic nerve in adult animals leads to disintegration of the muscle spindles in muscles of the hindlimbs. This is not the result of removal of γ motoneurons, because cutting the appropriate ventral roots does not produce this effect (Zelená and Soukup, 1974).

Whether this is a general phenomenon for specialized receptors or one that occurs just in these special cases is not known. These three cases involve the spinal and the cranial nerves; therefore, one might expect this to be a general phenomenon. It may be found, for example, that auditory nerve fibers induce the differentiation of the hair cells of the basilar membrane; we will not know until someone looks.

EFFECTS OF NERVE CELLS ON OTHER NERVE CELLS

It has been known for some time that some nerve cells influence others in ways other than through synaptic transmission. A phenomenon called **transneuronal degeneration** has been known for a long time, in which, in certain cases, after a fiber tract is transected, degenerative changes occur in the cells to which its fibers conduct their impulses. These latter neurons have not themselves been injured, but they begin to degenerate nonetheless. Such transneuronal changes are seen in cells of the lateral geniculate nucleus after a lesion of the retina, in cells of the pontine nuclei following lesions of the cerebral cortex or cerebral peduncles involving corticopontine fibers, in cells of the cochlear nuclei after destruction of the auditory nerve, and in ventral horn cells following sectioning of the dorsal roots. These transneuronal changes may involve moderate cell shrinkage, reduction in size of the nucleus or nucleolus, reduction in the Nissl substance, and perhaps disappearance of the cell altogether. Little is known about this phenomenon, except that it exists.

EFFECTS OF NERVE ON MUSCLE

Changes in muscle that result from denervation and reinnervation are many and can be profound. For example, if the nerve to a muscle is cut, the resting membrane potential of the muscle cells begins to drop (*i.e.*, they depolarize) within 2 hours. This change occurs sooner, the closer to the muscle the nerve is cut. This drop in potential is not related to impulse transmission or contractile activity, because these events stop immediately after the transection. Acetylcholine (ACh) is not involved because the miniature end-plate potentials continue during this fall in membrane voltage. It has been suggested that this depolarization may indicate that the nerve plays a role in regulation of electrogenic sodium pump activity in the muscle.

In the normal, innervated muscle, the transmitter substance ACh produces an effect only if applied to the region of the end-plate. The rest of the muscle membrane is insensitive to ACh. When the nerve has been cut, however, the sensitivity to ACh spreads over the muscle membrane away from the end-plate. The muscle becomes abnormally sensitive to ACh, a phenomenon termed **denervation hypersensitivity.** The same thing happens if the end-plate is treated with botulinum toxin, a deadly substance produced by bacteria that prevents the release of ACh from the motoneuron. This implies that ACh release may somehow regulate sensitivity of the muscle membrane to ACh.

Within 3 days after denervation, the concentration of acetylcholinesterase in the muscle cell around the motor end-plate drops by 50%, but it is restored to normal upon reinnervation of the muscle. After all cholinesterase has been destroyed in the end-plate by treatment with diisopropyl fluorophosphate (DFP), the levels gradually rise again in innervated but not in denervated muscles. Treatment with botulinum toxin does not alter cholinesterase concentrations. These observations indicate that the nerve somehow induces the synthesis of acetylcholinesterase in the muscle cell and that, however this is being done, acetylcholine is not involved in the induction.

The interaction of nerve and muscle is even more intimate than indicated above. If a muscle is denervated, it atrophies. Direct stimulation of the muscle slows the rate of atrophy while the nerve is regenerating but the nerve is required to keep the muscle viable. The dependence of muscle on innervation begins early in embryology. During development, myoblasts fuse to form myotubes that develop into muscle fibers. If myotubes do not become innervated, they do not differentiate into muscle fibers, but atrophy and are replaced by fat.

It has been known for a long time that muscles differ in their contractile properties. Some have rapid twitch contractions; some have slower twitch contractions. Some show tetanic fusion at higher frequencies of stimulation (motoneuron discharge); some show fusion at lower rates of stimulation. Some have steeper force–velocity relationships than others. These are the fast and slow muscles discussed in Chapter 14. The extensor digitorum longus (EDL) muscles of the foot are examples of fast muscles. The soleus (SOL) muscle of the calf of the leg is an example of a slow muscle. In the newborn animal, both muscles contract at the same speed. This is illustrated in Figure 18-1A. Shown on the left are isometric twitch contractions for SOL and EDL muscles in the newborn. As the animal grows older, the contraction speed of the EDL muscles increases, whereas that for SOL remains about the same (shown in Fig. 18-1A, right). At birth, the force–velocity relationships of the fast and slow muscles are nearly identical, as shown in Figure 18-1B, left, but by 100 days of age, the fast muscles (EDL) are contracting more rapidly for a given load, that is, their force–velocity curves are steeper (Fig. 18-1B, right). Both muscles would be fully innervated by that time.

About 20 years ago, it was noted that the motoneurons associated with fast muscles are phasically active at discharge rates between 30 and 60/sec, whereas those associated with slow muscles are tonically active and discharge at lower rates, 10 to 20/sec. Such a correlation between the discharge rate of the motoneurons supplying a muscle and the rate of its contraction suggested that the motoneuron might determine the contractile properties of the muscle. A most interesting experiment was done to test this suggestion. The EDL and SOL muscles were both denervated. If left in that condition, they both would have atrophied, but the nerve from the EDL muscle was grafted onto the SOL muscle and vice versa. Each nerve was able to form new, functional end-plates on its "wrong" muscle, and some amazing things happened, as shown in Figures 18-2 and 18-3. Figure 18-2A and C shows the twitch contractions (18-2A1 and 18-2C1) and responses to the repetitive stimulation (18-2A2–4 and 18-2C2–4) of EDL and SOL muscles that were denervated and then reinnervated with their own nerves again, as surgical controls. These muscles (S-EDL and S-SOL) are just like their untreated counterparts. However, those with **cross-innervation** (X-EDL, EDL with SOL nerve; X-SOL, SOL with EDL nerve) are different. X-SOL has a more rapid twitch contraction (Fig. 18-2D1) than

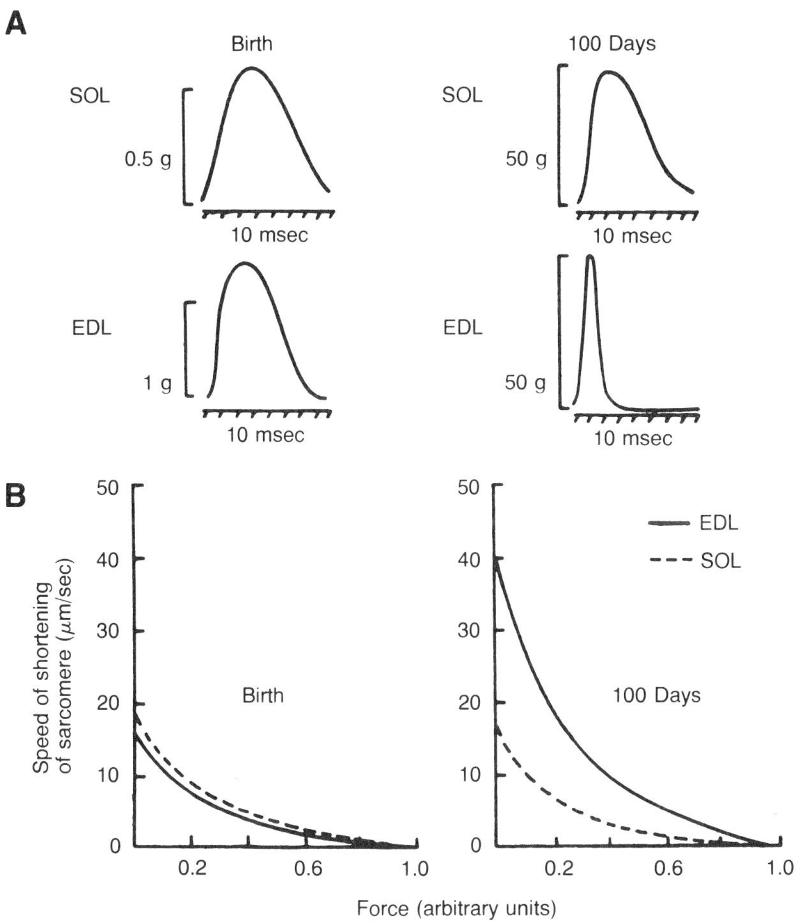

FIG. 18-1. A. Tension–time records of isometric twitch contractions for EDL and SOL muscles of the rat at birth and 100 days after birth. Note similarity of twitch contractions at birth and the faster EDL contraction at 100 days. **B.** Mean force–velocity curves for EDL and SOL at the same ages as in **A.** Note the similarity of the curves at birth and the steeper EDL curve at 100 days. (Close R: J Physiol (Lond) 173:74–95, 1964)

S-SOL; it is more like that of S-EDL. There is no fusion of tetanic contractions at 10/sec stimulation rates (Fig. 18-2D2) as there is in S-SOL (Fig. 18-2C2). In general, under the influence of the EDL nerve, the SOL muscle comes to behave more like the EDL muscle, that is, it becomes, in essence, a fast muscle. Likewise, the cross-innervated EDL slows its twitch contraction rate (Fig. 18-2B1) and the contractions fuse at a lower stimulus rate (Fig. 18-2B2). In short, it becomes a slow muscle. The changes in the force–velocity relationships are in the same direction. Figure 18-3, left, shows these relationships for the normal EDL muscle (N-EDL), for S-EDL, and for X-EDL. The relationship is less steep for X-EDL and is similar to those shown in Figure 18-3, right, for N-SOL and S-SOL. Figure 18-3, right, shows the force–velocity relationships for the normal SOL muscle (N-SOL), for S-SOL, and for X-SOL. The similarity between the X-SOL curve and those for N-EDL and S-EDL is striking.

The motoneurons do not even have to make functional contacts with the muscle to effect this change in contractility. If an EDL nerve is grafted onto an SOL muscle without denervating it first, the EDL nerve will not make functional contacts, as indicated by the lack of response in the muscle when the EDL nerve is stimulated. Nonetheless, the speed of contraction increases in the SOL muscle just as in Figure 18-2 and 18-3

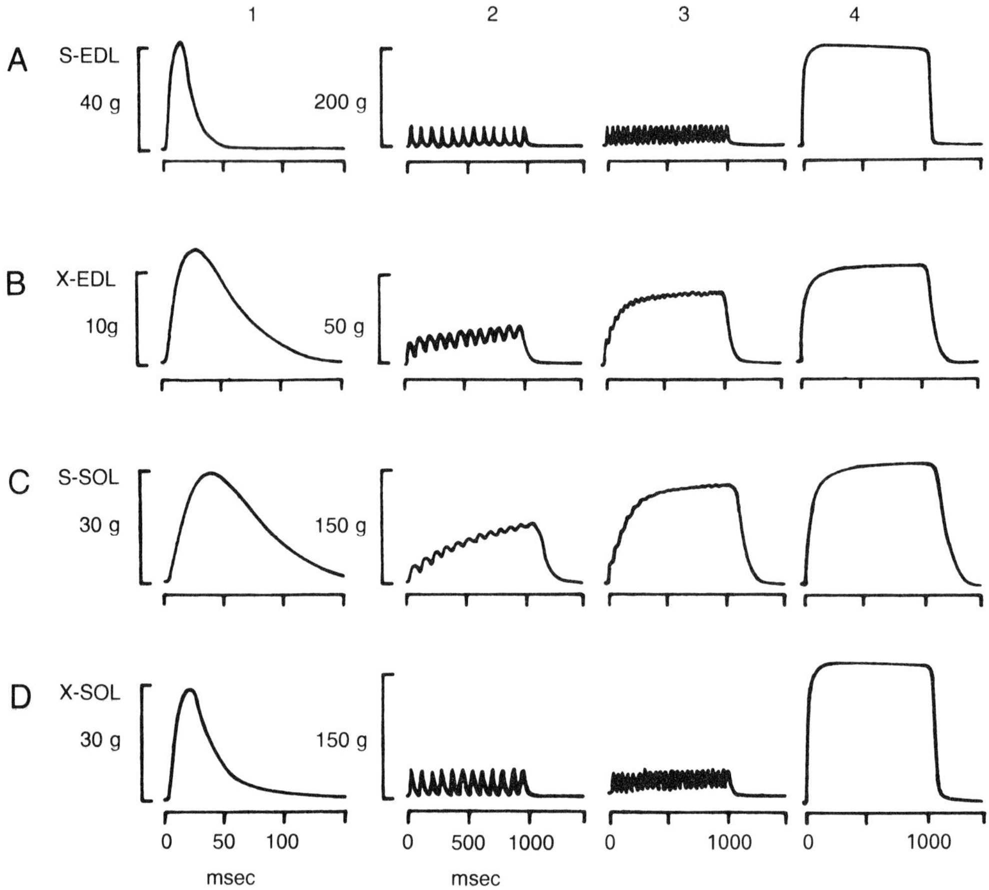

FIG. 18-2. Tension–time records of isometric contractions of self-innervated EDL **(A1)** and SOL **(C1)** and cross-innervated EDL **(B1)** and SOL **(D1)** muscles. Responses of the same muscles to repetitive stimulation at 10/sec **(2)**, 20/sec **(3)**, and 200/sec **(4)** are shown in the balance of the records. (Close R: J Physiol (Lond) 204:331–346, 1969

FIG. 18-3. Mean force–velocity curves for normal, self-innervated, and cross-innervated EDL and SOL muscles. (Close R: J Physiol (Lond) 204:331–346, 1969)

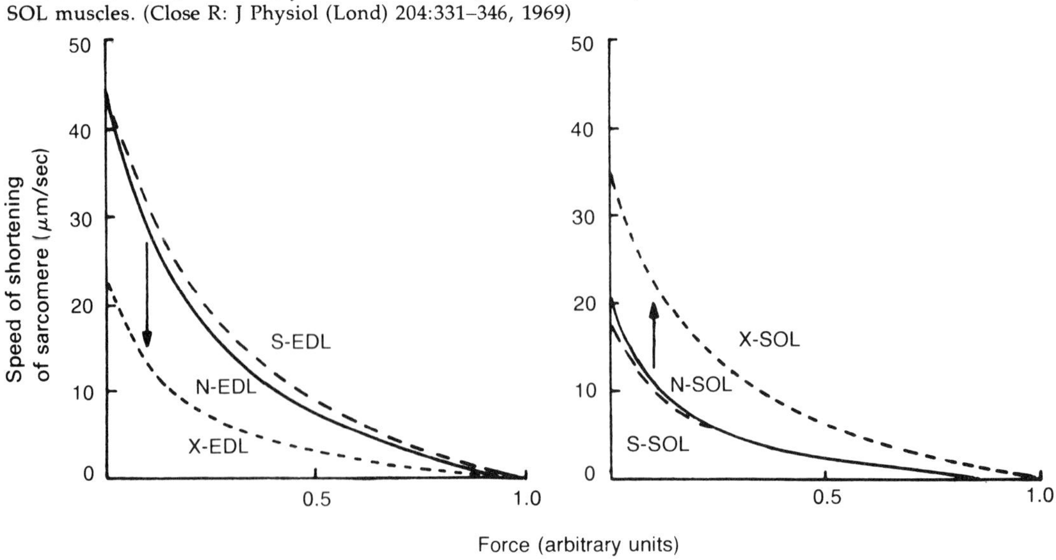

even though no effective end-plates are formed. Apparently, there must be some factor within certain motoneurons that causes some muscles to become fast muscles. The identity of this factor (substance) is unknown, but it is known that acetylcholine is not the factor. It is also known that nerve impulses themselves or the pattern of nerve impulses is not responsible for these changes in contractility.

In addition to the effect on contractility, the motoneurons seem to be able to regulate gene expression within the muscle. For example, the EDL and SOL muscles contain different myosin molecules. The myosin-ATPase activity of EDL is more than twice that for SOL (1.17 vs. 0.50 μmoles P_i/min/mg). In cross-innervated muscles, there is a change in this characteristic myosin-ATPase activity such that in X-EDL muscle it becomes lower (0.55 μmoles P_i/min/mg) and in X-SOL muscle it becomes higher (0.90 μmoles P_i/min/mg). In addition to this quantitative change, there is also a qualitative change in the myosin. Normal fast-muscle myosin contains two low-molecular-weight proteins not found in normal slow-muscle myosin; and slow-muscle myosin contains two such proteins not found in normal fast-muscle myosin. After cross-innervation, the muscles exchange these proteins so that those normally found in the fast muscle are found in the cross-innervated slow muscle (and vice versa), and there is a reduction in those proteins appropriate for a fast (slow) muscle. Because whether a cell will or will not make a certain protein is determined by gene action, it is suggested that this trophic effect is a regulation of gene expression.

AXOPLASMIC TRANSPORT

We do not know the identity of the trophic substance(s) at the receptors, at other nerves, or at the neuromuscular junction. But, we have some idea how these and other substances get to their site of action. Each part of a neuron is capable of synthesizing proteins with its own rate of production and spectrum of molecular species, but the major synthesis occurs in the cell body and the large dendrites. These proteins, along with transmitter substances and our neurotrophic substance, must be moved to their sites of action, which are primarily near the terminals. The somata of neurons export large quantities of substances; in fact, it has been estimated that ventral horn cells export their own weight in axoplasm in less than one day!

As indicated in Chapter 1, there are two forms of axoplasmic transport away from the soma: One carries materials at the rate of 410 mm/day **(fast transport);** the other carries materials at the rate of 1 to 12 mm/day **(slow transport).** In addition, the terminals of axons are capable of picking up proteins and transmitter substances or their metabolites and transporting them back to the soma, in a retrograde direction, at the rate of 40 to 100 mm/day **(retrograde transport).**

The mechanism of protein synthesis and its fast transport seems to be as follows: Polypeptide chains are released from polyribosomes into the lumen of the rough endoplasmic reticulum and eventually transferred to the Golgi apparatus. In the course of this transfer, carbohydrate groups may be added to proteins to form glycoproteins. The course of movement of the proteins and glycoproteins is shown in Figure 18-4. The smooth endoplasmic reticulum extends the length of the axon and connects, according to some investigators, by thin canaliculi with the synaptic vesicles. It also appears as a continuous system in the soma where the rough endoplasmic reticulum, Golgi apparatus, and smooth endoplasmic reticulum appear to be connected. The newly formed proteins and glycoproteins and perhaps other molecules follow the channels of the smooth endoplasmic reticulum, entering the axon and moving along its length. In the axon, the axolemma (the membrane of the axon) is supplied with a major fraction of the fast-transported material. This transfer to the axolemma may involve the lateral sacks of the smooth endoplasmic reticulum, the subaxolemmal plates. The remainder of the fast-transported material accumulates in the axon terminals, mainly in the synaptic vesicles and presynaptic membranes, but also in the mitochondria, and perhaps some occur in a free form. Some people think that the bulging at the end of the thin canaliculi of the smooth endoplasmic reticulum is the recycling or biogenesis of synaptic vesicles, but this is a point of conjecture. When transported proteins have been labeled,

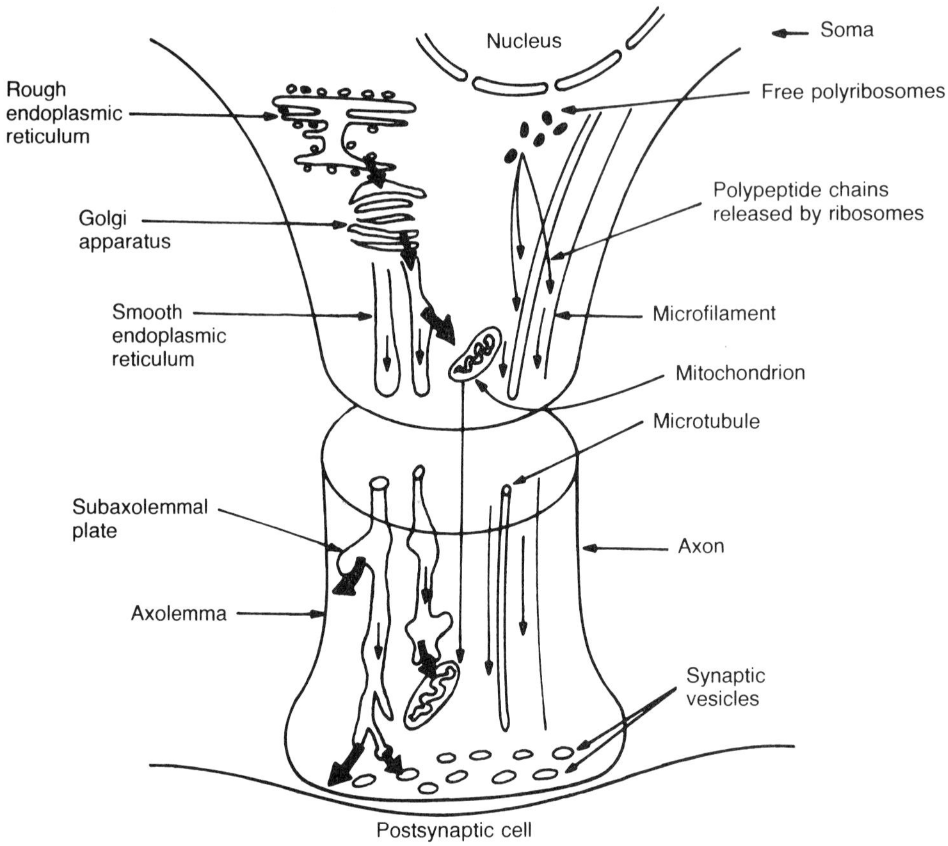

FIG. 18-4. A longitudinal section through a nerve cell showing the organization of the rough and smooth endoplasmic reticula and the Golgi apparatus and the course taken by proteins and other substances to the axon terminals. (Droz B: Brain Res 62:383–394, 1973)

label is sometimes found in the postsynaptic cell, that is, the protein or some subunit of the protein crosses the synaptic cleft and is picked up by the postsynaptic cell. This is perhaps the mechanism of interneuronal trophic effects.

There is some evidence that hydrolytic enzymes and soluble proteins enclosed in vesicles travel in the lumen of the channels, whereas plasma membrane components travel as a part of the walls of the channels. Therefore, not only the contents of the smooth endoplasmic reticulum but also its walls may be transported rapidly toward the nerve endings. Support for this general scheme comes from experiments with colchicine. Fast axoplasmic flow is abolished by treatment with colchicine, which disrupts the internal structure of the axon. This treatment has no effect on impulse transmission, but it depresses synaptic transmission.

The mechanism of slow axoplasmic transport is unknown, but it may involve diffusion or some more active transport mechanism. Whatever the mechanism, it may be guided by the microfilaments and microtubules that run the length of the axon. The total amount of material slow-transported is probably about four times that fast-transported, but only a fraction of it actually reaches the terminals. The majority is used in the axon.

Retrograde transport occurs presumably by the same mechanism as fast orthograde transport, but a given channel of the smooth endoplasmic reticulum probably cannot move materials in both directions at the same time. There is even evidence that specific substances may be transported in specific channels. Anatomists have begun to use retrograde transport to trace the locations of cell bodies connected to various axon terminals. An enzyme used by experimenters, horseradish peroxidase, is picked up by neuron terminals and transported back to the cell soma, where it can be visualized by developing with hydrogen peroxide and a chromagen. This has proved to be a powerful tool for tracing neuronal pathways, but as yet its limitations are not well worked out.

We do not know whether trophic substances are carried to the terminals by fast or slow transport, but at least now we know what the options are, if we can find out what the substances are.

SUGGESTED READING

Guth L: Trophic functions. In Hubbard JI [ed]: The Peripheral Nervous System. New York, Plenum, 1974

Vrbova G, Gordon, T, Jones R: Nerve-Muscle Interaction. London, Chapman and Hall, 1978

Zelená J, Soukup T: The differentiation of intrafusal fibre types in rat muscle spindles, after motor denervation. Cell Tiss Res 153:115–136, 1974

19

Development, Repair, and Recovery of Function

Anyone who has studied the development of an organism cannot help being impressed with how many opportunities there are for things to go wrong. The nervous system is no different from this point of view. This chapter begins with a brief discussion of the development of the nervous system, but this is not a chapter about embryology. No attempt is made to describe the development of individual nuclei; rather, some important generalizations about development are presented to allow the reader to compare results of experiments involving regeneration following damage and, perhaps, to better understand developmental anomalies. The events that follow damage to the peripheral nervous system are presented and compared with events following damage to the central nervous system. The concept of recovery of function following damage is discussed, providing examples, different interpretations, and possible causes.

DEVELOPMENT OF THE NERVOUS SYSTEM

Both the peripheral and central nervous systems are ectodermal in origin, developing from the neural plate, which first appears dorsally and rostrally in the embryo late in the third week of fetal life. Rapid growth of the margins of the single-layered neural plate causes a groove to form rostrocaudally, the neural groove. Further proliferation of the ectodermal cells causes the groove to deepen and finally to close over at its dorsal surface forming the neural tube. The junction of the developing neural tube with the general body ectoderm is thinner than the rest of the neural plate and is called the neural crest. As development proceeds, the neural tube and neural crest migrate into an internal position, being covered with surface ectoderm. Neural crest cells later develop into the dorsal root ganglia, the ganglia of the cranial nerves, and peripheral cells of the autonomic nervous system. The rostral part of the neural tube differentiates into the brain stem, diencephalon, and telencephalon, whereas the caudal part becomes the spinal cord.

From this point onward, the development of the nervous system is characterized by five processes: proliferation, migration, differentiation, interactions, and death. Proliferation of nerve cells occurs mainly in specific germinal zones that line the lumen of the neural tube. Later, these zones are found in the ependymal linings of the ventricles. Germinal cells that inhabit the germinal zones divide repeatedly, one daughter cell remaining in the germinal zone and the other migrating out into the developing nuclei. The cell remaining in the germinal zone gives rise to additional neurons and later some glial elements by further mitotic activity. The migrating cell has already lost its ability to undergo mitosis, but as yet the cell is undifferentiated.

There are both spatial and temporal gradients of proliferation in the germinal zone.

Not all types of neurons in the same tissue or in different tissues develop at the same rate; however, each distinct set of neurons originates on a fairly invariant timetable; the entire population of a set apparently completes the final cell cycle and becomes permanently postmitotic over a relatively short time. There appears to be an orderly sequence of production of neurons within a cytoarchitectonic region such that large neurons originate first, then intermediate neurons, and finally small neurons. One result of this sequence is that many structures develop from the inside outward. For example, in the cerebral cortex and cerebellum, the deeper, larger neurons develop and migrate first into position within the tissue; later, developing neurons must migrate past them into the outer layers. These later-developing neurons are statistically smaller than their predecessors. Other areas of the central nervous system, for example, the thalamus and hypothalamus, develop from the outside inward.

The differential origin of cells in different layers of the cerebral cortex leads to some interesting developmental anomalies in the rat and presumably also in man, though the timing probably differs. The rat has a gestation period of 28 days, during which neurons destined for cerebral isocortex originate on days 16 to 21. Neurons destined for deeper layers (layers V and VI) originate on days 16 and 17, whereas those destined for the superficial layers (layers II–IV) originate on days 18 to 21. X-irradiation with 150 to 200 r has, at best, a temporary influence on cells that are undergoing mitosis; recently postmitotic, migrating cells are killed; and long-term postmitotic, differentiated cells are not influenced. The actual threshold for damage to recently postmitotic cells may be as low as 60 r.

X-irradiation of the developing rat fetus with 150 to 200 r on day 20 or 21 of gestation leaves layers V and VI fairly intact, but layers II to IV are reduced to a thin band of disorganized cells. The large (Betz) cells of layer V are damaged by irradiation earlier, on day 17 of gestation, leaving their dendritic development abnormal. Neurons in the isocortex of such animals are scattered and jumbled, sideways and upside-down. Irradiation at this same strength before day 15 has little permanent effect on the isocortex, as does irradiation postnatally. This level of X-irradiation appears to damage neurons irreparably only at certain critical times. A similar pattern of disruption can be seen in the cerebellar cortex, with prenatal irradiation disrupting Purkinje cells' structure and orientation and reducing their numbers, and early postnatal irradiation markedly altering the granule cell layers. This treatment in infant rats causes them, as adults, to be impaired in horizontal jumping ability and climbing, where balance is important, among other effects (Bruner and Altman, 1973). Any specific relationship between these induced anomalies and naturally occurring developmental anomalies in these same tissues is unknown.

The spatial gradients within the germinal zone are responsible for separate origins of neighboring regions of the brain that are cytoarchitectonically distinct. The somatosensory cortex in animals and man develops before either the visual or auditory cortices, perhaps an example of ontogeny recapitulating phylogeny. In addition, phylogenetically older parts of the brain appear to arise earlier in development than phylogenetically newer parts. Thus, hippocampal development precedes development of neocortical areas in both animals and man. There is also a tendency for motor nuclei to begin and complete their histogenesis before sensory nuclei at the same level of the neuraxis.

The time of origin of a particular cell can therefore be seen to depend upon a number of factors. Different types of neurons within the same tissue and different tissues develop at different times and different rates. The position of the cell within the gradients of mitotic activity is a function of its size and the tissue in which it will live. Phylogenetic status of the neuron also appears to determine when it takes origin, older neurons appearing first. For most neurons in most tissues, histogenesis is a prenatal process, that is, the proliferative phase of development is completed before birth. A few neurons in the olfactory bulb, hippocampus, brain-stem nuclei, and cerebellar cortex take origin after birth. This contrasts with the histogenesis of glial cells, which, though it is thought to involve some of the same stem cells as neurogenesis, occurs both prenatally and postnatally.

Once a neuron reaches its target tissue, it begins to differentiate. In some cases, the cell's axon develops first and in others the dendrites develop first. In any case, neurons that migrated earlier also differentiate earlier. Thus, in the cerebral cortex, deeper lying neurons are already well differentiated at birth, whereas more superficial neurons are less well differentiated, and the most superficial neurons may not even be in their adult positions yet. The axon of the cell may grow in two different manners. In some neurons, as the cell migrates from the ependymal zone past already-migrated neurons, it may trail its axon behind it, presumably making synaptic contacts with cells it passes. This sort of developmental pattern is more likely to occur in small neurons, whose axons do not leave the structure in which the soma resides. Larger neurons, especially those that migrate early, send their axons out during the postmigratory differentiation.

The direction of the initial outgrowth of the axon and its growth toward particular postsynaptic sites on particular cells seem to be invariant in development. Sprouting of the axon from the cell normally occurs in the correct direction, that is, the direction of the cells it will contact. This direction is controlled by some intrinsic factor because it is unchanged when the cell is rotated. However, when the axon grows in the correct direction relative to the soma in the rotated condition, it is growing incorrectly with respect to its target cell. This condition is soon corrected when the axon turns around, suggesting that there are also external controls on axon growth.

During growth, the axon will extend, retract, branch, and eliminate branches as it grows toward its target. Even over long distances, the axon is able to find its target cells and make synaptic contact, sometimes with specific parts of the cells. For example, the cerebellar climbing fibers originate in the inferior olivary nucleus and contact the dendrites, not the soma, of the Purkinje cells. Axonal growth could be guided by electrical fields generated by or near the target cells, by differences in local chemical environments, or by the physical nature of the substrate through which the axon grows. It is difficult to see how electric fields could be used for guidance over long distances; an axon must surely pass through a number of different field strengths and orientations before arriving at its target. Chemical gradients may be more useful, but, except in certain circumstances, it is hard to see how these gradients could be created. If the physical substrate alone were to guide the axon, then it would have to possess a topologic map to its target before starting to grow. Perhaps a combination of these three factors will account for axonal guidance.

The growth of the primary afferent neurons is a special case worth considering. The cells of the neural crest send a process toward the periphery, where it contacts a particular receptor. Depending upon the receptor type, it may even induce the formation of the receptor structure, as in the case of taste receptors. Having made its peripheral contact, the cell then sends another process into the spinal cord where it makes contacts appropriate for the actions of the receptor it has contacted on the periphery. It is not known what factors lure the process to the periphery or to the spinal cord. Neither sensory stimulation nor reflex activity appears to be required because development proceeds normally in the anesthetized frog embryo and the nerves function normally when the anesthetic is withdrawn. A substance, isolated from the submaxillary gland, has an effect on developing neurons that has suggested to some investigators that it may play a role in guidance. This substance, called **nerve growth factor,** causes elongation of neurites of cells in culture, changes in their adhesion properties, and increased survival times of cultures of dissociated nerve cells. Nerve growth factor also influences the growth of certain nerve cells in young and adult animals, where it exerts its influences primarily upon sympathetic ganglion cells, increasing both their size and number, but it also affects dorsal root ganglion cells of certain types for a limited time during development. Whether there is a different nerve growth factor for all target cells, or even most target cells, is not known.

The onset of synaptogenesis within the nervous system also occurs according to a remarkably strict timetable. In each region of the central nervous system there is usually a minimum variation, less than one day, in establishment of a particular type of synaptic connection on all cells of a particular type. The incoming axons appear to compete for synaptic sites on cells: Those that are successful live on; those that do not form connections die. It appears that the nervous system comes equipped with many more nerve cells than it really needs. To survive, a cell must make a viable contact. It has been estimated that as many as 50% of the cells in the ciliary ganglion of the chick embryo die at the time synaptic contacts are being made with the iris. It is possible that this overproduction of neurons is a safety factor, assuring a sufficient number of viable neurons.

DEGENERATION AND REGENERATION

DEMYELINATION

The degeneration and death of developing neurons described previously are normal occurrences and do not reflect previous damage to the cell. Of the possible damages that can occur to axons, we will discuss only demyelination and crush or cut. In diphtheritic neuritis or multiple sclerosis, axons are demyelinated, but conduction remains saltatory in large myelinated fibers up to the time it stops altogether. On the other hand, conduction apparently becomes continuous, like that in unmyelinated fibers, in myelinated fibers less than 6 μm in diameter. Because of the demyelination, internodal capacitance increases and internodal transverse resistance decreases, resulting in decreased conduction velocity. Up to a 25-fold increase in conduction time can occur before conduction is blocked.

Repetitive activity in demyelinated axons leads to a progressive increase in internodal conduction time or total block of the spike, perhaps because of an accumulation of sodium in the intracellular fluid. This accumulation will also lead to a decrease in spike amplitude in demyelinated axons, though the reduction in the spike amplitude probably would have little effect on normal nodes. It has been speculated that the increase in intracellular sodium concentration is due to a deficiency in the sodium pump, but evidence for this speculation is not strong. Normal nerves conduct action potentials at a frequency of 200 per sec with little or no change in amplitude; however, demyelinated nerves show a rapid decrease in amplitude at frequencies as low as 10 to 25 per sec. This could perhaps account for the rapidly developing muscle weakness during exercise that is a common complaint of multiple sclerosis patients. It could also explain the fading of visual images when an object is looked at for some time.

ORTHOGRADE CHANGES FOLLOWING CRUSH OR TRANSECTION

When an efferent peripheral nerve is damaged by crushing or cutting it, a characteristic series of events occurs both distal (in the orthograde direction) and proximal to the damage (in the retrograde direction). In the orthograde direction, the endoplasmic reticulum becomes fragmented into rows of vesicles within 24 hours; the neurofilaments and neurotubules lose their longitudinal orientation and dissolve within 24 to 48 hours. Mitochondria swell. These events are probably the result of Ca^{2+} influx because they do not occur if the axons are kept in Ca^{2+}-free medium. The axon becomes irregular in shape and it fragments while the myelin sheath retracts from the axon at the nodes, creating an increase in the width of the nodes. Myelin breaks down into ellipsoids that contain axonal material that becomes degraded. The ellipsoids are then removed by Schwann cells or macrophages. The basement membrane that normally surrounds the axon and its myelin does not degenerate but remains, forming a tube, called the Schwann tube. Within the Schwann tube, Schwann cells proliferate, forming columns of cells within the distal stump of the nerve and apparently serve to guide regenerating axons to their termination sites.

In severed nerves, proliferating Schwann cells fill the gap between the cut ends in the first few days. Migration of Schwann cells occurs from both the distal and proximal ends, but primarily from the distal end, because the rate of growth is apparently higher. Axonal outgrowths arise from the proximal side of the traumatized zone and traverse the gap, guided by Schwann cells. Initially, the axons lie in the space between the basement membrane and the Schwann cells, but later the axon can be found lying in a gutter along the Schwann cell, forming a mesaxon. This is the beginning of the remyelination process; remyelinated fibers are seen as early as 7 days after a crush or 28 days after nerve section.

RETROGRADE CHANGES FOLLOWING CRUSH OR TRANSECTION

During these events, the soma of the axotomized neuron is also undergoing a similar sequence of changes. Not all cells undergo this exact sequence, but most experience at least some of these changes. The soma swells, the nucleus moves to an eccentric position in the cell, and the Nissl substance disappears (chromatolysis). There is certainly a decrease in the membrane potential at the cut site due to the membrane trauma. This lasts for hours and leads to a widespread cellular depolarization that may be an important cause of the neuron swelling through osmotic changes. There is a weakening of the attachment between neurons and glia.

There are also prominent changes in the structure and effectiveness of synapses on the axotomized neuron. Within a few days after axotomy, glia can be found insinuated between some of the synaptic terminals and postsynaptic sites on some cells. There is a concomitant decrease in sensitivity to some transmitter substances, perhaps due in part to the glial insinuation. There is also a change in enzyme concentrations in presynaptic terminals, for example, acetylcholinesterase concentration decreases. There is a general increase in axodendritic synaptic activity and a decrease in axosomatic synaptic activity, although not all axosomatic activity decreases and not all axodendritic activity increases.

There is an increase in ribonucleic acid (RNA) synthesis in most cells and a change in its form; free polyribosomes increase, perhaps accounting for the reduced Nissl substance. There is also an increase in synthesis of some proteins, but there need not be an increase in protein concentration because there is also an increase in proteolytic activity. Interestingly, there is not an across-the-board increase in protein synthesis. Synthesis of proteins associated with synaptic transmission, for example, dopamine β-hydroxylase or monoamine oxidase, usually decreases, whereas synthesis of "repair" proteins—membrane components—increases. Synthesis of the other major membrane component, lipids, also increases. There is no immediate effect of axotomy on the rate of axonal transport processes, but, after 1 to 2 days, the rate of axonal transport may decrease and then increase again as RNA and protein synthesis increases. Changes in rate of transport may be independent of changes in the nature of transported substances.

Effects on dendrites of axotomized cells are not as great as those on the somata, but they are of the same sort. In addition, there may be a reduction in the number, diameter, and length of dendrites of axotomized cells. The effects on both somata and dendrites are more prominent in young animals, and more cells do not survive to regenerate. The duration of these retrograde changes usually corresponds to the period of axon regeneration.

A sequence of events not dissimilar to that described previously for motoneurons also occurs in sensory neurons. Following transection of a sensory nerve peripheral to the dorsal root ganglion, there are chromatolysis of the cell bodies in the ganglion, increases in neurofilaments and glycogen granules in the axon central to the ganglion, changes in myelin structure central to the ganglion (including formation of lipid droplets and some shrinkage), swelling of the terminals, and aggregation of synaptic vesicles in terminals in the spinal cord. The rate of axoplasmic transport falls, at least for some materials, in the central axon. These changes, which occur in spite of the maintained connection of the central axon with the soma in the ganglion, are similar to what occurs retrogradely in cut motor axons, but they occur on a slower time scale. Over a period of months, some of these changes are reversed. The rate of axoplasmic transport increases and there is sprouting of the terminal axon segments in the spinal cord.

REGENERATION

The regeneration process in vertebrate peripheral nerves begins with an outgrowth of the severed axon from the proximal stump and an invasion of the distal stump. This is quite different from what sometimes happens in invertebrates in which the axon apparently grows from both proximal and distal stumps and the correct fibers rejoin. In vertebrates, the distal axon degenerates and s removed from the nerve. Axons arising from the cut proximal stump apparently invade the distal stump at random, growing straight ahead when possible. Therefore, the likelihood that an axon will regrow into its original Schwann tube is determined by the orientation of the cut ends. If they are aligned exactly as they were originally, then it is very likely that the axons will regrow appropriately; the more the orientation deviates from the original, the less likely it is that they will regrow appropriately. When the nerve is crushed, the Schwann tubes are not broken, and the regenerating axons will invade the same tubes they originally did.

During the regeneration process, axons increase in diameter, rapidly at first and then more slowly. This can be seen in Figure 19-1 for myelinated fibers, and in Figure 19-2 for unmyelinated fibers, by examining the curves for maximum conduction velocity. The maximum velocity of conduction, measured from the compound action potential, in both types of fibers drops rapidly after nerve damage: from 60 to 2 m/sec in myelinated fibers and from 2 to 1 m/sec in unmyelinated fibers. From 10 to 30 or 40 days after damage, the velocity increases from 2 to 40 m/sec in myelinated fibers and from 1 to 2 m/sec in unmyelinated fibers. The conduction velocity and, thus, the diameter of unmyelinated fibers is nearly normal at this time. This, however, is not the case with myelinated fibers. Remyelination begins within a week after nerve crush, but it takes up to a year for myelin to return to its full thickness, if it ever does.

Figure 19-1 also shows the proliferation of Schwann cells referred to earlier. Notice that there is a 13-fold increase in their numbers that recovers to about 700% by 220 days after transection of the sciatic nerve, implying that there is a considerable mortality of Schwann cells during the regeneration process. With the proliferation of Schwann cells and branching of the axons, the nerve increases its diameter during regeneration (Fig. 19-1), but later the diameter decreases as the Schwann cells die and some axon branches are retracted. Apparently, regenerated axons can maintain more than one axon in the peripheral nerve; after transection, regenerated nerves contain 1.7 times more fibers on the average than intact ones of the same type.

Unmyelinated axons branch considerably as they regenerate such that, at 30 days after a crush, they are seven times more numerous in the crushed than in the uncrushed cervical sympathetic trunk in the same animal (Fig. 19-2). By 180 days, all of the branches but one for each fiber have been retracted, and the number of unmyelinated axons is the same on both sides. Over the same period, there is only a twofold increase in the number of axons in the nerve proximal to the crush. Therefore, most of the branching occurs at the crush site. Interestingly, macrophages proliferate in the early stages of the degeneration–regeneration cycle, their numbers peaking at 5 days and returning to near normal at 100 days after nerve cut (Fig. 19-2), but there is still considerable cell mortality after this time.

The rate of regeneration is not constant but depends upon the nature of the damage and the method of measurement. Generally accepted values for rates of regeneration are 1 to 2 mm/day after a cut and 2 to 4 mm/day after a crush. However, these may be underestimates because of the tendency of the proximal part of the axon to degenerate partway back toward the soma. It must reinvade the region of the lesion before entering the distal stump. For nerve crush, the first *remyelinated* fiber is seen distal to the crush at 7 days, but the first *regenerating* fiber is seen at 4 days. With transection, the first *remyelinated* fiber does not appear distal to the cut until 28 days, but the first *regenerating* fiber is seen as early as 7 days. The amount of regeneration also depends upon the nature of the damage. With a crush, the fiber spectrum of the regenerated nerve is bimodal like that in Figure 12-4A (ignoring the unmyelinated fibers). After a cut the spectrum becomes unimodal with a flattening of the large fiber part of the curve. With a crush there is nearly a 100% regeneration, whereas regeneration in cut nerves always falls short of this mark.

It appears that with regeneration an axon contacts the same type of receptor on the periphery that it contacted before the damage. After a crush, the somatotopic organization is preserved because the axons regrow in the same Schwann tubes, which they follow to the same peripheral receptor. After a cut, the somatotopic organization can be disrupted. This may account, in part, for the deficit in tactile localization ability ob-

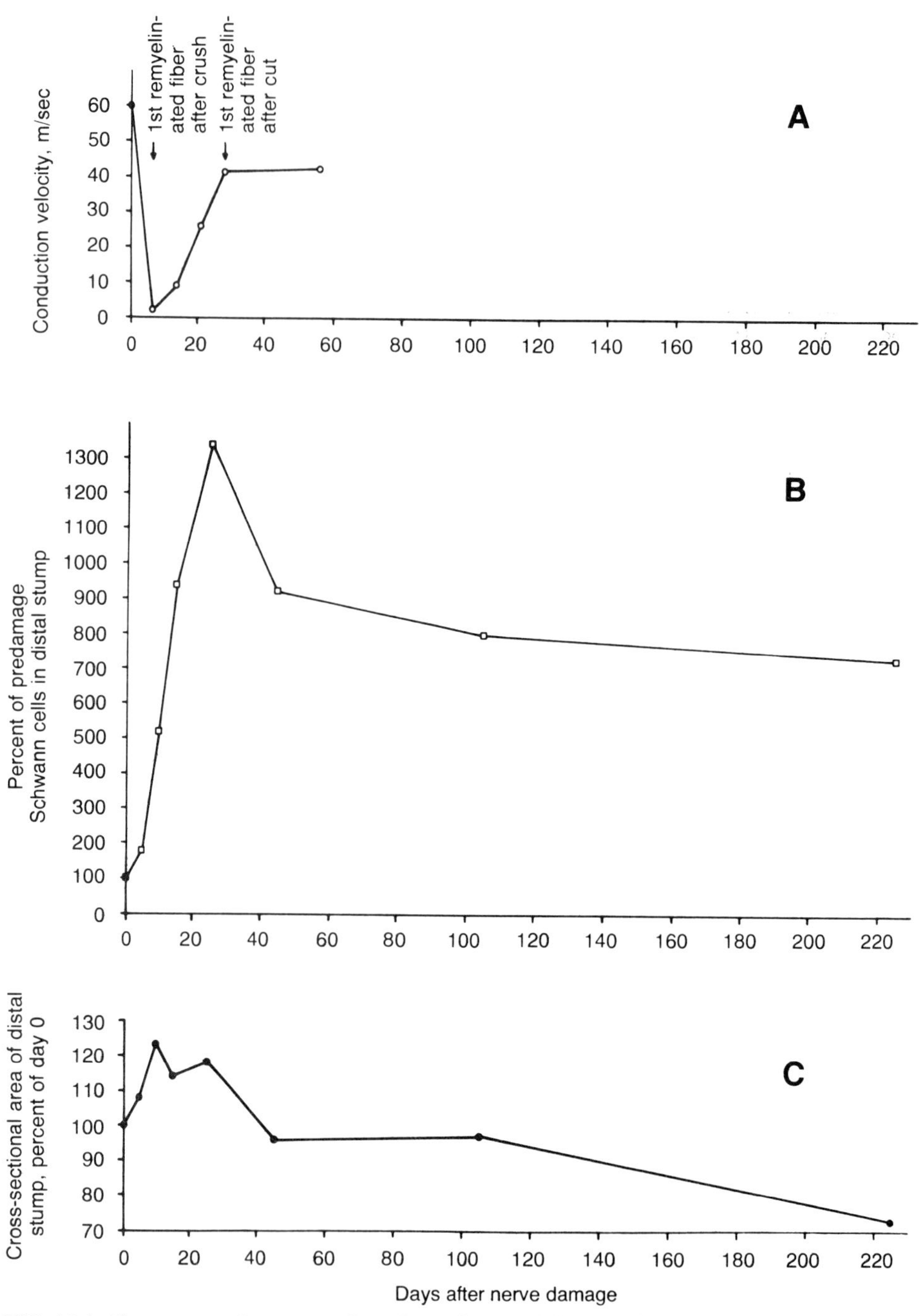

FIG. 19-1. Time course of recovery of myelinated axons following damage to the sciatic nerve. **A.** Conduction velocity of the largest fibers in the sciatic nerve 5 mm distal to crush site as a function of time after damage that occurred on day 0. (Jacobson S, Guth L: Exp Neurol 11:48–60, 1965) **B.** Changes in the number of Schwann cells distal to a transection of the sciatic nerve, expressed as a percent of the number of cells present before damage. **C.** Changes in cross-sectional area of the distal stump following transection of the sciatic nerve, expressed as percent of the area on day 0. (Abercrombie M, Johnson ML: J Anat 80:37–50, 1946)

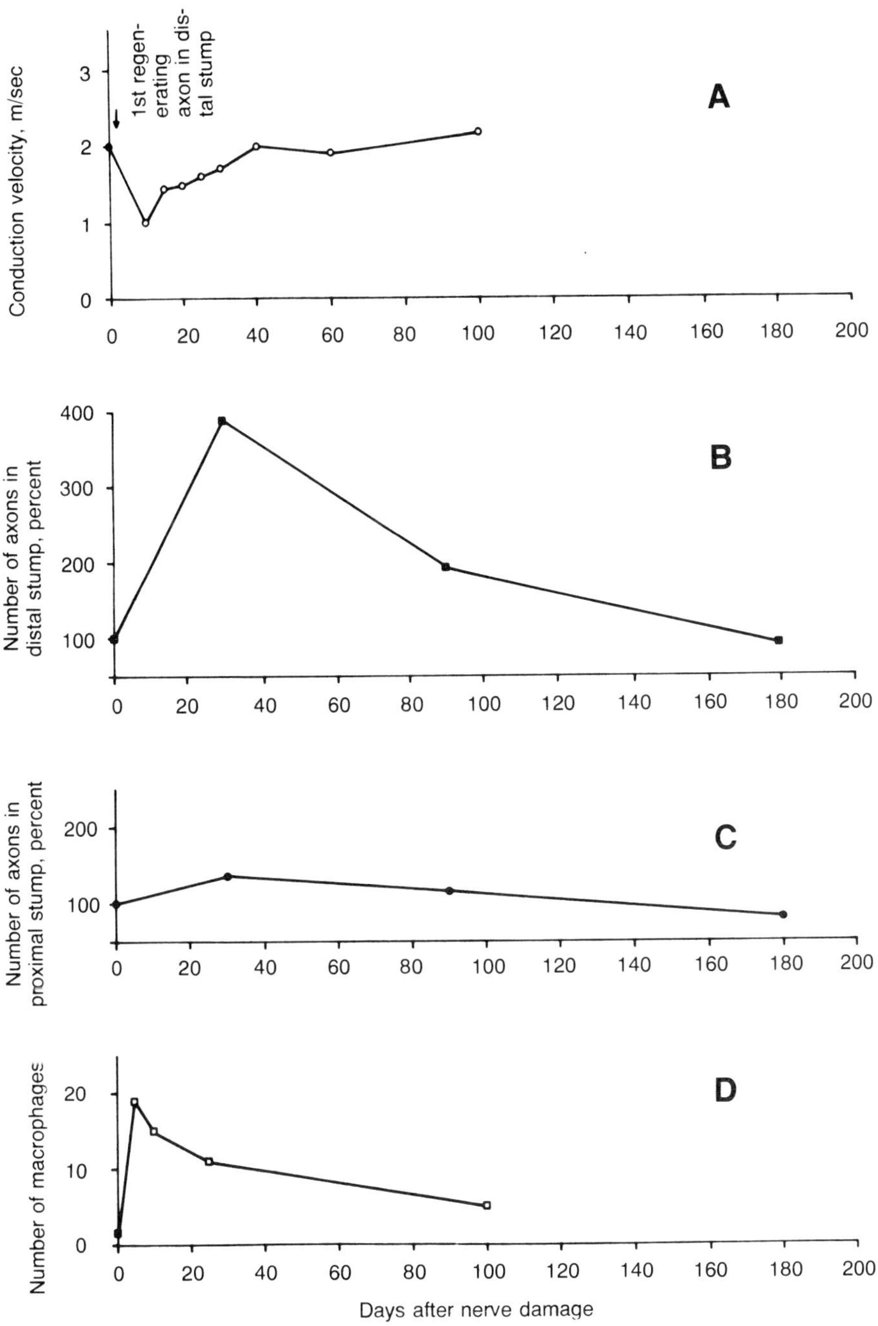

FIG. 19-2. Time course of recovery of unmyelinated axons following damage to sympathetic and parasympathetic nerves. **A.** Conduction velocity of the largest fibers in the cervical sympathetic trunk following crush as a function of time after damage that occurred on day 0. (Hopkins AP, Lambert EH: Brain 95:213–222, 1975) Numbers of axons in regenerating cervical sympathetic trunk as a function of time after crush are shown for the distal stump **(B)** and the proximal stump **(C)** expressed as a percent of the number in the undamaged, opposite sympathetic trunk. (Bray GM, Aguayo AJ: J Anat 117:517–529, 1974) **D.** Number of macrophages in regenerating abdominal vagus, expressed as a percent of the total cells, as a function of time after transection. (Abercrombie M, Evans DHL, Murray JG: J Anat 93:9–14, 1959)

served following transection and repair of the ulnar nerve in man (Ford and Woodhall, 1938). Tactile localization was reduced over the little finger; the patients could not recognize the aspect or the segment of the finger that was stimulated. They were not always certain which finger was touched. Two-point discriminations could not be made on the tip of the little finger, and sensitivity to passive movement of the terminal joint was reduced. There was also some alteration in motor function, for example, strong adduction of the thumb involved contraction of all of the interosseous muscles. When any of the intrinsic muscles of ulnar innervation contracted, all of them contracted together.

There was a decrease in stereognosis and some abnormality in pain and temperature senses such that gentle scraping of the ulnar skin sometimes caused pain, and heating only sometimes led to sensations of warmth, but otherwise touch, temperature, and pain sensations were normal. More recent investigations have shown that tactile thresholds increase after repair by suturing, and, after nerve crush, nociceptive C fibers responding to warmth increased their sensitivity. The density of these receptors was apparently normal. This observation of increased nociceptor sensitivity may explain the hyperpathia that occurs during degeneration in which the heat–pain threshold drops from the normal 45°C to 38°C. Under these conditions, objects just slightly warmer than skin temperature elicit painful sensations.

It is not known to what extent the regeneration process mimics the developmental process, but it is possible that similar mechanisms are involved. If so, some interesting observations may shed light on developmental processes. In any case, they give some idea of the limits of regeneration. Changes in skeletal muscle following removal of its innervation have already been discussed in Chapter 18. The hypersensitivity of the muscle to acetylcholine that develops followed denervation and the reinnervation by the muscle nerve are both blocked by recurrent, direct stimulation of the muscle after denervation. When the muscle has been denervated, it allows foreign nerves to reinnervate it, as we saw in the discussion of cross-innervation. The neuromuscular junction need not be physically disconnected; blocking synaptic transmission with botulinum toxin will also cause the muscle to allow cross-innervation. When the botulinum toxin is removed, it is found that both the original motoneurons and the foreign motoneurons can cause the muscle to contract. Muscle fibers are quite permissive in allowing foreign innervation. The frog sartorius muscle can be innervated by fibers in the vagus nerve; vagus stimulation, under these circumstances, causes muscle contraction, but, the contraction is different from normal (slower). The vagus nerve can also reinnervate a denervated superior cervical ganglion, and sympathetic preganglionic fibers can form effective synapses on skeletal muscle. These fibers normally contact other nerve cells, *not* muscle.

The transplantation of skin from one place to another in the human also results in reinnervation and some change in sensory thresholds. In patients who have lost a digit, surgeons can reconstruct the digit and cover it with skin they have removed from between the toes. Table 19-1 summarizes the results of psychophysical testing in such patients. The touch thresholds, two-point thresholds, and movement detection thresholds were measured for normal skin of the finger, transplanted skin of the finger, and normal skin of the foot. Touch thresholds for transplanted skin are much closer to those for normal finger skin than to those for foot skin. The same can be seen for both two-point and movement thresholds. Clearly, the sensitivity of the receptors to these stimuli is not determined by the source of the skin but by its position on the body, or, more accurately, by which nerve fibers innervate it.

Peripheral nerves have characteristic cutaneous receptive fields as we have seen. The receptive fields for adjacent nerves overlap to some extent depending upon where the field is on the body. If the area around the receptive field of a nerve is denervated, the nerve will sprout and reinnervate denervated areas, but only those within the regions of overlap with its own receptive field. It will not extend sprouts outside its receptive field. (This is unlike the behavior of motor fibers that will sprout and innervate other muscle tissue.) On the other hand, if the nerve itself is crushed and allowed to regenerate when those surround-

TABLE 19-1. TACTILE SENSITIVITY IN NORMAL AND TRANSPLANTED SKIN*

	FOOT	TRANSPLANT	FINGER
Touch threshold, mg	1500	500	300
Two-point threshold, mm	10–18	3–7	3–4
Direction of movement, mm	18	7	6

* Data from Dykes RW, Terzis JK, Strauch B: J Can Sci Neurol 6:437–439, 1979.

ing are cut and prevented from regenerating, the nerve will reinnervate not only its own receptive field but also the surrounding regions outside its receptive field. It seems that regenerating nerves may not be under the same constraints with respect to sprouting as neurons already innervating a target. These results have led to the following proposed scenario for peripheral nerve development: First, arriving neurons sprout locally at the target tissue under the influence of a sprouting stimulus from the target. Nerve endings associate with specific target sites and cause a reduction in the effectiveness of the sprouting stimulus. As a result, sprouting eventually ceases. When the mature nerve is cut, the sprouting stimulus is uncovered, causing nearby undamaged fibers to sprout.

We do not know if this scenario is accurate for development; it seems reasonable. In any case, this research does suggest a novel treatment for seemingly permanently anesthetic skin. Some physicians advocate removal of an anesthetic digit (*e.g.*, a finger) because it is constantly in the way and susceptible to damage. From the results reported previously, it is apparent that the nerves to surrounding tissues will not sprout into the anesthetic area. Perhaps if nerves innervating the surrounding, sentient tissue were crushed, they would reinnervate their own target tissues and also sprout into the anesthetic area. This sort of treatment has proved effective in rats (Diamond and Jackson, 1980).

Regeneration is not confined to sensory systems. For example, an extra limb bud can be grafted onto a tadpole. When the tadpole metamorphoses into a frog, the frog will have five legs. A graft in the thoracic region results in a sentient fifth limb that does not move. However, if the graft is made in the lumbar region, the limb is sentient and it moves. The animal moves each joint of the limb in unison with the corresponding joint on the adjacent normal limb. Appropriate reflex movements can be evoked from and in both the grafted and the adjacent limbs. It is apparent that the innervation of the graft does not result from simple sprouting of neurons to the adjacent limb because there is an increase in ventral horn cells in segments innervating the graft. It is not known whether specific neurons grew out to the appropriate muscle or whether neurons grew out randomly and their properties were specified by the muscle they contacted.

CENTRAL RESPONSES TO DAMAGE

It is apparent that peripheral neurons are capable of regeneration and that considerable reorganization in their properties and the effects of their activity is possible. Central axons do not seem to regenerate, at least in adults. There is a report of regeneration of pyramidal tract axons in newborn hamsters, though their course through the brain stem and spinal cord is altered. Motor performance in these animals was described as "normal" (Kalil and Reh, 1979). Usually, however, central fibers do not regenerate; the glial scar that forms after damage may prevent the penetration of axons even if they sprout. Some central neurons may also have a low potential for regeneration.

When afferent fibers to a neuron are damaged, other terminals on that neuron can sprout and fill the synaptic sites vacated by the damaged neurons. For example, when the fimbria of the hippocampus are cut, there is, within two days, a degeneration and dissolution of degenerating axons, the debris being removed within two months. Sprouting occurs in fibers of the medial forebrain bundle, filling the vacancy left by the fimbrial fibers from the septum. This sprouting does not restore the function of the degenerated fibers, but it may maintain the excitability of the hippocampal neurons by adding excitation to replace that lost because of the damage. It has been speculated that sprouting is stimulated by release of some substance from the postsynaptic neuron upon deafferentation, a release that is inhibited by normal innervation. However, sprouting does not always occur following deafferentation. It does not occur in the dorsal column nuclei following transection of the dorsal columns or in the lateral geniculate nucleus following removal of the visual inputs. Thus, it seems unlikely that sprouting can explain much of the recovery that occurs after lesions in the central nervous system. Clearly, sprouting does not occur in the spinothalamic tract following tractotomy even when pain sensations recur.

There are other changes that occur following deafferentation. There is a sharp reduction in the extent of the dendritic field of motoneurons following transection of the spinal cord. Neurons can even be reduced to having only two dendrites. Cutting the optic radiation causes the dendrites of neurons in the visual cortex to deviate from their normal vertical orientation, bending downward, seemingly in search of a new afferent input. There is, of course, no regeneration in either of these cases and little or no spontaneous recovery.

RECOVERY FOLLOWING CENTRAL DAMAGE

We know that there is recovery following damage to the central nervous system. Pain recurs following its abolition by various central lesions. Feeding behavior begins again following the aphagia induced by lateral hypothalamic lesions. Hyperemotionality that is induced by septal lesions also wanes with time. Recovery from brain damage requires variable lengths of time, from a minimum of minutes or hours following a mild concussion to years following left temporal lobectomy. Recovery time depends upon the following factors:

1. The nature, level, and extent of the damage
2. The rate of onset of the damage. Recovery is usually better following lesions of rapid onset than following lesions of slower onset, for example, tumors.
3. Age at the time of damage. In general, younger people suffer less deficit and recover faster than adults.
4. Extent and permanence of indirect trauma due to accessory complications such as edema and hypoxia
5. The measure of recovery

Often serial lesions produce much less or even no deficit when compared with a lesion of comparable size and location made all at once. A learned auditory discrimination task is lost following bilateral temporal lobe ablation in animals, but when ablation of one temporal lobe is followed at least 7 days later by ablation of the other temporal lobe, the learned ability is not lost. Likewise, in shuttle avoidance tasks in which the animal learns to move to another location at a light signal to avoid a shock, removal of both striate cortices results in loss of the learned avoidance. If the lesions of the cortices are done serially with a rest peroid in between, the avoidance ability is not lost. However, if the animal is kept in the dark during the interim between the serial lesions, the ability is lost. Apparently, some experience is required between the lesions to protect the ability from being lost, perhaps to transfer "knowledge" of the training to some other brain site.

Drugs can occasionally restore abilities lost following damage. For example, contact placing—the reflex placing of the foot on a surface when any part of the foot contacts the surface—is lost in animals following pyramidotomy or lesions of the motor cortex. The reflex can be restored temporarily by administration of amphetamines. It can also be restored permanently by a subsequent lesion of the contralateral ventrolateral funiculus or, in the case of a previous motor cortex lesion, a subsequent lesion of the contralateral motor cortex. The temporary remission of parkinsonian symptoms following administration of catecholamines has already been noted (Chap. 16).

Interestingly, contact placing responses are not lost following pyramidotomy if they were part of a presurgical training program. An animal trained to make placing responses to a light or sound signal before the pyramids are sectioned still makes the responses to the signal afterward. The same protection of index finger–thumb apposition and discrete grasping and releasing, normally lost after pyramidotomy, occurs when they are part of a presurgical training program. Both abilities are present in the postsurgical training situation, although there may still be impairments in other situations.

How then can we understand this type of recovery if there is no regeneration? A number of possible explanations have been given, including the following:

1. Sprouting leads to establishment of new neuronal networks. We have seen that this explanation probably does not have general applicability to recovery processes.

2. Damage leads to depression of activity at some distance from the lesion that recovers with time **(diaschisis)**. Damage to the nervous system, made experimentally or occurring naturally in a limited area, can lead to changes in structures at some distance. When thermocautery is used to coagulate brain tissue, the heat produced could alter the behavior of distant structures even though the neurons in them do not die. It is known that, in strokes, there is a marked, transient decrease in the blood flow and, presumably, the metabolic rate in brain areas distant from the lesion, even in the opposite hemisphere (Høedt-Rasmussen and Skinhoj, 1964).

3. Control of the behavior is taken over by another structure **(vicarious function)**. It is possible that more than one structure is capable of performing a certain function, but only one does so during normal development. When this one is damaged, the other may take over for it. As we shall see, this is apparently what happens in development of speech centers in one hemisphere (the dominant hemisphere) only. It is not known to what extent the nondominant hemisphere can take over speech production and perception when the dominant hemisphere is damaged in adults; it can take over completely when damage occurs in very young children (see Chap. 21).

4. Alternate movements are found to accomplish the lost behavior **(substitution)**. After recovery, the "same" behavior may reappear, albeit performed using different muscles, different contraction sequences, different limbs, or different sensory receptors. In a sense, this is not the same behavior, but a new one accomplishing the same goal.

5. Relatively ineffective synapses increase in effectiveness following removal of other synapses. Neurons in the medial aspect of the dorsal horn of the spinal cord normally respond to stimulation of the foot and toes in cats, but after deafferentation of the foot and toes, they begin to respond to stimulation of the leg. This change in receptive fields probably does not result from sprouting because it occurs too soon after deafferentation. Rather, it is likely that these neurons received synaptic input from leg receptors that was too weak to cause the neurons to discharge. When other synapses were removed, these normally weak synapses somehow increased their effectiveness (Devor and Wall, 1978).

6. Damage leads to irritation, perhaps denervation hypersensitivity (Chap. 18), which inhibits activity in some undamaged structure involved in production of the behavior; this irritation is reduced with time. This explanation is complementary to diaschisis. If one could somehow make cerebellar Purkinje cells irritable so that they discharged spontaneously in prolonged bursts of spikes, the cerebellar nuclei would be virtually completely inhibited, resulting in a marked deficit in some behaviors.

7. In some cases, motivation for the behavior is lost, but new and different motivations are found later. Aphagia following hypothalamic lesions could be due to a loss of motivation to eat, for example, a loss of response to reduction in blood sugar levels. Apparent recovery could occur when the animal responds to extreme deprivation of nutrients and cellular deterioration.

8. Naturally occurring lesions could be reversible. Early recovery could be due to reversal of vascular lesions or reoxygenation of tissues, inactive due to borderline hypoxia. With spinal cord trauma in dogs, a longitudinal incision in the dura can shorten recovery time up to 50%, presumably due to a reduction in local fluid pressure.

It is not possible to say which of these explanations is most important, which has the most general application. In some cases of recovery, it is possible to rule out some of these possibilities, but it is seldom possible to eliminate all but one. Braun (1978) has pointed out that one's interpretation of the recovery process depends upon the interpretation of the loss. Using as an example the recovery from aphagia following lateral hypothalamic lesions, he observed that if aphagia is thought to result from loss of motivation to eat, then reappearance of eating can be viewed as a response motivated by the extreme deprivation that eventually occurs; if aphagia results from disruption of visceral activity leading to gastric ulcers, then reappearance of eating can be seen as based upon recovery of balanced visceral activity and ulcer healing; if aphagia results from decreased numbers of catecholamine neurons, then reappearance of eating can be seen as being due to compensatory changes in the remaining catecholamine neurons and their receptors; and if aphagia is due to a temporary lack of motivation to eat caused by a decrease in the set point (the regulated point) for body weight, then recovery is really an epiphenomenon occurring when body weight is reduced to the new set point, at which point eating begins to maintain this value. Actually, if the body weight of an animal is reduced prior to a lateral hypothalamic lesion, aphagia does not develop. This suggests that the last possibility above is a reasonable explanation and that there is actually no recovery at all, because the body weight set point is never corrected (LaVere, 1975).

Recovery following brain damage is clearly a complicated process (or processes) that we are just beginning to understand. The foregoing discussion coupled with particular examples elsewhere in the text should give the reader some idea of the range of functions for which recovery is possible and some idea of the possible causes for the initial losses and later recovery.

SUGGESTED READING

Baker RE, Corner MA: Possible mechanisms underlying the development of central and peripheral cutaneous afferent connections. In Cuenód M, Kreutzberg GW, Bloom FE [eds]: Development and Chemical Specificity of Neurons, Progress in Brain Research, Vol. 51. Amsterdam, Elsevier, 1979

Braun JJ: Time and recovery from brain damage In Finger S [ed]: Recovery from Brain Damage New York, Plenum Press, 1978

Bruner RL, Altman J: Locomotor deficits in adul rats with moderate to massive retardation o cerebellar development during infancy. Behav Biol 9:169–188, 1973

Devor M, Wall PD: Reorganization of spinal corc sensory map after peripheral nerve injury. Nature 276:75–76, 1978

Diamond J, Jackson PC: Regeneration and collateral sprouting of peripheral nerves. In Jewet DL, McCarroll HR Jr [eds]: Nerve Repair anc Regeneration: Its Clinical and Experimenta Basis. St. Louis, CV Mosby, 1980

Dykes RW, Terzis JK: Reinnervation of glaborous skin in baboons: Properties of cutaneous mechanoreceptors subsequent to nerve crush J Neurophysiol 42:1461–1478, 1979

Ford FR, Woodhall B: Phenomena due to misdirection of regenerating fibers of cranial, spinal and autonomic nerves. Arch Surg 36:480–499, 1938

Goldberger ME: Recovery of movement after CNS lesions in monkeys. In Stein DG, Roser JJ, Butters N [eds]: Plasticity and Recovery o Function in the Central Nervous System. New York, Academic Press, 1974

Grafstein B: The nerve cell body response tc axotomy. Exp Neurol 48:32–51, 1975

Harris A: Inductive functions of the nervous system. Ann Rev Physiol 36:251–305, 1974

Høedt-Rasmussen K, Skinhoj E: Transneural depression of the cerebral hemispheric metabolism in man. Acta Neurol Scand 40:41–46, 1964

Hollyday M, Mendell L: Analysis of moving supernumerary limbs of *Xenopus laevis*. Exp Neurol 51:316–324, 1976

Horch K: Guidance of regrowing sensory axons after cutaneous nerve lesions in the cat. J Neurophysiol 42:1437–1449, 1979

Jacobson M: Developmental Neurobiology, 2nd ed. New York, Plenum Press, 1978

Kalil K, Reh T: Regrowth of severed axons in the neonatal central nervous system: Establishment of normal connections. Science 205: 1158–1160, 1979

LaVere TE: Neural stability, sparing, and behavioral recovery following brain damage. Psychol Rev 82:344 358, 1975

Silver J: Cell death during development of the nervous system. In Jacobson M [ed]: Handbook of Sensory Physiology, Vol. IX, Development of Sensory Systems. Berlin, Heidelberg, New York, Springer-Verlag, 1978

Varon S: Nerve growth factor and its mode of action. Exp Neurol 48:75–92, 1975

20

Cerebral Cortical Activity: Primary Evoked Potentials and the Electroencephalogram

PRIMARY EVOKED POTENTIALS

In the most general terms, an **evoked potential** is an electrical response recorded in some part of the nervous system in response to a stimulus. The stimulus *evokes* the response. The simplest example of an evoked potential is the axon spike caused by an electrical shock to the axon. Although the neurophysiologist most often uses such a shock in studying evoked potentials, the latter can also be initiated by more natural, adequate stimuli such as light flashes, taps, or clicks. Nearly *synchronous* activity in many parts of the nervous system will result in an electrical potential that can be recorded using either micropipette electrodes or larger, wire electrodes. The potentials are used by neurophysiologists to study how portions of the nervous system are interconnected. For example, we know that a point in one hemisphere is connected neurologically to the corresponding point on the opposite hemisphere, because stimulation at one point will evoke a change in potential at the other, the so-called transcallosal evoked potential.

Although evoked potentials can be recorded from many structures in the nervous system, they are of limited clinical use except during surgery. During brain surgery, knowledge of the various pathways in the nervous system allows the surgeon to pinpoint the site at which he may want to cut by recording the appropriate evoked potential. For example, one procedure for surgical relief of parkinsonism is to make a lesion in the ventrolateral nucleus of the thalamus. Because parkinsonism apparently results from malfunction of the basal ganglia, whose primary efferent pathway is through the ventrolateral nucleus, interrupting abnormal signals from the basal ganglia at the thalamus can produce some relief of symptoms. The surgeon can make the lesion by passing a small amount of current through an electrode placed in the nucleus. The current heats the tissue and destroys cells near the electrode. The surgeon will verify that the electrode is in the nucleus by recording the potentials evoked there by movement of the joints.

During neurosurgery in human patients, the cerebral cortex is exposed by removing a section of the calvarium covering the central fissure. A large electrode, actually a piece of 0.5-mm diameter silver wire, is placed on the postcentral gyrus about 10 cm lateral to

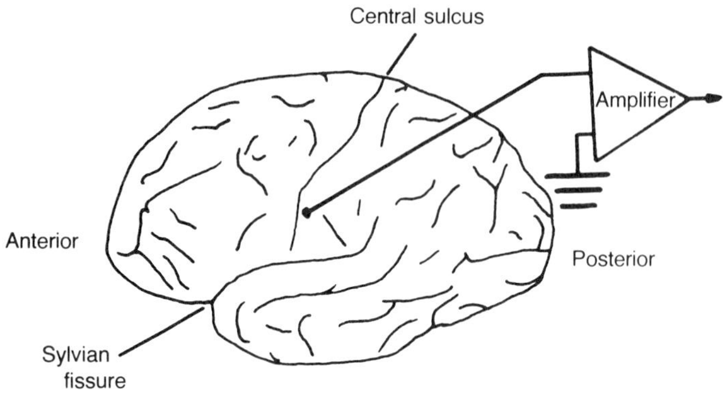

FIG. 20-1. The physical arrangement for recording evoked potentials from the surface of the postcentral gyrus of the cerebral cortex.

FIG. 20-2. Typical configuration of the potential evoked in the cerebral cortex by stimulation of the skin. The potential recorded from the surface first goes positive about 12 to 20 msec after the stimulus (indicated by the stimulus artifact) and has a characteristic "W" configuration.

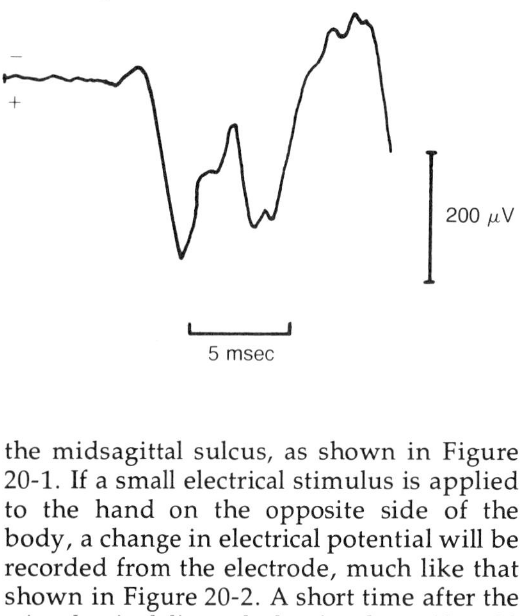

the midsagittal sulcus, as shown in Figure 20-1. If a small electrical stimulus is applied to the hand on the opposite side of the body, a change in electrical potential will be recorded from the electrode, much like that shown in Figure 20-2. A short time after the stimulus is delivered, that is, about 10 to 20 msec after the stimulus artifact, the potential at the electrode first becomes more positive and then more negative with respect to a second or indifferent electrode placed on some electrically inactive site, such as the ear lobe. In humans, the potential often has a characteristic "W" configuration, as shown in Figure 20-2. If the electrical stimulus is gradually increased in intensity, the amplitude of the recorded potential gradually increases until it reaches some maximum. At that point, further increases in intensity do not result in any change in response amplitude. The size of the maximal response varies from a few microvolts to several millivolts depending upon the exact recording site and the stimulus site. If the stimulus is repeated again and again, the same change in potential will be recorded each time, perhaps accompanied by additional activity on some trials. The basic form of the potential, however, is visible on each trial. This response of the brain to the external stimulus is called the **primary evoked response** or **primary evoked potential.**

Tapping at the same place on the skin evokes a response at the same site on the cortex, which is very similar in timing and shape to the one evoked by electrical stimulation. However, the recording electrode does not have to be moved very far on the cortex (only a few millimeters) before the recorded response gets much smaller and finally disappears. At this new recording site, however, it is possible to produce a primary evoked response by tapping a different area of skin close by the first area. Thus, it is possible to use the primary evoked response to map which areas of the cerebral cortex respond to stimuli on different parts of the skin, by associating the site on the cortex where the response of largest amplitude is recorded with the site on the skin where the stimulus was applied. As a stimulus is moved in a systematic way across the body, the site of maximum activity moves in a systematic way across the cerebral cortex. Mapping the cerebral cortical areas that respond to skin stimulation is possible, because the primary evoked response results from synchronous activity in

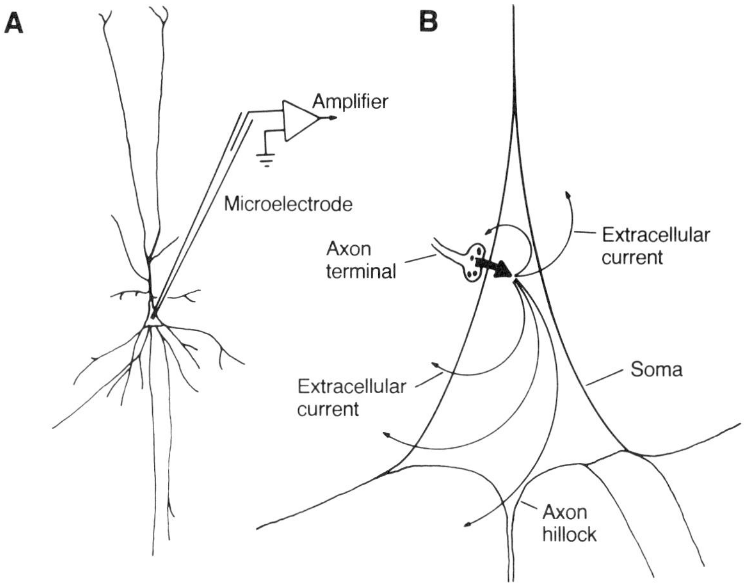

FIG. 20-3. A. The setup for recording the transmembrane potential of a cortical neuron using a micropipette. **B.** A synapse is diagrammed with the current flow patterns that occur during synaptic activity. **Important:** Some current flows in the extracellular fluid.

one of the fast-conducting pathways to the cerebral cortex, which shows a high degree of topographical organization. We have already mentioned such maps when we considered the somatotopic organization of the somatic cerebral cortex.

The area of the cortex in which these recordings were made, that is, the postcentral gyrus, is called the somatosensory cortex. If recordings are made instead from the occipital lobe, near the calcarine fissure, primary evoked potentials can be obtained by flashing a light in the patient's eye. This is one reason why this area is termed visual cortex. The configuration of the potential is essentially the same as that shown in Figure 20-2, except that it starts a little earlier. Clicks can evoke similar potentials in the auditory area of the cortex on the superior temporal lobe. However, stimuli applied to one sensory system do not produce primary responses in the cortical areas of a different sensory system: Clicks do not produce primary evoked responses in somatosensory cortex, nor do taps or light flashes produce them in auditory cortex.

Evoked potentials in the cortex can also be produced by stimulating appropriate regions of the thalamus. Evoked responses can be recorded in auditory cortex following stimulation of the medial geniculate nucleus, in visual cortex following stimulation of the lateral geniculate nucleus, and in somatosensory cortex following stimulation of the nucleus ventralis posterolateralis. With the thalamic stimulation, evoked potentials occur earlier, that is, with shorter **latency** (the time between the stimulus and the beginning of response), than when the sensory receptors are stimulated, primarily because the pathway from thalamus to cortex is shorter than from skin to cortex. It is possible to elicit the cortical primary evoked response in the appropriate area of cortex with an electrical stimulus applied anywhere along the pathway leading to it, whether it is applied to a peripheral nerve, along an ascending tract, at the thalamus, or even in the subcortical white matter. Of course, the closer to the cortex the stimulus is applied, the shorter the latency of the response.

How are these primary evoked responses generated? All electrical neural activity results from the fact that there is a separation of charge across the neuron's membrane. The exact magnitude of the resulting voltage varies from cell to cell, but it is usually within the range of 50 to 90 mV. Figure 20-3A illustrates the normal resting state of

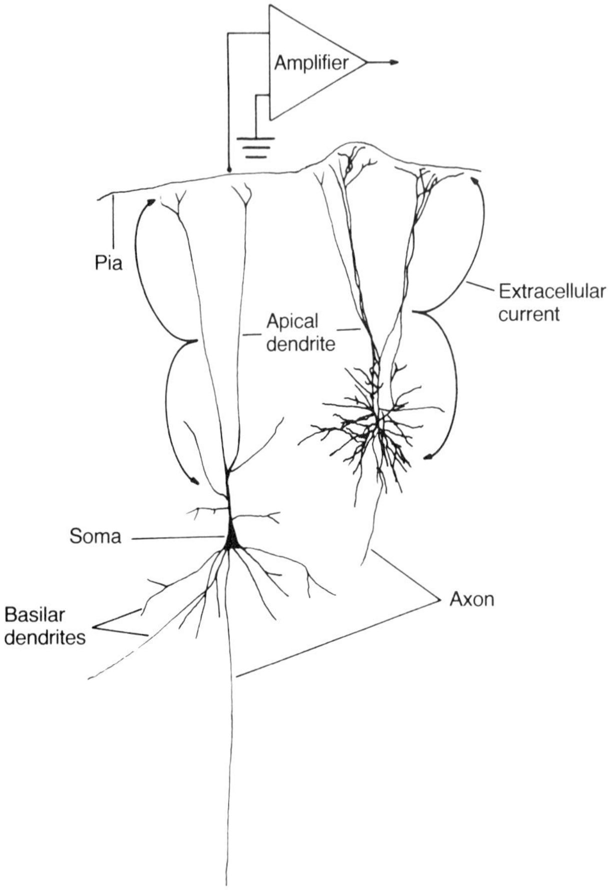

FIG. 20-4. The recording setup for evoked potentials again, this time with some typical cells indicated. Again, note that some current flows in the extracellular fluid in the vicinity of the recording electrode.

a neuron with a potential difference across the membrane such that it is negative inside with respect to outside. Whenever the neuron is excited, current flows through the membrane from outside to inside at active regions and back out of the cell at inactive regions. Remember that current flows only in closed circuits. Therefore, current that flows through the membrane also flows through the extracellular fluid, as shown by the arrows in Figure 20-3B.

In the cerebral cortex, most of the cells are lined up with their dendrites pointing up toward the surface and with their axons pointing away from the surface. When these cortical neurons are excited, the current crossing the membrane flows through the extracellular fluid (Fig. 20-4). This current flowing through the resistance of the cortex produces a voltage that we can measure if it is large enough. As we saw in Figure 20-3, some of this current will pass near the recording electrode. Only a small amount of current passes the electrode when only one cell is active and if that cell is 500 μm away from the electrode. However, in human cerebral cortex, cells are packed so closely together, with a density of 30 to 60 neurons per 10^6 cubic micrometers (30,000–60,000/mm^3), that more than 1000 neurons are within 300 μm of the recording electrode. If large numbers of these neurons close to the electrode are activated synchronously, as they are during the primary evoked response, the total extracellular current flow would be considerable and easily recorded.

What cellular events can contribute to the response? Actually, there are only two: the nonpropagated postsynaptic potentials or PSPs and the propagated, all-or-none action

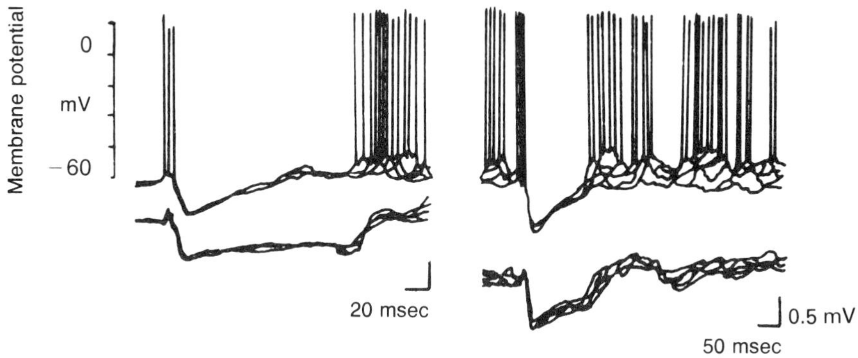

FIG. 20-5. A micropipette was used to make the records in this figure as shown in Figure 20-3A. The **upper record** in each pair of traces was made inside a cell, whereas the **lower record** in each pair was made just outside the cell. Note that synaptic potentials, EPSPs and IPSPs, are still seen outside the cell, but there is not even a hint of an action potential. Voltage calibrations are the same for both sets of records, and they apply to lower traces. (Humphrey DR: EEG Clin Neurophysiol 25:421–442, 1968)

potentials. The PSP has a voltage of only a few millivolts, whereas the action potential has a voltage of up to 120 mV. One might expect that the larger action potentials make a greater contribution to the evoked potential, but actually they do not. When recorded from outside the cell there is considerable decrement in potential with distance away from the cell through the extracellular fluid and the decrement for the action potential is much greater than for the PSPs. Figure 20-5 illustrates this phenomenon. The upper traces are recordings made with a fine pipette electrode inside a neuron in the cerebral cortex of a cat. The lower traces are recordings from another pipette electrode placed outside the neuron. In the intracellular recording, both action potentials and PSPs are clearly visible, but at a short distance away from the cell only the PSPs can be seen in the record, and these are essentially identical to those recorded inside the cell. Therefore, we must conclude that primary evoked response represents mainly the sum of all the PSPs generated in all of the cells in the proximity of the electrode. These PSPs can be either hyperpolarizing or depolarizing, that is, IPSPs or EPSPs, and they can be staggered so that they do not all start at the same time. The closer a cell is to the recording electrode, the more voltage it will contribute to the recorded response. Thus, the small cells that constitute the majority of cortical neurons and reside near the surface, contribute the most to the cortical primary evoked response, whereas the giant Betz cells, which are most conspicuous, fewer, and farther away, contribute less to potentials recorded at the cortical surface.

Recording evoked responses from the surface of the brain is of limited clinical use outside of a surgical suite. However, it is also possible to record evoked potentials from the scalp, though the potentials are much reduced in amplitude. Between the source of the potential and our recording electrode on the scalp are dura mater, cerebrospinal fluid, bone, muscle, skin, and perhaps hair, all of which reduce the amplitude of the primary response and, in the case of skin and muscle, may add some additional, unwanted electrical signals of their own. The evoked potential recorded from the scalp has an amplitude of less than 100 μV (or 0.1 mV), a small potential indeed. One way around this problem is to repeat the stimulus over and over again and sum up the individual responses. If the number of repetitions is large enough, then the sum or average response will contain the evoked response and not those unwanted signals. This gives the neurologist a fairly powerful tool for testing the continuity of the primary sensory pathways to the cortex. For example, if he suspects that there is a lesion of the auditory system he can try to record the evoked responses to clicks and compare his result with normal potentials, perhaps from the other side of the head, perhaps from another person who has no impairment.

Short-latency responses to clicks pre-

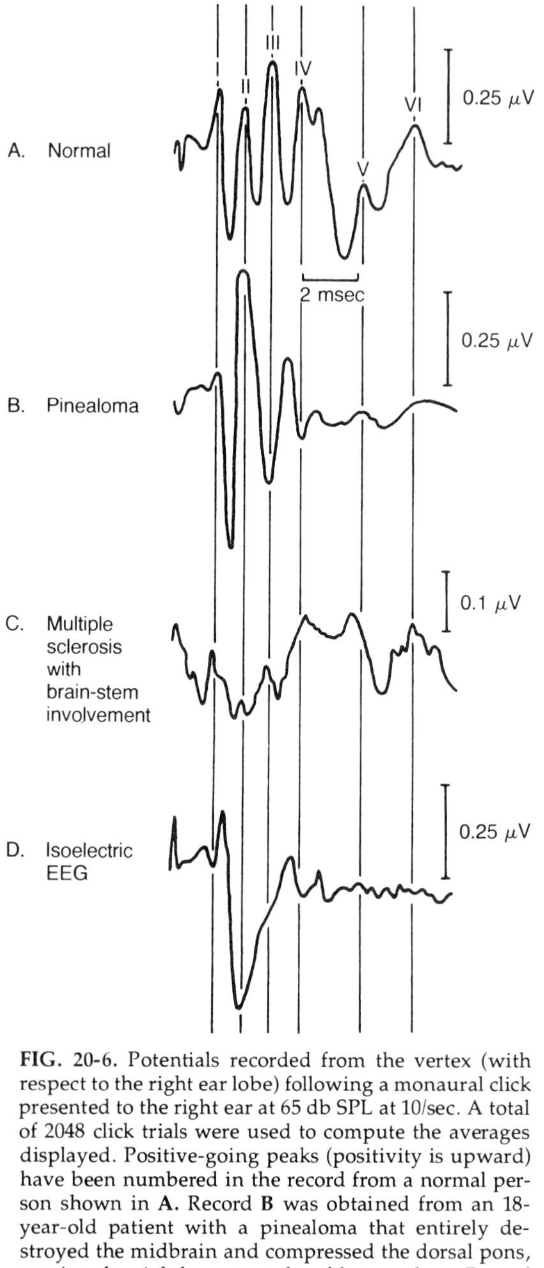

FIG. 20-6. Potentials recorded from the vertex (with respect to the right ear lobe) following a monaural click presented to the right ear at 65 db SPL at 10/sec. A total of 2048 click trials were used to compute the averages displayed. Positive-going peaks (positivity is upward) have been numbered in the record from a normal person shown in **A.** Record **B** was obtained from an 18-year-old patient with a pinealoma that entirely destroyed the midbrain and compressed the dorsal pons, sparing the eighth nerve and cochlear nucleus. Record **C** was obtained from a 35-year-old woman with multiple sclerosis involving the midbrain region. A 21-year-old woman without pulse or respiration was resuscitated with return of heart beat but with an isoelectric EEG. Evoked potentials from this patient are shown in **D.** (Starr A, Achor LJ: Arch Neurol 32:761–768, 1975)

sented to one ear can be recorded at the vertex with respect to ear lobe and educed from background activity by averaging 2000 or so such responses. An example of the response in a normal individual is shown in Figure 20-6A. There are seven very small potentials marked I to VII that apparently occur in all normal individuals with characteristic latencies for particular sound intensities. These potentials, often referred to as "Jewett bumps," are supposed by many investigators to be derived from brain-stem auditory centers, and their absence is thought to indicate the level of auditory system damage. For example, wave I is thought to be due to activity in the VIIIth cranial nerve, whereas waves II and III are thought to result from discharges in the cochlear nucleus and superior olive. Waves IV and V have been associated with the inferior colliculus, but the source of waves VI and VII is as yet unspecified. Not all investigators are convinced that these are the sources of the potentials, yet the potentials could serve as useful diagnostic tools if their auditory origin can be verified. They are not influenced by coma due to barbiturates, sedatives, hypoxia, diabetic ketoacidosis, uremia, concussion, or status epilepticus. The latency of wave I, normally 1.6 msec at 65 db SPL, is lengthened to 2.2 msec with a middle ear conduction loss of 20 db, but is unchanged with loss due to damage to the central auditory pathway. Figure 20-6B shows the same potentials in a patient, shown post mortem to have a pinealoma. Nearly complete loss of all components after wave III is obvious, whereas a delay in time of occurrence of waves II and III is apparent. Figure 20-6C was recorded from a patient with multiple sclerosis involving brain-stem structures. Wave I is of normal latency, but the rest are of reduced amplitude, and their shapes are somewhat altered from normal. Figure 20-6D was recorded from a patient with an isoelectric EEG and shows only wave I, the other waves being undiscernable. Shortly after this record was made the patient suffered a cardiac arrest and wave I also disappeared. It is apparent that these potentials could be useful in diagnosis, but care must be taken in regarding these as "auditory potentials." This caution is highlighted by the observation that the patient whose records are shown in Figure 20-6C had intact hearing "bilaterally to whispered speech" and yet had obvious abnormalities of these potentials.

Another example of the use of evoked potentials is shown in Figure 20-7. Potentials

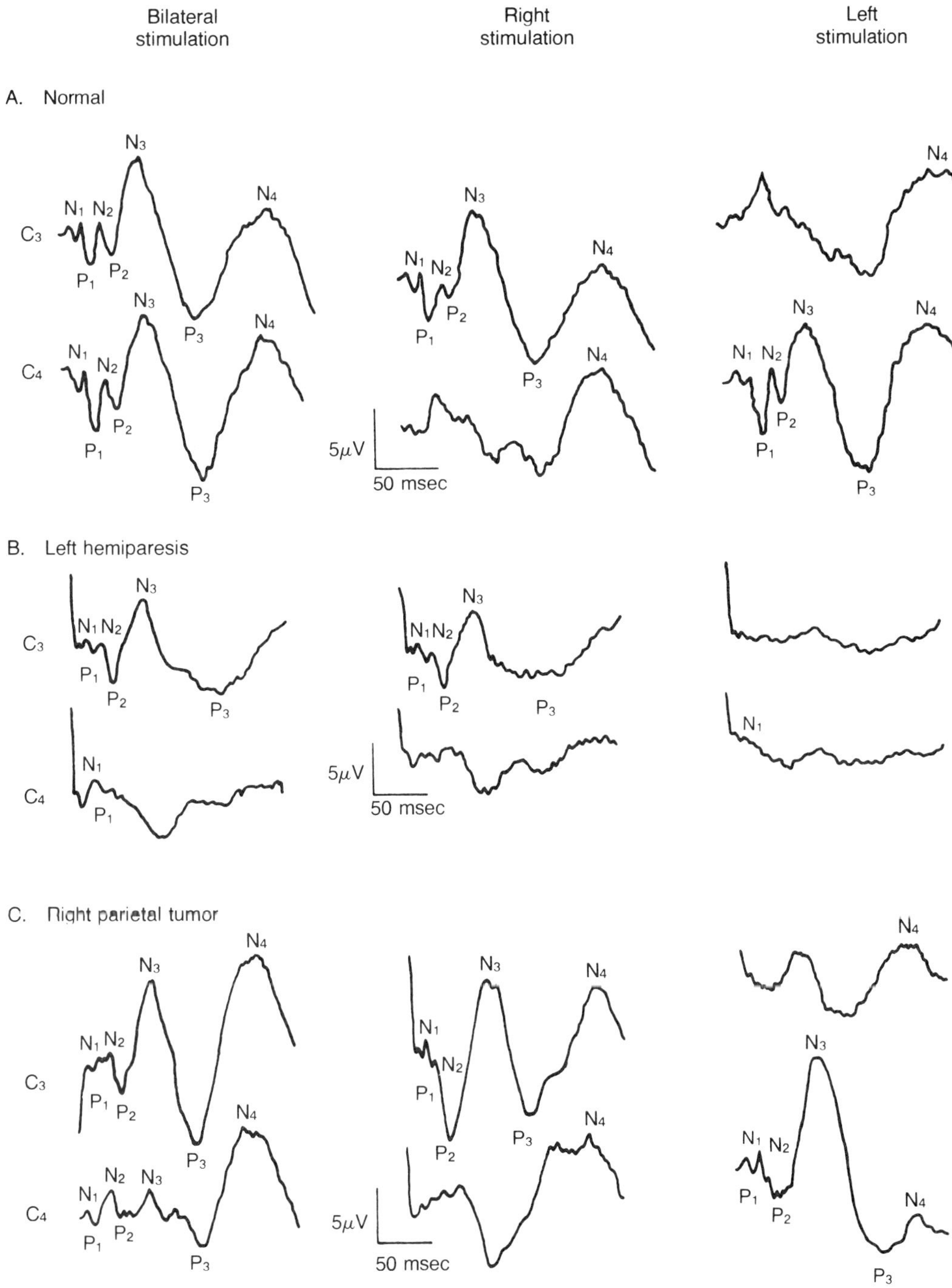

FIG. 20-7. Potentials evoked in the pericentral region of the cerebral cortex on the right, C_4, and left, C_3 (with respect to the earlobe), by bilateral, right, and left superficial radial nerve stimulation. The symmetry of responses to bilateral stimulation in a normal individual is shown in **A.** The records in **B** are from a patient with left hemiparesis. Note that responses to bilateral stimulation are similar to those evoked by right stimulation, but they are not symmetric. A right parietal tumor, **C,** results in a depression of P_2, N_3, and P_3 waves and enlargement of the N_3 component of the C_4 response to left stimulation. (Yamada T, Kimura J, Young S, Powers M: Neurology 28:218–223, 1978)

recorded from the region of the central sulcus on the right (C_4) and left (C_3 of Fig. 20-12) in response to stimulation of the superficial radial nerve on the right and left sides and both sides together are illustrated. The responses recorded from a normal individual are shown in Figure 20-7A. The potentials recorded from both sides following bilateral stimulation are very like those recorded only contralaterally following unilateral stimulation, consisting of a characteristic series of negative and positive deflections, the early portion of which is the W potential of Figure 20-2. Their diagnostic value lies in their specificity to somesthesia and in their bilateral symmetry. For example, the patient with left hemiparesis, whose records are shown in Figure 20-7B, shows normal responses to right radial nerve stimulation but abnormal responses to left radial stimulation and lack of symmetry in responses to bilateral stimulation. A similar pattern is evident in records from a patient with a right parietal lobe tumor (Fig. 20-7C), though the potentials are different in their abnormality. Presumably, these differences will be of significance diagnostically in the future when they are understood.

Primary evoked responses are often used to test the effect of drugs or certain training or therapeutic procedures on the central nervous system. Normally, the investigator compares evoked potentials before and after the drug is administered. This procedure in itself is sound, but it is very difficult to draw reliable conclusions about how a drug works from observed changes in the evoked response. Keep in mind that the evoked potentials are generated by *all* of the active cells in the neighborhood of the electrode, not just those whose activity may be enhanced or reduced by a particular procedure or drug.

THE ELECTROENCEPHALOGRAM OR EEG

The cells of the nervous system of a living human are seldom completely silent. They discharge spontaneously in the absence of any stimulus that can be detected. If there were enough of these cells discharging spontaneously at the same time, we might expect to be able to record their activity in the same way the activity of cortical cells was recorded during the primary evoked potential. In fact, we can record the spontaneous electrical activity of the human cortex from the scalp. The recording is called the **electroencephalogram** or, simply, the **EEG.** The EEG represents the "spontaneous," on-going activity of the cerebral cortex like the primary evoked response represents the "evoked" activity of the cortex. Some care should be exercised in interpreting the terms spontaneous and evoked. We call an event spontaneous because we are not deliberately stimulating the person at the time it occurs, but that does not mean there are no stimuli impinging on his receptors.

The EEG, like the evoked potential, is the sum of the many postsynaptic potentials in all of the active cells near the recording electrodes. However, unlike the evoked potential, it cannot be associated with any particular stimulus or event within the nervous system. In spite of this, the EEG is one of the most powerful tools the neurologist has at his disposal for diagnosing certain malfunctions of the cerebral cortex.

The EEG looks like a lot of wavy lines, and it is hard at first to imagine that they are of any value. But, let us look a bit closer (Fig. 20-8). First, the waves of each record occur at a number of different frequencies, but in each, there is one predominant frequency. The predominant rhythm or frequency is a useful index (Table 20-1). If the dominant frequency is between 8 and 14 per sec, it is called **alpha rhythm. Beta rhythms** are those between 14 and 50 per sec, **theta rhythms** between 4 and 8 per sec, and **delta rhythms** less than 4 per sec. Second, the records differ in terms of the amplitude of the activity, but amplitude is less important in characterizing the EEG than frequency. In all of these rhythms, the amplitude of the waves is inversely related to their frequency. The usual convention is to call high frequency–low amplitude waves, fast activity and low frequency–high amplitude waves, slow activity.

The precise pattern of the EEG, in terms of both amplitude and frequency, is influenced by a number of factors. The dominant frequency is a function of the age of the patient. At birth the beta and delta rhythms dominate, whereas in childhood theta rhythms are predominant. Somewhere be-

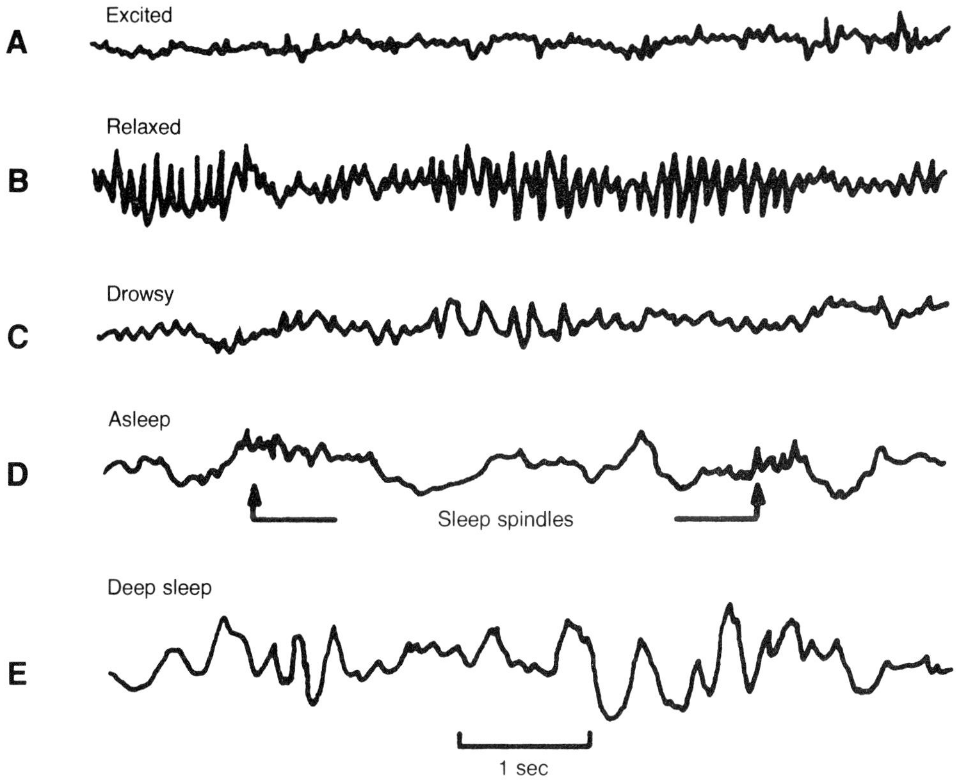

FIG. 20-8. Typical EEG patterns are shown for various states of consciousness. Note presence of sleep spindles in record **D.** (Penfield W, Erickson TC: Epilepsy and Cerebral Localization. Springfield, IL, Charles C Thomas, 1941)

TABLE 20-1. EEG RHYTHMS AND THEIR CHARACTERISTIC FREQUENCIES

EEG DOMINANT FREQUENCY (Hz)	RHYTHM
14–50	Beta
8–14	Alpha
4–8	Theta
<4	Delta

tween ages 14 and 19, an adult pattern becomes fully developed. That adult pattern is different for each individual, and the pattern is stable in the absence of disease or trauma. Normally, records from frontal and parietal regions show higher frequency, lower amplitude rhythms than do records from the occipital region.

The EEG of an awake, relaxed adult with eyes closed is usually an alpha rhythm, but some people never have alpha rhythm. A typical alpha rhythm is shown in record B of Figure 20-8. If the person with alpha rhythm opens his eyes or fixes his attention on something, the dominant frequency increases to the beta range and the amplitude decreases (Fig. 20-9). This phenomenon is called **alpha blocking** or **desynchronization** or **activation.*** When the person closes his eyes, the alpha rhythm usually returns. A lot of equipment is now available to "condition alpha waves," the idea being that because alpha rhythms are normally associated with a relaxed state, by increasing the amount of time spent with alpha rhythms, there will be an increase in relaxation. By using this equipment, one trains oneself to relax. It is a shame that so many people have spent so much money to achieve a state that is easily produced by closing the eyes and letting the mind wan-

* This is another example of confusion of terminology, resulting, this time, from usage of the same term in two different fields. Activation as defined here is the usage as employed by experimental physiologists. Clinical electroencephalographers employ the same term to signify any maneuver that produces a change in the pattern of electrical activity of the brain.

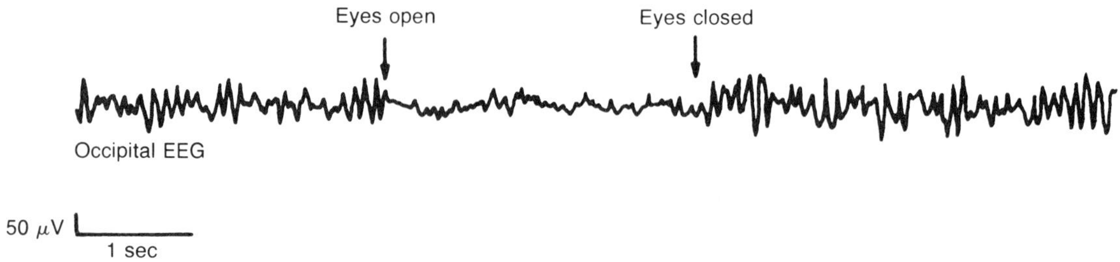

FIG. 20-9. An example of EEG activation or desynchronization produced by opening the eyes **(first arrow).** Normal relaxed alpha rhythm is converted to beta rhythm by this maneuver. Alpha rhythm is regained by closing the eyes **(second arrow).** (Curtis BA, Jacobson S, Marcus EM: An Introduction to the Neurosciences. Philadelphia, WB Saunders, 1972)

FIG. 20-10. The EEG of a normal 19-year-old before and after 130 sec of hyperventilation. Recordings are monopolar from frontal, pericentral, parietal, and occipital leads as shown in Figure 20-12. (Saunders MG: Am J EEG Technol 8:41–57, 1968)

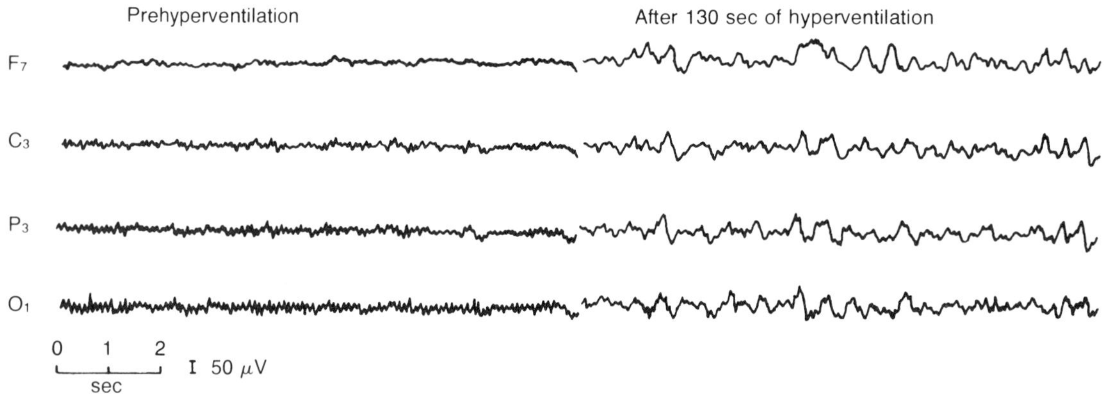

der, a state that can be trained without expensive equipment.

The EEG is also profoundly influenced by the metabolic condition of the brain. Brain tissue has the highest requirements for oxygen of any body tissue and, as might be expected, any change in oxygenation influences cellular activity and therefore the EEG. With cerebral hypoxia (reduced oxygen supply), there is a gradual, continuous decrease in the dominant frequency of the EEG especially in frontal regions as oxygen tension falls. There apparently is not a decrease in faster activity, but an increase in slower activity as indicated by frequency spectral analysis. Changes in the EEG pattern have been seen with reductions in cerebral venous oxygen partial pressure to 29 mm Hg.

Hypercapnia (increased carbon dioxide), by itself, usually results in an increase in the dominant EEG frequency when it develops gradually. This is true of moderate hypercapnia, which results in elevation of both total cerebral blood flow and local flow in different regions. Hypocapnia (reduced carbon dioxide) has the same effect on the EEG as hypoxia, as seen in Figure 20-10. In this figure are shown recordings from frontal, pericentral, parietal and occipital regions of the cortex, before and after 130 sec of hyperventilation to lower carbon dioxide levels. Notice the dramatic increase in slow activity. Hyperventilation is used clinically to "activate" the EEG (in the clinical sense). This normal pattern of change is not reliably seen unless hyperventilation is followed by a period of reduced oxygen. The combination of hypocapnia and hypoxia produces delta rhythms in about 79% of cases of individuals less than 35 years old, when oxygen falls to 75% and carbon dioxide to 38% of resting levels; hypoxia alone or hyperventilation alone may not produce delta rhythms, even when oxygen levels are reduced to 58% or carbon dioxide levels are reduced to 30% of resting levels. Individuals over 35 may not show this delta activity in response to hypoxia and/or hypocapnia or they may show it at more extreme values. The threshold may be lowered (*i.e.*, delta activity may occur at higher levels of oxygen and carbon dioxide) in females during menstruation or in any person during periods of hypoglycemia. The opposite, an increased threshold, may occur during hyperglycemia. Reduction of cerebral circulation and thus of local oxygen concentration is, of course, produced by hyperventilation in addition to decreased carbon dioxide concentrations. Hypoxia or hypocapnia often triggers epileptic attacks in people prone to them and therein lies the usefulness of these maneuvers to the electroencephalographer. Often, attacks occur naturally with low frequency, and it is difficult to trap them during an EEG recording session.

Changes in dominant EEG frequency also occur with phenytoin (an antiepileptic drug) poisoning, profound hypoglycemia, barbiturate overdoses, and hepatic disease. The changes are similar to those occurring during hyperventilation, but recovery to normal is not as rapid when the conditions are reversed. A general increase in theta activity often accompanies pernicious anemia, panhypopituitarism, Cushing's and Addison's diseases, vitamin B deficiency, and, in fact, a wide range of disorders involving altered states of consciousness and mood.

The EEG is frequently used clinically and experimentally to indicate the state of arousal of the patient. Typically, the EEG of a person who is deeply asleep (the threshold for arousal is high) shows delta rhythms with a dominant frequency of 3 per sec or less. An example of delta rhythms in sleep is shown in Figure 20-8E. As the person awakens, short bursts of activity at 10 to 14 per sec start to appear in the record. These bursts are called sleep spindles because the appearance of the envelope of the wave form is spindle-shaped. Some sleep spindles are seen in Figure 20-8D. As sleep gradually becomes lighter, the interval between spindles becomes shorter until they become alpha rhythms or the waking rhythm in B. Further arousal of attention desynchronizes or activates the EEG, as in A. A similar change in the EEG occurs in animals and presumably also in humans during recovery from barbiturate anesthesia. As the depth of anesthesia is lessened, the frequency of the EEG increases.

For a long time, it was thought that outward signs of arousal and activation of the EEG were inextricably linked, that is, whenever the EEG was activated the animal was aroused and whenever the animal was aroused the EEG was activated. We now know that this is not always the case. A classic example of a mismatch between EEG activation and behavior occurs in **paradoxical sleep.** During paradoxical sleep the person is behaviorally deeply asleep, as evidenced by the high threshold for arousal by peripheral stimulation, but his EEG is typical of the awake state. The nervous system is quite active during this stage of sleep, which recurs several times during a sleep period and which is the time when dreaming occurs. Paradoxical sleep is characterized by **rapid eye movements (REM)** that occur in bursts and by mild muscle jerks, yet there is a marked hypotonia, seen most easily in neck muscles, that apparently results from decreased skeletomotor and fusimotor activity.

Isolation occurs, to a certain extent, as a result of any hospitalization. Figure 20-11 shows an extreme case of what happens to the EEG during isolation. There was a reduction in alpha activity and an increase in slower activity in this healthy person following 14 days of complete isolation. The effects of partial isolation would, of course, be less dramatic.

Another use of the EEG in the clinic is for locating damaged areas of the cerebral cortex. Nervous tissue that has been damaged, for example by local asphyxia or trauma, may discharge abnormal, irregular bursts of spikes that are seen in the EEG as slow activity often with a characteristic form. This abnormal discharge may produce symptoms in the patient, such as seizures. Most EEG recordings are made between two electrodes placed on the scalp rather than between one electrode on the scalp and one on the ear or some other inactive site. Recordings from two active electrodes are called **bipolar** recordings, whereas recordings from one active and one indifferent electrode are called **monopolar** recordings. There are conventional sets of electrode positions, called leads, as shown in Figure

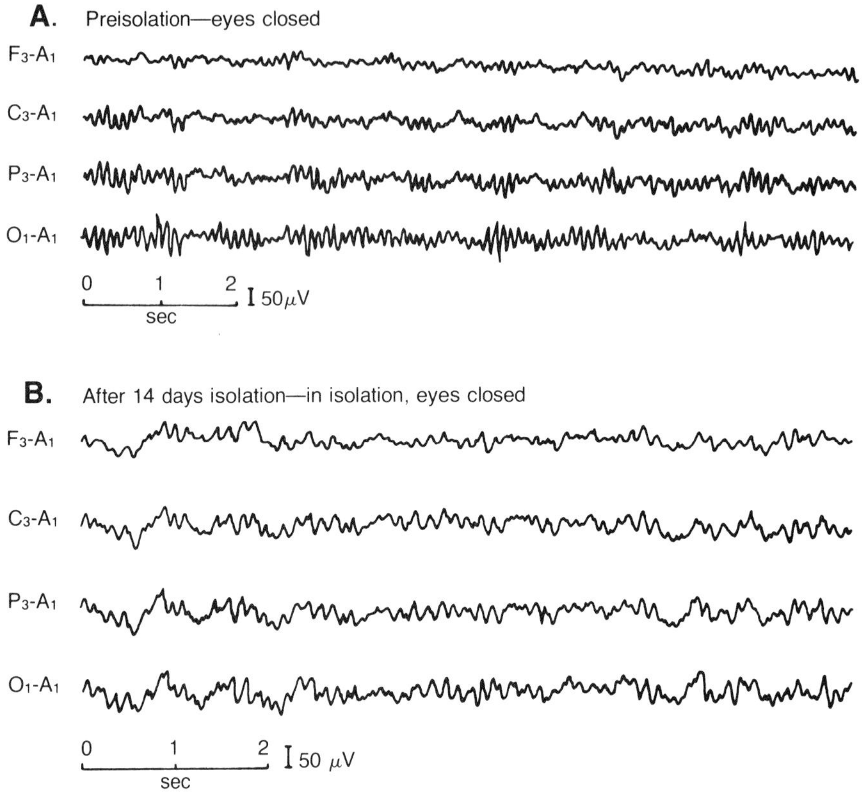

FIG. 20-11. The EEG of a normal volunteer before **(A)** and after **(B)** 14 days of complete isolation in an experimental isolation chamber. Note increase in slow activity. (Saunders MG: Am J EEG Technol 8:41–57, 1968)

FIG. 20-12. A projection of the head demonstrating the standard positions of the International Federation ten-twenty electrode placement system. (Curtis BA, Jacobson S, Marcus EM: An Introduction to the Neurosciences. Philadelphia, WB Saunders, 1972)

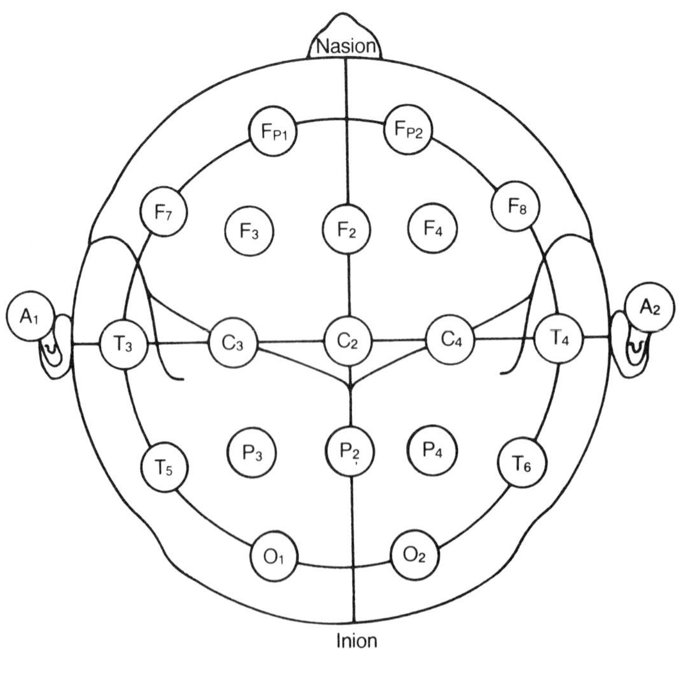

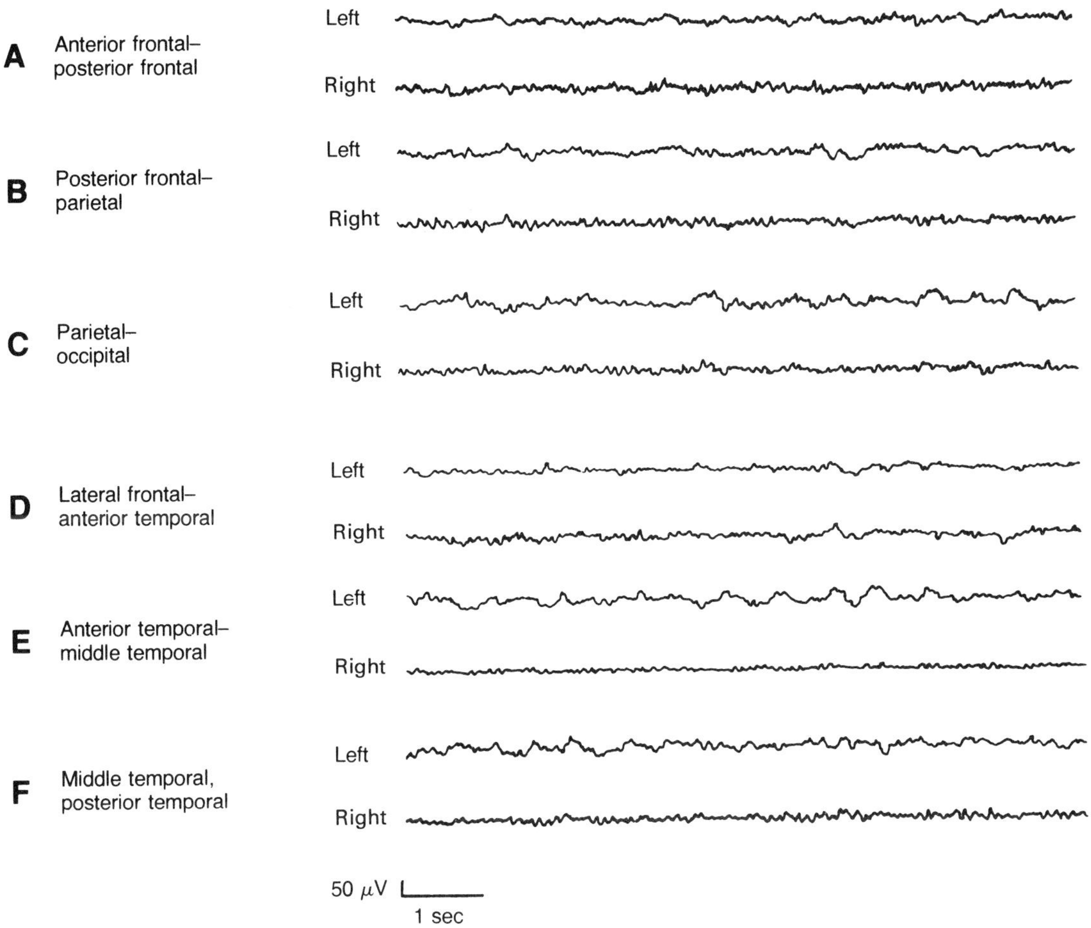

FIG. 20-13. Focal 2- to 5-Hz slow activity in the left temporal-parietal area. This record is from a 42-year-old patient 3 months after a partial resection of a glioma arising in the middle-posterior temporal and posterior parietal area. (Curtis BA, Jacobson S, Marcus EM: An Introduction to the Neurosciences. Philadelphia, WB Saunders, 1972)

20-12. The advantage of bipolar recording is that activity can be sampled from two sites in the brain at the same time. The disadvantage of bipolar recording is that from that single record it is impossible to tell which of the sites is the source of any pathologic signs. EEG electrodes are normally disk or cup-shaped pieces of metal 5 to 10 mm in diameter. The electrodes are normally coated with a conducting paste and then taped in place (to ensure good contact with the scalp). The whole procedure is painless, and many patients find it a pleasant and interesting experience. A physician should tell the patient what to expect *before* he orders an EEG. Far too many people make life rough for the encephalographer (and the patient) simply because of the anxiety that can accompany ignorance.

Abnormal activity is localized by comparing EEG activity from a pair of electrodes on one side of the head with the activity from the corresponding pair on the opposite side of the head. Figure 20-13 shows typical EEG traces as the neurologist would see them. The upper trace in A was made from a pair of electrodes on the left side of the head, one electrode over the anterior frontal cortex (for example position F_{P1} of Fig. 20-12) and the other over the posterior frontal cortex (for example position F_3 of Fig. 20-12). The lower trace is from the corresponding electrode positions on the right side of the head (F_{P2} vs. F_4). The second pair of traces (B) was made over the posterior frontal and parietal cortices (positions F_3 and P_3 of Fig. 20-12), and so on. Now look for differences between left and right in each pair of traces.

TABLE 20-2. THE EPILEPSIES AND THEIR SYMPTOMS

EPILEPSY	SYMPTOMS
Psychomotor (temporal lobe)	Stereotyped behavior often with emotional outbursts, partially responsive to environment, amnesic to behavior during seizure
Petit mal	Fixed stare, unconsciousness, unresponsiveness, lack of activity
Grand mal	Myoclonus, progressive myoclonus, loss of erect posture, unconsciousness

Notice that activity is slower on the left side than on the right, a sign of abnormal activity on the left. Next, localize the specific site of the lesion by comparing the cortical records from the left side with each other. Notice that in pairs B and C there is slow activity. These two sets of recordings have in common an electrode in parietal cortex; therefore one would conclude that parietal cortex was involved in the lesion, because frontal cortex records in A are normal on the left side. Again, notice that in E and F, involving the middle temporal lobe, there is also some abnormal slow activity. The neurologist would conclude that this patient has some lesion localized in the posterior parietal–middle temporal region. These records were in fact made from a patient who suffered from a glioma, a tumor of the brain tissue, in the predicted region.

Some lesions of the cerebral cortex are termed **epileptogenic,** that is, they produce epileptic attacks. Epilepsy is characterized by paroxysmal disturbances of the functions of the brain that may be manifested in one of three ways as summarized in Table 20-2. In **psychomotor epilepsy,** the seizure often takes the form of a stereotyped behavior such as chewing or tapping the finger, sometimes accompanied by an emotional outburst. These attacks are most often caused by a lesion of the temporal lobe (this is also called **temporal lobe epilepsy),** and the patient normally has no memory of the attacks and may not be aware of any problem. **Petit mal** attacks are characterized by the lack of activity on the part of the patient, who may only stare fixedly. During the attack, there is usually a loss of responsiveness and consciousness, but the patient seldom falls down. The third form of epilepsy, the best known, is the **grand mal** seizure. The patient may have a characteristic preseizure, visual, auditory or other experience called an **aura,** and then suddenly there will be a **myoclonus,** a rhythmic contraction in some part of the body, perhaps the hand. This specific myoclonus may spread to include the whole arm (progressive myoclonus), then become generalized so that the whole body is involved in a generalized seizure. The patient normally collapses and is entirely unconscious during the seizure.

It is possible to distinguish the various forms of epilepsy by studying the EEG, but a discussion of the diagnostic procedure is beyond the scope of this presentation. Suffice it to say that all forms of epilepsy are characterized by the appearance of **spikes** in the EEG. These spikes are much longer in duration (15–80 msec) than the action potential of a single cell, so they are undoubtedly generated by nearly synchronous activ-

FIG. 20-14. Focal spike discharge **(arrows)** from the left temporal area of a 4-year-old boy with focal seizures manifested as psychomotor automatisms and repetitive twitching of the right side of the face and hand. Etiology unknown. (Curtis BA, Jacobson S, Marcus EM: An Introduction to the Neurosciences. Philadelphia, WB Saunders, 1972)

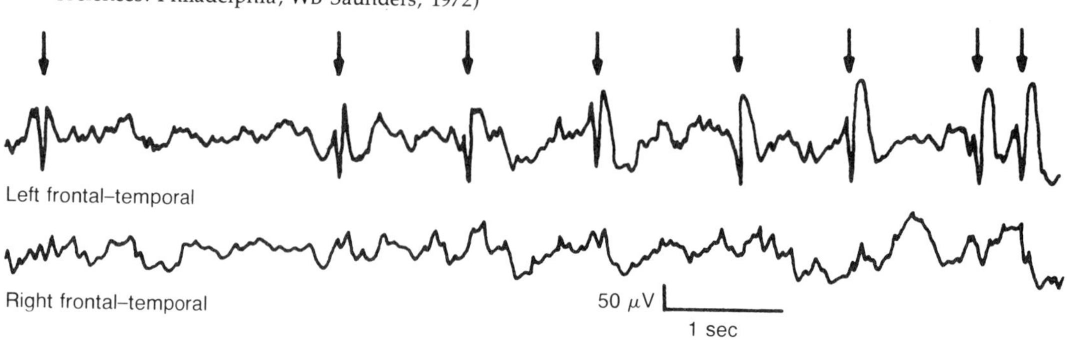

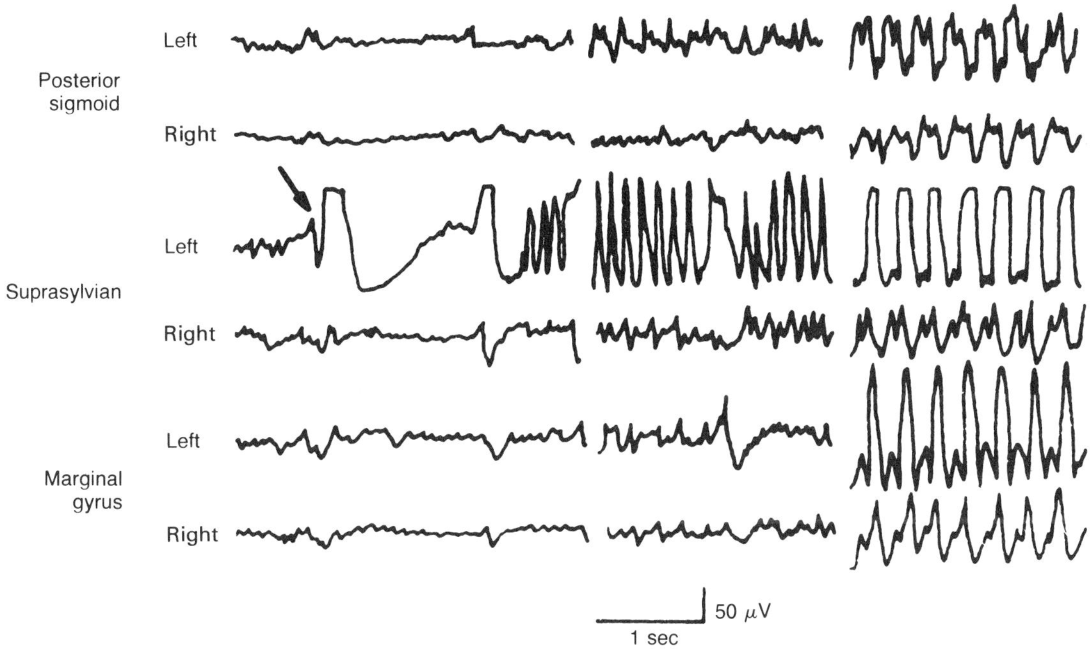

FIG. 20-15. Generalization of a focal spike discharge in records from a cat. Note that discharge begins in the left suprasylvian area and then spreads to somatosensory and visual cortex on both the left and right hemispheres. (Marcus EM, Watson CW, Goldman PL: Arch Neurol 15:521–532, 1966)

ity in a large number of neurons. Recordings in both humans and animals have shown that these sharp waves are concomitant with high-frequency, abnormal bursts in cerebral cortical neurons. Figure 20-14 shows records from the temporal cortex of a patient with a psychomotor disturbance. Typical spikes are indicated by the arrows. The spikes frequently are followed by longer duration waves (Figs. 20-14 and 20-15); together the spike and longer wave are referred to as the **spike and dome complex.** Spikes are a good indicator of a pathologic condition, but sometimes a patient may be monitored for many hours and still no spikes appear. This is especially true in mild psychomotor disturbances. The detection of spikes can be accomplished without reading miles of chart paper by recording the EEG activity on a tape recorder at a slow speed and then playing it back at high speed. Spikes are readily detected by listening for clicks in a speeded up record. When one is located, that section of tape is printed for permanent record. This way, many hours of records can be scanned in just a few minutes. However, it is not always possible to find spikes even when the abnormal behavior is present.

In the EEG record, it is sometimes possible to see the development of generalized seizures. The seizure typically starts with abnormal activity in the particular area of the cortex where the lesion is located. In Figure 20-15, notice that the spike, indicating abnormal discharge, first appears in the left suprasylvian area, at the arrow, grows in amplitude and frequency, and then begins to spread to the other recording sites. This spread of the paroxysmal discharge is correlated with the spread of the muscle contractions (progressive myoclonus). Presumably, the seizure spreads across the body as the abnormal discharges spread across the sensorimotor cortex. By paying attention to the first movement, it is often possible to predict where the lesion is located by virtue of the somatotopic or topographic organization of the cortex. It can be simply a matter of looking up the site of the first movement on a topographic map of the cortex. Often, the preseizure aura also gives a clue; for example, visual auras are often associated with lesions of visual cortex.

The EEG is used to determine whether a person who appears comatose is dead or alive. At present, one of the legal requirements for determining clinical death is the

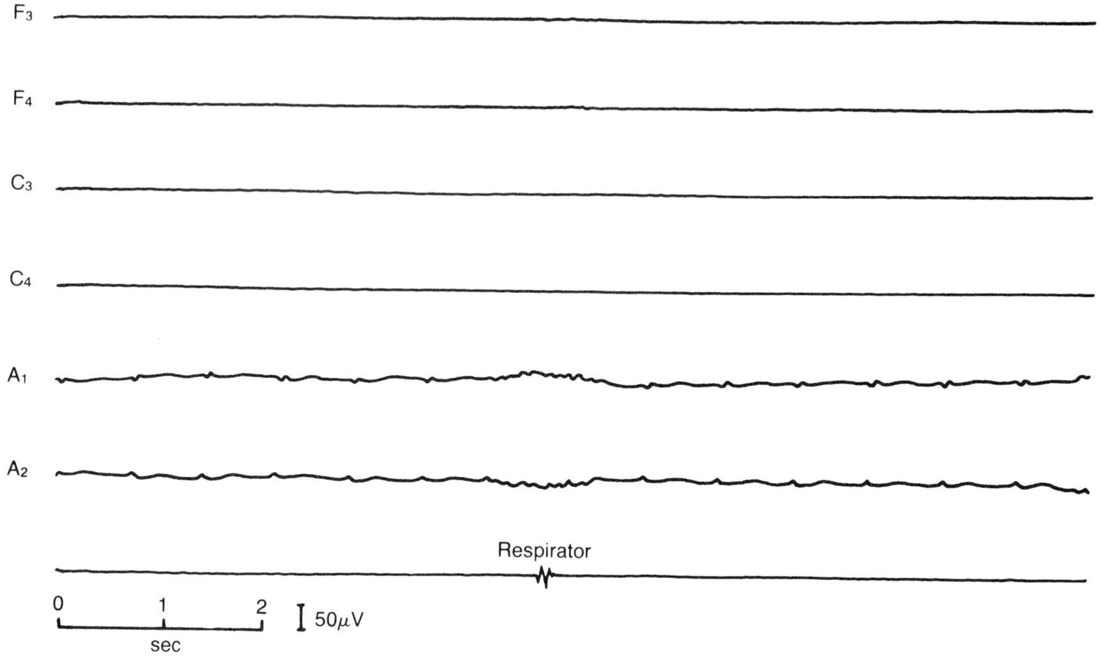

FIG. 20-16. The isoelectric or flat EEG. A clinical sign of death in some specific situations. (Saunders MG: Am J EEG Technol 8:41–57, 1968)

absence of electrical activity in the cerebral cortex—the EEG is flat. Figure 20-16 shows an example of an isoelectric or flat EEG. An artifact, due to heart beat, is easily seen in records taken from leads A_1 and A_2, on the ears, with respect to ground. Small artifacts, due to artificial respiration, can be seen on almost all traces. Otherwise, there is no activity at all. There may soon be a change in this legal definition, because there have been several patients with flat EEGs who have not only survived but survived without symptoms of brain damage. Defining death is a thorny clinical, legal, and ethical problem that will not be easily solved.

SUGGESTED READING

Andersen P, Anderson SA: Physiological Basis of the Alpha Rhythm. New York, Appleton-Century-Crofts, 1968

Kooi KA, Tucker RP, Marshall RE: Fundamentals of Electroencephalography, 2nd ed. Hagerstown, MD, Harper and Row, 1978

Kooi KA, Marshall RE: Visual Evoked Potentials in Central Disorders of the Visual System. Hagerstown, MD, Harper and Row, 1979

21

Activities Involving the Cerebral Hemispheres

In this chapter, we consider some of the other functions of the part of the nervous system above the spinal cord. We deal with functions that are thought to be uniquely human and functions known to be shared with other animals. As time progresses, there appear to be fewer capacities in the former category and more in the latter; recent work with language capacities of gorillas and chimpanzees are cases in point. These are the capacities of the human organism about which we want to know most, but unfortunately they are the capacities about which we can say least. One usually leaves discussions of consciousness, emotion, and learning with a sense of incompleteness and dissatisfaction because we understand so little about these phenomena. Yet, some of the experiments have yielded results that everyone finds fascinating. We normally assume that these are functions of the cerebral cortex, but the cerebral cortex does nothing by itself and, as we shall see, many subcortical structures cooperate in producing these behaviors.

CONSCIOUSNESS

The term consciousness is frequently used, but a satisfactory definition is difficult to find. It has something to do with an awareness of one's self and of the environment, and it seems to have two aspects: arousal state and content. The arousal state concerns whether the person is awake or asleep or stuporous or comatose; these are states that we can usually distinguish by the nature of the EEG record, as we saw in Chapter 20. We also distinguish between the contents of consciousness—how the person behaves, whether he perceives his environment, and whether he learns and remembers.

The state of arousal of an individual is determined not by his cerebral cortex, but by some lower centers, including the reticular formation of the brain stem. There is no lesion, experimental, clinical, or accidental, involving only the cerebral cortex, that produces unconsciousness in man; yet very small vascular lesions of the brain stem can produce coma. Brain-stem transections at or below the midpontine level produce animals that show regular periods of wakefulness as determined by the EEG pattern; higher lesions do not. It is known that a lesion of the median raphe nuclei of the brain stem produces permanent insomnia that is relieved by administration of serotonin. A lesion of the mesencephalic tegmentum, on the other hand, produces an animal that is never awake. Stimulation nearly anywhere in the central gray core, including the periaqueductal gray matter and mesencephalic tegmentum, will awaken a naturally sleeping animal. The region from which this kind of arousal is produced is called the **ascending reticular activating system** and extends throughout the reticular areas of the medulla and pons and upward into the hypothalamus, subthalamus, and ventromedial thalamus.

The arousal evoked by stimulation in the reticular activating system includes both behavioral effects and desynchronization of the EEG. Even animals made permanently asleep by transections of the neuraxis at midbrain or low diencephalic levels can usually be aroused by such stimulation above the transection, but in these animals the arousal does not outlast the stimulus as it does normally. Behavioral arousal and EEG desynchronization usually occur together, but they can be dissociated under appropriate experimental conditions. EEG desynchronization is most easily produced by stimulation in the anterior part of the nucleus reticularis pontis oralis, whereas behavioral arousal is most easily produced by stimulation in the posterior hypothalamus. A lesion in this region of the posterior hypothalamus produces an animal whose EEG becomes desynchronized when its toes are pinched; however, there is no behavioral arousal in such an animal. On the other hand, a lesion in the region of the nucleus reticularis pontis oralis produces an animal that becomes behaviorally aroused by toe pinch, but whose EEG is not desynchronized.

The hypothalamus is also involved in regulating the temporal patterns of sleep. Animals normally have regular daily times of sleep and wakefulness. With certain hypothalamic lesions, an animal will still sleep and is awake for about the same total number of hours per day, but the pattern is one of abnormally short periods of sleep, seemingly distributed at random throughout the day.

The system for controlling arousal state is by no means simple or well understood. It certainly involves brain stem, hypothalamic, and posterior diencephalic structures and possibly also some parts of the prefrontal cortex. It involves connections between these areas that produce behavioral and EEG arousal as well as sleep. We have already seen that a lesion of median raphe nuclei removes the ability to sleep. A lesion of the rostral hypothalamus results in a hyperactive animal that is constantly awake, whereas stimulation in this area puts an awake animal to sleep. Whether these waking and sleeping centers exert their effects by inhibiting each other or by a direct effect on cerebral cortex and the behavioral arousal mechanism or both is unknown. What is known about the content of consciousness is discussed in the next sections.

EMOTIONAL BEHAVIOR

Emotion is another of the behaviors for which there is really no satisfactory definition. It has both unobservable internal and observable external aspects. It is a cognitive process in that one must perceive the causative situation and evaluate it in light of past experience and cultural variables. For example, a particular situation can be potentially beneficial or deleterious to one's self, family, or country. The person may not even be aware that the evaluation is occurring. Emotion is either pleasant or unpleasant and need not be the same to every individual. It is expressed outwardly in the form of facial expressions, gestures, vocalizations, body postures, and other movements or it may be expressed in the form of an absence of movement. There may be concomitant autonomic activity resulting in changes in heart rate, blood pressure, piloerection, sweating, and flushing. Movements of emotion can propel the individual toward another object, as in attacks, or away, as in flight. Finally, emotional behavior can result in excitement and alertness or depression, dullness, and sluggishness.

The initiation and regulation of emotional behavior by the brain is thought to involve the limbic system. Knowledge of the limbic system is quite old; it was named by the surgeon, Broca, in the last century. Actually, little research was done to link the limbic system with emotion until about 1937 when the neuroanatomist, Papez, published a proposed mechanism of emotion involving the limbic system. Figure 21-1 is a summary diagram of most of the parts of the limbic system and their interconnections. The word limbic means "in a form of a ring." The system is given this name because the various parts are organized into rings of interconnected structures. The major parts of the limbic system are as follows: (1) structures of the temporal lobe of the cortex: the amygdala, hippocampus, and parahippocampal cortex; (2) other cortical structures: the orbital and cingulate cortices; (3) anterior and dorsomedial thalamic nuclei; (4) the hypothalamic structures: the hypothalamus proper, septum, and preoptic area; (5) the mammillary bodies; (6) the habenula; (7) the interpeduncular nuclei; and perhaps others. The limbic system re-

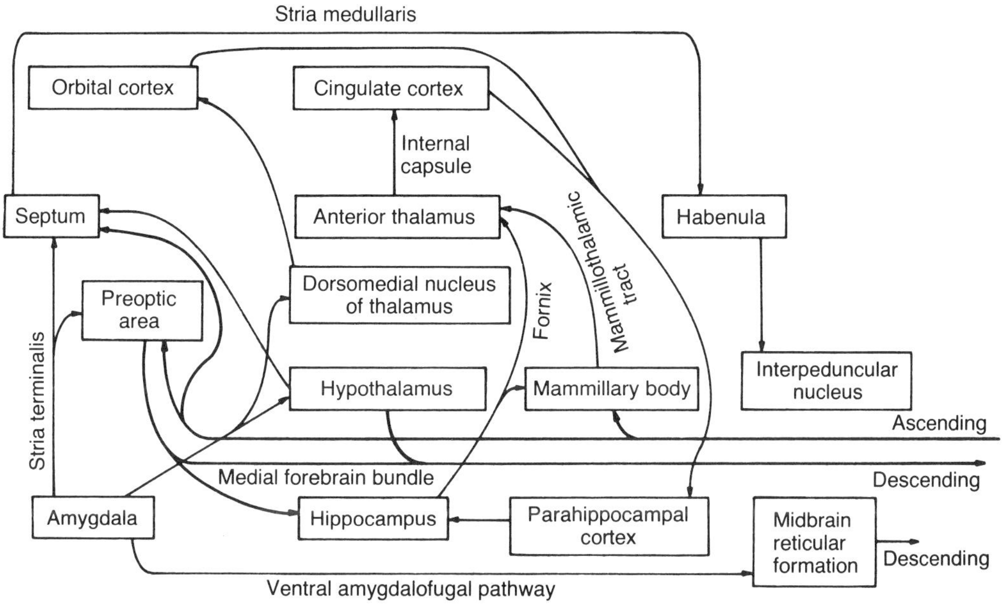

FIG. 21-1. Interconnections between structures of the limbic system.

ceives input from enteroceptors and exteroceptors. It is intimately related to the olfactory system, and it also receives input from every sensory modality. It sends its output to various autonomic nuclei in the brain stem and, through the hypothalamus, influences every part of the body through release of hormones from the pituitary gland.

It has already been noted that removal of structures of the hemisphere above the mammillary bodies results in sham rage, a rage that is typical of normal aggressive behavior except in its lack of direction toward the offending object. The rage is most intense if the lesion is made immediately above the mammillary bodies, less if the hypothalamus is spared, and least if only the neocortex is removed. If a lesion is made in the ventromedial hypothalamic nuclei, a similar rage results but, unlike sham rage, the attacks are well directed. Similarly, a lesion in the septal area makes a normally placid animal savage. Interestingly, a subsequent lesion of the amygdala makes the animal tame again. Bilateral removal of the amygdala without a concomitant septal lesion leads to decreased aggressive behavior in normally savage animals.

Stimulation in the ventromedial and other areas of the hypothalamus elicits aggressive or attack behavior or what appears to be stalking and prey-killing behavior in animals that begins when the stimulus is turned on and ends when it is turned off. Aggressive behavior is also elicited by stimulation in the amygdala, but, unlike that due to hypothalamic stimulation, it develops more slowly and outlasts the stimulus by some period of time. In addition to aggressive behavior, amygdalar stimulation also leads to cessation of movements, changes in spinal reflex activity, controversive head and eye movements, swallowing, licking, chewing, changes in heart and respiration rates, changes in gastrointestinal motility, micturition, defecation, pupillary dilation, and piloerection. These changes are all characteristic of emotional responses, though not necessarily of aggressive behavior. In humans, stimulation of the amygdala leads to sensations of fear, disturbances of mood, a sense of unreality, and distortions of bodily perceptions.

Bilateral removal of the temporal lobe leads to a constellation of effects that are called the **Klüver-Bucy syndrome.** The symptoms include the following:

1. Visual agnosia—inability to recognize seen objects
2. Compulsive exploratory behavior—everything is examined with the mouth or by smell

3. Passivity, unresponsiveness, and decreased emotional responsiveness
4. Lack of fear
5. Intensification of sexual activity—increased frequency and directed toward the same sex or even different species
6. Changes in dietary patterns

Attempts have been made to localize the structures whose removal produced each of these symptoms. There has been little success in such efforts.

Stimulation in the region of the medial forebrain bundle or the preoptic area produces a sensation described as pleasurable by humans. Apparently, animals also find it pleasurable because they will press a lever in order to receive an electrical stimulus in this area, some people call the pleasure center. They will elect to press the lever and receive the shock rather than eat when they are hungry, drink when they are thirsty, or engage in sexual activity with a receptive female. In fact, rats will cross an electrified grid that they normally would not cross, in order to press the lever and receive the shock. Obviously, the sensation is a powerful one in influencing behavior.

It is probable that the hypothalamus cannot, by itself, initiate directed emotional behavior, but requires the modulating, directing, and regulating influence of the rest of the limbic system. As we have seen, stimulation of various parts of the limbic system can activate all of the autonomic and behavioral concomitants of emotional behavior, but as yet we do not know how or where the behavior is initiated or what parts of the system play what roles in what behaviors. It is clear that the limbic system plays an important role in emotional behavior.

LEARNING AND MEMORY

Learning is usually defined as a relatively permanent change in behavior as a result of practice or experience. There is a vast psychologic literature dealing with the kinds of learning and their characteristics, which we will not attempt to go into here. Animals can learn certain responses to stimuli just by associating the stimuli with other stimuli that normally elicit the desired response (classical conditioning). For example, if an animal is presented with a puff of air directed at the eye, it blinks. Repeated pairings of a brief light flash or tone and a puff of air effect some change in the nervous system such that the light flash or tone, by itself, evokes the blink. Another kind of learning is called instrumental or operant conditioning. In instrumental conditioning, an animal must perform some task in order to get a reward or avoid punishment. Thus, an animal will learn new behaviors in order to get a reward or relief from pain. This phenomenon is familiar to every animal trainer. We now know that animals will learn complex behavior patterns in order to receive electrical stimulation in parts of the hypothalamus, particularly the preoptic area, the pleasure center.

Some theorists claim that human learning can be explained in terms of classical and instrumental conditioning, whereas others maintain that there is something more, something unique about human learning ability. This something, if it exists, has yet to be identified. Much of what we know about learning has been obtained from animals, raising the question of the applicability of the results to humans. It has already been noted that humans may differ even from monkeys in the indispensibility of the cerebral cortex in sensory functions, so it should be cautioned that there may be profound differences between man and animals, even in elementary learning processes. Because animal evidence is all that is available in many cases, we will treat it as if it also applied to humans.

In general, the following principles seem to emerge from studies on learning:

1. Ablation of the cerebral cortex has no effect on classical conditioning. The results of early studies were taken to indicate that classical conditioning could not occur in the absence of cerebral cortex; we now know this is untrue. Classical conditioning can be demonstrated in a part of the spinal cord isolated by transection, indicating that even the spinal cord is capable of this sort of learning.

2. If the task to be learned requires a sensory capacity that is abolished by a lesion in the cerebral cortex, then no amount of training is successful in teaching the task. For example, some visual discrimination learning requires a visual capacity that is abolished by a lesion of the visual cortex. Visual

discrimination learning of this kind is impossible following such a lesion. (However, recent evidence suggests this point may have to be reexamined. Look back at Chapter 7.)

3. Retention is impaired, but retraining is possible for instrumental conditioning if lesions (that do not abolish a needed sensory capacity) are made in primary cortical sensory areas. For example, the primary somesthetic area is not required for somesthesia, and somatic discrimination learning is possible following a lesion to this area. On the other hand, it is known that parietal lobe lesions (not necessarily restricted to the primary somesthetic area) interfere with the ability of humans to discriminate the shape of objects either by manipulating them (astereognosis) or by viewing them. Attempts to retrain this ability have failed.

4. If a number of sensory modalities are involved in the learning process, then a bigger cortical lesion is needed to interfere with learning than if a single modality is involved. In fact, the amount of impairment is a function of the amount of cortical tissue removed and is independent (to some extent) of where on the hemisphere it is removed. This has been termed the law of mass action. This would follow whether learning were a localized function or were distributed across the surface of the cortex.

5. Lesions that involve both primary sensory cortex and association cortex of one modality may cause considerable, lasting impairment of learning in that modality (a notable exception is the modality of smell).

6. The temporal pole and the junction between temporal and occipital cortices seem to be important for learning visual discrimination tasks.

7. Prefrontal cortex seems to be involved in learning ordered responses where time is a critical feature. This is seen most readily in delayed response learning, where the person or animal is required to delay a response until some time after the cues are presented. Monkeys with prefrontal lesions can find a raisin they have seen placed in a covered well if they are allowed to do so within a short time, but they cannot if they are required to wait more than a few minutes. This is an easy task for normal monkeys.

8. When learning involves the cortex on one side only (*e.g.*, when cues are presented in only half of the visual field), the corpus callosum participates in transfer to the other cortex, at least for some learned responses. If the optic chiasm is transected midsagittally, the image from each eye is transmitted only to the ipsilateral hemisphere. After such a lesion, an animal can perform a visual discrimination task learned with one eye covered, using either eye to sense the objects. If a transection of the corpus callosum is done with the transection of the optic chiasm, then the task can be performed only with the eye uncovered during training. The other eye can be used to *relearn* the task. Apparently, the learning normally occurs bilaterally by way of the corpus callosum.

With instrumental conditioning, animals can change the behavior of neurons in the same way they change their overt behavior. These changes in the discharges of neurons, as a result of conditioning, could be brought about by making or changing some overt movement or behavior. We know that neurons in the CNS are responsive to sensory input from the periphery, sometimes evokable by an appropriate movement. A neuron, responsive to stimulation of a particular area of skin, may discharge if the animal brings the area into contact with some object, even its own body. In fact, in some of these conditioning experiments, movements or changes in movements have been observed concomitant with changes in neural activity. Clearly, the animal could be stimulating itself. It is also conceivable that a neuron's discharge could be altered by itself, that is, in isolation from any movement or sensation. Evidence suggests that this actually does not happen (Wyler, Burchiel, Robbins, 1979). Work is in progress to find some way to use this control over nerve cells to run prosthetic devices for lost limbs. As yet, the work has just begun.

Attempts have been made to record both evoked potentials and discharges of single cells or small groups of cells during training of animals in order to find neural concomitants of learning. There are changes in evoked potentials that occur while an animal is learning a particular task. Unfortunately, these changes are difficult to interpret for several reasons. It is not known what events (postsynaptic potentials) are responsible for producing the various parts (positive and negative deflections) of the evoked potential, if, indeed, a single event is responsible for each part. Because the evoked potential reflects activity in all neurons neighboring the recording electrodes, we cannot say with certainty which neurons we are studying. Learning has been defined as a change in behavior; usually this means a change in movement. We cannot, as yet, separate the neural events, parts of an evoked potential, that are associated simply with the production of a movement from those associated with the learning process itself.

Interpretations of single-cell recordings during learning are even more difficult. The problem of separating changes due to motor activity from changes due to learning itself is also inherent in single-cell recordings. In addition, we cannot follow the behavior of a single cell long enough to observe it both before and after learning has occurred, and, even if we could, we could not be sure it was, in fact, the same neuron. The neurons that are near the recording electrode after learning has occurred may behave differently either because they have "learned" or because they are different neurons.

Memory is the ability to recall events or tasks learned or experienced minutes, days, or years before. It is customary to divide memory into two types, **immediate recall** or **short-term memory** and **long-term memory.** Short-term memory usually has a duration of minutes to perhaps hours, whereas long-term memory has a duration from minutes (or hours) to years. It is not possible to say precisely when a given memory crosses the border from short-term into long-term memory or even if short- and long-term memory involve the same continuous process or two different processes.

Animals given electroconvulsive shocks or other treatments to interrupt brain activity within about 5 minutes after a training session do not remember the task they were trained to perform when tested some time later. When no treatment is given, the same animals remember the task 5 minutes and even weeks after the training sessions. If the same treatment is given to the animal 4 hours after training sessions, it has no effect at all on their ability to remember the task even weeks later. It thus appears that there is a period shortly after an event when the memory is vulnerable to disruption; then something happens to make the memory trace resistant to erasure. It is this event that constitutes the conversion from short-term to long-term memory.

Clinically, it is found that immediately following electroshock therapy or some brain concussions there is no memory of the therapy or the concussion or of events that occurred some time preceding it. In man, this lack of memory or amnesia may encompass longer periods than in animals, sometimes days, weeks, or even years, but more remote memories are usually intact. The patient, under these circumstances, is still capable of forming new long-term memories, but there are conditions where this ability is also impaired.

The **amnesic syndrome,** or Korsakoff's psychosis, is an impairment of the ability to convert short-term memory into long-term memory, without impairment of immediate recall and without elimination of already formed long-term memories, and it results from bilateral damage to the hippocampal formation of the temporal lobes. Some pathology is usually also found in the mammillary bodies, a major projection site of the hippocampus. The uncus, parahippocampal cortex, mammillary bodies, and amygdala do not seem to play a role in this syndrome, nor do bilateral lesions of the fornix, the output pathway from the hippocampus, produce impairment of memory. The patient can recall bits of information for minutes (immediate recall), but if he is distracted these are lost. He can also recall events that happened prior to the damage to his brain (long-term memory).

The amnesic syndrome can sometimes result from thiamine deficiency or bilateral occlusion of the posterior cerebral arteries that supply the hippocampus. It also results from surgical removal of one temporal lobe (temporal lobectomy) when the other has been damaged. Temporal lobectomy without prior damage to the other hippocampus does not produce any memory impairment. General symptoms of the amnesic syndrome are indicated in the following case history:

> A 29-year-old patient had been incapacitated by intractable seizures since the age of 16. As a treatment, the mesial surfaces of both temporal lobes were resected to about 8 cm posterior of temporal

pole. Following this surgery, the patient no longer experienced seizures, but he also no longer recognized the hospital staff nor could he find his way around the hospital. He seemed not to be able to recall the day-to-day events of his hospital stay. He did not recall the death of his favorite uncle three years earlier, but could recall some trivial events just before his admission to the hospital. His earliest memories were clear and vivid. Even after three years, this patient was unable to remember a new address (though he remembered the old one) or where he had put objects he habitually used. There was no decrease in his IQ, in fact, there was a slight increase. His understanding and reasoning were normal, as were psychologic test results for perception, abstract thinking, motivation, and personality. He could retain a three-digit number or a pair of unrelated words for several minutes; if he was distracted they were immediately forgotten. (Scoville and Milner, 1957)

The memory storage process apparently depends upon the integrity of the hippocampus, but we know little about the location of long-term storage of information. Some cases of temporal lobe epilepsy exhibit seizures preceded by auras consisting of memories of past events. Typically, the same past event is played back to the patient just prior to each seizure, serving as a signal that the seizure is impending. During surgery to excise the **focus** (the pathologic cortical area responsible for the seizure), the cortical surface of the temporal lobe is stimulated electrically to locate the site of the focus. When the site is located and stimulated, the memory of the aura is played back again to the patient in an interesting way. When the stimulating current is turned on, the memory begins to be recalled by the patient and the events in the memory continue in sequence, as they originally happened, until the current is switched off. If, after a moment, the stimulus is turned on again, the memory is picked up again where it left off before. It is as if a tape recorder were being turned on and off. Removal of the focus abolishes the seizures with their auras, but does not eliminate the memory that was part of the aura. It is unknown whether the memories remain because of bilateral storage at conjugate sites (the site of the focus and the same site on the contralateral hemisphere) or whether the memories are actually stored elsewhere. No single site for storage of memory traces has yet been found in the central nervous system.

The nature of the storage process is as much a mystery as its location. It is clear that long-term memory is not a result of activity in reverberating circuits (circuits in which activity is transmitted continuously around a closed loop pathway), but short-term memory may be. Electroconvulsive shock, deep coma due to overdoses of sedative drugs, and complete cessation of electrical activity, all of which would stop reverberation, do not interfere with already formed long-term memories, but they do destroy short-term memories and disrupt their conversion to long-term memories. Many claims have been made about the involvement of specific, single ribonucleic acids (RNA) or other specific proteins in memory, but in general the claims remain unsubstantiated. It is noteworthy that drugs that block protein synthesis will also block transformation of short-term into long-term memory. Also, a variety of CNS stimulants have been shown to improve learning in animals and restore learned behaviors that have been lost as a result of CNS lesions. The process must certainly involve biochemical changes in cells, perhaps in formation of new or more permanent or more effective synaptic junctions.

PERSONALITY

It has been known for over 100 years that the prefrontal lobes are involved in determining and regulating personality. Seizures brought on by abnormalities of the prefrontal lobes often involve transient changes in personality, with compulsive behavior and the release of social inhibitions that may persist for several weeks following the seizures. Bilateral removal of the prefrontal lobes results in a reduction in emotional responsiveness and anxiety, but no change in perception. For example, patients with prefrontal lobotomies still report feeling pain, but they say it no longer bothers them. The patients become impulsive and distractable; they lack concern over the consequences of their actions, and they are unable to plan ahead. Following lobotomy, a man urinated in the corner of the room. When told not to repeat this action, he agreed, but shortly was back in the corner again. A woman, who had planned and prepared meals for her family for many years, was unable to do so following a lobotomy, although she was able to perform the individual activities involved when told what to do next.

Prefrontal lobotomy patients sometimes have difficulty postponing gratification. Although they are distractable, they show a tendency to persevere in activities and seem unable to shift their responses to suit a change in environment or circumstance. Their thinking often becomes rigid and concrete with some deficits in abstract reasoning. These symptoms are illustrated in the following case history:

> A 60-year-old housewife and fashion designer was admitted to the hospital with a history of several years of fatigue, loss of ambition, lack of enthusiasm, and a tendency to cry readily over minor problems. A depression of mood and a tendency toward introspection had also developed. She also reported loss of appetite and weight. Neurologic examination was normal except for slowness of speech and thought processes. Thyroid function tests indicated hypothyroidism, for which she was treated and released.
>
> After discharge, the emotional and personality symptoms continued and worsened. She also developed difficulty in walking, unsteadiness of gait, difficulty climbing stairs, and getting out of chairs. Her motor and mental activities became slower and she procrastinated in making decisions. There was a progressive deficit in memory and episodic blurring or fogging of vision.
>
> At age 67, she was readmitted to the hospital with slowness of speech and gait, slight disorientation for date and year, exaggerated deep tendon reflexes, and no significant sensory findings, except a slight decrease in position sense of the toes. Shortly, she developed headaches, vomiting, increasing somnolence, a Babinski sign, and sluggish pupil responses. Cerebrospinal fluid pressure was elevated, as was fluid protein. Bilateral carotid arteriogram revealed a butterfly-shaped meningioma in the anterior cranial fossa that was removed. Histologic examination indicated that the tumor was benign. The patient showed immediate improvement at the conclusion of surgery. Pupils were equal in size and reactive to light. Two months later she could recognize the doctor by name, but did not know the place or time. Assistance was still required when walking. There was also some impairment of recent memory. The development of symptoms indicated an involvement of prefrontal lobes by the tumor, compressing them and producing alterations of mood and personality. Continued growth of the tumor compromised premotor and perhaps motor areas resulting in disturbance of gait, possibly due to compression of the anterior cerebral arteries, and later possibly also the temporal lobes were compromised, resulting in memory loss. (Curtis, Jacobson, Marcus, 1972)

In the 1940s and 1950s prefrontal lobotomies were frequently performed in mental institutions and prisons on patients whose behavior was considered undesirable and intractable. The procedure made them docile and carefree, but the alterations in their personalities were severe. At one point, it became so fashionable to have a lobotomy performed that it actually became an office procedure. Only a small incision in the orbit above the eye is required. Some physicians did as many as 1000 **leukotomies** per month during one period. Fortunately, anxiety and intractable behaviors are now controllable on a temporary basis by the use of tranquilizers, and lobotomies are seldom performed. Some states allow them only in cases of uncontrollable, incapacitating anxiety or fear or for relief of the suffering from pain in terminal illness, where it has been shown to a review board that the patient is unresponsive to any other form of treatment.

SPEECH AND OTHER UNILATERAL FUNCTIONS

Thus far, everything that has been said about the nervous system applies equally to both sides, that is, the nervous system is

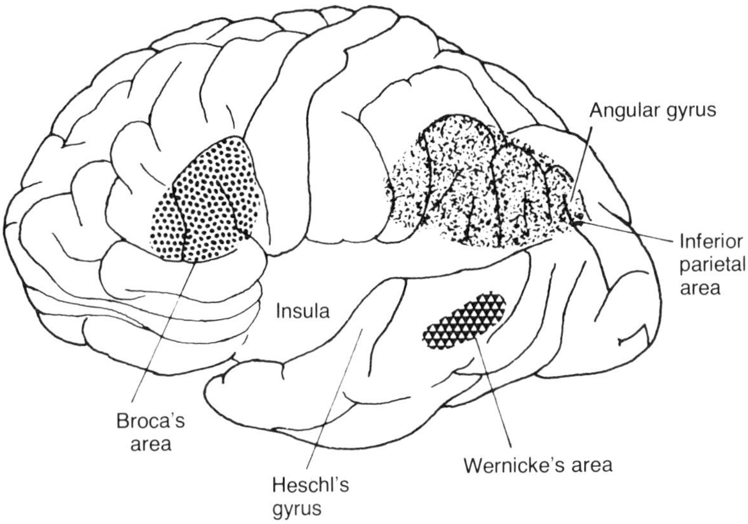

FIG. 21-2. A drawing of the lateral aspect of the dominant hemisphere of the human brain showing the approximate locations of Broca's, Wernicke's, and the inferior parietal speech areas. Note that the temporal lobe has been pulled out, exposing the insula beneath. (Geschwind N: Sci Am 226(4):76–83, 1972)

bilaterally symmetric. However, there are some cortical functions that are not served equally by both hemispheres. In one cerebral hemisphere, there is a region, called **Broca's area,** that is involved in speech (Fig. 21-2). Broca's area (areas 44 and 45) is located in the frontal cortex just anterior to the face area of the precentral gyrus. Actually, there are two additional areas of the same hemisphere that are involved with speech. These are the inferior parietal lobule, consisting of the angular and supramarginal gyri (areas 39 and 40), and **Wernicke's area** (area 22), located on the posterior aspect of the superior temporal gyrus just behind the auditory cortex. The location of these three areas is seen in Figure 21-2. These areas are found in only one hemisphere, and their presence *defines* the **dominant hemisphere.** The dominant hemisphere is usually the one opposite the favored hand (in most individuals, the left hemisphere), but, in a few cases, it is the hemisphere on the same side as the favored hand (92% of right-handed people are left hemisphere dominant, 50%–60% of left-handed people are left hemisphere dominant).

Electrical stimulation during neurosurgery in any of these three areas leads to arrest of speech, hesitation or slurring of speech, distortion, repetition, inability to name, misnaming, and vocalization. Vocalization can also be elicited from the motor cortex where it always takes the form of a sustained or interrupted cry.

Various types of speech disorders result from damage to the speech areas. The general term for these disorders is **aphasia.** Lesions involving Broca's area and adjacent cortex produce a **motor** or **expressive aphasia,** in which the patient does not or cannot speak. What words are used are uttered slowly and with great effort. Usually, difficulties also show up in writing words. In expressive aphasia, it appears that the patient has lost his motor programs for making correct and properly timed sequences of movements of lips and tongue although he apparently still knows what to say. A lesion of Wernicke's area or the inferior parietal lobule produces a **receptive aphasia** in which the patient cannot understand spoken language or written language **(alexia),** but is capable of spontaneous speech. Many times, lesions of the inferior parietal lobes of the dominant hemisphere also produce what is known as Gerstmann's syndrome. This syndrome may include one or more of the following symptoms: **dysgraphia,** a deficit in writing without motor or sensory deficits in the upper extremities; **dyscalculia,** a deficit in the performance of calculations; **left–right confusion;** and **finger agnosia,** errors in finger recognition. It is seldom that aphasias present themselves simply as described above. Usually, a given aphasia is a mixture of expressive and receptive difficulties. A number of classification schemes have been invented, but no one of them can handle all cases. The following case history illustrates aphasia:

> A 19-year-old soldier was struck in the head at the left temple by a piece of shrapnel. He remained conscious and remembered everything that happened. When admitted to the hospital 4 days later, he was speechless. Shortly thereafter he began to make articulate noises that seemed not to be related to words. For instance, he would utter "ho-nus" when asked his name or "ong" when shaking his head in the negative. He could understand and follow simple commands, but was slow to follow two or three consecutive orders (complete inability to follow commands is **apraxia**). As he improved he was able to say the alphabet and days of the week, but pronounced the words and letters poorly. He could write his own name and address, but not that of his mother. He could not count aloud, but could write the numbers up to 21. When asked to write a simple phrase of dictation, he frequently failed to finish the phrase. Seven months after the injury he still had great difficulty in evoking appropriate words during spontaneous speech. Pronunciation was poor; writing was done only with difficulty. Seven years later he still hesitated in searching for appropriate words and showed defective enunciation and influency in writing. (Head, 1926)

The devastating losses in language abilities resulting from even small lesions of speech centers of the dominant hemisphere suggest that a dominant hemispherectomy should abolish language altogether. Surgeons were surprised to find that this procedure does not result in complete aphasia, but in some verbal loss, especially in responses to written commands. Deficits are fewer in writing than in speech and least in responses to verbal commands. Speech abilities are recovered to a great extent over a period of 8 months. Why losses due to hemispherectomy are smaller than predicted is one of the enigmas of neuroscience, yet it should be recalled that the influence of hemispherectomy on movement is also less than expected.

In a few cases of intractable seizures, physicians have elected to section the corpus callosum by itself or in combination with the anterior commissure and the hippocampal commissure in order to stop the spread of the seizures from one hemisphere to the other. In many cases, this procedure has been successful, and it has given the scientist an opportunity to study the abilities of each hemisphere in isolation. The separation of the two hemispheres creates, in some senses, two minds within the same body. The patient, sometimes called a **split-brain patient,** is able to get around well and can do most, if not all, of the things he did before, but some things he does in a subtly different way. For example, in performing tasks that require the cooperation of both hands, the patient is severely impaired. If asked to match a pile of blocks by building a new pile next to it, the patient finds one hand putting a block in place, while the other one takes it away or moves it somewhere else. He can only do the task successfully if he sits on one hand, letting the other one do the work. Split-brain patients show no impairment in intellectual functioning. In fact, in the one case where adequate pre- and postoperative testing was performed, the patient showed improvement in standardized memory tests, short-term memory, and learning rate. Apparently, separating the hemispheres does not disrupt these functions. Why they improved in this one case is a matter of conjecture, and whether this is a consistent result of the surgery awaits further tests.

Sectioning the corpus callosum surgically has some rather interesting effects on sensation in the modalities of somesthesia, audition, and vision. The ability to localize the site of a stimulus to the skin is not impaired in split-brain patients, but if the testing procedure is set up in such a way that each hemisphere is tested separately, then it can be shown that a hemisphere can only localize stimuli on the contralateral body surface. Thermal sensitivity and position sense of a hemisphere are likewise limited to the contralateral side of the body. Complex discriminations of solid shapes with no limit to the number of alternatives are performed only by the contralateral hemisphere, but if the alternatives are easily discriminated (as tested using the contralateral hemisphere) and few in number (*e.g.*, cubes vs. spheres), then the ipsilateral hemisphere can discriminate them as well. By what pathways the sensory information reaches the ipsilateral hemisphere in the split-brain patient is unknown. When the discriminations are learned by one hemisphere only, the other hemisphere shows no indication that it "knows" of the learning, that is, there is no intermanual transfer of tactile discriminations.

There is no loss of auditory sensitivity after the brain is split, and the ability to localize the source of a sound is unimpaired. The patient can also respond properly, using either hand, to a verbal command directed at either ear. He cannot, however, fuse two sounds, one presented to each ear. A normal person, presented with "pro" to the right ear and "duct" to the left ear in quick succession, hears "product." The split-brain patient hears "pro" with the left hemisphere and "duct" with the right. The left hemisphere-dominant patient's verbal report will be "pro" only, but he will write "duct" using his left hand.

Under conditions where the brain has been surgically split, it is possible, provided that the eyes do not move, to direct visual stimuli to each hemisphere independently because of the pattern of crossing of optic nerve fibers in the optic chiasm. Objects in the right visual field are seen by the left hemisphere; those in the left visual field are seen by the right hemisphere; and the macula is *not* represented bilaterally. Following the commissurotomy, objects in the right visual field of a patient with left hemisphere dominant can be correctly named by the patient, those in the left cannot, presumably because of the location of speech areas. On the other hand, a photograph shown to either hemisphere can be correctly pointed out using the contralateral hand. The patient is unable to make same–different discriminations between photographs presented one to each hemisphere.

Split-brain patients have difficulty with **stereopsis** (depth perception) when an object lies immediately in front of or behind the fixation point. This is because the images fall on the retina so that they are transmitted to different hemispheres, and determining whether to converge or diverge the eyes is impossible. In Figure 21-3, the eyes are fixated on point A; the images of points B and C fall on the temporal retinae and nasal retinae, respectively, and therefore are transmitted to both hemispheres. So in the case of either point B or point C, neither hemisphere would have both images to compare, the basis upon which decisions about convergence and divergence are normally made. When both images of an object fall on the retinae so that they are transmitted to the same hemisphere (as in the case of point D in Fig. 21-3), there is no problem.

The question arises whether the nondominant hemisphere has any verbal capabilities at all. To test this, a word was flashed in the opposite visual field, and the patient was asked to pick the word out of a number of others. The nondominant hemisphere can do this, at least for some kinds of words. It has no difficulty in recognizing nouns and adjectives. Apparently, the nondominant hemisphere does have language skills, but these are not manifested normally, because it has no access to the speech apparatus. They are clearly seen, however, if written responses are required.

The nondominant hemisphere appears to be better at visual form perception than the dominant one, at least for complex forms and faces. This is shown by the following tests. Split-brain patients were asked to copy line drawings that suggested spatial perspective, for example, a cube. Performance was consistently better with the left hand than with the right hand despite the fact that all patients were right handed and had little experience drawing with their left hands. Evidence indicates that the left hand receives its major motor control from the right, in these cases, nondominant hemisphere. Assembling complex puzzles is also much easier for these patients when they use their left hands.

This superiority of the nondominant hemisphere for form perception also shows up when no fine motor coordination is required by the test. Two photographs, each of a different face, are cut along the vertical midline of the face. The left half of one face is put together with the right half of the other, forming a composite face. If a split-brain patient fixes his gaze on the junction between the two half-faces, the left half-face is seen by the right hemisphere and the

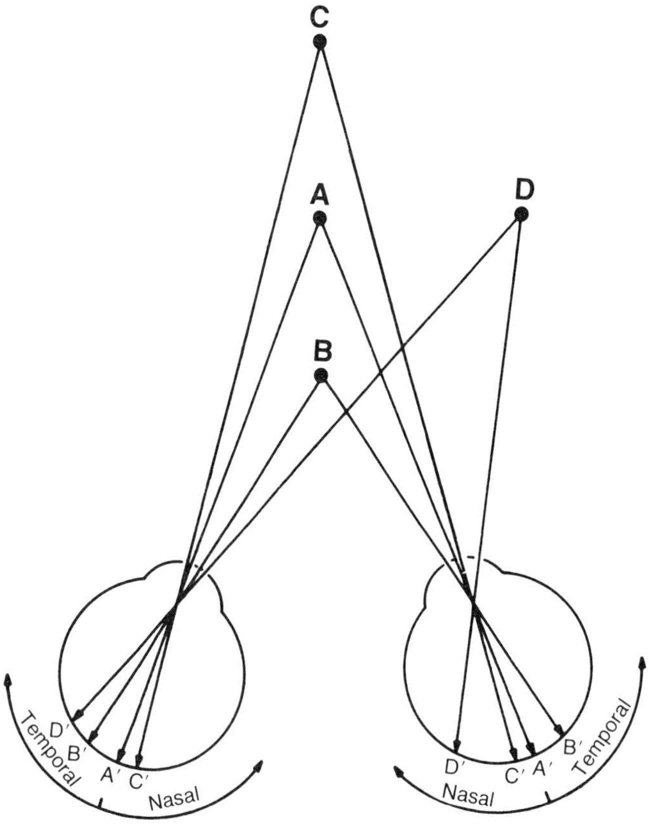

FIG. 21-3. The images of an object immediately in front of **(B)** or behind **(C)** the fixation point **(A)** fall on both temporal retinae **(B′)** or both nasal retinae **(C′)** and therefore are transmitted to different hemispheres. The image of an object anywhere else **(D)** falls on one nasal and one temporal retina **(D′)** and therefore is transmitted to only one hemisphere.

right half-face is seen by the left hemisphere. If the composite face is flashed briefly so that the eyes will not have time to move, then neither hemisphere is aware of the half-face in the ipsilateral visual field. The patient, asked to point out which of the original faces he saw in the brief flash, nearly always selects the one, half of which was seen by the right, nondominant hemisphere; if asked to describe the face he saw, he describes the face, half of which was seen by the dominant hemisphere and never reports seeing two halves of different faces.

In spite of what was earlier said about lesions of the inferior parietal lobe of the dominant hemisphere (Gerstmann's syndrome), the calculating ability of the nondominant hemisphere appears to be superior to that of the dominant one. The test is to give the right and left hemispheres addition and subtraction problems and require an answer to be selected from among several alternatives by pointing, the test not requiring the use of language. Problems can be presented to only one hemisphere at a time by flashing them in only the left or right visual field when the eyes are not moving. The superiority of the nondominant hemisphere, shown in this test in terms of number of correct responses, does not show up in tests requiring verbal responses. This is presumably the reason for the dyscalculia of dominant hemisphere lesions; the ability is normally tested using verbal responses.

The nondominant hemisphere appears to be better at some sorts of tests of creativity involving making associations between concepts, similar to the Miller Analogies Test you may have taken. Still other aspects of creativity seem to be the province of the dominant hemisphere.

Apparently, each hemisphere has a sense of self, recognizing the individual's name and supplying it when requested. Each hemisphere has its own system of subjectively evaluating current events, planning for future events, setting response priorities, and generating personal responses. Both hemispheres are capable of the same emotional responses. A picture of a nude person of the opposite sex evokes the same emotional response whether it is shown to the dominant or nondominant hemisphere of a split-brain patient. The emotional responses and evaluations of people and things by the two hemispheres can also come into opposition with each other. There are reports of a man who shook his wife with the left hand and came to her rescue with the right and of a man who pulled down his pants with one hand and pulled them up with the other.

In split-brain patients, it has been observed that when the two hemispheres agree on evaluations of people and other matters, the patients outwardly appear calm and tractable, but when the two hemispheres disagree, they are outwardly hyperactive, agitated, and aggressive. It would appear that the two hemispheres are also capable of reading differences in each other. In one experiment, words were flashed tachistoscopically to one hemisphere or the other, and the patient, in this case a 15-year-old boy, was asked to "do what the word says." When the word "kiss" was flashed to the right (mute) hemisphere, the patient immediately responded, "Hey, no way, you've got to be kidding." When asked what the word was he responded, "nurse." When "kiss" was flashed to the left (verbal) hemisphere, he responded in the same tone, "No way. I'm not going to kiss you guys." How the verbal hemisphere could read the emotional content of the word in both exposures is unknown, but clearly it did (Gazzaniga, LeDoux, Wilson, 1977).

The dominant hemisphere clearly has the major role in complex motor functions as indicated by the existence of a preferred hand, but the nondominant hemisphere is perfectly capable of controlling its half of the body on its own. There is even some indication of ipsilateral control of muscles other than finger muscles; however, it is not known to what extent this control is the result of cross-cueing, that is, using small compensatory changes in the midline postural muscles as indicators of motor performance, and to what extent there is direct control by sensory feedback to the ipsilateral hemisphere. In some surgical cases, an entire hemisphere has been removed down to the thalamus, and in these cases both sides of the body move about equally well. The two hemispheres do compete with each other in split-brain patients. Such a patient can easily build a simple jigsaw puzzle with either hand, but has great difficulty using both hands, because as one hand puts the pieces in place, the other removes them. Recall that complex puzzles are only constructed with ease by the hand contralateral to the nondominant hemisphere because of its spatial abilities. The two hemispheres normally work together, communicating with each other by way of the commissures, to produce normal behavior, both in terms of movement and sensation and in terms of covert processes like calculating and reasoning. It is only when one hemisphere is not functioning or when the two are functioning independently that we can see that they are not equal.

It is not known how this asymmetry in the cerebral hemisphere comes about. Some investigators believe that the dominance of one hemisphere develops as a result of experience in early life. One theory links the development of language skills to reinforcement of handedness by parents, but the existence of left dominant, left-handed people seems to contradict this theory. Other investigators maintain that the asymmetry is part of the heredity of the individual and that it merely shows itself gradually as behavior develops. Clearly, there are some asymmetries in handedness and in neural responses to speech sounds in infants. These would appear to be innate. Yet, some verbal asymmetries have not been found in boys until 5 to 7 years of age and in girls until 9 to 11 years of age. Whether this late appearance is innate or learned, the difference in time of onset in the sexes may help to explain the greater resistance of girls to permanent damage to language function caused by early brain trauma. It may be that either hemisphere can become dominant, but only one does under normal circumstances.

There are clear structural differences between the two hemispheres that may underlie these differences in hemispheric functions. There are, of course, the larger "speech areas" in the dominant hemisphere. In addition, auditory primary sensory and association areas appear to be larger in the dominant hemisphere than in the nondominant, whereas the temporoparietal cortex appears to be larger in the nondominant hemisphere. In right-handed people, most of whom are left hemisphere dominant, the frontal lobes are more often wider in the right and the occipital lobes more often wider in the left hemisphere. There are many more structural asymmetries in the brain, but we do not know which may be associated with dominance. Structural asymmetries have also been found in fossil human and protohuman brains, in all of the living great apes, and in some of the lesser apes and monkeys. Again, the relationship of these asymmetries to language is unknown; in fact, we are only just becoming aware of the extent of language capabilities in animals.

Such asymmetries are not unique to the brains of mammals. Birds also show asymmetries in areas associated with the production of song, and there is a clear hemispheric dominance in the control of song. The lateral asymmetry in birds is maintained down to the motoneurons that innervate the syrinx. This dominance is interesting in light of the fact that the bird's brain is so different in structure from the mammalian brain.

SUGGESTED READING

Burkland CW, Smith A: Language and the cerebral hemisphere. Neurology 27:627–633, 1977

Curtis BA, Jacobson S, Marcus EM: Introduction to the Neurosciences. Philadelphia, WB Saunders, 1972

DeJong RN, Itaboshi HH, Olsen JR: Memory loss due to hippocampal lesions. Arch Neurol 20:339–348, 1969

Gazzaniga MS: The Bisected Brain. New York, Appleton-Century-Crofts, 1970

Gazzaniga MS, LeDoux JE, Wilson DH: Language, praxis, and the right hemisphere: Clues to some mechanisms of consciousness. Neurology 27:1144–1147, 1977

Geschwind N: Specializations of the human brain. Sci Am 241:180–199, 1979.

Glickstein M: Neurophysiology of learning and memory. In Ruch TC, Patton, HD [eds]: Physiology and Biophysics. I. The Brain and Neural Function, 20th ed. Philadelphia, WB Saunders, 1979

Head H: Aphasia and Kindred Disorders of Speech. Cambridge, University Press, 1926

Klüver H, Bucy PC: "Psychic blindness" and other symptoms following bilateral temporal lobotomy in Rhesus monkeys. Am J Physiol 119:352–353, 1937

Olds J, Milner P: Positive reinforcement produced by electrical stimulation of septal area and other regions of rat brain. J Comp Physiol Psychol 47:419–427, 1954

Papez JW: A proposed mechanism of emotion. Arch Neurol Psychiat 38:725–743, 1937

Penfield W: The neurophysiological basis of thought. Mod Perspectives Psychiat 1:313–349, 1971

Rosenzweig MR, Bennett EL [eds]: Neural Mechanisms of Learning and Memory. Cambridge, MA, M.I.T. Press, 1976

Scoville WB, Milner B: Loss of recent memory after bilateral hippocampal lesions. J Neurol Neurosurg Psychiat 20:11–12, 1957

Tsukada Y, Agranoff BW [eds]: Neurobiological Basis of Learning and Memory. New York, Wiley, 1980

Wyler AR, Burchiel KJ, Robbins CA: Operant control of precentral neurons in monkeys: Evidence against open loop control. Brain Res 171:29–39, 1979

22

The Clinical Implications of Neurophysiologic Concepts

Most neurologists find that the most frequent complaint they hear about is headaches. Most headaches are probably due to nervous tension, anxiety, or fatigue and can be treated adequately with aspirin or other drugs. Much less common are headaches that result from tumors, some of which can be treated by surgery. The second most frequent neurologic problem is stroke. Usually, for stroke victims, the procedure, after the patient is out of danger, is to treat the patient with physical therapy. The physical therapist's job frequently is to make the person comfortable and to regain, as much as possible, functions lost due to the stroke. In general, the treatment of other maladies of the nervous system is similar.

However, the implicit assumption in the way we treat nervous disorders seems to be that the patient has lost *the* tissue that performed a particular function and that nothing can restore the tissue or the function. In a way, this attitude is surprising in a scientific age, but, in another way, it is not. If the nervous system is viewed as a set of structures, each with a function that it and it alone can serve, then there is nothing to be done for the patient. For example, if the pyramidal tract is viewed as the only structure that initiates and controls voluntary movements, then its destruction must be assumed to have the inevitable consequence of eliminating voluntary movements. Or, if the spinothalamic tract is viewed as the only pain pathway, then its destruction must eliminate pain sensation from the areas it serves.

This concept, which we will call the "essential component" concept, of the nervous system pervades most neuroanatomy and neurophysiology textbooks and if not stated explicitly, it is at least implied. It seems natural for it to be this way, because the ideas of somatotopic organization and localization of function seem to be so comfortable—that is the way we build our machines.

We have already examined the idea of somatotopic organization in some detail. It might be valuable to examine the idea of localization of function in some detail to see just what we are claiming when we say a function is localized to a particular structure. The term localization appears to be used in several different ways by different people. For some, functions are localizable to an entire hemisphere or to a particular nucleus, but, with the recent increase in interest in neurochemistry, more and more people are talking about localization to particular subcellular organelles. Functions can be localized to a particular circumscribed region of the brain, as motor functions of speech are localized to Broca's area, or they can be localized to systems distributed over large regions of the brain, as emotional behavior is localized to the limbic system.

And, what is a function? Laurence and Stein (1978) have pointed out that the term function is at times used to specify means and, at times, to specify ends, most authors failing to be explicit about which of these contexts they are using. In the context of ends, functions refer to a goal they accomplish (eating, thinking), the effects they have within a particular context (inhibition), or the role they have within some larger system (contrast enhancement in vision). In the context of means, functions refer to the way in which a goal is accomplished, describing the actual behavior of an organism (it pulls with upper arm and shoulder muscles). These are not exclusive contexts; they may not even be related. There are usually a number of means to achieve any goal, and the same means may lead to different goals in different situations.

It is difficult to speak of localization when by function we mean a goal. Because goals can usually be achieved by a number of means, they must have numerous localizations, or must they? The more general or complex a goal, the less easily it can be localized. No one has trouble speaking of the localization of language or movements, but it is doubtful that anyone would argue strongly for localization of book writing. However, it was only in the early 1800s that the phrenologists argued for localization of conscientiousness, adhesiveness, and marvelousness. Perhaps future neuroscientists will smile to themselves in a similar way about localization of language. If by function we mean a means, then saying a function is localized indicates nothing more than that a particular biochemical or electrophysiologic process exists and can be used. Such localization is not particularly useful to our understanding of brain. Still, the idea of localization of function is pervasive in neuroscience and so is its derivative, the essential component concept.

Yet, there is nothing in our knowledge of the nervous system that requires this essential component concept to be true! The notion that specific behavioral processes are related to specific subregions of the brain is based in part upon the assumption that deficits resulting from removal or damage to a specific structure reflect what the structure normally does. (One cannot help but be reminded of the popular joke about the boy who concluded that grasshoppers hear with their legs on the grounds that his trained grasshopper failed to respond to the command "jump" after its legs were removed.) In fact, we have seen in Chapter 19 and elsewhere that this is not necessarily the case; the deficits may reflect what the remaining tissues of the region or even tissues at some distance from the damaged structure do. Care should be taken, for example, in concluding that the hypothalamus plays a role in vision simply because tumors there (over the optic chiasm and tract) commonly produce visual impairments. Great physiologists even in the last century knew that the assumption that deficits reflect normal processes, probably was not valid.

There is certainly nothing in the structure of the nervous system that requires the essential component concept. Many colleagues are fond of saying that in the nervous system, "everything is connected to everything." In a way, that is true! If you follow any pathway far enough, you can get from one structure to any other structure of the nervous system, though you may have to go through a mechanical linkage to do it (the exteroreceptors are a notable exception). There is certainly nothing in neurophysiology that compels one to think in terms of "essential components." Stimulation of any structure always has more than one consequence, and stimulation in several different places at different levels can have the same consequence. With respect to behavior, ablation of most central nervous system structures above the brain stem does not eliminate behaviors, though it may alter them in profound ways. Cutting the pyramidal tract does influence movements, but it does not eliminate them. Cutting the spinothalamic tract does influence pain sensitivity, but it does not eliminate it.

What then is the alternative to the essential component concept, and what are its implications for clinical practice? Knowledge of the way the nervous system has evolved tells us that the structures that evolved early are among the only essential components. These are the motoneurons, the receptors, and their reflex connections. Almost everything else added later serves only a modulating function—it only modulates the essential activities of the essential components. It is the pattern of this addition and modulation that makes a monkey, a monkey, and a man, a man. Let us call this the "modulating component" concept. From time to time, new components were added to the system or parts of older components were specialized, allowing new behaviors to develop. In these cases, ablation of these new or specialized components eliminates those new behaviors.

The visual system offers an example for illustration of the implications of the modulating component concept. With damage to the striate cortex, cortical blindness results, the usual interpretation being that the striate cortex "produces" vision and its removal "eliminates" vision. This is the essential component concept. Suppose instead that vision is actually a subcortical event produced by a number of visual structures or pathways, including the superior colliculus and the lateral geniculate nucleus. The visual cortex allows vision to be more flexible or perhaps to achieve some new aspects not present without the cortex. In the process of corticalization, the subcortical visual structures received an input from the cortex and came to depend upon the cortical input to maintain their excitability levels. We have seen time and time again how important summation is to normal neuron discharges. With cortical damage, the visual cortical input to the subcortical structures is eliminated and the neurons in these structures drastically reduce their firing or stop altogether, as spinal motoneurons do during spinal shock. Certainly, this scenario is consistent with what we know of the behavior of neurons. With the essential component concept, there is no treatment for this disorder; vision is permanently, irreparably lost. On the other hand, if the foregoing reasoning, based on the modulating component concept, is sound, then an appropriate prothesis to restore at least some visual abilities would be any device that increases the excitability in the subcortical structures or pathways, whether or not it excites fibers running out of the visual cortex.

Some interesting results obtained in cats are suggestive that this interpretation is correct and they also suggest a possible treatment. In cats, unilateral removal of the superior colliculus results in homonymous hemianopsia, complete to the vertical meridian, ipsiversive circling movements, and deficits in contralateral movements of the eyes, all of which are somewhat compensated over several weeks time. Unilateral removal of area 17, the primary visual cortex, has only minimal and transient effects or none at all. However, a lesion involving the entire occipitotemporal cortex from the splenial sulcus to the rhinal fissure, including both primary and supplementary visual areas, results in complete contralateral hemianopsia with no compensation occurring with a 1-year period. Thus far, there is nothing new in these observations. However, if this lesion of the cortex is followed by another to the contralateral (with respect to the cortical lesion) superior colliculus, there is a marked return of the visual function that was lost following the cortical lesion, and the deficit that would normally result from the collicular lesion alone is less severe. Table 22-1 gives a qualitative summary of the results one obtains from such an experiment.

One way of understanding these results is as follows: Visually guided behavior is a function of both subcortical and cortical centers. Removal of the visual cortex eliminates a descending (corticotectal) facilitation of the ipsilateral superior colliculus, leaving an inhibition from the contralateral superior colliculus and possibly elsewhere and resulting in an imbalance in the system. The result is that the discharges of the ipsilateral superior colliculus cease and with them visually guided behavior. Destruction of the contralateral colliculus disinhibits the ipsilateral one, allowing a return of its functioning. The reason for the less severe deficiencies due to the collicular lesion itself is not clear. If this interpretation is correct (there are other possible interpretations), then a possible treatment for hemianopsia resulting from cortical damage would be to stimulate the superior colliculus ipsilateral to the cortical damage. To date this has not been attempted in humans, but 10 to 15 years ago it would not even have been considered. It would have been assumed that there was nothing to be done for the benefit of the patient.

Work with patients suffering from cortical blindness has shown that repeated measurement of visual threshold leads to a reduction in thresholds and increased contrast sensitivity in the damaged visual field and in the contralateral homologous area.

TABLE 22-1. SUMMARY OF VISUAL DEFICITS FOLLOWING CORTICAL AND CORTICAL + COLLICULAR LESIONS*

DEFICITS AFTER RIGHT CORTICAL LESION	DEFICITS AFTER SUBSEQUENT LESION OF THE LEFT SUPERIOR COLLICULUS
Total left hemianopsia	Response to stimuli in left field
Normal right field	Response to stimuli in right field diminished, but improving to near normal
Follows visual stimuli only on right	Following only on left initially, later also on right with left favored
Blink to lateral threat on right only	Blink to threat on left only initially, later also on right
Eye movements and pupils normal	Pupils normal; eye movements to right absent initially, improve to almost normal, normal to left

* Sprague JM: Science 153:1544–1547, 1966

Improvements were seen only with specific training; no improvement was seen between sessions. Even though no specific procedures other than visual sensitivity measurements were performed, improvements in flicker–fusion thresholds, acuity, and color vision were also observed. The reasons for these improvements are not clear, but it is possible that systematic stimulation itself leads to increased excitability of the remaining visual pathway.

If the nervous system is viewed in the modulating component way, one will be led to the conclusion that there may be certain modalities of sensation and perhaps certain motor functions that cannot be replaced once lost, but there are others, perhaps the majority, in which another structure can take over the same modulating job or a new strategy can be developed to accomplish the behavior (perhaps using different movements, different muscles, or different central nervous system structures). To a certain extent this happens naturally. The recovery of pain sensation following tractotomy and the recovery of motor function following a stroke are examples of this process at work.

A physician should keep an open mind to this possibility and be alert to recognize cases in which this kind of "repair" may be possible. There may be some course of action that will speed up the process or perhaps allow it to happen. At least, bear in mind the extent to which your view of how the nervous system is put together and how it functions determines what you do for the patient.

SUGGESTED READING

Laurence S, Stein DG: Recovery after brain damage and the concept of localization of function. In Finger S [ed]: Recovery from Brain Damage. New York, Plenum Press, 1978

Glossary

The following is a list of commonly used terms and the meanings they have for neurophysiology.

A band. Anisotropic or dark band in striated muscle; contains actin and myosin.

A fiber. A myelinated nerve fiber with conduction velocity in the range from 1 to 120 m/sec; a class of fibers divisible into α, β, γ, and δ subgroups.

Absolute refractory period. Time after an action potential during which the membrane cannot initiate another spike no matter how strong the stimulus.

Accommodation. In the eye: adjustment of the eye for near vision by contraction of ciliary muscle; in membranes: elevation of critical firing level with prolonged small depolarization.

Acetylcholine. An acetic acid ester of choline, a transmitter substance at many peripheral nervous system synapses and perhaps some central synapses.

Acetylcholinesterase. An enzyme present in nervous tissue, muscle, and erythrocytes that catalyzes hydrolysis of acetylcholine to choline and acetic acid.

Actin. A protein of the thin myofilament, localized to the I band of the sarcomere.

Action potential. The all-or-none, conducted voltage response of a nerve or muscle membrane that is used to communicate information from one cell to another, *syn.* Spike.

Activation. In EEG: reduction in amplitude and increase in frequency of the EEG accompanying alerting, *syn.* Alpha-blocking, Desynchronization; in membranes: opening of voltage-gated ionic channels.

Acuity. Clarity of vision measured as the minimum distance between two distinguishable points at a standard distance.

Adaptation. Decline in response of a sensory neuron to a maintained stimulus (see also light adaptation and dark adaptation).

Adequate stimulus. The form of stimulus to which a receptor is most sensitive.

Adipsia. Absence of drinking or abnormal avoidance of drinking.

Adrenergic synapse. A junction between two cells that employs as its transmitter substance one of the catecholamines, epinephrine, norepinephrine, and perhaps isoproterenol.

Afferent. Pathways leading to; in the case of peripheral nerves, those conducting to the central nervous system.

After-depolarization. A membrane potential more positive than the resting membrane potential that occurs following termination of the spike, *syn.* Depolarizing after-potential.

After-hyperpolarization. A membrane potential more negative than the resting membrane potential that occurs following termination of the spike, *syn.* Hyperpolarizing after-potential.

Agnosia. Loss of the power to recognize the import of sensory stimuli.

Agraphesthesia. Inability to recognize letters traced on the skin.

Akinesia. Absence of movement.

Alcoholic cerebellar degeneration. Degeneration of the cerebellum due to chronic over-consumption of alcohol.

Alexia. Inability to read.

Algesia. Suffix meaning pain; examples: hypalgesia, reduced pain sensation; hyperalgesia, heightened pain sensitivity; analgesia, no pain sensitivity.

All-or-none. Independence of action potential amplitude from stimulus strength; also refers to tendency of spikes to travel over the entire membrane of a cell, *syn.* All-or-nothing.

All-or-nothing. Independence of action potential amplitude from stimulus strength; also refers to tendency of spikes to travel over the entire membrane of a cell, *syn.* All-or-none.

Alpha adrenergic effects. A constellation of effects produced by circulating norepinephrine or norepinephrine released from postganglionic sympathetic nerve terminals. Also produced by epinephrine and isoproterenol but effects are smaller in magnitude.

Alpha blocking. Disappearance of alpha rhythms from the EEG, *syn.* Activation, Desynchronization.

Alpha–gamma coactivation. The tendency for α and γ motoneurons to be activated together.

Alpha motoneuron (α motoneuron). A motoneuron whose axon is an Aα fiber, *syn.* Skeletomotor neuron.

Alpha rhythms. EEG records characterized by high-voltage waves occurring at 8 to 14 per sec.

Alpha spasticity. A tonic contraction of one muscle or a group of synergistic muscles at a joint, caused by excitation of alpha motoneurons innervating the muscles.

Amnesic syndrome. Inability to remember past events; defect in formation of new long-term memories.

Amplification. A circumstance in which the output signal is greater than the input signal.

Anesthesia. The lack of tactile sensation.

Angina pectoris. Pain due to infarction of the coronary blood vessels, referred to the chest and upper arm.

Anhidrosis. An abnormal deficiency of sweat.

Annulospiral ending. The termination of a group Ia afferent fiber in the equatorial region of a muscle spindle, *syn.* Primary muscle spindle ending.

Anomaloscope. A color-matching device used to detect anomalous trichromacy.

Anomalous rectification. A decrease in the ionic conductance of the cell membrane with depolarization of the membrane.

Anomalous trichromacy. Color vision involving three pigments but one is abnormal, producing a weakness in response to that primary color.

Anorexia. Lack or loss of the appetite for food.

Antagonist muscle. A muscle that acts in opposition to another at a joint.

Antidromic. In the direction opposite that normally taken by action potentials in the nervous system.

Aphagia. Abstention from eating.

Aphasia. Impairment of communication by language in any form; expressive aphasia—inability to speak or write; receptive aphasia—inability to understand spoken or written language.

Apraxia. Inability to carry out motor acts on command in the absence of paralysis.

Areflexia. Absence of reflexes.

Argyll Robertson pupil. Pupil shows miosis of accommodation, but no light reflex.

Ascending reticular activating system. A group of interconnected nuclei of the brain stem responsible for producing desynchronization of the EEG.

Asthenia. Weakness, lack of strength.

Astereognosis. Inability to recognize objects by feeling them.

Astigmatism. Unequal curvature of the refractive surfaces of the eye as a result of which a beam of light is not sharply focused on the retina.

Ataxia. Awkwardness and lack of fluidity in motor behavior associated with loss of control mechanisms of the cerebellum.

Athermesthesia. Loss of temperature sensation.

Atopognosis. Loss of ability correctly to locate a sensation.

Athetosis. Basal ganglion disease characterized by slow, sinuous movements.

Atrophy. A wasting away; a diminution in the size of a cell, tissue, or organ.

Audibility curve. A graph of a person's threshold for detection of various pitches in the range of human hearing, *syn.* Threshold of hearing curve.

Audiogram. A plot of a patient's hearing ability, either an audibility curve or a hearing loss curve.

Audiometry. The testing of the sense of hearing.

Audition. The act of hearing or the ability to hear.

Aura. Sensations or feelings preceding an epileptic seizure.

Autogenic inhibition. Depression of the excitability of an α motoneuron by the groups Ia and Ib afferent fibers that innervate the same muscle as the α motoneuron.

Autonomic nervous system. The portion of the nervous system concerned with regulation of the activity of cardiac muscle, smooth muscle, and glands.

Autonomous zone. The part of the receptive field or dermatome of a nerve or root not shared with other nerves or roots.

Axoaxonic synapse. The synaptic junction between two axons thought to mediate presynaptic depolarization or presynaptic inhibition.

Axodendritic synapse. A synaptic junction in which an axon's bouton is the presynaptic element and a dendrite is the postsynaptic element.

Axosomatic synapse. A synaptic junction in which an axon's bouton is the presynaptic element and a soma is the postsynaptic element.

Axon. The straight, relatively unbranched process of a nerve cell or the efferent process of a nerve cell, *syn.* Nerve fiber.

Axon hillock. The place where the axon arises from the soma of a neuron; thought to be the site of initiation of the spike.

Babinski sign. Dorsiflexion of the toes on stimulating the sole of the foot, sign of a pyramidal tract lesion.

Ballism. Basal ganglion disease characterized by violent, flinging movements of the limbs due to contraction of proximal limb muscles.

Bell-Magendie law. The notion that sensory fibers enter the spinal cord through dorsal roots, motor fibers exit the spinal cord through ventral roots.

Best frequency. The frequency of an auditory stimulus that gives the response of highest rate in an auditory neuron.

Beta adrenergic effect. A constellation of effects produced by circulating epinephrine, or isoproterenol released from postganglionic sympathetic nerve terminals (if they exist). Also produced by norepinephrine but effects are smaller in magnitude.

Beta rhythms. EEG records characterized by low-voltage waves occurring at 14 to 50 per sec.

Binasal hemianopsia. Hemianopsia or loss of vision involving the nasal visual fields of both eyes.

Bipolar. Having two poles; with respect to electrophysiology, stimulating or recording through two electrodes, *cf.*, Monopolar.

Bitemporal hemianopsia. Hemianopsia or loss of vision involving the temporal visual fields of both eyes.

Bouton terminaux. A swelling of an axon near its termination; the presynaptic structure in most synapses, *syn.* End bulb, Synaptic knob, Terminal.

Bradykinesia. Slowness of movement.

Brightness. A quantitative measure of the intensity of light, the amplitude of its waves, or the number of photons.

Broca's area. Areas 44 and 45 of the frontal cerebral cortex that play a fundamental role in production of speech.

Brown-Séquard syndrome. Ipsilateral paralysis and loss of discriminatory and joint sensation and contralateral loss of pain and temperature sensation due to damage to one-half of the spinal cord.

Caloric test. A test of vestibular function involving the induction of nystagmus by putting warm or cold water in the external auditory meatus.

Capacitance. The ability of the nerve membrane to separate and store charge.

Cardiac muscle. Striated muscle found in the heart.

Causalgia. A burning pain due to injury of a peripheral nerve.

C fiber. Unmyelinated primary afferent neurons.

Channel. A passage in the membrane through which ions can flow, *syn.* Pore.

Chemically gated channel. A normally closed ionic channel that is opened by action of a chemical transmitter substance.

Cholinergic synapse. A junction between two cells that employs as its transmitter substance acetylcholine.

Chorea. Basal ganglion disease characterized by rapid, complex, jerky movements that are involuntary.

Chromatic aberration. Colored rings resulting from different amounts of refraction by a lens of light of different wavelengths.

Clasp-knife reflex. Sudden release of tension of a spastic muscle that occurs near the maximum length as the muscle is gradually lengthened, *syn.* Lengthening reaction.

Clonus. The alternating contraction and relaxation of a rapidly extended muscle in spasticity, *syn.* Myoclonus.

Coding. Process by which features of a stimulus or information about an event is expressed in terms of nerve impulses or, in some cases, graded electrotonic potentials.

Cogwheel rigidity. The form of rigidity of parkinsonism, in which the muscle lengthens in a series of little jerks when it is stretched.

Cold fibers. Cutaneous primary afferent fibers that have cooling as an adequate stimulus and respond to cooling the skin with an increase in frequency of discharge.

Collateral inhibition. Inhibition produced in a group of neurons by activity in some neurons of the group that excite inhibitory interneurons by way of collaterals of their axons; sometimes inaccurately used as *syn.* for Recurrent inhibition.

Color blindness. In vision, inability to detect or weakness in response to one or more of the three primary colors.

Color opponent cells. Visual neurons in which one part of the receptive field (*e.g.*, the center) is sensitive to light in one part of the visible spectrum (*e.g.*, red light), whereas another part of the field (*e.g.*, the surround) is sensitive to another part of the spectrum (*e.g.*, green light).

Complex cells. Neurons in visual cortex that are sensitive to bars of light moving in particular directions across the retina.

Compound action potential. The response of a peripheral nerve to an electrical stimulus; represents the sum of the action potentials of all active fibers in the nerve.

Conduction deafness. Hearing loss due to impairment of movement of the tympanum, the ossicles, or the membrane of the oval window.

Conductivity. The capacity of living matter to conduct action potentials.

Cones. Visual receptors in the retina specialized for photopic and color vision.

Conjugate eye movements. Refers to rotation of the eyes in the same direction at the same time.

Consensual light reflex. Constriction of the pupil of the eye opposite that into which a light is shown.

Contralateral. On the opposite side.

Control system. A mechanism that regulates the output of a device.

Convergent eye movements. Refers to rotation of the eyes toward each other.

Critical firing level. The value of the transmembrane voltage to which a nerve or muscle cell must be depolarized in order for an action potential to be evoked.

Cross-bridge. The connection of the head of the myosin molecule with the thin filament in the A band of the sarcomere; according to the cross-bridge theory, the force-generating apparatus of the muscle.

Crossed-extension reflex. Contraction of contralateral extensor muscles concomitant with initiation of a withdrawal reflex.

Cross-innervation. Refers to the transplanting of one nerve onto a foreign muscle and the transplanting of the nerve from that muscle onto the muscle of the first nerve.

Cross-projection. The head of the myosin molecule projecting at right angles past the thin filaments; according to the electrostatic theory, the site of charge separation resulting in an electric field.

Crude touch. Touch sensations of higher threshold and poor localizability.

Cutaneous nerve. A nerve, most fibers of which innervate the skin.

Dale's principle. The concept that a neuron can synthesize only one chemical transmitter substance.

Dark adaptation. An increase in the sensitivity of visual receptors as a function of time in the dark.

Decerebrate rigidity. A spasticity resulting from functional disruption of brain-stem activities at the midcollicular level.

Decibel. A unit used to express the ratio of two sound pressures in hearing, equal to $^1/_{10}$ the common log of the ratio of pressures.

Decomposition of movement. Lack of fluidity in movement characterized by the breaking down of composite movements into their component parts, a symptom of cerebellar disease.

Delayed rectification. During a spike, the change in potassium conductance due to membrane depolarization that occurs *after* the change in sodium conductance.

Delta rhythms. EEG records characterized by high-voltage waves occurring at less than 4/sec.

Dementia. Loss of intellectual function.

Dendrite. Process of a neuron specialized to act as a receptor; the afferent process of a neuron.

Dendroaxonic synapse. The synaptic junction between a dendrite and an axon in which the dendrite is thought to be the presynaptic element.

Dendrodendritic synapse. The synaptic junction between two dendrites.

Dendrosomatic synapse. The synaptic junction between a dendrite and a cell soma in which the dendrite is presumed to be the presynaptic element.

Denervation hypersensitivity. Elevated response of a nerve or muscle membrane receptor to a transmitter substance following resection or removal of its afferent nerve supply.

Depolarization. A change in the transmembrane potential of a cell in the direction of the isoelectric point (*e.g.*, zero voltage).

Depolarization phase. The earliest positive-going portion of the nerve or muscle spike, *syn.* Rising phase, Upstroke.

Depolarizing after-potential. A membrane potential more positive than the resting membrane potential that occurs following termination of the spike, *syn.* After-depolarization.

Depth of field. The range of distances from an observer over which images are in focus for a given strength of lens.

Dermatome. The area of skin innervated by a dorsal root.

Desynchronization. Reduction in amplitude and increase in frequency of the EEG accompanying alerting, *syn.* Activation, Alpha-blocking.

Deuteranomaly. Color vision involving three pigments but the green one is abnormal, leading to reduced green sensitivity.

Deuteranope. A person who lacks response to green light, "green color-blind."

Diaschisis. A loss of function due to depression of activity at some distance from a lesion.

Dichromatism. Color vision involving only two pigments.

Difference threshold. The smallest change in the magnitude or quality of a stimulus that can be detected by an observer.

Diffusion. The process of becoming widely distributed that occurs because of molecular concentration differences only.

Diopter. A measure of the strength of a lens, the reciprocal of the focal length of the lens expressed in meters.

Diphtheritic neuritis. A neuritis occurring in the period after an infection by diphtheria bacteria.

Direct light reflex. Constriction of the pupil when light is shown into the same eye.

Doctrine of Specific Nerve Energies. The concept that says that the modality of a sensation is determined not by the stimulus that elicits it, but by the nerve fiber that is excited by the stimulus.

Doll's eye maneuver. A test of the vestibulo-ocular reflex in which the head is rotated from side to side and the rotation of the eyes in the opposite direction is observed.

Dominant hemisphere. The cerebral hemisphere that contains the speech centers.

Dream sleep. A stage of deep sleep characterized by desynchronized EEG patterns, REM, and dreaming, *syn.* Paradoxical sleep, REM sleep.

Dynamic fusimotor neuron. A γ motoneuron whose activity increases predominantly the dynamic response of primary spindle endings to muscle stretch.

Dynamic index. The difference in rate of discharge of a spindle receptor during active stretching and maintained stretch.

Dynamic response. The response of a primary spindle ending that signals rate of change of muscle length during stretch.

Dyscalculia. Impairment of ability to solve mathematical problems.

Dysdiadochokinesia. Impairment of ability to perform rapid alternating movements, a symptom of cerebellar disease.

Dysesthesia. A persistent, painful sensation, produced by gentle stimulation, that often occurs after destruction of CNS pathways.

Dysgraphia. Inability to write properly.

Dyskinesia. Impairment of the ability to move, resulting in fragmentary or incomplete movements.

Dysmetria. A condition in which there is improper measuring of distance in movement, disturbance of the power to control the range of movement, a symptom of cerebellar disease.

Dyssynergia. Disturbance of coordination in closely related muscles.

Efferent. Pathways leading from; in the case of peripheral nerves, those conducting away from the central nervous system.

Electrical equivalent circuit. A collection of electrical components assembled in a particular configuration that behaves like the cell membrane.

Electrically excitable motor cortex. That area of the cerebral cortex, the stimulation of which leads to movements, *syn.* Motor cortex.

Electrical synapse. The junction between two nerve cells at which communication is by direct transfer of charge not by release of a transmitter substance, *syn.* Electrotonic synapse.

Electrochemical equilibrium. A balance between chemical and electrical driving forces such that there is no net movement of ions across the cell membrane.

Electroencephalogram. A recording from the scalp of the changes in electrical potential in the brain, primarily in the cerebral cortex, *abbr.* EEG.

Electrogenic pump. An energy-requiring process in which there is a net transfer of charge across the membrane resulting in a membrane voltage.

Electromyogram. A recording of the electrical activity of muscle during contraction, *abbr.* EMG.

Electrotonic synapse. The junction between two nerve cells at which communication is by direct transfer of charge, not by release of a transmitter substance, *syn.* Electrical synapse.

Emmetropia. The normal condition of the eye with respect to refraction.

End bulb. A swelling of an axon near its termination; the presynaptic structure in most synapses, *syn.* Bouton terminaux, Synaptic knob, Terminal.

End-plate potential. The depolarizing postsynaptic potential in the striated muscle that leads to the muscle spike.

Enteroceptor. A receptor that senses some aspect of the condition of the environment inside the body.

Epileptogenic. Producing or capable of producing seizures.

Equilibrium potential. The value of the transmembrane voltage at which the net driving force for an ion or a membrane event (*e.g.*, an EPSP or IPSP) is zero.

Evoked potential. An electrical response of a group of neurons produced by a stimulus to sensory receptor or neural pathway.

Excitability. The ability to generate action potentials.

Excitatory postsynaptic potential. A depolarizing change in the transmembrane potential of a neuron due to synaptic activity that tends to increase the probability of discharge of the neuron, *abbr.* EPSP.

Extensor thrust reflex. An automatic increase in the contraction of physiologic extensor muscles of the leg when the plantar surface of the foot contacts some non-noxious object.

Exteroceptor. A receptor that senses some aspect of the condition of the environment outside the body.

Extrafusal muscle fiber. The regular contractile fibers that produce the shortening of a muscle; they lie outside the muscle spindle.

Facilitation. The addition of EPSPs in which the resultant is more than the algebraic sum of the individual EPSPs, cf., Temporal summation.

Falling phase. The return of the membrane potential from the peak overshoot of the spike back to the resting potential, *syn.* Repolarization phase.

Far point. The remotest point at which an object is clearly seen when the eye is at rest.

Far-sightedness. A pathologic condition of refraction in which the eyeball is too short for the refractive power of the lens and images focus behind the retina, *syn.* Hyperopia.

Fasciculations. A small, local contraction of muscles visible through the skin; represents spontaneous discharge in one or more muscle fibers innervated by a motoneuron.

Fast axoplasmic transport. The active movement of substances down the axon of a neuron in the orthograde direction at up to 410 mm/day.

Fast muscle. Relative term, referring to the speed of twitch contraction and relaxation and to the relatively high rates of stimulation at which tetanic fusion occurs.

Feedback. The return of some of the output of a system as an input so as to exert some control over the process performed by the system.

Feedback inhibition. A situation in which the output of a neuron (or set of neurons) is used to inhibit (perhaps through an interneuron) further inputs to the neuron (or set of neurons).

Feedforward inhibition. A situation in which the output of a neuron (or set of neurons) is used to inhibit neurons subsequent to it in a particular pathway.

Finger agnosia. Inability to recognize or

indicate on command the fingers on one's own hand or the hands of others.

Flaccidity. Weakness, laxness, softness.

Flexion reflex. Automatic contraction of the flexor muscles of a limb so as the remove the limb from a noxious stimulus, *syn.* Nocifensive reflex, Withdrawal reflex.

Flexor reflex afferent fibers. Nerve fibers, stimulation of which evokes a flexion reflex, Aδ and C fibers and groups II, III and IV of muscle.

Flower-spray endings. The termination of group II afferent fibers on the nuclear chain fibers of muscle spindles, *syn.* Secondary muscle spindle endings.

Flux. Movement of ions due to concentration forces, *syn.* Diffusion.

Focal length. The distance from the center of a lens to the point of focus of light from a distant object.

Focus. The location of a group of cells in the cerebral cortex whose abnormal discharge initiates seizures.

Follow-up length servo mechanism. A process by which movements can be initiated indirectly by inputs to γ motoneurons rather than α motoneurons.

Fovea. The central region of the retina specialized for detail vision, *i.e.*, for acuity.

Frequency theory. A theory that says the frequency of a sound wave is encoded by the auditory receptors in terms of their rate of discharge.

Frontal eye fields. Premotor areas of the cerebral cortex from which contraversive eye movements are evokable by electrical stimulation.

Fused tetanic contraction. A tetanic muscle contraction in which there is no trace of the individual twitches that have been summed.

Fusimotor neuron. A motoneuron whose activity results in contraction of intrafusal muscle fibers, *syn.* γ Motoneuron.

Gamma bias. Refers to the ongoing discharge of fusimotor neurons, *syn.* Gamma tone.

Gamma motoneuron (γ motoneuron). A motoneuron whose axon is an Aγ fiber, *syn.* Fusimotor neuron.

Gamma spasticity. A tonic contraction of one muscle or a group of synergistic muscles at a joint, caused by excitation of the gamma motoneurons innervating the muscles.

Gamma tone. Refers to the ongoing discharge of fusimotor neurons, *syn.* Gamma bias.

Gate theory of pain. A theory that says the perception of pain depends not only upon activity in nociceptors, but also upon the balance between activity in nociceptors and large myelinated cutaneous afferent fibers.

Generator potential. A nonpropagated change in the membrane potential of a receptor that leads to the generation of action potentials within the receptor itself, *cf.*, Receptor potential.

Golgi tendon organ. A receptor located at the muscle–tendon junction that signals developed tension in the muscle.

Grand mal attacks. Epileptic seizures characterized by myoclonus, progressive myoclonus, loss of erect posture, and unconsciousness.

Gustation. The sense of taste.

H band. The lighter region in the center of the anisotropic or A band, from which the thin filaments are absent.

Hearing loss curve. A plot of the threshold of hearing for a patient as deviations from normal for different frequencies of sound.

Hemianopsia. Loss of vision in either the nasal or temporal half of the visual field.

Hering-Breuer reflex. The nervous mechanism that tends to limit inspiratory excursions, mediated by stretch receptors in the intercostal muscles whose activity leads to inhibition of inspiratory neurons in the brain stem.

Herpes zoster. An acute inflammatory disease of the dorsal root ganglion caused by the virus of chickenpox and characterized by small vesicles occurring on the skin supplied by the affected nerve.

Hertz. Cycles per sec, *abbr.* Hz.

Hodgkin cycle. The regenerative sequence in which depolarization leads to increased conductance, leading to sodium ion influx and further depolarization.

Homonymous hemianopsia. Hemianopsia involving either the left or right halves of the visual fields of both eyes.

Homonymous muscle. The muscle of origin of the nerve fibers being considered.

Horner's syndrome. Sinking in of the eyeball, ptosis of the upper eyelid, constriction of the pupil, anhidrosis, and flushing of the affected side of the face caused by paralysis of the cervical sympathetic nerves.

Hue. A quality of light correlated with its wavelength. The color of the light.

Hypalgesia. Diminished pain sensation.

Hypercomplex cells. Neurons in visual cortex that are sensitive to bars of light moving in particular directions across the retina and that require the bar to be less than a certain maximum length.

Hyperphagia. Ingestion of a greater than optimal quantity of food.

Hyperopia. A pathologic condition of refraction in which the eyeball is too short for the refractive power of the lens and images focus behind the retina, *syn.* Farsightedness.

Hyperpathia. Abnormally exaggerated response to painful stimuli.

Hyperpolarization. From the resting potential, a change in the transmembrane potential of a cell away from the isoelectric point (*i.e.*, zero voltage).

Hyperpolarizing after-potential. A membrane potential more negative than the resting membrane potential that occurs following termination of the spike, *syn.* After-hyperpolarization.

Hyper-reflexia. Exaggerated reflexes.

Hyperstimulation analgesia. A reduction or elimination of pain sensation brought about as a result of strong stimulation outside a damaged area.

Hypertonia. A condition of excessive muscle tone; increased resistance to passive stretch.

Hypesthesia. Reduced cutaneous sensation.

Hypophysectomy. Surgical removal or other destruction of the pituitary.

Hyporeflexia. Weakening of the reflexes.

Hypotonia. A condition of diminished muscle tone.

I band. The isotropic or light band of striated muscle; contains only actin filaments.

Immediate recall. Memory of learned material or responses having a duration of minutes to perhaps hours, *syn.* Short-term memory.

Impedance matching device. A mechanism that compensates for differences in sound transmission through different media; in the ear, through air and perilymph.

Inactivation. Closure of the voltage-gated ionic channels.

Inhibitory postsynaptic potential. A hyperpolarizing change in the membrane potential of a neuron due to synaptic activity that tends to decrease the probability of discharge in the neuron, *abbr.* IPSP.

Integrate. To combine signals from a number of sources.

Integrative synapse. A synaptic junction at which the critical firing level is reached only by the summation of EPSPs from many sources; a point of integration.

Intention tremor. An involuntary trembling that is heightened when a movement is attempted.

Intermediate zone. The part of a dermatome or receptive field outside the autonomous zone.

Intrafusal muscle fiber. The contractile tissue of the muscle spindle; it lies inside the spindle.

Ionotropic transmission. Synaptic transmission in which the transmitter substance produces a change in ionic conductance of the postsynaptic membrane directly by interaction with a postsynaptic receptor.

Iontophoresis. The introduction by means of an electrical current of ions of soluble salts into the tissues of the body.

Ipsilateral. On the same side.

Irradiation. Spread of the flexion reflex to involve additional muscle groups and additional movements with stronger stimulation.

Isometric contraction. A contraction during which the muscle does not change length.

Isotonic contraction. A contraction of a muscle under constant load.

Klüver-Bucy syndrome. Behavior disturbances resulting from bilateral temporal lobe damage; characterized by a tendency to examine objects orally, depression of emotional reactions, and lack of sexual inhibitions.

Labeled lines. The notion that particular modalities and submodalities have their own special pathways to the brain and activity induced anywhere along one of these pathways is interpreted as a stimulus of the appropriate modality or submodality.

Latency. The time between application of a stimulus and appearance of a response.

Lateral inhibition. Refers to the inhibition of the discharge evoked by stimulation within a cell's excitatory receptive field that occurs when an area outside that receptive field is stimulated; alternatively inhibition of an element in a sensory system caused by activity in an adjacent element of the same type.

Left-right confusion. Confusion of laterality.

Lengthening reaction. Sudden release of tension of a spastic muscle that occurs near the maximum length as the muscle is gradually lengthened, *syn.* Clasp-knife reflex.

Leukotomy. The operation of cutting the white matter in the oval center of the frontal lobe of the brain, *syn.* Lobotomy.

Light adaptation. A reduction in sensitivity of visual receptors as a function of time in the light.

Light reflex. Constriction of the pupils when a bright light is shown into an eye.

Limen. The psychologic term for threshold.

Linear function or relation. The relationship between two variables such that the equal changes in one result in equal changes in the other; an equation of the form $y = ax + b$.

Lobectomy. Excision of a lobe.

Lobotomy. Incision into a lobe, cutting all the fibers in the white matter, *syn.* Leukotomy.

Logarithmic function or relation. The relationship between two variables such that equal percentage changes in one result in equal changes in the other; an equation of the form $y = a \log x + b$.

Long-term memory. Recall of learned responses or material having a duration of minutes to years.

Loudness. The "perceived intensity" of a sound related to both the amplitude of the sound wave and its frequency.

Lower motoneuron syndrome. A group of symptoms resulting from disease of either the motoneuron or the muscle or both.

Macula lutea. An irregular yellowish depression in the retina surrounding the fovea.

Macular sparing. Refers to the presence of visual sensation in the entire macula in hemianopsias resulting from occipital cortex lesions.

Masking. An increase in the threshold for perception of a given stimulus caused by the presence of another stimulus.

Mask-like face. Refers to the lack of spontaneous facial expressions in the patient with basal ganglion disease, particularly parkinsonism.

Maximal response. The largest electrical response obtainable from a nerve, tract, or nucleus.

Maximal stimulus. The stimulus strength that just yields the maximal response.

Membrane potential. The electrical potential that exists across the cell membrane as a result of inhomogeneous ion distributions.

Meniere's disease. Deafness, tinnitus, and vertigo resulting from accumulation of endolymph in the labyrinth.

Metabotropic transmission. Synaptic transmission in which the transmitter substance causes activation of a second messenger that causes the change in postsynaptic membrane potential.

Miniature end-plate potential. A tiny, spontaneous postsynaptic potential recorded near the end-plate in muscle fibers, *abbr.* MEPP.

Miosis. Constriction of the pupil of the eye.

Modality. One of the basic senses: somesthesia, vision, audition, gustation, and olfaction.

Monopolar. Having a single pole; with respect to electrophysiology: stimulating or recording through one active electrode and one indifferent (or reference) electrode, *cf.*, Bipolar.

Monosynaptic reflex. Reflex involving only one synapse within the central nervous system.

Motor cortex. That area of cerebral cortex, the stimulation of which leads to movements, *syn.* Electrically excitable motor cortex.

Motor end-plate. The specialized terminal of a motoneuron that forms a synaptic contact with the muscle membrane.

Motor unit. An alpha motoneuron and the muscle fibers it innervates.

Multiple sclerosis. A disease in which there are multiple patches of demyelination in the white matter of the central nervous system. These are repaired and new patches appear in different places in subsequent attacks.

Multi-unit smooth muscle. Smooth muscle containing few tight junctions, but richly innervated; responds as individual motor units, not as a single unit.

Muscarinic effect. The subset of actions normally produced by acetylcholine that can also be produced by muscarine.

Muscle nerve. A nerve most fibers of which innervate a muscle.

Muscle spindle. A fusiform mechanoreceptor found mixed with extrafusal muscle fibers and in parallel with them.

Myelinated fiber. A nerve fiber wrapped by a series of Schwann cells, resulting in greater conduction velocity.

Myoclonus. Clonus.

Myofibril. A muscle fibril; one of the slender threads in a muscle composed of numerous myofilaments.

Myofilament. Any of the small filaments that comprise a myofibril; either a thick or myosin filament, or a thin or actin filament.

Myogenic. Of muscle origin.

Myopia. A pathologic condition of refraction in which the eyeball is too long for the refractive power of the lens and images focus in front of the retina, *syn.* Near-sightedness.

Myosin. The protein of the thick myofilament, localized to the A band of the sarcomere.

Myotatic reflex. An automatic contraction of a muscle elicited by stretching it, *syn.* Stretch reflex, Tendon jerk reflex.

Near point. The nearest point at which the eye can distinctly perceive an object.

Near-sightedness. A pathologic condition of refraction in which the eyeball is too long for the refractive power of the lens and images focus in front of the retina, *syn.* Myopia.

Negative feedback loop. A circuit in which part of the output is used to reduce the input to the circuit.

Nernst equation. A mathematical formula stating the voltage across a cell membrane that results from a difference in ion concentration inside and outside the cell.

Nerve. A collection of axons or nerve fibers.

Nerve cell. A cell specialized for excitability and conductivity, *syn.* Neuron.

Nerve deafness. Hearing loss due to damage to auditory receptors or auditory pathways of the central nervous system.

Nerve fiber. The straight, relatively unbranched process of a nerve cell, *syn.* Axon.

Nerve growth factor. A substance isolated from submaxillary glands that has the property of stimulating growth of sympathetic ganglion cells and, under certain circumstances, dorsal root ganglion cells.

Nervous system. The neurons and associated cells of the body.

Neuralgia. Paroxysmal pain that extends along the course of one or more nerves.

Neurogenic. Of nerve origin.

Neuromuscular junction. The synaptic contact between an α motoneuron and the muscle fiber it innervates.

Neuron. A cell specialized for excitability and conductivity, *syn.* Nerve cell.

Neurotrophic effect. Interactions between nerve cells or between nerve cells and other types of cells in which the nerve fibers initiate or control molecular and/or functional modification in the other cells.

Nicotinic effect. The subset of actions normally produced by acetylcholine that can also be produced by nicotine.

Nociceptor. A receptor whose adequate stimulus is strong enough to produce damage.

Nocifensive reflex. Automatic contraction of the flexor muscles of a limb so as to remove the limb from a noxious stimulus, *syn.* Flexion reflex, Withdrawal reflex.

Nodal synapse. The junction between any part of a nerve cell and a node of Ranvier of a nerve fiber.

Nonelectrogenic pump. An ion pump whose operation does not result in a net transfer of charge into or out of the cell.

Norepinephrine. A substance secreted as a transmitter substance by sympathetic postganglionic nerve terminals and as a hormone by the adrenal medulla.

Nuclear bag fiber. An intrafusal muscle fiber with nuclei accumulated in an equatorial swelling.

Nuclear chain fiber. An intrafusal muscle fiber with nuclei arranged in a line throughout its relatively uniform-diameter central region.

Nyctalopia. Congenital night-blindness caused by a lack of rod functioning in the retina.

Nystagmus. A slow deviation of the eyes either horizontally, vertically, rotatory or mixed, followed by a rapid return to the starting position. The sequence is repeated.

Obligatory synapse. A synaptic junction at which a single presynaptic action potential initiates a postsynaptic action potential.

Occlusion. In neurophysiology, the inability of two action potentials to occupy the same region of membrane at the same time; thus an antidromic impulse blocks a concomitant orthodromic impulse in the same fiber by occlusion.

Off-response. The discharge of a neuron initiated when a stimulus is turned off.

Olfaction. The sense of smell.

Olivocochlear bundle. A bundle of efferent nerve fibers originating in the superior olive and ending on hair cells in the basilar membrane. They are inhibitory in function.

On–off response. The discharge of a neuron initiated both when a stimulus is turned on and when it is turned off with silence in between.

On-response. The discharge of a neuron initiated when a stimulus is turned on.

Opisthotonos. A form of spasm in which the head and the heels are bent backward and the body bowed forward.

Orthodromic. Conduction in the direction normally taken by action potentials.

Otolith. Literally: stone in the ear; a calcium carbonate crystal found in the otolith organs of vertebrates, *syn.* Statoconium.

Otolith organ. A vestibular organ containing otoliths, the utricle, or saccule.

Overshoot. Refers to that portion of the action potential where the membrane polarity is reversed, *i.e.*, where the membrane potential is positive inside with respect to outside.

Pacemaker cell. A cell that is rhythmically, spontaneously active, initiating activity in other cells in the same rhythm.

Pallesthesia. The sensation of vibration.

Papilla. A small, nipple-shaped projection or elevation, as on the tongue.

Paradoxical sleep. A stage of deep sleep characterized by desynchronized EEG patterns, REM, and dreaming, *syn.* Dream sleep, REM sleep.

Paralysis. Loss of function in a part of the body due to lesion of the neural or muscular mechanisms controlling it.

Parasympathetic nervous system. The division of the autonomic nervous system made up of ocular, bulbar, and sacral segments.

Paresis. Weakness, partial paralysis; adjectival form: paretic.

Paresthesia. An abnormal sensation of burning, prickling, or tingling.

Parkinsonism. Basal ganglion disease characterized by hypokinesia, tremor at rest, and muscular rigidity.

Past-pointing. An error in pointing to a target in the direction of a previous rotation, *e.g.*, in a Bárány chair.

Petit mal attacks. Epileptic seizures characterized by fixed stare, unconsciousness, unresponsiveness, and lack of activity.

Phantom limb pain. Pain referred to a limb that has been removed.

Photophobia. Abnormal visual intolerance of light.

Photopic. Pertaining to vision in the light.

Physiologic extensor muscle. Antigravity muscle.

Pitch. The quality of a sound determined by the frequency of its waves.

Place theory. A theory that says pitch is encoded in terms of the place on the basilar membrane that gives maximum vibration in response to a given frequency of sound.

Polarized. Embued with poles; experiencing a separation of charge; refers to difference in potential across a cell membrane.

Polydipsia. Excessive drinking persisting for long periods of time as in diabetes mellitus.

Polymodal nociceptor. A receptor that responds to more than one type of noxious stimulus, *e.g.*, noxious heat and noxious mechanical stimuli.

Polysynaptic reflex. A reflex involving more than one synapse in the central nervous system.

Pore. A passage in the membrane through which ions can flow, *syn.* Channel.

Postganglionic fiber. Nerve fibers originating in and running peripheral to an autonomic ganglion.

Postrotatory nystagmus. Nystagmus in the direction opposite to that of and due to a previous rotation, *e.g.*, in a Bárány chair.

Postsynaptic element. The component of a synapse that receives the transmitter substance and/or conducts impulses in the efferent direction with respect to the synapse.

Postsynaptic inhibition. Decrease in the probability of firing of a neuron because of the IPSPs generated in it.

Postural fixation. Assumption of unusual body positions as in basal ganglion disease.

Power function or relation. The relationship between two variables such that the equal percentage changes in one result in equal percentage changes in the other; an equation of the form $y = x^a$.

Preganglionic fiber. Nerve fiber originating in the central nervous system and running to an autonomic ganglion.

Presbycusis. Decrease or loss of sensitivity to high frequencies of sound with advancing age.

Presbyopia. Hyperopia due to loss of elasticity of the lens at about age 40.

Presynaptic element. The component of a synapse that releases the transmitter substance and/or conducts impulses in the afferent direction with respect to the synapse.

Presynaptic inhibition. Decrease in the probability of firing of a neuron due to decrease in transmission to it that results from depolarization of afferent terminals on it.

Primary afferent fiber. The first order fibers of a sensory system; those entering the dorsal roots of the spinal cord.

Primary evoked potential. The change in potential recorded in a primary sensory cortical area following stimulation of the receptors associated with that area.

Primary muscle spindle receptor. The termination of a group Ia afferent fiber in the equatorial region of a muscle spindle, *syn.* Annulospiral ending.

Protanomaly. Color vision involving three pigments, but the red one is abnormal leading to reduced red sensitivity.

Protanope. A person who lacks responses to red light; "red color-blind."

Psychomotor epilepsy. Seizures characterized by stereotyped behavior often with emotional outbursts and partial responsiveness, *syn.* Temporal lobe epilepsy.

Psychophysics. The science dealing with the quantitative relationships between stimuli and sensations.

Quadrantanopsia. Blindness in one quarter of the visual field.

Quantum. In optics: a unit of light; in synapses: the minimum amount of transmitter substance that can be released, probably the contents of a single synaptic vesicle.

Rapidly adapting. A rapid decline to zero of a response of a sensory neuron to a maintained stimulus.

Receptive field. The area of the periphery whose stimulation influences firing of a neuron.

Receptor. In sensory system: a structure specialized to be sensitive to certain forms of energy; in synaptic transmission: the site of binding of a transmitter substance with postsynaptic membranes.

Receptor potential. The nonpropagated change in membrane potential of a receptor that does not lead to action potentials in the receptor, but does generate them synaptically in another cell, *cf.*, Generator potential.

Reciprocal inhibition. Interconnections of neurons arranged so that pathways that excite one group of motoneurons inhibit the antagonist motoneurons.

Reciprocal innervation. Interconnections of neurons arranged so that pathways that excite one group of motoneurons inhibit the antagonist motoneurons and those that inhibit a group of motoneurons excite the antagonist motoneurons.

Rectification. In synapses: the property of allowing transmission through a pathway in only one direction; in membranes: a change in ionic conductance with a change in membrane potential.

Recurrent inhibition. Inhibition of an element produced by its own output through excitation of an inhibitory interneuron, *cf.*, Collateral inhibition.

Red muscle. Dark-red-colored muscle tissue, composed of fibers rich in myoglobin; slow muscle fibers.

Referred pain. Pain due to damage to an internal organ that is referred to a structure on the surface of the body.

Reflex. A relatively stereotyped movement or response elicited by a stimulus applied to the periphery, transmitted to the central nervous system, and then transmitted back out to the periphery.

Refractive index. A measure of the amount of bending of light on entering a medium; the speed of light in a vacuum/speed of light in the medium.

Reinnervation. Refers to the reattachment of a nerve fiber to a muscle or another nerve fiber after the original connection has been severed.

Relative refractory period. The period after a spike when greater than normal stimuli are required to excite a nerve or muscle cell.

REM sleep. The stage of sleep in which dreaming is associated with mild muscle jerks and rapid eye movements (REM), also characterized by a desynchronized EEG, thus the *syn.* Dream sleep, Paradoxical sleep.

Renshaw inhibition. A form of collateral inhibition of α motoneurons involving a special inhibitory interneuron, the Renshaw cell.

Repolarization phase. The return of the membrane potential from the peak overshoot of the spike back to the resting potential, *syn.* Falling phase.

Resistance. The opposition by a conductor to the passage of an electric current.

Resting membrane potential. The membrane potential of a cell that is not active, *i.e.*, not generating spikes; the average membrane potential.

Retrograde axoplasmic transport. The active movement of substances up the axon of a cell (toward the soma) in the retrograde direction at up to 100 mm/day.

Rhizotomy. Interruption of a spinal root within the spinal canal.

Rigidity. Stiffness of a limb due to increased tone in both flexors and extensors, *cf.*, Spasticity.

Rinne's test. A hearing test in which a tuning fork is placed on the mastoid process to distinguish conduction deafness from nerve deafness.

Rising phase. The earliest positive-going portion of the nerve or muscle spike, *syn.* Depolarization phase, Upstroke.

Rods. Visual receptors in the retina specialized for scotopic vision.

Saccade. An abrupt, rapid, small eye movement; usually occurs in a series during scanning; also occurs as a part of nystagmus.

Saltatory conduction. Conduction of the nerve spike where the spike jumps from node to node.

Sarcomere. The serially repeating unit of muscle that gives it its striated appearance.

Saturation. Homogeneity or purity of wavelength of light.

Scanning speech. Speaking characterized by irregular volumes and speech rhythms; a symptom of cerebellar disease.

Scotoma. An area of depressed or absent vision within the visual field, surrounded by an area of normal vision.

Scotopic. Pertaining to vision in the dark.

Second messenger. A substance, activated by interaction of a synaptic transmitter substance with the postsynaptic receptor that causes either a change in membrane ionic permeability or activation of an electrogenic pump, leading to a change in postsynaptic membrane potential.

Secondary muscle spindle receptor. The termination of group II afferent fibers on nuclear chain fibers of muscle spindles, *syn.* Flower-spray endings.

Sham rage. An outburst of behavior in an animal with a lesion somewhere above the tectum, resembling anger, but lacking direction.

Short-term memory. Recall of learned responses or material having a duration of minutes to hours, *syn.* immediate recall.

Simple cells. Neurons in visual cortex that are sensitive to narrow bars of light oriented in a particular direction across the retina, but not sensitive to movement of the bar.

Single-unit smooth muscle. Smooth muscle containing many tight junctions that contracts as a unit and responds to stretch.

Skeletomotor neuron. A motoneuron whose axon is an Aα fiber; contacts extrafusal muscle fibers, *syn.* Alpha motoneuron.

Slow axoplasmic transport. The movement of substances down the axon of a neuron in the orthograde direction at up to 12 mm/day.

Slow muscle. Relative term, referring to the speed of twitch contraction and relaxation and to the relatively low rates of stimulation at which tetanic fusion occurs.

Slowly adapting. A slow decline without complete cessation of a response of a sensory neuron to a maintained stimulus.

Smooth muscle. Muscle of the linings of internal organs and blood vessels that lacks cross-striations and is caused to contract by autonomic discharges.

Sodium–potassium pump. Mechanism for extrusion of sodium and uptake of potassium by cells against the concentration gradients for these ions, *syn.* Sodium pump.

Sodium pump. Mechanism for extrusion of sodium and uptake of potassium by cells against the concentration gradients for these ions, *syn.* Sodium–potassium pump.

Soma. Cell body.

Somatosomatic reflexes. Reflexes involving somatic stimuli and somatic responses.

Somatotopic organization. Pertaining to the orderly mapping of parts of the body onto the cerebral cortex and other parts of the nervous system.

Somatovisceral reflexes. Reflexes involving somatic stimuli and visceral responses.

Somesthesia. Consciousness of the body and bodily sensations resulting from activity in enteroceptors and exteroceptors.

Space constant. Distance along the membrane at which an imposed transmembrane voltage falls to 1/e of its initial value.

Spasticity. Resistance of a limb to passive stretch due to increased tone in either flexors or extensors (usually extensors), but not both.

Spatial summation. Algebraic addition of generator potentials elicited by stimuli at two different points.

Spherical aberration. Formation of rings around images due to unequal refraction in the center and on the periphery of a lens.

Spike. The all-or-none, conducted voltage response of a nerve or muscle membrane that is used to communicate information, *syn.* Action potential; a 15–18 msec deflection characteristic of epileptic but not normal EEG.

Spike and dome complex. An EEG phenomenon, consisting of a rapid (15–18 msec) deflection with a return to baseline, followed by a much slower wave; a characteristic pattern, repeated frequently in epileptic cortex.

Spinal shock. A condition following functional disconnection of the spinal cord from higher centers, which is characterized by areflexia, anesthesia, and lack of movements.

Split-brain patient. A patient who has had his corpus callosum sectioned.

Static fusimotor neuron. A γ motoneuron whose activity increases the static responses of both primary and secondary spindle endings.

Static response. The response of spindle endings that signals maintained length of a muscle.

Statoconium. Calcium carbonate crystal found in the otolith organs of vertebrates, *syn.* Otolith.

Stereopsis. Depth perception.

Stereotaxic coordinates. A Cartesian system in which points in the brain are referenced by coordinates in horizontal, sagittal, and frontal planes.

Stretch reflex. An automatic contraction of a muscle elicited by stretching it, *syn.* Myotatic reflex, Tendon jerk reflex.

Striated muscle. Any muscle whose fibers are divided by transverse bands into striations.

Subliminal fringe. A group of neurons that is excited during a reflex, but which does not reach critical firing level and does not discharge a spike.

Submodality. Any division of one of the modalities, example: touch is a submodality of somesthesia.

Substitution. Recovery of function due to use of alternate movements.

Subthreshold stimulus. A stimulus whose strength is too low to initiate a response.

Supramaximal stimulus. A stimulus whose intensity is greater than that which just gives a maximal response.

Suprathreshold stimulus. A stimulus that is of sufficient strength to give a response.

Surround inhibition. The inhibition of a cell's discharge that results from stimulation of an annular area around the excitatory receptive field.

Sympathetic nervous system. The division of the autonomic nervous system made up of thoracic and lumbar segments.

Sympathetic tone. Refers to the ongoing discharge in sympathetic nerve fibers that leads to a resting contraction of vascular smooth muscle.

Sympathectomy. The transection, resection, or other interruption of transmission in some portion of the peripheral sympathetic pathways.

Synapse. The site at which neurons make functional contact.

Synaptic cleft. Space between pre- and postsynaptic cells at a chemical synapse across which the transmitter substance must diffuse.

Synaptic delay. The time required for release of a chemical transmitter substance, its diffusion across the synaptic cleft, its interaction with the postsynaptic receptor, and the initiation of a change in postsynaptic membrane potential.

Synaptic knob. A swelling of an axon near its termination; the presynaptic structure in most synapses, *syn.* Bouton terminaux, End Bulb, Terminal.

Synaptic vesicles. Small, membrane-bound sacs in the presynaptic terminals that contain the transmitter substance.

Synergist muscle. A muscle that has the same action at the same joint as another muscle.

Tabes dorsalis. A syphilitic infection of the dorsal root ganglion.

Temporal lobe epilepsy. Seizures characterized by stereotyped behavior often with emotional outbursts and partial responsiveness, *syn.* Psychomotor epilepsy.

Temporal summation. Algebraic addition of generator potentials elicited by two stimuli applied at the same point in rapid succession.

Tendon jerk reflex. An automatic contraction of a muscle elicited by stretching it, *syn.* Myotatic reflex, stretch reflex.

Terminal. A swelling of an axon near its termination; the presynaptic structure in most synapses, *syn.* Bouton terminaux, End bulb, Synaptic knob.

Tetanic contraction. Sustained contraction of a muscle without intervals of relaxation.

Thalamotomy. The production of a circumscribed lesion in the thalamus.

Theta rhythms. EEG records characterized by high-voltage waves occurring at 4–8 per second.

Thick filament. The larger diameter myofilament of the myofibrils of striated muscle.

Thin filament. The smaller diameter myofilament of the myofibrils of striated muscle.

Threshold. Minimal stimulus required for a response or sensation.

Threshold of hearing curve. A graph of a person's threshold for detection of various pitches in the range of human hearing, *syn.* Audibility curve.

Tic douloureux. Excruciating episodic pain in the dermatome of the trigeminal nerve often precipitated by gentle stimulation of certain trigger points, *syn.* Trigeminal neuralgia.

Time constant. The time over which the transmembrane voltage passively falls to 1/e of its initial value.

Tinnitus. A sensation of ringing, buzzing, roaring, or clicking in the ears, not of external origin, in some cases audible to people other than the patient.

Tonotopic representation. A distribution of sensitivity in auditory structures such that the range of audible tones is represented in sequence across the structure.

Tractotomy. Section of a tract.

Transmitter substance. A compound released at a synapse from the presynaptic element that effects a change in potential of the postsynaptic cell.

Transneuronal degeneration. Refers to the wasting of a nerve cell when the fibers that innervate it are severed.

Tremor at rest. An involuntary trembling that is suppressed or reduced when a movement is attempted.

Trichromatic theory. Theory of color vision that says there are three fundamental color sensations and three different color receptors; color sensation is the result of activity in this ensemble, *syn.* Young-Helmholtz theory.

Trichromatism. Color vision involving three pigments.

Trigeminal neuralgia. Excruciating episodic pain in the dermatome of the trigeminal nerve often precipitated by gentle stimulation of certain trigger points, *syn.* Tic douloureux.

Tritanope. A person who lacks response to blue light.

Tropomyosin. A filamentous protein that is part of the thin myofilament of striated muscle.

Troponin. A globular protein that is part of the thin myofilament of striated muscle.

Tuning curve. A plot for auditory neurons of the threshold stimulus strength against the frequency of the auditory stimulus.

Twitch contraction. The all-or-none response of a muscle or muscle cell to a single brief stimulus.

Two-point threshold. The minimum distance between two stimuli to the skin at which they can be perceived as two stimuli instead of one.

Unfused tetanic contraction. A tetanic contraction in which individual twitch contributions can still be seen.

Unmyelinated fiber. A nerve fiber without myelin surrounding it.

Upper motoneuron syndrome. A group of symptoms resulting from removal of supraspinal influences on spinal mechanisms.

Upstroke. The earliest positive-going portion of the nerve or muscle spike, *syn.* Depolarization phase, Rising phase.

Vertigo. A sensation as if the world were revolving around the person or the person is revolving in space.

Vestibulo–ocular reflex. Refers to the automatic movement of the eyes in the direction opposite to that in which the head is rotated.

Vicarious function. Recovery of function due to assumption of control by another neurologic structure.

Visceral afferent fibers. Fibers carrying sensory information from visceral organs to the central nervous system.

Viscerosomatic reflexes. Reflexes involving visceral stimuli and somatic responses.

Viscerovisceral reflexes. Reflexes involving visceral stimuli and visceral responses.

Visibility curve. A plot of the threshold for vision against the wavelength of light in the stimulus.

Vision. The act of seeing; sight; sensations induced through photoreceptors.

Visual axis. A line perpendicular to a tangent to the cornea through the centers of the lens and the fovea.

Visual field. The total extent of the visual world seen by one eye at rest.

Voltage clamp. A device for fixing the transmembrane voltage of a cell at a constant value.

Voltage-gated channel. A normally closed ionic channel that is opened by a change in transmembrane voltage (usually a depolarization).

Warm fibers. Cutaneous thermoreceptors that increase their discharge rate with increasing skin temperature.

Weber fraction. The ratio of the just-noticeable-difference in stimulus strength to the standard stimulus strength.

Weber-Fechner function. The magnitude of the sensation evoked by a stimulus is proportional to the logarithm of the stimulus strength.

Weber's test. A hearing test using a tuning fork employed to distinguish conduction deafness from nerve deafness.

Wernicke's area. Area 22 of the temporal cerebral cortex that plays a fundamental role in reception and comprehension of speech.

White muscle. A paler colored muscle consisting of fibers lacking high myoglobin concentrations; fast muscle fibers.

Withdrawal reflex. Automatic contraction of the flexor muscles of a limb so as to remove the limb from a noxious stimulus, *syn.* Flexion reflex, Nocifensive reflex.

Young-Helmholtz theory. Theory of color vision that says there are three fundamental color sensations and three different color receptors; color sensations are the result of activity in this ensemble, *syn.* Trichromatic theory.

Z-line. The boundary of the sarcomere and point of attachment of thin filaments of adjacent sarcomeres.

Common Abbreviations

ACh	acetylcholine
A	ampere
C	capacitance
cm	centimeter
CNS	central nervous system
C	concentration
g	conductance
g_x	conductance of ion "x"
i	current
db	decibel
EEG	electroencephalogram
EMG	electromyogram
ϵ_x	equilibrium potential of ion "x"
EPSP	excitatory postsynaptic potential
Hz	hertz
IPSP	inhibitory postsynaptic potential
P_i	inorganic phosphate
i_x	ionic current of ion "x"
JND	just-noticeable-difference
kHz	kilohertz
kV	kilovolt
V_{max}	maximum velocity of shortening
MLF	medial longitudinal fasciculus
MΩ	megohm
V_m	membrane potential
m	meter
m/sec	meters per second
μF	microfarad
μm	micrometer
μV	microvolt
mA	milliampere
mg	milligram
ml	milliliter
mm	millimeter
mM	millimole
msec	millisecond
mV	millivolt
MEPP	miniature end-plate potential
min	minute
M	molar
NE	norepinephrine
nm	nanometer
VPL	nucleus ventralis posterolateralis of the thalamus
VPM	nucleus ventralis posteromedialis of the thalamus
Ω	ohm
pF	picofarad
dV/dt	rate of change of voltage
R	resistance
$\dot{V}_E$	respiratory flow rate
V_r	resting membrane potential
sec	second
SPL	sound pressure level
λ	space constant
TEA	tetraethylammonium
TTX	tetrodotoxin
τ	time constant
V	volts or voltage

Index

Page number followed by t indicates table; page number followed by g indicates glossary definition.